THE THEORY OF CATERING

10TH EDITION

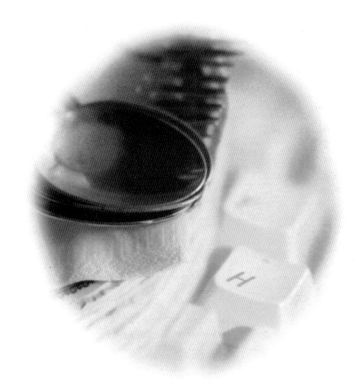

Professor
David Foskett
Victor Ceserani
Ronald Kinton

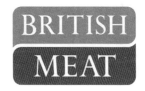

BRITISH
MEAT

Hodder & Stoughton

A MEMBER OF THE HODDER HEADLINE GROUP

Orders: please contact Bookpoint Ltd, 130 Milton Park, Abingdon, Oxon OX14 4SB. Telephone: (44) 01235 827720. Fax: (44) 01235 400454. Lines are open from 9.00 – 6.00, Monday to Saturday, with a 24 hour message answering service. You can also order through our website www.hodderheadline.co.uk.

British Library Cataloguing in Publication Data
A catalogue record for this title is available from The British Library

ISBN 0 340 850418

First published 1964

Tenth Edition published 2003

Impression number	10 9 8 7 6 5 4	
Year	2008 2007 2006 2005 2004	

Typeset by Fakenham Photosetting Ltd
Printed & Bound in Italy.

CONTENTS

PART 1 The Hospitality Industry

PART 2 Trends and Influences

PART 3 Food commodities, nutrition and science

PART 4 Planning, production and service

PART 5 Organisation and business development

PART 6 Legislation

FOREWORD FOR 'THE THEORY OF CATERING'

If you were to ask what the phrase 'The Theory of Catering' means to any serious catering professional, they would tell you that, when they were studying at Hotel and Catering School, it was their bible along with 'Practical Cookery'.

Twenty years ago I arrived at Ealing Hotel School armed with all the books on my reading list and 'The Theory of Catering' was the one which became most dog-eared over my years of study. Indeed it still has a place on the bookcase in my office today.

The profession, which is now described as Hospitality, is an extremely technical one, where the successful caterer needs considerable practical knowledge and many different skills. Today, more than ever, it is essential that those working in the industry have not only a solid training, but that they keep themselves up to date throughout their career, adopting a programme of Continuing Professional Development. Changes in trends and influences, as well as legislation, mean that today's professional needs to stay abreast of the fast changing environment.

Throughout my career, one of the key principles I have followed is never to ask a member of staff to do something I could not do myself. I have, therefore, armed myself with the skills and knowledge, both technical and practical, to enable this to be the case. If a new piece of equipment is delivered, I am there with the rest of the staff for the briefing on its operation. This has had the effect of raising my own credibility within my team, as they are fully aware that I know what I am talking about.

'The Theory of Catering' gives those studying for, or working within, the world of Hospitality a focal point to which to refer when in need of an answer. As well as giving an overview of the industry as a whole, it also follows the food chain through its natural path, from commodity and its science through delivery from the supplier, storage, preparation, production and final service to the waiting customer.

These are just some of the many topics covered in a simple to follow and practical way, written by practitioners who have been there and done it.

The World of Hospitality is a wide and varied one and if you work hard and have the determination and ambition to achieve you can, quite literally, go almost anywhere.

Alistair Telfer MBA DMS FHCIMA President HCIMA 2001–2003

July 2002

As a deeply committed caterer I am delighted to write this foreword. I have long had admiration for Ronald, Victor and David who work tirelessly to support and promote our exciting and rewarding industry.

Like many of you I joined the catering industry because of my passion for providing good food and service. It can be an extremely hard industry to work in, the hours can sometimes be long and sometimes even when you are doing your best, customer feedback can be tough. But, despite this it is also a truly enriching industry. Looking around at the different avenues you can work in makes it a remarkable business to join. From working in the finest hotels to field based kitchens for the forces to running your own enterprise anywhere in the world, where else would you get this range of different businesses? You could even say our industry is now fashionable? With footballers, filmstars and fashion models opening their own restaurants. Turn on the television and you will likely see a programme dedicated to the food business and just look at the wealth of subjects our industry covers. For the wannabe entrepreneur and the dedicated food professional, at whatever stage you are in your career in this business, with *The Theory of Catering* by your side you cannot go wrong. It is full of valuable information, which the authors have gathered over many years from their different experiences in the business. It is not a book to be read and put on the shelf, but one that should be continually referred to as you move through this fascinating business.

Caroline Mortimer, Managing Director European Business Development, Compass Group

INTRODUCTION TO THE TENTH EDITION

As travel, tourism, recreation and hospitality become increasingly important in the economic life of the vast majority of countries, so the need for well trained operatives and managers continues to grow.

This book is designed to meet the needs of those training for, or involved in, the catering industry (often referred to as the hospitality industry).

The tenth edition has been revised and updated to keep in line with the continuing changes both in industry and catering education. As in previous editions we have not attempted to write a completely comprehensive book, but rather have set out an outline as a basis for further study. In this way we hope to assist students at all levels and, for those who wish to study at great length, further references and websites are suggested where appropriate.

Obtaining employment and building a career
With the decision made to come into catering, it is to be hoped that prior to or during the course, students will have worked in the industry and seen some of the different types of work available. If possible, they will have obtained experience in a variety of different establishments (hotels, hospitals, industrial, restaurants). **People do best at that which interests them most, so try to find out what appeals to you**.

Having got on the ladder, you need to consider the following points when trying to get up it:

○ Do not get off one ladder until you have got onto another one; in other words make certain you have a job to go to before leaving present employment.
○ It is generally advisable to stay with your first employer for at least one year, and to spend at least a year in subsequent jobs.
○ It is desirable to keep in continuous employment; gaps do not present employers with a view of a stable employee.
○ Advancement is more likely if you keep within one area of catering (contract, hospital, restaurants) so that experience gained can be of benefit to employers.
○ However, some careers, such as teaching, need people experienced in several aspects of the industry.
○ Know where you are going and have attainable goals. However, if a real mistake has been made and a move has been wrong then a change may be for the best.

In evaluating the need to progress, these factors need to be considered apart from the money: value of new experience, establishment's reputation, conditions and hours of work, opportunities for advancing in existing establishment, facilities offered for self-development, such as further courses, overseas experience, etc.

If possible, when leaving college or any employment, endeavour to leave in such a way that you can return at any time. The catering industry needs people who are loyal, prepared to work hard and to enjoy their work together as a team.

ACKNOWLEDGEMENTS

We are greatly indebted to the following for their helpful advice and contributions to this edition:

James Stirling Gallacher OBE (Compass Group UK)

Michael Stapleton, UK Corporate Affairs Manager (Compass Group UK)

William J Vickers, Marketing and Food Services Director (Compass Group UK)

Jonathan Wilde, Group Marketing Manager (SODEXHO Catering and Support Services)

Peter Hazzard, Food Services Director (SODEXHO)

Peter Webb, Neal Martin, Commercial Manager, Hotel Services, P & O Princess Cruises

Adele Fisherman School Meals Services

Edward Griffiths for Planning a Function

David Stockton, British Airways

John Gray, British Meat

John Cousins for an overview of Food and Beverage Service

Paul Hambleton, Thames Valley University for the Chapter on Computers

The Dairy Council

Sea Fish Authority

British Egg Information Services

British Hospitality Association

Food Service Intelligence

AVAB

Photographs appear courtesy of:

Charvet Premier Ranges Ltd; Welbilt UK Ltd; Cowlothern; Rational UK; Bonnet UK; M & J Seafoods; Westminster Kingsway College; The Dairy Council; Russums; Multinational UK Ltd; Savoy Group; Ron and Eve Jones; British Meat; PKL Group (UK)

PART 1

The Hospitality Industry

CHAPTER 1

AN OVERVIEW OF THE UK AND GLOBAL HOSPITALITY INDUSTRY

THE UK HOSPITALITY INDUSTRY

The UK hospitality industry is a significant growth area employing over 2 million people – 7% of the total workforce. The industry operates in a wide range of sectors, its activities impact on the daily lives of almost every member of society. People working in hospitality provide food, drink and accommodation to meet the needs of the domestic and international leisure and tourism market. They also provide hospitality services in offices, factories, department stores, hospitals, prisons, sports centres, leisure centres, clubs and so on. The hospitality industry therefore does not just include the commercial or profit sectors where payment is made directly by the customer, but also the non-profit sector where payment is made indirectly.

This adds up to some 300,000 approx catering outlets in the UK serving almost 9 billion meals a year, for which they charge about £20 billion for the food, but not for the drinks.

It is a £43 billion industry which services a £6 billion tourism industry and is also the backbone of all types of public services, where over a third of this workforce is employed. In all contributes £21.5 billion is taxation to the Treasury and fuels a massive diverse supply chain. The industry is also a job creator some 310,000 new jobs will need to be filled by 2009 and it will lead the way as an agent of social inclusion. It is an integral, essential contributor to national, regional and local economies and sustains some 261,000 small and micro businesses.

The multiple retailers are beginning to see the catering market both as a threat to their existing business and an opportunity for some additional growth. It is important not to make too much of this at current levels, but there will probably come a time when eating out accounts for a greater share of the food £ than buying food for cooking at home; indeed the USA passed this watershed in 1995.

A common approach is to look at the structure of the industry in terms of the nature of the service offered by different types of outlet, and that is the way that the tables on pages 3–5 are constructed. They show that the largest sectors, in terms of numbers of outlets, are hotels and pubs, both of which have about 60,000 places at which to eat, followed by the leisure sector. This latter sector is, in fact, a microcosm of the catering industry itself since it is comprised of a wide variety of outlets from sports clubs and stadia to theme parks, historic properties, cinemas and so on. Indeed, many researchers are unsure whether to include the leisure sector within the catering market, since it consists of a large number of outlets each of which serves only small quantities of food. However, this sector will be amongst those showing fastest growth over the next few years.

Like hospitality and tourism all leisure markets benefit from improving economic conditions. For many people real disposable income has grown and the forecasts are that it will continue to grow. On average, people were approximately a third more wealthy at the end of the 1990s than we were at the beginning. In wealthy economies leisure and pleasure sectors outperform the economy. Generally as people become wealthier, their incremental income is not usually spent on upgrading the essentials but on pleasure and luxury items. However, whenever there is a downturn in the economy, the leisure sectors have suffered disproportionately.

The leisure sector is worth approximately £60.3 billion and is forecast to grow by a further 10 billion by 2003. It has been described as the biggest, fastest growing industry in the UK. Within the leisure sector, some areas have slowed down, some are consolidating and concentrating on core businesses. One of the most useful ways of categorising the leisure sector is to separate it into popular leisure activities. Some examples are theatre, ten pin bowling and cue sports, casinos, bingo and health and fitness.

In terms of meals served, the table shows that the most significant sectors are food service, which accounts for approximately 23% of the market, followed by pubs, staff catering and healthcare at approximately 13%. An expected rise in household incomes of 3.4% per annum in real terms between 1999 and 2009, this will result in a rise of 3.7% is spent on eating out. As a result, spending on catering will account for a slightly greater share of personal disposable income by 2009. Traditionally catering activity has been divided into either profit or cost sector markets. The profit sector includes such establishments as restaurants, fast food chains outlets, cafés, takeaways, pubs and leisure and travel catering outlets while the cost sector refers to catering outlets for business and industry, education and healthcare. Recent developments have blurred the division between profit and cost orientated establishments.

Despite its complexity, the catering sector represents one of the largest sectors of the UK economy and is fifth in size behind retail food, cars, insurance and clothing. It is also an essential support to tourism, another major part of the economy, and is one of the largest employers in the country.

Food, market values and distribution

Five main types of food are used in the catering industry:
- fresh food (meat, fish, vegetables);
- ambient food (groceries, hot beverages; confectionery and snacks);
- chilled food (meat, fish and dairy products);
- frozen food (ice cream, desserts, vegetables, potatoes); and
- drink (alcoholic and non-alcoholic drink)

Drink and fresh food account for almost three quarters of total expenditure.

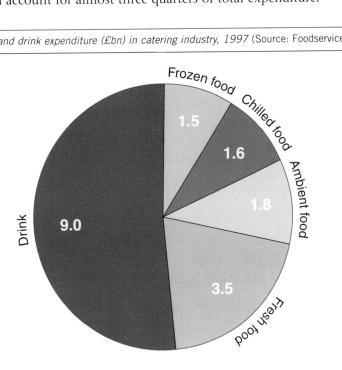

Figure 1.1 *Food and drink expenditure (£bn) in catering industry, 1997* (Source: Foodservice Intelligence)

Frozen food — 1.5
Chilled food — 1.6
Ambient food — 1.8
Drink — 9.0
Fresh food — 3.5

Alcoholic drink accounts for 80 per cent of the £6.24bn spent on drinks, while fresh meat products account for 38 per cent (£1.14bn) of fresh food. (Prices in constant 1998 prices.)

Food sales

In 2000, food sales in the profit sector accounted for 90 per cent of total food sales.

Food sales in profit and cost sectors (£m), 2000

	2000	%
Restaurants	4,184	19
Quick Service	5,954	27
Pubs	3,159	14
Hotels	4,882	22
Leisure	1,964	9
Staff Catering	862	4
Healthcare	586	2
Education	602	2.5
Services	146	0.5
TOTAL	**22,337**	

Source: Foodservice Intelligence

Figure 1.2 *Food sales in profit and cost sectors (%), 2000*

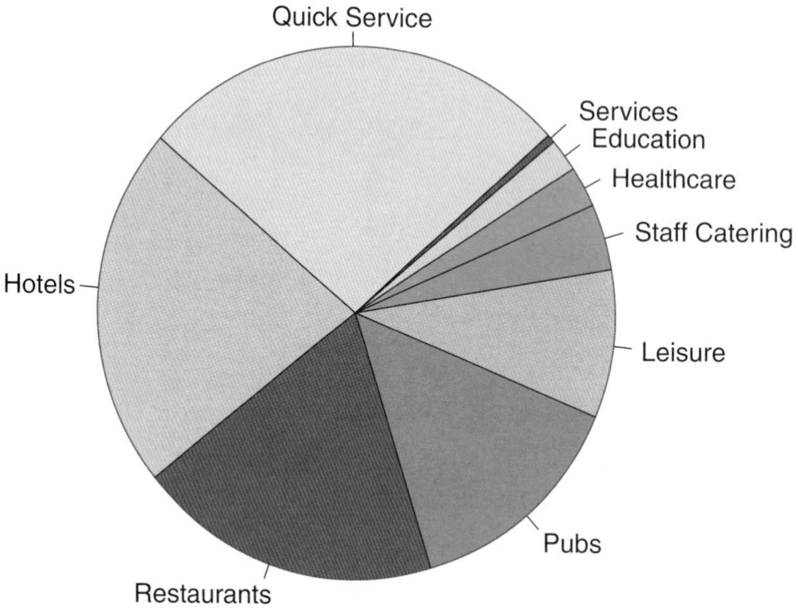

Between 1996 and 2000, the number of meals served and the value of food purchases increased in the profit sector but declined in the cost sector.

Number of meals served (m), 1996 and 1999–2000

	1996	1999	2000	%
Restaurants	609	660	676	8
Quick Service	1,930	1,908	2,007	23
Pubs	1,036	1,139	1,095	13
Hotels	628	671	677	8
Leisure	506	542	541	6
Staff Catering	988	1,032	1,049	13
Healthcare	1,087	1,070	1,086	13
Education	1,274	1,204	1,211	14
Services	233	225	227	2
TOTAL	**8,291**	**8,452**	**8,569**	

Source: Foodservice Intelligence

In 1998, the UK eating-out market was worth £15.1bn with fast food accounting for nearly one-third and restaurants just over two-thirds. These proportions are little changed from 1995.

UK eating-out by market by sector (£m), 1996–2000

	1996	1997	1998	1999	2000
Restaurants	3,986.0	4,108.5	4,123.8	4,131.0	4,183.7
Quick Service	6,015.4	6,001.9	6,089.5	6,091.8	5,953.9
Pubs	3,030.0	3,196.0	3,268.7	3.343.6	3,159.3
Hotels	4,530.7	4,628.1	4,659.9	4,771.5	4,881.5
Leisure	1,894.4	1,940.6	1,974.5	2,047.2	1,963.6
Profit	**19,456.5**	**19,875.1**	**20,116.4**	**20,385.1**	**20,142.0**
Staff Catering	844.3	853.9	862.8	860.8	862.1
Healthcare	621.8	619.3	603.4	589.4	585.6
Education	662.1	636.1	614.8	598.1	601.9
Services	154.6	147.0	148.2	145.8	145.7
Cost	**2,282.8**	**2,256.3**	**2,229.2**	**2,194.1**	**2,195.3**
TOTAL	**21,739.3**	**22,131.4**	**22,345.6**	**22,579.2**	**22,337.3**

Source: Foodservice Intelligence

Number of outlets in profit and cost sectors, 1996 and 1999–2000

	1996	1999	2000
Restaurants	25,300	25,397	25,392
Quick Service	29,677	28,527	28,846
Pubs	57,404	53,261	51,633
Hotels	48,529	48,696	48,413
Leisure	18,299	18,707	18,850
PROFIT SECTOR	**179,209**	**174,588**	**173,134**
Staff Catering	21,780	20,952	20,960
Healthcare	28,798	30,443	30,915
Education	34,580	34,436	34,650
Services	2,968	3,055	3,064
COST SECTOR	**88,126**	**88,986**	**89,589**
TOTAL	**267,335**	**263,574**	**262,723**

Source: Foodservice Intelligence

Meals served

Over 8,500m meals were served in 2000, the majority in the profit sector.

Number of meals served (m), 1996 and 1999–2000

	1996	1999	2000
Profit sector	4,709	4,920	4,995
Cost sector	3,582	3,531	3,574
TOTAL	**8,291**	**8,451**	**8,569**

Source: Foodservice Intelligence
Note: Prices are expressed in constant 2000 prices

Figure 1.3 *Number of meals served (m), 1996 and 1999–2000* (Source: Foodservice Intelligence)

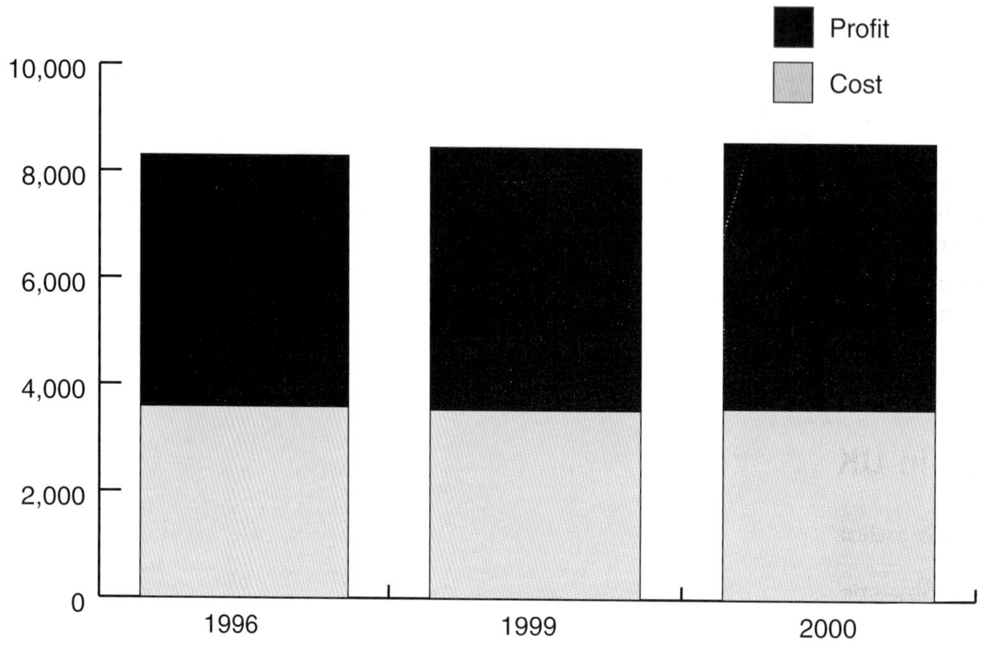

While there is a clear overlap with tourism, the hospitality industry consists of all these business operations which provide for their customers any combinations of the three core services of food, drink and accommodation. There are however a number of sectors within the hospitality industry that can be regarded separately from tourism, for example industrial catering, and those aspects of hospitality that attract only the local community.

Restaurants in the UK have approximately 40% of the commercial market while small establishments employing less than 10 staff form the majority of the industry. The South-east of England has the highest concentration of catering and hospitality outlets. Rapid expansion has taken place in the hospitality industry during the 1980s, throughout all sectors. Within the hotel sector, room stocks have increased by some 40 percent. This period of growth has been fuelled by the need for the large companies to maintain competitive advantage and by the provision of a suitable environment for growth. However the key feature of the UK hospitality industry is the extent of the fragmentation of ownership. The hotel sector is predominantly independently owned.

These properties come in all shapes, sizes and locations. More than three-quarters of them have fewer than 20 rooms and are invariably family-run. The UK hospitality industry has some of the highest failure rates for the hospitality business especially during the recession years of the 1990s.

The hotel sector, despite its disparate nature, can be divided into distinct categories, such as luxury, business, resort, townhouse and budget properties. Each category has its own characteristics. Business hotels, as the name suggests, are geared to the corporate traveller. Emphasis therefore tends to be on functionality. These hotels will usually have a dedicated business centre, up-to-date communication technology in the rooms and ample conference and meeting facilities. Business hotels are more likely to be chain operated, often with a strong brand element. Townhouses, meanwhile, are notable for their individuality, intimacy and emphasis on service. These hotels invariably are small and, as the name suggests, located in converted town houses with a domestic feel that is emphasised by their decor. The fastest growing sector is budget hotels, where the accommodation units are co-located with a food source operation such as a Steak House or Little Chef.

Formal dining and buffet set-ups, traditional fare and theme restaurants, room service and public bars: clearly the provision of food and beverage (F&B) varies greatly between establishments. Again some general differences can be discerned between the various hotel categories. Upmarket hotels are likely to provide a full range of F&B services, usually with at least one à la carte restaurant, 24 hour room service and a well-stocked bar. Townhouse properties, in contrast, generally provide little or no food, while budget hotels are characterised by the presence of a family restaurant. This is often a stand-alone, branded outlet that also draws custom from the surrounding area.

Recently many hotels have been re-examining the place of Food and Beverage in their operation. While many townhouses open with no restaurant at all, other hotels believe that Food and Beverage provision is an essential guest service. This has led hotels to consider alternative methods of running a restaurant, such as contracting out to a third party or introducing a franchise operation.

The economics of running a restaurant in an hotel show why this has taken place. While Food and Beverage receipts traditionally provide about 20% to 30% of an hotel's total revenue, over three-quarters of this will be absorbed by departmental expenses, including payroll costs of approximately a third. An hotel's room department typically provides 50% to 60% of revenue, but departmental costs accounts for only 25% to 30% of this.

Tourism in UK economy, 1999

Economic indicator	Tourism share (%)
Gross Domestic Product	3.6
Consumer spending	5.7
All exports	4.4
Service exports	24.3

Source: Tourism Intelligence Quarterly

Overseas visitor spending in UK and UK residents' spending abroad (£m), 1995–99

	1995	1996	1997	1998	1999
Overseas visitor spending in UK	11,763	12,290	12,244	12,671	12,498
UK resident spending abroad	15,386	16,223	16,931	19,489	22,020

Source: IPS, ONS

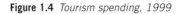

Figure 1.4 *Tourism spending, 1999*

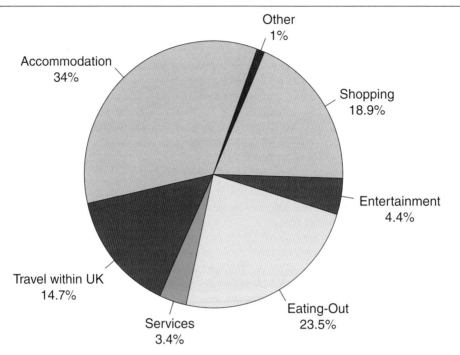

Businesses today find themselves competing in a world economy for survival, growth and profitability. Managers working in the industry have to learn to adjust to change in line with market demands for quality and value for money, and increased organisational attention will have to be given to profitability and professionalism.

The globalisation of the hospitality industry and tourism industry has advanced under the pressures of increased technology, communication, transportation, deregulation, elimination of political barriers, sociocultural changes and global economic development, together with growing competition in a global economy. An international hospitality company must perform successfully in the world's business environment. There are a vast number of influences in the external international environment which greatly affect the multinational organisation.

The travel, tourism and hospitality is the world's largest industry. According to the World Travel and Tourism Council (WTTC), the annual gross output of the industry is greater than the Gross National Product (GNP) except the United States, and Japan. Worldwide the tourism hospitality industry employs over 112 million people.

The leading five tourist destination countries in 1999 (USA, Italy, France, Spain and the UK) account for over 41% of world tourism arrivals, the leading 20 account for over two-thirds. These figures illustrate the continuing dominance of Europe as an international tourism destination with seven European destinations of the leading ten. New countries, notably China and Poland have entered the leading ten destinations for tourism arrivals since 1993. The UK remains a major recipient of world tourism and currently ranks behind only USA, Italy, France and Spain.

○ Monetary and fiscal policies and exchange controls – some countries may limit the amount of money that can be withdrawn from their country as well as impose large payments for international transactions (e.g. joint ventures, entry in the country).

○ Financial and investment markets, individual consumer and corporate interest rates, the availability of credit, exchanges, etc.

○ Taxation and tariffs – taxes on individuals, corporations and imported goods, imposed by the host country/government.

○ Trade/industrial factors – import/export measures of activity in commerce etc. These can serve as indices in determining the state of the economy (e.g. prosperity, depression, recession, recovery).

○ Labour markets – the level of unemployment, welfare spending etc.

In many countries, especially in emerging tourism destinations, the hospitality and tourism industry plays a very important role in the national economy, being the major foreign currency earners.

As the world economy continues to become more inter-dependent, increasing amounts of business travel will occur. Therefore the global economic environment plays a significant role in the internationalisation opportunities for hospitality and tourism companies. Global economic policies and developments play a critical role in the hospitality and tourism industry.

One of the principal challenges confronting tomorrow's industry will result from the transition to the Information age. The convergence of computing, telecommunications and content will shape the way and pace at which people live and work. Above all, it will change the nature of the exchange process between providers and their customers. The latter will have more choice. The information super highway will offer numerous ways to find out whether a hospitality company, restaurant etc delivers on its promises. Dissatisfied clients will be able to vent their feeling to an internet-connected community of thousands. Companies will in turn be expected to systematically accumulate information about the customer.

THE HOSPITALITY INDUSTRY: PRODUCT AND SERVICE

The hospitality product consists of tangible and intangible elements of food, drink and accommodation together with the service, atmosphere and image that surround and contribute to the product.

The hospitality industry contains many of the characteristics of service industries with the added complications of the production process. It is the production process which is the complicated element as it focuses on the production and delivery often within a set period of time.

The need to provide the appropriate environment within which hospitality can be delivered means that most hospitality businesses need a substantial amount of investment in plant and premises. This creates a high fixed cost/low variable cost structure. The variable costs in servicing a room are minimal although the hotel itself, particularly in the luxury hotel market, has a high fixed cost. In general the financial break-even point for hospitality businesses often is reasonably high. Exceeding this level will result in high profits, but low volumes will result in substantial losses.

Hospitality services suffer from fluctuation in demand. This demand will fluctuate over time and by the type of customer. Forecasting business is therefore often difficult because of the mixture of patterns and variables which can affect demand, making planning, resourcing and scheduling difficult.

Hospitality cannot be delivered without customers, who are involved in many aspects of the delivery of the hospitality service.

Achieving a satisfactory balance between demand patterns, resource scheduling and operational capacity is a difficult task for managers in hospitality. Managing customer demand to achieve optimum volume at maximum value is extremely complex. Too few customers could mean financial ruin. Too many customers without the required capacity or resources, often means that the customers' experience suffers leading to dissatisfaction. Scheduling of resources is also difficult, if too many staff are on duty to cover the forecast demand, then profitability suffers. Insufficient staffing creates problems, with servicing and staff morale. Forecasting is therefore a crucial function which contributes to the successful operation of the hospitality business.

The ability to deliver a consistent product to every customer is also an important consideration. Staff must be trained in teams to deliver a consistent standard of product and service. This means being able to cater not just for individual customers but to the needs of many different groups of customers all with slightly different requirements. The success of any customer experience will be determined at the interaction between the customer and the service provider.

The service staff have an additional part to play in serving the customer. They are important in the future selling process, they should be trained to use the opportunity to generate additional revenue.

From this analysis we are able to identify four characteristics of the hospitality industry which makes it a unique operation.

Firstly, hospitality cannot be delivered without customers, who provide the source of revenue for the continued financial viability of the operation. The customer is directly involved in many aspects of the delivery of the hospitality service, and is the judge of the quality of the hospitality provided.

Secondly, achieving a satisfactory balance between demand patterns, resource scheduling and operations is a particularly difficult task in the hospitality industry.

Thirdly, all hospitality operations require a combination of manufacturing expertise and service skill. It operates in many cases twenty-four hours a day. To deliver a consistent product to each individual customer requires teams of people well trained to deliver to a set standard every time.

Fourthly, no matter how well planned the operation is, how good the design and environment may be, if the interaction between the customer and the service provider is not right this will have a detrimental effect on the customer experience of the total product and a missed opportunity to sell future products. Good interaction between customers and service providers can also increase present sales, for example a waiter can 'up sell' by suggesting in a positive way additions to the meal, perhaps items in which the customer may not even have considered but is delighted by the recommendation or subtle persuasion.

TYPES OF CATERING ESTABLISHMENTS
Commercial Catering
HOTELS AND RESTAURANTS

The exact number of hotels in the UK is uncertain but there are approximately 22,000 registered with the Tourist Boards (BHA 2000). Their turnover makes up about 1% of UK GDP (BHA 1999) and they employ about 220,000 people, or about 13% of these employed in the hospitality industry (HTF 2000). There are around 7,000 available in five star hotels in the UK and 43,000 in four star hotels. The majority (over 80%) of these rooms are in group-owned hotels. The presence of international chains is high in the five star market. In the UK there are more hotel bedrooms (74,000) in the mid market three star category than in any other category (BHA 2000). The independent hotelier traditionally dominates this market.

In some cases special types of meal service, such as grill rooms or speciality restaurants, may limit the type of foods served – e.g. smörgasbord or steaks will be provided.

Wine bars, fast foods, take-away
QUICK SERVICE

Customer demand has resulted in the rapid growth of a variety of establishments offering a limited choice of popular foods at a reasonable price, with little or no waiting time, to be consumed either on the premises or taken away.

Delicatessen and salad bars

Offer a service (usually lunch) based on a wide variety of bread and rolls e.g. panini, focaccia, pitta, baguette and tortilla wraps. Fresh salads, home-made soups and one hot "chef's dish of the day" may be available.

A chilled food selection – from which customers can pick and mix can provide the basis for a day-long service including breakfast.

A 'made to order' sandwich counter and a baked jacket potato bar with a good variety of fillings are very popular components of some bars.

PRIVATE CLUBS

These are usually administered by a secretary or manager appointed by a management committee formed from club members. Good food and drink with an informal service in the old English style are required in most clubs, particularly in the St James's area of London.

Night clubs and casinos usually have the type of service associated with the restaurant trade.

CHAIN-CATERING ORGANISATIONS

There are many establishments with chains spread over wide areas and in some cases overseas. Prospects for promotion and opportunities are often considerable, whether it is in a chain of hotels or restaurants. These are the well-known hotel companies, restaurant chains, the popular type of restaurant, chain stores and the shops with restaurants, which often serve lunches, teas and morning coffee, and have snack bars and cafeterias.

LICENSED-HOUSE (PUB) CATERING

There are approximately 61,000 licensed houses in the UK and almost all of them offer food in some form or another. To many people the food served in public houses is ideal for what they want, that is, often simple, moderate in price and quickly served in a congenial atmosphere.

There is great variety in public-house catering, from the ham and cheese roll operation to the exclusive à la carte restaurant. Public-house catering can be divided into four categories:

○ the luxury-type restaurant;
○ Gastro Pubs – there is a growing trend for well qualified chefs to work in pubs and develop the menu according to their own specialities, making good use of local produce;
○ the speciality restaurant, e.g. steak bar, fish restaurant; carvery, theme;
○ fork dishes served from the bar counter where the food is consumed in the normal drinking areas;
○ finger snacks, e.g. rolls, sandwiches.

Licensed retailing is a vast sector of the hospitality industry which is experiencing rapid change. Movements in organisations' structures and size, of mergers and divestment ownerships and

The Evolution of the Pub

Period	Character of a Pub	Consumer Group	Products	Pub Implementations
Up to late Sixties	○ Drinking place	Men	○ Bitter (Mainly cask) ○ Spirits ○ Basic Food	○ Down-market ○ Basic facilities of the community ○ Home-grown entertainment ○ 'Ordinary' to working class men, not to other groups in society

Late Sixties to middle Seventies	○ The Themed pub	Men
		Youth
			○ Bitter
			○ Loss of cask
			○ Lager
			○ Spirits
			○ Basic Food
				○ Youth market
				○ Mass market
				○ Insensitive developments
				○ High tech. entertainment
				  – Jukebox
				  – Fruit machines
				  – Sound/light
				○ One bar pubs

Middle Seventies to 1990	○ Targeted concept	Men Youth Women	○ Bitter ○ Growth of cask ○ Lager ○ Soft drinks ○ Wine ○ Substantial growth in food	○ Retailing revolution ○ Pub is the hero ○ Targeted concepts ○ Introduction of service standards

1990's	○ Leisure experience	Men
		Youth
		Women
		Families
		Older people
			○ Increasing low/ non alcohol products:
			  ○ beers ○ soft drinks
			  ○ wines ○ coffee
			  ○ spirits
			○ Increasing food sales
			○ Increasing premium/ special products
			○ greater range of packaged products
			○ more premium cask ales
			○ more premium lagers
			○ Increasing leisure facilities – games and accommodation
				○ Signage/branding revolution
				○ Concept types will crystallise
				○ Greater consumer recognition
				○ Opportunity to sign and label pubs better
				○ More open retail format
				○ The term pub will become less relevant
				○ 'Pubs' will become more ordinary to society as a whole

Source: Whitbread Market Research

management skills have been driven by two macro influences. Firstly the impact of Beer Orders, forcing restrictions on the linkages between brewing and the licensed retail outlet ownerships, has brought about substantial restructuring of the industry. Subsequently five types of pub operators or retailers emerged as a result of the Beer Orders:

1 National retailer with brewing interest.
2 National retailer with no brewing interests (either de-merged or fully independent).
3 Regional or local retailer with brewing interests.
4 Regional or local retailer with no brewing interests.
5 Totally independent operator or free-houses.

Pub food is the most rapidly growing source of pub revenue and accounts for approximately 20% of total sales.

Beer remains the cornerstone of the pub, but different beers such as cask and speciality draught ales, stout and premium lagers are driving sales. Sales of soft drinks, wines, tea and coffee continue to grow.

Successful pubs are now diversifying to become significant leisure and retail outlets using sophisticated management controls, technological systems and marketing skills. A wider range of customer needs will be catered for, alcohol will continue to play an important part but food, entertainment and leisure facilities will become an increasing trend. Many pubs will specialise in particular markets by developing brands or concepts to attract target groups.

Further information:

British Institute of Innkeeping
Wessex House
80 Park St, Camberley, Surrey
GU15 3PT

Speciality restaurants

Moderately priced speciality eating houses are in great demand and have seen a tremendous growth in recent years. In order to ensure a successful operation it is essential to assess the customers' requirements accurately and to plan a menu that will attract sufficient customers to give adequate profit. A successful caterer is the one who gives customers what they want and not what the caterer thinks the customers want. The most successful catering establishments are those which offer the type of food they *can* sell, which is not necessarily the type of food they would *like* to sell.

Well-cooked fish and chips have always been popular in the UK and probably always will be; and it is interesting to note that one of the most successful speciality restaurant developments in the USA (the home of speciality restaurants) was the English fish and chip shop, complete with the food served in a bag made from an early copy of *The Times* newspaper.

COUNTRY HOTELS

Country house hotels have been and are being developed in many tourist areas, many are listed buildings, stately homes or manor houses.

CONSORTIA

A consortium is a group of independent hotels who purchase products and services such as marketing from specialist companies providing members of the consortium with access to international reservation systems. This enables the group to compete against the larger chains.

MOTELS/TRAVEL LODGES

These establishments are sited near motorways and arterial routes. They focus on the business person who requires an overnight stop or the tourist who is on a driving holiday. These properties are reasonably priced, they consist of a room only with tea and coffee making facilities. Staffing is minimal and there is no restaurant. However there will be other services close by often managed by the same company. The growth and success of the budget hotel sector has been one of the biggest changes to affect the hospitality industry in recent years.

TIMESHARE VILLAS/APARTMENTS

A timeshare owner purchases the right to occupy a self catering apartment, a room or a suite in a hotel, a leisure club for a specified number of weeks per year over a period of years or indefinitely.

HEALTH FARMS

Often a luxury hotel where the client is able to access a number of specialist health treatments for those who are stressed, over worked or wish to lose weight.

GUESTHOUSES

Guesthouses are to be found all over the UK. The owners usually live on the premises and let their bedrooms to passing customers. Many have regular clients. Guesthouses usually offer bed, breakfast and evening meal. They are small privately owned operations.

FARMS

Farmers recognising the importance of the tourism industry in the countryside, formed a national organisation called the Farm Holiday Bureau. Most members have invested to transform basic bedrooms to meet the required standards. The National Tourist Board inspects every member property to ensure good value and quality accommodation. In most cases the accommodation is on or nearby working farms.

YOUTH HOSTELS

The Youth Hostels Association runs hostels in various locations in England and Wales. These establishments cater mainly for single people and for those groups travelling on a tight budget. In some locations there are a number of sports facilities.

SEA FERRIES

Ferries cross the English and Irish Channels. As they compete in a competitive travel market against airlines, and in the case of the English Channel, Eurostar and Le Shuttle, they have invested in the total travel experience, offering very good restaurant and leisure facilities, fast food restaurants, shopping, bars and lounges.

AIRLINE SERVICES

Airline catering is a specialist operation. See Chapter 8 page 296.

AT THE AIRPORT

Airports offer a range of hospitality services catering for millions of people every year. They operate 24-hours a day, 365 days a year. Services include themed restaurants, speciality restaurants, coffee bars and seafood bars often with a shopping arcade.

Public Sector Catering (Cost Sector)

Hospitals, Universities, Colleges, Schools, Prisons, Armed Forces, Meals on Wheels, etc.

This has been known for many years as **Welfare Catering** which was characterised by its non-profit making focus, minimising cost by achieving maximum efficiency. However, with the introduction of competitive tendering, many public sector operations have been won by contract caterers who have introduced new concepts, and commercialism with the public sector. This sector is more commonly known as the cost sector.

PRISONS

Catering may be run by contract catering or by the Prison Service. The food is usually prepared by prison officers and inmates. The kitchens are also used to train inmates in food production, to encourage them to seek employment on release. Prisons have lost their Crown Immunity which prevented prosecution through poor hygiene and negligence.

THE ARMED SERVICES

These include feeding armed services staff in barracks, in the mess and in the field. Much of the work is specialist especially field cookery. However the forces like every other section of the public sector are looking to reduce costs and increase efficiency. They too have been forced to look to market testing and competitive tendering by the Ministry of Defence, resulting in contract caterers taking over many service operations.

Welfare catering

The fundamental difference between welfare catering and the catering in hotels and restaurants is the hotel or restaurant is run to make a profit and provide a service. The aim of welfare catering is to minimise cost and cover overheads by achieving maximum efficiency. The standards of cooking should be equally good, though the types of menu may be different.

Hospital catering is classified as welfare catering, the object being to assist the nursing staff to get the patient well as soon as possible. To do this it is necessary to provide good quality food that has been carefully prepared and cooked to retain the maximum nutritional value, and presented to the patient in an appetising manner.

NATIONAL HEALTH SERVICE

NHS Trusts have a duty of care to ensure that best value is achieved for the catering operation and cost effectiveness is achieved.

The scale of catering services in the NHS is enormous. Over 300 million meals are served each year in more than 300 NHS Trusts across approximately 1200 hospitals. The NHS spends in the region of £500 m per annum in food.

The staffing structure of the catering department depends on the size of the hospital and who runs the catering services. However the normal approach may include the following:

- ○ **Catering Managers** plan menus, obtain supplies and supervise the preparation, cooking and service of the meals, and are also responsible for training and safety. They visit the wards to advise on the service of food to the patients, and control the provision of the catering facilities for the doctors, nurses and other hospital employees.
- ○ **Assistant Catering Managers** assist and deputise for the catering managers with all or part of their duties, or they may be responsible for a small hospital.
- ○ At one time the **Kitchen Manager** was called the **Kitchen Superintendent**. This is now changing but they are still responsible to the catering manager or the assistant catering manager for the running of one or more hospital kitchens. Cooks are graded according to

experience and technical qualifications. In larger hospitals a **Head Cook** would be in charge of a kitchen under the control of the kitchen superintendent or catering manager.

Dining room supervisors are in charge of the staff serving in the staff restaurant and they are responsible to the catering manager.

People interested in being of service to the community and gaining job satisfaction do find this aspect of catering rewarding. Conditions, hours of work and pay as well as promotion prospects are factors which contribute to making this a worthwhile career.

All NHS hospitals are managed by Trust Boards, some of which have chosen to appoint a **Hotel Services Manager**, who has responsibility for the management of catering, domestic, portering and other services and this provides an extended career path and an opportunity to develop new skills.

In July 2000 the NHS plan set out a work programme for the NHS to improve standards of food. This is seen as essential in enabling the NHS to deliver a quality service, and to put patients at the heart of health care.

CATERING SYSTEMS WITHIN THE NHS

These are many different methods of providing catering services within the NHS. Some hospitals cook food in traditional kitchens and send it to the wards to be served to patients. Some buy in chilled or frozen foods that are regenerated (reheated) in mobile trolleys and some have ward kitchens in which a certain amount of preparation and finishing is undertaken. Even within these three broad categories of catering systems there are numerous variations, for example, hot plated, cold plated and bulk services.

The NHS Menu Group included experienced NHS Catering and dietetic professionals, along with nurses and representatives of the private sector caterers who were nominated by the Hospital Caterers Association, dieticians by the British Dietetic Association and nurses were nominated by the Chief Nursing Officer.

THE NHS PLAN

This sets out a long-term strategy for modernising and improving health services around the needs and expectations of patients. The Better Hospital Food programme attempts to improve the standards for patients in the following ways:

○ Providing a 24-hour NHS catering service with a new NHS menu designed by leading chefs. This covers breakfast, drinks and snacks, light lunchtime meals and an improved two course evening dinner.

○ A national franchise for NHS catering aims to ensure hospital food is provided by organisations with a national reputation for high quality and customer satisfaction.

○ Hospitals are to have ward housekeepers "to ensure that the quality, presentation and portion size of meals meets patients' needs; that patients particularly the elderly, are able to eat the meals on offer; and that the service patients receive is genuinely available around the clock".

○ Dieticians advise and check on nutritional values in hospital food. Patients views should be measured as part of the Performance Assessment Framework and the quality of food will be subject to inspections.

Patients who are able, are encouraged to eat at normal meal times and the normal mealtime service caters for the needs of the majority of patients. The NHS plan recognises the need to provide meals outside normal periods for patients who cannot eat at the usual mealtimes or are prevented from eating at the breakfast, lunch and/or dinner services.

The 24-Hour Catering Service comprises of three elements:

○ The Ward Kitchen Service

○ The Snack Box

○ The Light Bite

These are all available on request (subject to certain clinical considerations). These represent the minimum level of service required.

The Ward Kitchen Service

A ward-based kitchen service from which patients can obtain light refreshments such as tea/coffee/cold drinks, toast/preserves, biscuits and fruit, at any time of the day or night.

The Snack Box

This offers a number of items presented in a box, making up a replacement meal for patients who have missed a meal, or where patients would prefer a lighter alternative to the meals on offer throughout the Mealtime Service. There should be at least three alternative boxes:

1 A childrens box.

2 A snack box.

3 Sandwich snack box.

The Light Bite

Some patients may want a more substantial hot alternative and the Light Bite should be offered in these circumstances. These meals are designed to be quick and easy to prepare and serve to patients at ward level, and likely to be of pre-prepared microwaveable type. This means patients should be able to get nutritious, tasty hot food at any time of the day or night.

Further information:

NHS Estates Information Centre
www.nhsestates.gov.uk

Hospital Caterers Association
www.hospitalcaterers.org

British Dietectics Association
www.bda.uk.com

DIETICIANS

In many hospitals a qualified dietician is responsible for:

○ collaborating with the catering manager on the planning of meals;

○ drawing up and supervising special diets;

○ instructing diet cooks on the preparation of special dishes;

○ advising the catering manager and assisting in the training of cooks with regard to nutritional aspects;

○ advising patients.

In some hospitals the food for special diets will be prepared in a diet bay by diet cooks.

DIETS

Information about the type of meal or diet to be given to each patient is supplied daily to the kitchen. The information will give the number of full, light, fluid and special diets, and with each special diet will be given the name of the patient and the type of diet required.

THE MAIN HOSPITAL KITCHEN

In the majority of hospitals all the food, except diets is cooked in the main kitchen. In this kitchen all meals for patients, staff and visitors is prepared. In hospitals a staff restaurant is provided and there may be a snack bar for out-patients which may come under the control of the catering officer.

HOSPITAL ROUTINE

Hospital catering has its own problems, which often make it very difficult to provide correctly served meals. Wards are sometimes spread over a wide area, and, in a large hospital where there are long distances for the food to travel, provision of modern trolleys is essential to keep the food hot. The routine of a hospital is strictly timed and meals have to fit in with the mainstream business of making people well.

THE USE OF TECHNOLOGY

To get over some of the problems associated with conventional food production and distribution systems, some hospitals have invested in either cook chill or cook freeze catering systems or a combination of both. In some instances the production of the food is contracted to a food manufacturer where the skills of the hospital caterer are required to maintain standards and ensure the hygiene and regeneration systems are maintained. These systems remove the need to transport hot food over long distances at a specific time. This has always been a challenge for the professional caterer. The cost catering sector has, therefore, been strongly influenced by the introduction of technology into the kitchen, blending it with traditional expertise.

SCHOOL MEALS SERVICE

School meals play an important part in the lives of many children, often providing them with the only hot meal of the day. This was recognised as early as 1879 when a formal school meals service was first introduced, and came under government control in 1906. By 1944 the Education Act, which regarded the midday meal as the main meal of the day, required all maintained schools to provide a meal, conforming to strict nutritional and price guidelines, to anybody who wanted one. The school meals service continued to serve the community, without substantial change until 1980, when government policies sought to change the rationale and organisation of the service by way of the 1980 Education Act. This Act removed the obligation to provide school meals except where children were entitled to a free meal. At the same time minimum nutritional standards were abolished, along with the fixed charge, allowing those who continued with a service to serve and charge what they liked.

In April 2001, for the first time in over 20 years, minimum nutritional regulations were re-introduced by the DFES www.dfes.gov.uk, designed to bring all schools up to a measurable standard set down in legislation. From this date, Local Education Authorities and all schools with delegated budgets for the provision of school meals, are responsible for seeing that the compulsory minimum nutritional standards for school lunches are met. From this date there is also a duty to provide a paid meal, where parents request one, except where children are under five years old and part-time. This does not affect the LEA's or the school's duty to provide a free meal to those children who qualify for one.

The new regulations are based on the five food groups as set out in the "Balance of Good Health":
- fruit and vegetables;
- starchy foods;
- meat, Fish and other non-dairy sources of protein;
- milk and dairy foods;
- foods containing fat/sugar.

The regulations cover the first four groups only, and specify the following requirements:

Nursery schools

Food must be available from each of the first four groups

Primary schools

One option must be available from each of the first four food groups and:

○ fruit and a vegetables must be available every day; fruit based desserts must be available twice a week;

○ food from the starch group that is cooked in oil must not be on offer more than three days a week;

○ red meat must be served at least twice a week and fish at least once a week.

Cheese dishes may be included in the meat/fish protein group.

Secondary schools

Two options must be available from the first four food groups and:

○ A fruit and a vegetable must be available every day

○ Where a food from the starch group is cooked in fat or oil, an alternative starchy food not cooked in this way must also be available

○ Red meat must be served at least three times a week and fish at least twice a week

Although the regulations do not say that the meals have to be hot, it is strongly recommended that some school food should be hot, especially in the winter months. In addition drinking water should be available free of charge every day.

In special schools, because the ages are often mixed, either primary or secondary school standards may be complied with.

Further information and guidance is available on www.dfee.gov.uk/schoollunches.

School meals are generally organised in one of three ways; by a Direct Service Organisation (DSO), which is the catering arm of a local authority; by a private contractor or by an in-house provision controlled by individual schools. Each of these providers must be responsible for all aspects of the catering service including; control of finances; menu planning; food purchasing; kitchen planning; monitoring of the nutritional regulations and general administration. Supervision of the individual units is undertaken by catering managers, cook-supervisors or in the case of smaller units a cook-in-charge. The service is mainly staffed by part-time female operatives, who find that working in the school meals service can be fitted in with their domestic responsibilities. Due to the increased complexity of nutritional, hygiene and health and safety regulations, the traditional role of "school cook" has been replaced by a more professional approach to the catering function. All staff receive some form of training, often to a high level, so that the strictest standards of personal and kitchen hygiene can be maintained.

All schools offer a multi-choice menu, usually in secondary schools, operated as a cash cafeteria system, taking into consideration the wide-ranging needs of children from various cultural and religious backgrounds. In addition to these foods crisps, drinks, fresh fruit, yoghurts, cakes and biscuits, and a selection of freshly prepared rolls, sandwiches and salads can also be purchased. As well as the set menu, many senior schools offer fast food options such as burgers, pizzas, jacket potatoes and a pasta bar. At break time, hot hand-held savouries such as bacon rolls, sausage rolls and pizzas are also available. A breakfast service can also be found in many schools where there is a need, to provide for children who go to school without any breakfast. Additives, colourings and GMO foods are avoided where possible.

School lunches are seen as part of a whole-school approach to healthy lifestyles and social training. Some examples of this can be seen by the co-operation between caterers and teaching staff in a greater understanding of healthy eating messages, and the role, particularly in primary schools, that midday supervisors play in promoting good behaviour and table manners.

TYPICAL SCHOOL MENU

1 **Pizza-pasta bar:** vegetable lasagne; tomato and mascarpone pasta spirals; South Sea rice; coleslaw.

2 **Main servery:** hotpot; cauliflower cheese; jacket wedges; jacket potatoes; chips; apple crumble and custard.

3 **Baguette Bar:** variety of filled baguettes and sandwiches; hot bacon and sausage.

Plus: fresh fruit, yogurts, freshly baked cakes, pastries and cookies, drinks selection.

SAMPLE MENU				
MONDAY	**TUESDAY**	**WEDNESDAY**	**THURSDAY**	**FRIDAY**
Italian meat balls	Barbeque pork	Roast Chicken	Lamb Hot Pot	Breaded plaice
Vegetable pasty	Cheese tortellini	Vegetable chilli	Omelette	Mushroom and pepper Pasta bake
Fish Cakes	Kedgeree	Sweet and Sour Cod Balls	Fisherman's Pie	Sausages
Croquette potatoes	Spicy jacket wedges	Roast Potatoes	New Potatoes	Jacket potatoes
Pasta spirals	Wholemeal rolls	Rice	Sauté Potatoes	French stick
French beans	Red cabbage	Cabbage	Courgettes	Broccoli
Mixed veg	Peas	Sweetcorn	Cauliflower	Carrots
Baked beans	Baked beans	Baked beans	Baked beans	Baked beans
Salad	Salad	Salad	Salad	Salad
Coleslaw	Coleslaw	Coleslaw	Coleslaw	Coleslaw
Chocolate sponge	Lemon and coconut tart	Rhubarb crumble	Raspberry delight	Fresh fruit salad
Chocolate sauce	Cream	Custard		Cream

Primary schools: all pupils

These guidelines provide figures for the recommended nutrient content of an average school meal provided for over a one-week period. In practical terms this is the total amount of food provided, divided by the number of children eating it, averaged over a week.

	ENERGY	FAT	SATURATED FATTY ACIDS	CARBOHYDRATE	NME SUGARS	NSP	PROTEIN	IRON	CALCIUM	VIT A (retinol equivalents)	FOLATE
	30% of EAR	Not more than 35% of food energy *	Not more than 11% of food energy*	Not less than 50% of food energy*	Not more than 11% of food energy*	Not less than 30% of Calculated Reference Value**	Not less than 30% of RNI	Not less than 40% of RNI	Not less than 35% of RNI	Not less than 30% of RNI	Not less than 40% RNI
		Max *	Max *	Min	Max *	Min	Min	Min	Min	Min	Min
	MJ/kcal	G	g	g	g	g	g	mg	mg	micro-grams	micro-grams
MIDDLE 9–13 years	2.46 MJ 589 kcal	22.9	7.2	78.5	17.3	4.7	10.9	4.9	287	168	72

Sodium should be reduced in catering practice.

There is no absolute requirement for sugars or fats (except essential fatty acids).
** The Dietary Reference Value for non-starch polysaccharides is 18g for adults, and children should eat proportionately less, based on their lower body size. For pragmatic reasons, this has been calculated for these guidelines as a percentage of the energy recommendation, to give the Calculated Reference Value. The calculated NSP guidelines per 1,000 kcal.

Abbreviations:
DRV Dietary Reference Value
EAR Estimated Average Requirement
NME SUGARS Non-milk extrinsic sugars
NSP Non-starch polysaccharides
RNI Reference Nutrient Intake

Middle schools: all pupils

These guidelines provide figures for the recommended nutrient content of an average school meal provided for over a one-week period. In practical terms this is the total amount of food provided, divided by the number of children eating it, averaged over a week.

	ENERGY	FAT	SATURATED FATTY ACIDS	CARBOHYDRATE	NME SUGARS	NSP	PROTEIN	IRON	CALCIUM	VIT A (retinol equivalents)	FOLATE
	30% of EAR	Not more than 35% of food energy*	Not more than 11% of food energy*	Not less than 50% of food energy*	Not more than 11% of food energy*	Not less than 30% of Calculated Reference Value**	Not less than 30% of RNI	Not less than 40% of RNI	Not less than 35% of RNI	Not less than 30% of RNI	Not less than 40% of RNI
		Max*	Max*	Min	Max*	Min	Min	Min	Min	Min	Min
	MJ/kcal	G	g	g	g	g	g	mg	mg	micro-grams	micro-grams
MIDDLE 9–13 years	2.46 MJ 589 kcal	22.9	7.2	78.5	17.3	4.7	10.9	4.9	287	168	72

Sodium should be reduced in catering practice.

There is no absolute requirement for sugars or fats (except essential fatty acids).

** The Dietary Reference Value for non-starch polysaccharides is 18g for adults, and children should eat proportionately less, based on their lower body size. For pragmatic reasons, this has been calculated for these guidelines as a percentage of the energy recommendation, to give the Calculated Reference Value. The calculated NSP guidelines per 1,000 kcal.

Abbreviations:
DRV Dietary Reference Value
EAR Estimated Average Requirement
NME SUGARS Non-milk extrinsic sugars
NSP Non-starch polysaccharides
RNI Reference Nutrient Intake

FURTHER INFORMATION

Information on school meals policy may be obtained from the DfEE, Sanctuary Buildings, Great Smith Street, Westminster, London SW10 3BT, Pupil Welfare and Opportunities Division Area 4E8.

RESIDENTIAL ESTABLISHMENTS

Under this heading are included schools, colleges, halls of residence, nursing homes, homes for the elderly, hostels, where all the meals are provided. It is essential that in these establishments the nutritional balance of food is considered, and it should satisfy all the residents' nutritional needs, as in all probability the people eating here will have no other food. Since many of these establishments cater for students, and the age group which leads a very energetic life, these people usually have large appetites, and are growing fast. All the more reason that the food should be well cooked, plentiful, varied and attractive.

The food service management sector

Food Service Management covers such areas as feeding people at work in business and industry, catering in schools, college and universities, hospitals and healthcare, welfare and local authority catering and other non-profit making outlets.

Work in the traditional sectors, called cost, non-profit making, 'non-commercial' catering or 'social' catering continues but, because contractors are developing their interests in commercial catering, the term food service management describes more accurately the total contract catering industry.

Definitions in this sector are becoming increasingly blurred as contract catering enterprises move into other areas, including catering for members of the public in such outlets as leisure centres, department stores, airports, railways stations, public events and places of entertainment. Contractors are also providing a range of other support services such as housekeeping and maintenance, reception, security, laundry, bar and retail shops.

Catering for industry (industrial catering)

The provision of staff dining rooms for industrial workers has allowed many catering workers employment in first-class conditions. Apart from the main lunch meal, tea trolley rounds and/or vending machines may be part of the service. In some cases a 24-hour service is necessary and it is usual to cater for the social activities of the workers. Not only are lunches provided for the manual workers but the clerical staff and managerial staff will in most cases have their meals from the same kitchen and dining-room. There is ample scope for both men and women in this branch of the industry.

Many industries have realised that output is related to the welfare of the employees. Well-fed workers produce more and better work and because of this a great deal of money is spent in providing first-class kitchens and dining-rooms and in subsidising the meals. This means that the workers receive their food at a price lower than its actual cost, the rest of the cost being borne by the company.

Further information can be obtained from:

European Catering Association (ECA GB)
Bourne House
Horsell Park
Woking Surrey GU21 4HY
www,ecagb.co.uk.

Many companies are increasingly competing with a global economy, competition is fierce, this has led them to cut costs meaning that many organisations are moving towards a nil subsidy for meals consumed at the place of work.

Criteria for establishing a catering operation

A company is not committed to providing any catering facility if:

○ there are suitable facilities available within easy access of the employee's place of work;
○ these facilities offer a reasonable choice of food;
○ the times of opening are suitable to employer and employees.

If the above criteria are not met and the demand for catering services exist then a catering facility should be established.

Criteria for type of catering facility

Companies with 50 or more employees based on site should provide a full range of catering services, covering main meals, snacks etc. Such facilities should include a kitchen, ancillary areas, servers and dining rooms.

Companies employing less than 20 people based on site should have facilities to allow people to operate a self catering service. This would be designed to operate on a completely self-catering basis.

HOLIDAY CENTRES

Holiday centres around the UK provide leisure and hospitality facilities for families, single people and groups of people. Many companies have invested large sums of money in an effort to increase the quality of the holiday experience. Centre parcs have developed sub-tropical pools with other sporting facilities. Included in the complex are a range of different restaurant experiences. These centres are examples of all year round holiday centres encouraging people to take breaks from home, weekend breaks etc.

MOTORING SERVICES

Many motoring services provide food court type facilities for travellers, offering a comprehensive range of meals on a 24-hour basis.

DRIVE INS

Drive Ins are a relatively new concept in the UK. Drive Ins are an American import, the most notable being the McDonald's Drive Ins now located in many parts of the UK. Customers stay in their vehicles and drive up to a microphone in order to place a request. This is then relayed to a fast food service point and as the car moves forward in a queue the order is ready and waiting at the service window.

LUNCHEON CLUBS

Clerical staff in large offices are provided with lunching facilities, usually called a luncheon club or staff restaurant. These are often subsidised and in some instances the meal may be supplied without charge. The catering is frequently of a very high standard and the kitchen or kitchens will provide meals for the directors, which will be of the very best British fare or international cuisine.

Business lunches are served in small rooms so that there is privacy; the standard of food served will often be of the finest quality since the company will probably attach considerable importance to these functions. The senior clerical staff may have their own dining-room, whilst the rest of the staff will in some cases have a choice of an á la carte menu, a table d'hôte menu, waitress service or help-yourself and snack-bar facilities.

Luncheon clubs are provided by most large offices belonging to business firms, such as insurance head offices, petroleum companies, banks, etc. When luncheon facilities are not provided, many firms provide their employees with luncheon vouchers.

Large stores also provide lunching arrangements for their staff as well as the customers' restaurants.

Transport catering
RAILWAY

Meals on trains may be served in restaurant cars and snacks from buffet cars. The space in a restaurant car kitchen is very limited and there is considerable movement of the train, which causes difficulty for the staff.

Two train services run by separate companies are running through the **Channel Tunnel**. One is Euro Tunnel's Le Shuttle train, which transports drivers and their vehicles between Folkestone and Calais in 35 minutes. Food and drink is limited to that bought on dry land before the train departs.

Foot passengers wishing to ride from Waterloo to Paris or Brussels travel on Eurostar Trains. Eurostar sees the airlines as its direct competition; therefore it provides airline catering standards on board the train for first and premier class passengers. Meals are served by uniformed stewards and stewardesses in an environment similar to airline's club class. This food is included in the ticket price.

MARINE

The large liner's catering is of similar standard to the big first-class hotels and many shipping companies are noted for the excellence of their cuisine. The kitchens on board ship are usually oil-fired and extra precautions have to be taken in the kitchen in rough weather. Catering at sea includes the smaller ship, which has both cargo and passengers, and the cargo vessels which include the giant tankers of up to 100,000 tonnes.

Other aspects of catering
THE SERVICES

Catering for the armed services is specialised and they have their own training centre; details of catering facilities and career opportunities can be obtained from career information offices. Contract caterers are being increasingly used by the services.

Contract catering

The number of outlets operated by contractors declined marginally from 17,865 in 1999 to 17,830. By far the most important market in contract catering is business and industry where the number of outlets is increasing. The total number of meals continue to grow by just over 8% in 2000 to 1,471 million. The commercialisation of the contract catering market continues with the majority of contracts 66% being some form of fixed price/profit sharing agreement. The number of cost plus contracts has declined from 53% of the market to 33% in 2000.

Branded outlets is another growth area which also reflects the commercial influence of contracting.

There are many catering concerns that are prepared to undertake the catering for businesses, schools or hospitals, leaving these establishments free to concentrate on the business of educating or nursing, etc. By employing contract caterers and using the services of people who have specialised in catering, organisations can thus relieve themselves of the worry of entering a field outside their province. Contract caterers are used by nearly every type of organisation, including the armed forces. The arrangements made will vary.

Contracts

No two services or clients' requirements are the same, therefore contracts differ from company to company.

Some examples of the types of contracts available are:-

Executive Lease

The contractor provides a senior executive who will direct the client's catering operation. Normally the whole operation remains the responsibility of the client and the staff are employed by the client.

The aim is for the contractor and the executive to bring a level of expertise, which the client is unable to provide. The senior executive will be involved in implementing the systems managers and in the policy making.

The contractor will provide a manager for the unit; all staff are employed by the client on their terms and conditions. This differs from executive lease as the manager will not normally play a part in the policy making process.

Management

The client employs the contractor to supply a total catering service using the contractor's own on-site management and staff. The client also provides all the facilities and equipment.

The contractor submits a monthly account to the client, this identifies all the expenditure and income associated with the operation. The difference between the expenditure and income, including the contractor's fee, will be payable to or from the contractor.

Fixed Price

The contractor works to an annual budget fixed with the client. If the contractor overspends, she/he pays. However, if she/he under spends she/he retains the difference.

Concession

The contractor undertakes to manage an operation and rely for profit on his or her ability to maintain income levels over expenditure levels.

Contractor's Charges

Contractors generally offset their administration costs and gain their profits from three sources.
- Fees charged.
- Cash spent by customers and discounts from food and materials supplied to the client's operation.

Fee

The fees can be made up in a number of ways:
- a set annual figure charged on a weekly or monthly basis;
- a percentage of takings or costs;
- a combination of both with different percentages applying to various sections of costs;
- a per capita or per meal charge.

With over 60 companies registered in the UK contract catering is one of the biggest and most diverse sectors in the industry. COMPASS and SODEXHO are two of the largest food organisations in the UK with 8,400 locations. These include Little Chef, Travelodge and motorway service stations.

Size of contract catering market by number of meals (m) served, 1995 and 1998–2000

	1995		1998		1999		2000		% change
	m	%	m	%	m	%	m	%	1995–2000
Business and industry	465	42.7	512	39.3	545	40.1	583	39.6	25.3
State education	172	15.8	238	18.3	222	16.3	218	14.8	26.7
Independent schools	99	9.1	92	7.1	93	6.8	92	6.3	(0.7)
Catering for the public	134	12.3	150	11.5	140	10.3	145	9.8	18.8
Healthcare	81	7.4	155	11.9	198	14.6	237	16.1	192.5
Ministry of Defence	92	8.4	100	7.6	102	7.5	135	9.2	46.7
Local authorities	18	1.7	40	3.1	44	3.2	44	3.0	144.4
Oil rigs, training centres, construction sites	28	2.6	16	1.2	17	1.2	17	1.2	(39.2)
TOTAL	1,089	100.0	1,303	100.0	1,361	100.0	1,471	100.0	35.0

Source: British Hospitality Association Contract Catering Survey, 2001

Structure of the contract catering market by number of outlets, 1995 and 1998–2000

	1995		1998		1999		2000		% change
	Number	%	Number	%	Number	%	Number	%	1995–2000
Business and industry	7,574	48.5	8,410	46.3	8,766	49.1	8,930	50.0	17.9
State education	4,957	31.7	5,727	31.6	5,005	28.0	4,621	25.9	(6.7)
Independent schools	578	3.7	568	3.1	597	3.3	585	3.3	1.2
Catering for the public	971	6.2	1,328	7.3	1,218	6.8	1,253	7.0	29.0
Healthcare	397	2.5	822	4.5	923	5.2	971	5.5	144.5
Ministry of Defence	393	2.5	467	2.6	502	2.9	623	3.5	58.5
Local authorities	451	2.9	573	3.2	582	3.2	580	3.3	28.6
Oil rigs, training centres, construction sites	311	2.0	256	1.4	272	1.5	267	1,5	(14.1)
TOTAL	15,632	100.0	18,151	100.0	17,865	100.0	17,830	100.0	14.0

Source: British Hospitality Association Contract Catering Survey, 2001

PARTNERSHIP

Where the client and customer are partners in the operations and share the costs and revenues.

OUTSIDE CATERING

When functions are held where there is no catering or where the function is not within the scope of the normal catering routine, then certain firms will take over completely. Considerable variety is offered to people employed on these undertakings and often the standard will be of the very highest order. A certain amount of adaptability and ingenuity is required, especially for some outdoor jobs, but there is less chance of repetitive work. The types of function will include garden parties, agricultural and horticultural shows, the opening of new buildings, banquets, parties in private houses, etc.

Franchising

Franchising is where a manager pays a licence fee and makes whatever he/she can above an agreed percentage on the food he/she sells. Various catering concessions and outside contracting arrangements at clubs, leisure centres, colleges and offices are similar to franchising. A form of franchising is also practised in the pub business in addition to other systems like the managed pub.

Many companies who supply caterers with products like soft drinks, ice-cream or coffee distribute their products by means of purchased operators. Some suppliers providing food and drink to caterers have 'brand franchises' sometimes backing their product with appropriate equipment and advertising material to ensure that caterers prepare, present and promote the products in a consistent way.

Operating styles vary considerably from pizza, hamburgers, baked croissants to full menu restaurants, coffee shops and pancake houses. Despite all the differences, all the franchise schemes work on the same basic principle. An established catering company offers a complete package of experience, operating systems and on-going marketing support sufficient to enable outside operators to set up and operate their own units within the chain. The investor makes an initial franchise payment and then pays a continuing royalty or commission which is often expressed as a percentage of gross turnover. All investment in property, buildings and equipment is borne by the franchise; in some cases the franchise might play some part in securing the property.

Franchising has several advantages:

○ Firstly it allows for many to be set up nationally and by doing so maximises on economies of scale in purchasing promotional material in the development of the brand image.

○ The franchisee gains because the opportunity is shared to invest in a pretested catering concept, backed by advertising, research and development, training and other resources which may otherwise be beyond their finance parameters.

○ The banks also show an interest in franchising, in many ways they see it as a reasonably safe investment.

○ The oldest franchising schemes in the UK are Wimpy, established in the mid 1950s and KFC, which started in the early 1960s. Many of the most active franchise schemes are based on a fast-food style of menu and operating system. Now there is a growing market involving wider menus, medium spend restaurants, mainly licensed. Examples include Pizza Express Chain, and Dutch Pancake Houses.

Catering at sea

Major changes and developments have occurred and are occurring with ferry and shipping companies, particularly those dealing with cruises.

The standards of service, quality of food and hygiene is of the highest and the training schemes offered are most exceptional. For those wishing to make a career in this area of catering, the opportunities are of a first class nature. On becoming a crew member, in addition to the responsibilities associated with their work all personnel are knowledgeable on safety aspects such as life saving equipment, life jackets, life, life rafts, emergency signals etc.

The sea ferries offer a variety of food in all weather conditions, for example P&O have:

1 First base – a self service of burgers, fries etc which appeal to the younger generation.

2 Routemaster – a restaurant for freight and coach drivers and couriers which is plate service.

3 International Food Court with a wide range of international, speciality and English dishes where passengers can choose from a snack to a three course meal with wine.

4 Langan's Brasserie – an exclusive restaurant offering the finest quality of food freshly prepared and cooked.

5 Weather conditions affect crossings, passengers and crew, for example, a meal served in the Brasserie or elsewhere would be completed in 75 minutes.

The numbers of persons using the ferries is increasing despite the convenience of the Channel Tunnel. This may partly be due to the pleasure of the experience of eating on board ship.

Cruise companies are increasing rapidly their number of cruise liners and the size of their ships. This means the job opportunities and promotion prospects are excellent and training is also provided. The benefit of travel all over the world and producing and serving customers at the very highest standards in hygienic conditions makes it a most interesting and worthwhile career. As an example of working conditions, staff may work for three months and then have, say two months off. On board hours of work could be 10 hours a day for 7 days a week. This appeals to many people who wish to be producing food at its best in excellent conditions.

Figure 1.5 shows a Purser's dept F & B.

CRUISE SHIPS

Cruise ships are floating luxury hotels. In the 1980s there was a huge growth in the US cruising market. As a result cruise companies commissioned a number of re-builds. This growth continued throughout the 90s, as more and more people became interested in cruising as a lifestyle.

In 2001 P&O cruises and Royal Caribbean cruises merged to combine forces to create the world's largest cruise vacation group with the most modern fleet among the major cruise companies. This represents 41 ships and some 75,000 berths. With a further 14 ships planned by 2004, offering over 30,000 additional berths.

Demographic changes and consumer interest for leisure activities coupled with high levels of customer satisfaction, support a positive long term outlook for the cruise industry.

Each cruise ship takes an average of 1810 passengers in approximately 77,000 tons with 850 crew members.

On board there are two main traditional restaurants with a number of different food outlets reflecting the change of customer lifestyles, their needs and wants from the leisure markets. These include a French style bistro, self-service buffet option, branded fast food outlets. Many new customers prefer less formal dining. Their preference is for deck barbecues at lunchtime, themed buffets, e.g. Neptune buffet featuring a range of shellfish. People want to stay beside the pool and eat rather than dine in the traditional restaurant. This demonstrates how modern cruise ships cater for a wide clientele with a wide range of tastes. On board the customer will also

Figure 1.5 *The Purser's Department.*

Purser's Department
Food and Beverage

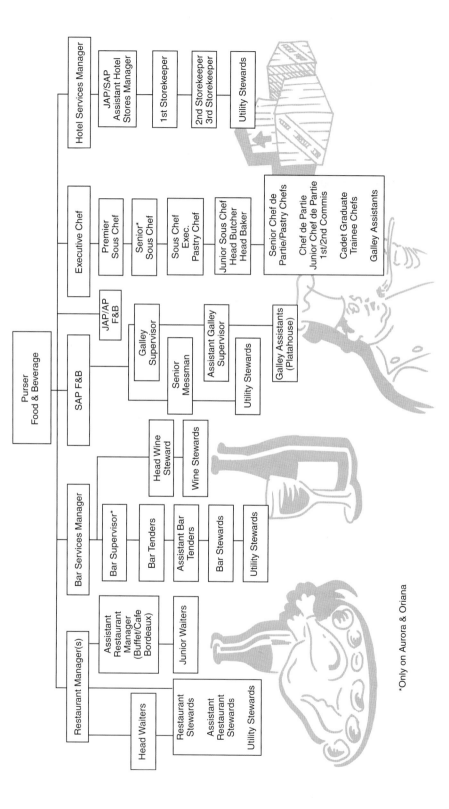

*Only on Aurora & Oriana

experience champagne and caviar bar, coffee and chocolate bar, pub style sports bar, club style bars etc.

Each cruise ship is positioned to cater for slightly different needs and markets within the cruise market.

The similarity between all ships is the dinner menu which is often a well balanced traditional style menu.

The difference between cruise ships is what happens on the decks, public rooms and the style of entertainment. In future some ships will have business centres, cyber cafes.

The food and beverage provision is computerised and requires the careful management of logistics. Raw materials, fresh fruit and vegetables, and meat supplies are sourced through key provision ports around the world. Meat, fruit and vegetables are sourced from the United States, Australia and New Zealand. Container ships are also sent to ports to meet the cruise ships on their arrival for re-stocking. As with every other operation all food orders from guests are placed into the computer to see what the guests are buying and a pye chart is printed out to examine the popularity for dishes. This assists with future ordering and cuts down on waste. In 2001 P&O cruises spent £12 million on food, £20 million on food and drink, 12 tonnes of food and drink were consumed daily.

A separate kitchen team looks after the mess rooms from a separate galley with approximately 8–10 staff. These staff work from a different set of menus.

Food hygiene and safety must meet not only UK standards but the US standard as well.

Staff work a 10 hour day, 7 days a week while at sea, then take extended time off before their next sailing.

Apart from the food, beverage and accommodation staff and the captain crew, there will be on board for every voyage a full engineering team, maintenance team and medical team.

Corporate hospitality

The purpose of corporate hospitality is to build business relationships and to raise corporate awareness. Corporate entertaining is also used as a means of thanking or rewarding loyal customers.

Companies are increasingly recognising the increasing importance of relationship marketing and corporate reputation.

Reasons for spending money on corporate hospitality:
1 Building relationships with potential customers.
2 To reward customers/thank you for loyalty.
3 As a marketing tool/raise company or product profile.
4 Increase business/sales.
5 To achieve closer informal contact in a relaxed environment.
6 To raise and keep up the company's profile/public relations.
7 Repeat business/retention of clients or customers.
8 Keep the customers happy/to entertain them, act as a sweetener.
9 To talk about business/networking.
10 To achieve better communication interaction/improved understanding.
11 Expected to do it.
12 To reward/boost staff or team morale.
13 Social benefits/opportunity to relax.

The corporate hospitality market has grown from £600 million in 1997 to £700 million in 1999. (Source: Corporate Hospitality & Event Association).

The main reasons for this growth is company expansion and increased budgets for corporate hospitality. These companies with increased budgets are generally committing to bigger or more superior events and increased spending per head or holding more frequent events.

An emerging trend is for companies to use corporate hospitality in a more targeted way rather than taking a broad brush approach. Companies are therefore being more selective about invitees and matching them to appropriate events.

90% of corporate hospitality is aimed at current customers or clients. There is also a trend towards using corporate hospitality to motivate employees, in an increasingly competitive corporate environment in encouraging companies to invest in their own workforce.

Recipients of corporate hospitality are more likely to accept invitations from current suppliers rather than from potential suppliers.

USING THE INTERNET AS A BUSINESS TOOL

As in all areas of business, the internet is playing an increasingly important role in corporate hospitality. The internet is used to source information. Bookings can also be made on-line.

Websites detail comprehensive corporate hospitality information on events throughout the year. On-line services allow customers to book an event directly offering real benefits to the customer. These include:

○ official hospitality in official locations;
○ cost efficient by booking direct from source;
○ time efficient;
○ one-stop shop service from initial enquiry through the event;
○ for many caterers, access to any established name, with the attendant back-up of media, advertising and merchandising material, is a strong argument for franchising.

Some references to economics elsewhere in the book

Topics for Discussion

1 Give your impressions of the food that was served at your previous schools with suggestions for improvement.

2 Explain the importance of food for the hospital patient with suggestions for the types of food to be offered.

3 Industrial catering is an important aspect of the catering industry; discuss why this is so and give examples of menus for three different dining rooms.

4 Discuss what you think persons travelling on aircraft would like to eat and explain how it may, or may not, be feasible to provide.

5 How do you think changes in the industry will occur over the next 10 years? Explain why you think they will happen.

6 Each student in the group to obtain a number of menus from each type of catering and pool for group discussion.

7 What impact, if any, do you think organic foods will have on menus?

Contd.

8   What essential differences attract staff to the various aspects of the industry, consider for example pay, conditions of work, career prospects etc?

9   Establishments such as motorway facilities should meet special needs, explain what they are and how they are met and select another area of catering and state what those needs are and how they are achieved.

CHAPTER 2

EMPLOYMENT IN THE HOSPITALITY INDUSTRY

EMPLOYMENT OPPORTUNITIES

Employment opportunities exist within the widely differing aspects of the industry, and careers within the various sectors will vary according to the type and size of the establishment. Most organisations will provide any or all of the following areas for employment:

- kitchens; (food preparation);
- restaurants; (food and beverage service);
- food Service Areas, Lounges;
- bars;
- sports and Leisure Facilities;
- administration;
- reception;
- accommodation and Housekeeping.

Jobs exist at all levels of employment: managers, chefs, commis chefs, restaurant managers, receptionists, housekeepers, bar stewards, pub managers, maintenance staff, sports instructors, purchasing officers, porters, financial managers, administrative and clerical staff.

The law now governs most aspects of the employment relationship, from the time an employer decides to recruit a new employee to the time the employee leaves.

EMPLOYEES OF A COMPANY

People employed under a contract of service and not those people who are working under a contract for service, who are self employed.

Workers

Workers who are not necessarily employees have levels of protection. A worker is an individual who works under a contract of employment where the individual undertakes any work or services for another party to the contract whose status is not that of a client or customer.

Legislation that protects 'workers'.

- Race, sex and disability discrimination.
- Health and Safety Legislation.
- National Minimum Wage.
- Working Time Regulations 1998.
- Part-time Workers Regulations 2000.

AGENCY WORKERS

These are temporary workers supplied to a client normally through an employment agency.

TEMPORARY EMPLOYEES

There is no distinction made in law between temporary workers and permanent employees. Some rights depend on employees having accumulated two years' continuous service with their employers. Once an employee has completed that qualifying period of service then he or she is entitled to these rights bestowed by the law whether or not the employer considers him or her to be a permanent employee.

CASUAL WORKERS

The hospitality industry employs many casual workers to help them through the peak periods of demand, especially in functions and in banqueting.

The question of whether casual workers can accumulate continuous service, and qualify for statutory rights given to employees, is impossible to answer in definite terms. In one case, the Court of Appeal upheld a tribunal ruling that regular casuals were not employees and so did not have the same rights as their full-time colleagues, because:

a their engagements were terminable without notice;

b the casual workers had the right to decide whether or not to accept work;

c there was no obligation on the company to provide work;

d it was the view of both parties that the casual workers were independent contractors;

e it is the recognised custom and practice in the hospitality industry that workers are engaged under contracts for services (i.e. they are not employees).

SEASONAL WORKERS

People who are only employed on a seasonal basis may qualify for certain statutory rights.

If a seasonal worker is employed on a part-time basis out of season, and there is no break in employment between the full-time and the part-time work, the service is classed as continuous.

FIXED TERM CONTRACTS

In July 2002 the EU Directive on fixed-term contracts came into force.

Employees on fixed-term contracts should not be treated less favourably than similar permanent employees in their terms and conditions of employment unless there is an objective reason to justify less favourable treatment. This does not relate to pay and pensions but to benefits such as annual leave, sick pay, access to social and recreational facilities.

PART-TIME WORKERS

The Part-time Workers Regulation came into effect on 1 July 2000 as a result of the EU Directive which seeks to remove any discrimination against and improve the quality of part-time work.

Human Rights Act in employment

The Human Rights Act 1998 came into force which prohibits discrimination and provides the right of freedom of expression; thought, conscience and religion; respect for private and family life.

This applies to employers in organisations of any size from the time of recruitment through the period of employment to termination.

It is illegal to dismiss an employee on the following grounds:

○ Political opinion.

○ Dress codes (e.g. that may discriminate against certain religious groups).

○ Religion.
○ Trade Union Membership.
○ Employers may infringe employees' rights to privacy through any monitoring or surveillance activities adapting such as e-mail or internet access.

EMPLOYMENT TRIBUNALS

Employment tribunals, previously known as industrial tribunals, were first created by the Industrial Training Act 1964 to deal with employers' appeals against assessment to levy by industrial training boards. Their scope, though, was radically extended in 1971 and again in 1974.

Their function now is also to provide the informal and speedy method for employees to enforce their rights against employers for breaches of the following acts:

Equal Pay Act 1970
Health and Safety at Work Act 1974
Sex Discrimination Acts 1975 and 1986
Race Regulations Act 1976
Transfer of Undertakings (Protection of Employment Regulations 1981)
Employment Rights Act 1996

For most purposes the tribunal will be comprised of the chairman and two other members who are appointed by the Secretary of State for employment, and will be drawn from lists proposed by the employers' organisations and employees' organisations. Under new rules brought in with the Trade Union Reform and Employment Rights Act 1993 the chairperson may also sit alone to hear some cases.

Appeals against the decisions of tribunals, on points of law, may be made to the Employment Appeal Tribunal, and from there to the Court of Appeal. The final arbiter in legal matters in the UK is the House of Lords.

All decisions of appeal courts in the UK (i.e. the Employment Appeal Tribunal and Court of Appeal) on points of law which establish a legal precedent (i.e. a principle of legal importance) are binding on the law courts unless and until they are overturned.

RIGHTS IN EMPLOYMENT

The Employment Rights Act 1996, consolidated all the legislation in the individual, as opposed to collective rights of employees that were formally contained in the following:

Redundancy Payments Act 1965
Contracts of Employment Act 1972
Trade Union and Labour Regulations Act 1974
The Employment Protection Act 1975
The Employment Protection Consolidation Act 1978
The Wages Act 1986
Trade Union Reform and Employment Rights Act 1993

The Collective Rights in these Acts remain.

Most have been incorporated into the Trade Union and Labour Relations (Consolidation) Act 1992. Also included are the Working Time Regulations 1998 and the Data Protection Act 1998. *See page 42 for further legislation.

ENFORCEMENT OF EMPLOYMENT RIGHTS

Employees make an application to the employment tribunal. This may be done by obtaining a form from the local job centre. A copy of the completed form is automatically sent to ACAS, who may choose to get involved by approaching the "Applicant" (employee) and the "Respondent" (employer). All claims should be made within three months of termination of employment.

Contd. p 42

Recruitment and selection

The purpose of recruitment is to select the staff you require who will best fit your organisation. The employer's freedom, however, to select the preferred candidate is to some extent limited. The Race Relations Act 1976, Sex Discrimination Act 1975, Rehabilitation of Offenders Act 1974, Trade Union Reform and Employment Rights Act 1993, the Disability Discrimination Act 1995 and rules in employment of overseas workers all impose restrictions.

Racial discrimination

Employers may not discriminate against employees or job applicants on racial grounds. Therefore you cannot treat a person less favourably on racial grounds than he or she treats or would treat other people.

It is unlawful, under the Race Relations Act 1976, to publish, or cause to be published, an advertisement which indicates an intention to discriminate on racial grounds. It is also unlawful to discriminate against people on racial grounds in the arrangements for determining who should be selected for a job, the terms on which employment is offered or by refusing to offer a person the job because of his or her racial group.

Discrimination in employment is also unlawful. There must be equal opportunities for promotion, training, transfer, facilities and services.

People must also not suffer segregation and victimisation on racial grounds.

Sex discrimination

The Sex Discrimination Act 1975 outlaws discrimination on grounds of sex and on the grounds that a person is married. There is nothing, however, that prevents an employer from discriminating against single people, provided he or she makes no distinction between men and women.

Job advertising must also not discriminate on the basis of sex. It would not be unlawful to advertise for a steward provided that the advertisement clearly stated that the job was open to men and women.

Rehabilitation of offenders

The Rehabilitation of Offenders Act 1974 provides that certain offences will become 'spent' after a specific period of time. The effect of this is that the offender is allowed to treat the spent conviction as never having existed, and if the employer later discovers the existence of the spent conviction he or she cannot use it as grounds for dismissing an employee or excluding a job applicant from employment.

Workers from overseas

A person who is a European Community national is allowed to enter the UK to obtain employment without a work permit or other prior consent.

Nationals of EC member states have the right to the same treatment as British citizens as regards pay and conditions, union rights, social security and industrial injury benefits and facilities for vocational training and retraining and of national employment services.

For this reason hospitality companies in the UK regularly recruit from the European Union to overcome skill and staff shortages.

Workers from the EFTA states, for example Finland, Iceland and Norway, are free to work in the UK.

Commonwealth citizens and foreign nationals

People from the Commonwealth and outside the European Union must obtain work permits, which must be for a specified occupational area in a named company.

Hotel and catering employees who have managed to secure a senior post in the UK have to apply for work permits. The senior posts must be one of the following:

- hotel or restaurant managers;
- senior chefs;
- senior restaurant staff;
- senior receptionists.

Applicants must have at least five year's experience outside the UK. Two years of which must be in a supervisory position. They must be coming to work in a UK organisation under the category 'high class' as specified by the Department of Education and Employment. The price and the range of food and wine offered to customers should reflect the need for the establishment to recruit high calibre staff from overseas www.workpermits.gov.uk.

Asylum and Immigration Act 1996

The Act was introduced to ensure that only those who are legally entitled to work in the UK are offered employment. Employers who employ illegal immigrants face a fine for each person who is employed illegally. Therefore employers must make certain checks before employing a person. For example, employers could ask for one of the following to confirm status:

- national insurance number;
- document issued by previous employer;
- passport describing the holder as having the right of abode in the UK;
- a birth certificate issued in the UK or the Republic of Ireland;
- a letter from the Home Office confirming status;
- an official work permit.

Equal Pay Act 1970

The Equal Pay Act 1970 gives men and women the right to equal pay. The right applies when the work of a woman is of the same or broadly similar nature to the work of the man, and when the work, although it may be different, has been given equal value under a job evaluation scheme. When the work of a woman is not the same or similar to the work of a man, but has been rated as equivalent under a job evaluation scheme, the woman may still claim equal pay with a man if the work she is doing requires effort, skill and problem solving of equal value to what a man is doing in the same employment.

The Disability Discrimination Act 1995

The Act applies to all organisations which employ fifteen or more people. This Act is very similar to the Sex Discrimination and Race Relations Acts, and protects disabled people against discrimination. Guidance notes on the definition of disability have been issued by the HMSO entitled 'Guidance on matters to be taken into account in determining questions relating to the definition of disability'.

The Act makes it unlawful to discriminate against a disabled person in the recruitment process, in the terms upon which a job is offered, in the opportunities offered for promotion training, transfer or any other benefit, or in the dismissal of a disabled person.

The Disability Discrimination Act 1995 will be enforced by October 2004. This will require employers with 15 or more staff to ensure that discrimination does not occur in the work place or in relation to recruitment and dismissal. Further information: Disability Rights Commission (DRC) 08457 622633 www.drc-gb.org

STAKEHOLDER PENSION SCHEMES

Companies employing more than 5 staff are required by law to set up pension schemes for all employees both full and part-time. Fines up to £50,000 can be imposed for non-compliance.

Employee associations

INDEPENDENT TRADE UNIONS

There are only a small number of trade unions which operate in the hospitality industry.

Trade unions must be certified as independent by the certification officer. The certification of independence is only granted if the trade union is:

a not under the domination or control of an employer;

b not liable for financial support by an employer.

The certification officer takes into account the history of the union and its collective bargaining record, its organisation and structure and its membership base.

Whether a trade union is recognised or not is entirely dependent on the employer. Recognition means the employer is willing to negotiate with the union on employment matters.

Staff associations

Apart from trade unions no other type of employee association has legal standing in the UK. They are however referred to within the European Social Charter.

The Trade Union and Labour Relations (Consolidation) Act 1992, imposes a duty on all employers who recognise independent trade unions for the purpose of collective bargaining to disclose to representatives of these unions all information relating to the undertaking which is both:

i information without which the representatives would be impeded in carrying on collective bargaining to a material extent, and

ii information which should be disclosed to them for the purposes of collective bargaining, in accordance with good industrial relations practice.

The duty to disclose only arises where a trade union representative makes a written request for information which he or she believes the trade union needs for the purposes of collective bargaining.

Employees who are members of an independent trade union which is recognised by the employer are allowed to take reasonable time off during working hours to take part in any activities of that union or any other activities where the employee is acting as a representative of that union.

The Fixed Term Employees (Prevention of Less Favourable Treatment) Regulations 2002 apply to "employees" and not to the extended category of "workers" (do not apply to agency workers). They intend to curb the abuse of fixed term contracts and to limit their successive renewal. The regulations provide that fixed term employees should not be treated less favourably than comparable permanent employees in their terms and conditions of employment unless there is objective justification.

The regulations do not cover:

○ pay;

○ Occupational pension schemes.

The Working Time Regulations 1998

From 1 October 1998, the regulations impose the following duties on employers.

1 A maximum average working week of 48 hours, over 7 days. Any worker can agree to work in excess of the limit, provided that the agreement is in writing. It must be possible for the worker to terminate the agreement.

2 Rules for rest breaks require a daily rest of 11 hours consecutively in every 24-hour period worked. 24 hours rest in every 7 days, averaged over 2 weeks. 20 minutes when working more than 6 hours, or a period to be agreed.

The regulations also specify paid holidays. There are also rules for night work shifts.

Exceptions:

There are exceptions for those working:

○ in the air, rail, road, sea, inland waterways;

○ sea fishing;

○ trainee doctors;

○ armed forces, police, etc.

The Health & Safety Executive will monitor the implementation of the regulations by employers.

The British Hospitality Association (BHA) has produced a Standard Workforce Agreement for their members.

A.C.A.S – Advisory, Conciliation and Arbitration Service

ACAS's staff are employment relations experts. Their job is to help people to work together effectively. This ranges from setting up the right structures and systems to finding a way of settling disputes when things go wrong.

ACAS has a wealth of experience working with employers, employees, trade unions and other representatives.

ACAS was founded in 1974; it is a public funded body, run by a council of 12 members from business, unions and the independent sector.

Aims of equal opportunities

Equal opportunities aims to remove discriminatory barriers and put in place arrangements to help disadvantaged groups catch up. This approach is underpinned by legislation.

The United Kingdom as a member of the European Union has implemented several directives applicable to all member states including the Equal Treatment Directive, the Equal Pay Directive and the Parental Leave Directive by passing the following acts:

The Sex Discrimination Act 1975
The Race Relations Act 1976
The Disability Discrimination Act 1995

Equal opportunities legislation takes a similar approach in many countries. First, it makes direct discrimination illegal. This means treating men and women differently, preferring one ethnic group to another, or not employing disabled people. Discrimination at work is usually quite obvious when it occurs and it is illegal even if discrimination is seen as in the best interests of the individual (e.g. worry about a women coping in an all male kitchen). Secondly, it makes indirect discrimination illegal. This means putting in place requirements which are applied to all applicants or employees but which have the effect of excluding more of one group than another. If these requirements cannot be justified they are illegal. Typical examples based on cases coming before industrial tribunals in the UK.

○ Putting a minimum age limit of 28 for joining a management training scheme (excludes more women than men because women are more likely to be away from work to look after children at this stage in their lives).

○ Requires fluent English for a kitchen porter's job (excludes people for whom English is not a first language which is not a necessary requirement for the job).

○ Having less favourable terms for part-timers than for full timers (a higher proportion of women work part-time than men).

EQUAL OPPORTUNITIES

○ Developing an overarching Equal Opportunities policy statement covering all groups.

○ Introduce policies forbidding sexual and racial harassment, together with supporting procedures.

○ Introduce recruitment, selection, appraisal and promotion policies and procedures, supported with management training.

○ Advertise all vacancies, use up-to-date job descriptions and person specification and select by job related criteria.

○ Private targeted training e.g. assertiveness training, management courses for women and ethnic minorities, disability awareness.

○ Make work as accessible as possible for different groups (e.g. flexible hours, help with childcare, make buildings as accessible as possible for disabled people).

○ Introduce workforce monitoring to enable further equal opportunities, plans and initiatives.

ADOPTING AN EQUAL OPPORTUNITIES APPROACH

○ Open the pool to get the best quality people.

○ Makes clear the qualities to look for in recruitment and promotion.

○ Develops individuals who may have been overlooked in the past.

○ Makes sure all legal requirements are met.

○ Motivates all staff.

However, positive discrimination is also unlawful but positive action is allowed and encouraged.

Source: HCIMA May 1999

Employment growth by sector

	1999	2009	% annual growth 1999–2009
Hotels	222,100	267,300	1.9
Restaurants	410,700	503,600	2.1
Pubs and bars	271,800	350,700	2.6
Contract catering	129,000	150,100	1.5
Hospitality services	636,800	683,700	0.7
TOTAL	**1,670,400**	**1,955,300**	**1.6**

The total of 1.67 million includes people working in the industry who are not hospitality classified, such as marketing and administration jobs.

Looking at purely hospitality classified occupations, the 1999 total of 1.53 million staff is expected to increase by 1.6% each year reaching 1.79 million employees by 2009.

Source: Hospitality Training Foundation Skills and Employment Forecasts 2000

Some references to employment in the book.

Topics for Discussion

1 Outline the function of an employment tribunal.
2 Discuss the reasons why the hospitality industry is poorly represented by trade unions.
3 Discuss some of the legislation which protects people from employment discrimination.
4 Why is it important to any organisation to develop good industrial relations?
5 Do you believe that the current employment legislation is adequate, inadequate or prohibits the development of the hospitality industry?

*[contd. from page 36] **Employment Act 2002 covers maternity leave and pay and gives special rights to working parents.**

PART 2

Trends and Influences

CHAPTER 3

FOOD AND SOCIETY

TASTE

Why do we eat what we eat, select one dish from the menu in preference to another, choose one particular kind of restaurant or use a take-away? Why are these dishes on the menu in the first place? Is it because the chef likes them, the customer or the consumer wants them, or is this the only food available? What dictates what we eat?

Catering reflects the eating habits, history, customs and taboos of society but it also develops and creates them. You have only to compare the variety of eating facilities available on any major street today with those of a short while ago.

Taste affects food choice, and is based on biological, social and cultural perspectives. The perception of taste results from the stimulation of the taste cells which make up the taste buds. Taste is not specific to individual foods, but to the balance between four main types of chemical compound. These compounds correspond to four sensations (see page 418–420).

Some factors which affect what we eat
THE INDIVIDUAL

Everyone has needs and wishes these to be met according to his or her own satisfaction.

○ **Tastes** and **habits** in eating are influenced by three main factors: upbringing, peer group behaviour and social background. For example, childrens' tastes are developed at home according to the eating patterns of their family, as is their expectation of *when* to eat meals; teenagers may frequent hamburger or other fast-food outlets; and adults may eat out once a week at an ethnic or high-class restaurant, steakhouse or pub.

○ Degree of **hunger** will affect what is to be eaten, when, and how much to eat – although some people in the western world overeat and food shortages cause under-nourishment in poorer countries. Everyone ought to eat enough to enable body and mind to function efficiently; if you are hungry or thirsty it is difficult to work or study effectively.

○ **Health** considerations may influence choice of food, either because a special diet is required for medical reasons, or (as the current emphasis on healthy eating shows) because everyone needs a nutritionally balanced diet. Many people nowadays feel it is more healthy not to eat meat or dairy products. Others are vegetarian or vegan on moral or religious grounds.

RELATIONSHIPS

Eating is a necessity, but it is also a means of developing social relationships. The needs and preferences of the people you eat with should be considered. This applies in the family or at the place of study or work. School meals can be a means of developing good eating habits, both by the provision of suitable foods and dishes and by creating an appropriate environment to foster social relationships. Canteens, dining rooms and restaurants for people at work can be places where relationships develop.

Often the purpose of eating, either in the home or outside it, is to be sociable and to meet people, or to renew or provide the opportunity for people to meet each other. Frequently there is a reason for the occasion (such as birthday, anniversary, wedding, awards ceremony), needing a special party or banquet menu – or it may just be for a few friends to have a meal at a restaurant.

Business is often conducted over a meal, usually at lunchtime but also at breakfast and dinner. Eating and drinking help to make work more enjoyable and effective.

EMOTIONAL NEEDS

Sometimes we eat not because we need food but to meet an emotional requirement:

○ for sadness or depression – eating a meal can give comfort to oneself or to someone else; after a funeral people eat together to comfort one another;

○ for a reward or a treat, or to give encouragement to oneself or to someone else; an invitation to a meal is a good way of showing appreciation.

IDEAS ABOUT FOOD

People's ideas about food and meals, and about what is and what is not acceptable, vary according to where and how they were raised, the area in which they live and its social customs.

Different societies and cultures have had in the past, and still have, conflicting ideas about what constitutes good cooking and a good chef, and about the sort of food a good chef should provide. The French tradition of producing fine food and highly respected chefs continues to this day – whereas other countries may traditionally have less interest in the art of cooking, and less esteem for chefs.

What constitutes people's idea of a snack, a proper meal or a celebration will depend on their backgrounds, as will their interpretation of terms such as lunch or dinner. One person's idea of a snack may be another person's idea of a main meal; a celebration for some will be a visit to a hamburger bar; to others, a meal at a fashionable restaurant.

The idea of what is 'the right thing to do' regarding eating varies with age, social class and religion. To certain people it is right to eat with the fingers, others use only a fork; some will have cheese before the sweet course, others will have cheese after it; it is accepted that children and often elderly people need food to be cut up into small pieces, and that people of some religions do not eat certain foods. The ideas usually originate from practical and hygienic reasons although sometimes the origin is obscure.

IMAGES OF FOOD

Fashions, fads and fancies affect foods and it is not always clear if catering creates or copies these trends.

○ Nutritionists inform us what foods are good and necessary in the diet, what the effect of particular foods will be on the figure and how much of each food we require. This helps to produce an 'image' of food. This image changes according to research, availability of food and what is considered to constitute healthy eating.

○ What people choose to eat says something about them as a person – it creates an image. We are what we eat, but *why* do we choose to eat what we do when there is *choice*? One person will perhaps avoid trying snails because of ignorance of how to eat them, or because the idea is repulsive, whilst another will select them deliberately to show off to guests. One person will select a dish because it is a new experience, another will choose it because it was enjoyed when eaten before. The quantity eaten may indicate a glutton or a gourmand; the quality selected, a gourmet.

The food itself

Crop failure or distribution problems may make food scarce or not available at all. Foods in season are now supplemented by imported foods, so that foods out of season at home are now available much of the time. It means that there is a wide choice of food for the caterer and the customer.

○ Food is available through shops, supermarkets, cash and carry, wholesalers and direct suppliers. People at home and caterers are able to purchase, prepare, cook and present almost every food imaginable due to rapid air transport and food preservation. Food spoilage and wastage are minimised; variety and quality are maximised.

○ It is essential that food looks attractive, has a pleasing smell and tastes good. Food which is nutritious but does not look, smell or taste nice is less likely to be eaten. With cooking, these points must be considered, but it should be remembered that people's views as to what is attractive and appealing will vary according to their background and experience.

RESOURCES

Money, time and facilities affect what people eat – the economics of eating affects everyone.

○ **How much money** an individual is able, or decides to spend on food is crucial to what is eaten. Some people will not be able to afford to eat out, others will only be able to eat out occasionally, but for others eating out will be a frequent event. The money that individuals allocate for food will determine whether they cook and eat at home, use a take-away (e.g. fish and chips, Chinese), go to a pub, eat at a pancake house, or at an ethnic or other restaurant.

○ The **amount of time** people have to eat at work will affect whether they use any facilities provided, go out for a snack or meal, or bring their own food to work.

○ The **ease of obtaining food**, the use of convenience and frozen food and the facility for storing foods, has meant that in the home and in catering establishments the range of foods is wide. Foods in season can be frozen and used throughout the year, so if there is a glut then spoilage can be eliminated.

INFLUENCES

The media influences what we eat – television, radio, newspapers, magazines and literature of all kinds have an effect on our eating habits (see the table on page 47).

○ Healthy eating, nutrition, hygiene and outbreaks of food poisoning are publicised; experts in all aspects of health including those extolling exercise, diet and environmental health, state what should and should not be eaten.

○ Information regarding the content of food packets and the advertising of food influences our choice. Knowledge about eating and foods is learnt from the family, through teachers, at school meals, at college, through the media and through the experience of eating at home and abroad.

The following examples illustrate how these factors can affect what people eat: A TV programme shows the effects of a drought in Africa, in a region where political factions are at war, thus preventing food distribution. Money is given by people morally concerned that others are starving, so air transport is used to deliver foods that have been preserved to provide adequate nutrition. The food should also be in keeping with the religious beliefs and cultural background of those in need.

Another example is related to planning a menu. The first thing to consider is who it is for; therefore it must not conflict with the consumer's religious beliefs or ethnic origin. The price must be affordable and the items on the menu obtainable. To illustrate further: let us say that a restaurant owner has advertised in the local paper, and a family decide to go to this restaurant to celebrate an anniversary. The food they select will be in keeping with their taste, and it may include dishes they are familiar with or new dishes on the menu (which, perhaps, are prepared off the premises and reheated in the owner's new technological equipment). Some of the items available on the menu may have been flown in from countries which have a climate that allows the production of foods not grown here. In addition, it might so happen that the restaurant is part of a pub which was, say, an original coaching inn named after Bonnie Prince Charlie – so perhaps Scottish dishes are always available, particularly on special occasions such as Burns night, when the local Scots celebrate and eat haggis which is traditional, nutritionally beneficial and flown down from Scotland. (Also, the host and his wife may have relations in Ireland and Wales, so perhaps national dishes of these countries feature on the menu as well.)

We are all creatures of habit conditioned by customs and restrictions, as much in what we do or do not eat, as in what we will or will not wear. Variety is not only the spice of life: it is the ingredient which makes catering and cooking so fascinating.

Influences on what people eat

MEDIA	TRANSPORT	RELIGIOUS

TV
books
newspapers
journals
	transport of foods by:
	    sea
	    rail
	    air
	transport of people
		taboos
		festivals

GEOGRAPHICAL	**HISTORICAL**	**ECONOMIC**

climate
indigenous:
    fish
    birds
    animals
    plant life
	explorations
	invasions
	establishment of trade routes
		money to purchase
		goods to exchange

SOCIOLOGICAL	**POLITICAL**	**CULTURAL**
family school work place leisure fashion and trends	tax on food policies on food 'mountains' export and import restrictions	ethnic tribal celebrations
PSYCHOLOGICAL	**PHYSIOLOGICAL**	**SCIENTIFIC**
appearance of food smell taste aesthetics reaction to new foods	nutritional healthy eating illness additives	preservation technology

These influences are separated for convenience but in reality overlap. Only when sufficient food is available for survival can pleasure from food develop.

FOOD CHANGES IN BRITISH SOCIETY

In the past, inns catered for people travelling by coach, with coffee houses in the towns. Later, with the development of railways, the hotel and catering industry expanded rapidly.

The twentieth century has brought sweeping changes in eating patterns and health. A hundred years ago, most people ate plenty of fibre from bread and potatoes, but they lacked an adequately varied diet. Diseases caused by a lack of vitamins and minerals were common. Today, the problems are different. Many people eat too much meat, dairy produce and sugar, and too little fibre for good health. New methods of farming and food processing, food selling and storage have helped to alter what we eat.

1900s

As the population grew rapidly at the turn of the century, so food imports rose. By 1914 British farmers met less than a quarter of the country's food needs.

New manufacturing processes created new products; people began to eat less bread and potatoes as the new shops brought in cheap cod packed in ice. Flour, margarine and tinned condensed milk were cheap and popular; biscuits, jam, chocolate and cheese also began to be factory-made. Such products were often cleaner and purer than those previously available, but sometimes of less nutritional value. In towns the first grocery store chains appeared and new co-operative retail societies also flourished. Eating out was limited to fish and chip shops, chop houses and pubs.

Beneath the outward prosperity of Edwardian England were various social problems. One-third of the population was poor and undernourished, a situation that led eventually to school medical inspections and clinics.

1930s

The First World War had brought home just how dependent Britain was on imported food, and how unfit the nation was – thousands of men had been graded unfit for active service. Measures were taken to boost British food production such as subsidies and import restrictions. However, cheap meat, wheat and butter from abroad encouraged farmers to specialise in milk, eggs and vegetables.

More of almost every type of food was eaten, but even so researchers found that less than half the population could afford a healthy diet. Rickets, tuberculosis, anaemia and physical underdevelopment were common among the poor, leading eventually to the introduction of free school milk and infant welfare clinics to help combat these problems.

A number of companies started to dominate food processing and retailing during the 1930s, and shops increasingly sold preprepared brand-name goods. Eating out also became more popular with the introduction of milk bars and modestly priced Restaurants such as Lyons Tea Shops and ABC (Aerated Bread Company) Tea Shops.

1950s

The Second World War had created food shortages but rationing and other Government action meant that on average the nation's diet was better than before the war. When rationing ended, consumers bought foods that had been in short supply. However, only half the population ate a cooked breakfast, and breakfast cereals became fashionable.

At the time, health experts were concerned to ensure that people were eating a balanced diet, with sufficient vitamins and protein. However, these years of plenty were laying down the foundations for increasing obesity and heart disease. Other changes were that shops began to convert to self-service due to rising labour costs. Chinese restaurants became popular for eating out due to their cheapness, because they offered a take-away service, and because people were becoming more adventurous in their choice of foods.

1970s

By now UK farmers produced two-thirds of the nation's food, due to increasing use of technology and pesticides, fertilisers and hormones. Joining the EC gave farmers new subsidies and guaranteed prices, which resulted in overproduction of some foods. Most people began the day with a cereal breakfast and approximately 18% ate nothing. Fewer midday meals were taken at home. Tea shops went out of fashion and were replaced by burger bars. There was growing interest in foreign food. Health experts' attention shifted from the problems of inadequate nutrition to the new health risks of eating too much of certain types of food.

1980s

Supermarkets continued to expand and, due to air-cargo transport, almost every type of food became available. The demand for ethnic dishes continued, leading to the opening of many ethnic restaurants. **Nouvelle cuisine** became fashionable, but it tended to give way to healthy eating which was popularised not only in **haute cuisine** but also in the home and school meals. British chefs and cooking were now earning respect. The microwave oven greatly affected people's eating habits at home, and supermarkets responded by popularising products which could be cooked or reheated in the microwave. The 1970s saw the expansion of the use of the freezer; in the 1980s it was the expansion of the use of the microwave.

1990s

Increasing numbers of customers became aware of and required healthy eating, demanding, for example, lighter dishes, less fat, sugar and salt. Food additives also came under closer scrutiny. Severe cases of food contamination have made the national press, causing concern to the caterer and public alike. The majority of the cases were caused by Salmonella, Listeria and staphyolococcal organisms. As a result, hygiene codes of practice came under close examination and legislation has been passed in Parliament resulting in the Food Act of 1991.

Legislation from the EC caused caterers to be increasingly aware of laws affecting the industry. These particularly affect safety at work and temperature of foods.

Considerable attention was paid to 'green' issues, the production and use of organic foods and all environmental issues, in particular the control of waste. There was a trend towards more informal eating with bistros and theme restaurants (particularly US Theme restaurants such as Exchange Diner, TGI Friday) and also restaurant branding (such as Café Flo and Café Rouge); there was a move away from French menu terminology. Travel inns lodges increased alongside motorway service stations and some hotels subcontracted their restaurants.

Dishes on menus reflected the great variety of foodstuffs available and imaginative and attractive presentation results.

However, certain foodstuffs were giving rise for concern:

○ beef (mad cow disease);
○ nuts and certain other foods (causing allergy in a small number of people);
○ sweetbreads.

There was an increasing demand for vegetarian dishes.

2000 ONWARDS

The late 1990s have set many patterns for change which will develop in the next decade.

The increase on TV of celebrity chefs has greatly enhanced the awareness of cooking and the original presentation of dishes, publicised the catering industry and created interest in the use of less traditional foods. The effects of plate presentation will continue to affect the service of food, enabling foods to be served at the right temperature and more quickly. Greater attention to presentation and plate appeal will continue to be required of kitchen staff.

Demand for popular catering, pub catering and large seater restaurants may well increase because customers expect value for money, good service and clean premises as well as prepared food. Inner city and shopping eating places will continue to increase since a wide variety of foods is offered at reasonable prices which can be served in a short space of time. Food courts in shopping centres, railways stations, airports and the service of meals and snacks in supermarkets will develop even further. Themed restaurants and various catering brands with transform the British restaurant scene.

The definition of the hospitality industry will become increasingly blurred with more and more companies expanding their operations combining recreation, sport and leisure activities with hospitality. For example, football clubs such as Chelsea operate a leisure complex with conference facilities, hotel accommodation and football.

'Eating on the hoof' and 'grazing' will continue to increase. Snacking and the eating of ready-made foods from supermarkets, sandwich bars or petrol stations will become even more popular. Children have grown up to such a lifestyle and are less likely to sit down as part of a family traditional meal.

The delivery of ready-made dishes from a variety of establishments to the home such as pizzas or curries will increase since it fits into the family pattern or lifestyle of mothers who work, TV programme scheduling and so on. Ordering by the use of the internet with delivery from all kinds of shops and establishments will expand, as will demand for organic foods.

As the population of more elderly people increases, more concessions for this age group will be made, especially to use facilities at quieter times. Childrens' demands will be given greater consideration – a generation brought up on McDonalds will expect special treatment in the future.

Fashions or trends in foods will continue. The introduction of 'exotic' and unusual foods such as ostrich and alligator will develop further because there will be a demand to satisfy the palates of the greatly increased number of people travelling abroad and having new experiences. Cruising, once the domain of the wealthy and the elderly, is rapidly becoming very popular with all age groups. Many very large cruise ships are going to enable thousands of people to enjoy ship-board meals and novel onshore eating experiences. Eurostar trains have enabled many more people to sample European cuisine, thus affecting their demand in this country. Observing travelator food restaurants in Japan or experiencing the carving of grilled giraffe in Africa will affect expectations. Restaurants providing foods from almost every country of the world will continue to expand and will offer menus from more than one culture or country.

Traditions will inevitably be tested: chefs' uniforms will continue to become more trendy, waiters' attire more varied and informal. More British chefs will continue to be respected and women given greater opportunities to achieve. Menu structures will be much less formal and the use of prepared foods for all kinds of establishments will be accepted. Butchery, fishmongery, baker, pâtisserie and vegetable preparation may well continue to be an off-site function leaving the kitchen to assembly and presentation areas. The creativity of the chef will be in even greater demand.

The challenge of doing business in the 21st century requires the manager to increase productivity, faster and at a higher quality and at a lower cost, thus increasing profits.

Pressures such as these are felt acutely in both the hospitality and food service industries, where delivering a unique yet satisfying guest experience has to be balanced against improving operations, reducing costs and boosting that all important bottom line.

The internet has become a tool for communicating. The appropriate software empowers people and businesses. Advanced computer technologies, internet connectivity, and lines of business applications and processes and Web services are available to managers.

Restaurant and hotel guests now demand more choice. They want to be able to communicate on the device of their own choice, whether it's a mobile phone, wireless, PDA (Personal Digital Assistant) or PC (Personal Computer). They want to communicate at a time that is convenient to them and not just during the hotel or restaurant's hours of operation.

This requirement of flexibility is essential whether you are the hotelier, restaurateur or one of their business partners.

The challenges facing the hospitality industry can be organised with five key categories:

○ deep and rich customer relationships;

- employee productivity;
- operating efficiency;
- connected commerce communities;
- business value.

Advanced computer technology will assist in all five areas.

It is predicted that the Internet will be used further. It will allow restaurants to develop additional revenue per customer. It will enable a customer to place an order more easily, using a variety of devices – such as mobile phones so that an order is ready and waiting when the customer pulls up to the drive-though window. Or offering collateral products or services that appeal to the customer demographics of a particular hotel or restaurant. Employee productivity can be directly addressed. High turnover creates an increased demand for training that can now be provided in line and at a pace that suits the learner. Such self paced training can save businesses money and result in a more productive and efficient workforce. Online training will help employees add to their base of knowledge and build on their skills sets, which will assist in building a better informed and knowledgeable workforce.

Operating efficiency means that multiple parties such as hotel/restaurant guests, suppliers, credit authorisation services and others, will collaborate on business transactions and communicate data across a broad spectrum of devices and applications.

Business systems will interact with other businesses.

New technology will enhance efficiency and increase profits at nearly every point in the booking and check in processes.

Booking over the internet will be made simpler with availability within a group of hotels checked and the customer notified of the nearest location and duties.

Hotels will be able to collect a whole range of data on guests staying in their hotels, e.g. preferences in terms of rooms, room service utilisation etc.

Food production methods and patterns of trading are influenced by the European Union and particularly by the Common Agricultural Policy (CAP). The Treaty of Rome, signed by the six original members of the Common Market (Germany, France, Belgium, Luxembourg, Italy and The Netherlands) established subsidies to support their collective farming community. These countries all experienced severe food shortages in the years immediately following the Second World War. Today this system, known as CAP determines what subsidies are paid to farmers for their crops and animals, what chemicals can be used in food production, the conditions under which animals are reared and transported and the levies and taxes that are placed on foods that are imported from outside the EU. Food production in the UK is now a part of a world system that is strongly affected by cheaper production methods and competition from overseas, particularly outside the EU.

CAP both supports and protects farmers from the realities of world trade; they are guaranteed a price for all the commodities they produce.

The success of supermarkets and the range and variety of foods on their shelves demonstrates how successful the world trade in food has become. The disadvantage however is the ease by which plant or animal disease can travel around the world. Rigorous precautions have to be taken to maintain the safety of all food imports.

After the 2001 general election the new Labour administration created a new department to replace the Ministry of Agriculture, Fisheries and Food, this department is known as **DEFRA**: Department for Environment Food and Rural Affairs.

The aims and objectives of the Department are:

Sustainable development

○ To create a better environment at home and internationally, and the sustainable use of natural resources.

○ Economic prosperity through sustainable farming, fishing, food, water and other industries that meet consumers' requirements.

○ Thriving economies and communities in rural areas and a countryside for all to enjoy.

Objectives

○ To protect and improve the rural, urban, marine and global environment and conserve and enhance biodiversity, and to lead to the integration of these with other policies across Government and internationally.

○ To enhance opportunity and tackle social exclusion through the promotion of sustainable rural areas with a dynamic and inclusive economy, strong rural communities and fair access to services.

○ To promote a sustainable, competitive and safe food supply chain which meets consumers' requirements.

○ To improve the enjoyment of an attractive and well-managed countryside for all.

○ To promote sustainable, diverse, modern and adaptable farming through domestic and international action and further ambitious CAP reforms.

○ To promote sustainable management and the prudent use of natural resources both domestically and internationally.

○ To protect the public's interest in relation to environmental impacts and health, including diseases which can be transmitted through food, water and animals, and to ensure high standards of animal health and welfare.

DEFRA is responsible for the following

1 Animal Health and Welfare.
2 Environment.
3 Exports and Trade.
4 Farming.
5 Fisheries.
6 Food and Drink.
7 Horticulture.
8 Plants and Seeds.
9 Rural Development.
10 Sustainable Development.
11 Water.
12 Wildlife and Countryside.

Research by the Food Service Intelligence suggests that the traditional three meals a day is now in terminal decline in the UK. The research group suggests that Britons are rapidly becoming a nation of snackers, fuelled by the increasing availability of food service outlets (for example, high streets, motorway services) and the strong branding and cheap rapid service of the major chains providing a nationwide service.

The research company also predicts that the away-from-home food market will account for 50% of the total food expenditure by 2020 as lifestyles change and consumers spend increasingly less time at home preparing meals. In fact, it predicts that food service will become an increasingly round the clock business as old ways of working disappear in the 21st century. Manufacturers will concentrate more on the food service sector in the future as they begin to see the major opportunities for profits it offers them.

The Food Standards Agency is responsible for Food Safety and Quality in the UK. Further information HCIMA Technical brief 44.

http://foodstandards.gov.uk

Some references to trends in society and food elsewhere in the book

Kitchen design	205	Sensory evaluation	417
Kitchen developments	308	Influences	54

Topics for Discussion

1 The food preferences of the group and how they have evolved.
2 Healthy eating: what is your opinion regarding this topic?
3 The value of conducting business during a meal such as breakfast or lunch.
4 The group's ideas about food.
5 Influences on what we eat.
6 Potential future changes in British society that could affect eating habits.

CHAPTER 4

INFLUENCES OF ETHNIC CULTURES

CULTURAL VARIETY

The races and nations of the world represent a great variety of cultures each with their own ways of cooking. Knowledge of this is essential in catering because:

○ There has been a rapid spread of tourism, creating a demand for a broader culinary experience.

○ Many people from overseas have opened restaurants using their own foods and styles of cooking.

○ The development of air-cargo means perishable foods from distant places are readily available.

○ The media, particularly television, has stimulated an interest in worldwide cooking.

A few years ago it was necessary for a caterer to be knowledgeable about traditional classical French cooking; today they must also be aware of the foods and dishes of many other races. It is not within the scope of this book to deal in depth with gastronomy, but it is hoped that this brief introduction will stimulate an interest in terms and food associated with ethnic cooking.

RELIGIOUS INFLUENCES

Throughout the world religion always has, and still does, affect what many people eat. Some people's diets are restricted daily by their religion; others are influenced by what they eat on special occasions. Fasts, feasts, celebrations and anniversaries are important happenings in many people's lives. It is necessary for those involved in catering to have some basic knowledge of the requirements and restrictions associated with religions.

Christian

For most Christians, eating habits are not affected – though some will be vegetarians, usually for moral reasons, and some may refrain from eating meat on Fridays. Some sects, for instance Mormons, have many rules and restrictions regarding eating and drinking, for example complete abstinence from tea, coffee and alcohol, and an emphasis on wholesome eating. Many Christians refrain from eating certain foods during Lent – usually something they like very much. Other religious days often observed are:

○ Shrove Tuesday: the day before the start of Lent, when pancakes are on many menus, traditionally to use up ingredients prior to Lent.

○ Good Friday: hot cross buns are often eaten as a reminder of Christ's crucifixion.

○ Easter Sunday: simnel cakes are made with marzipan and chocolate, and Easter eggs (decorated boiled or chocolate eggs) are eaten as a symbol of new life and the Resurrection.

○ Christmas (25 December): celebrated with feasting, with roast turkey today often replacing the traditional roast beef and boar's head, followed by Christmas pudding and mince pies.

Muslim

Muslims celebrate the birth of Mohammed at the end of February or early in March. Alcohol and pork are traditionally forbidden in their diet. Only meat that has been prepared according to Muslim custom by a *halal* butcher is permitted. During *Ramadan*, which lasts for one month and is the ninth month of the Muslim calendar, Muslims do not eat or drink anything from dawn to sunset. The end of the fast is celebrated with a feast called *Idd-ul-Fitar*, with special foods. Muslims from Middle Eastern countries would favour a dish like lamb stew with okra; those from the Far East, curry and rice.

Hindu

Most Hindus do not eat meat (strict Hindus are vegetarians) and none eat beef since the cow is sacred to them. *Holi* is the festival which celebrates the end of winter and the arrival of spring. *Raksha Bandha* celebrates the ties between brothers and sisters at the end of July or in August, and *Janam Ashtami* celebrates the birth of Krishna, also in August. *Dussehra* is the festival of good over evil; *Diwali* is the festival of light, celebrating light over darkness, held in October or November. Samosas (triangles of pastry containing vegetables), banana fudge and vegetable dishes of all kinds, as well as favourite foods, are eaten to celebrate.

Sikh

The Sikhs do not have strict rules regarding food but many are vegetarians. *Baisakhi* day in April celebrates the new year and is the day Sikhs are baptised into their faith.

Buddhist

Strict Buddhists are vegetarians and their dishes vary since most live in India and China, where available foods will be different. *Vesak* in May is the festival to celebrate the life of the Buddha.

Judaism

The religion of the Jews has strict dietary laws. Shellfish, pork and birds of prey are forbidden. Acceptable foods are fish with scales and fins, animals that have 'cloven hoof' and birds killed according to the law. Strict Jews eat only meat that has been specially slaughtered, known as *kosher* meat.

Milk and meat must neither be used together in cooking nor served at the same meal, and three hours should elapse between eating food containing milk and food containing meat.

The Jewish Sabbath, from sunset on Friday to sunset on Saturday, is traditionally a day of rest. In the evening plaited bread called *chollah* is broken into pieces and eaten. *Matzo*, an unleavened crispbread, is served at Passover as a reminder of the exodus of the Jews from Egypt. *Pentecost* celebrates the giving of the Ten Commandments to Moses on Mount Sinai; cheesecake is now a traditional dish served at this celebration. *Hanukkah*, the Jewish Festival of Lights in December, is a time of dedication when pancakes and a potato dish, potato *latkes*, are usually eaten.

ECLECTIC CUISINE

This is the mix of modern national styles and flavourings from different countries which has developed over recent years. Its origins can be traced to Australian chefs who have been influenced by the Pacific Rim. These various styles, ideas and methods are today drawn from a variety of sources throughout the world.

Transportation has greatly assisted the development of eclectic cuisine.

Further development on this theme has been the introduction of matching serving dishes and plates to the food with the effect of enhancing the overall presentation. Such a concept stretches the chef's creativity and imagination, pioneering into new dimensions of food presentation, making the dishes ever more attractive, adding colour, flair and fashion to dining out.

Modern restaurants place great emphasis on decor, space, fashion and overall design. The chef's role is to match the food style and presentation to the new era of food styles. Examples of these styles are:

○ French Thai;
○ American Japanese;
○ Indian with French presentation;
○ Australian/Pacific Rim.

NATIONAL COOKING STYLES

British

From the UK and Ireland come some of the finest raw ingredients in the world, and there is also a legacy of a large number of regional recipes including a vast repertoire of puddings.

French

France is the recognised home of classical cooking, which has been built up by the craftsmanship, love and respect for food of many famous chefs over the years. Each region of France has its specialities and a gastronomic tour can provide a wide education in food and good eating. French chefs were the first to use a variety of cooking styles and ingredients.

Italian

The food and cooking of Italy, according to reports dating back to the Sixteenth century, was considered elegant and the first cookbook – *Apuus* – was compiled in the heyday of the Roman Empire. The Italians brought their culinary skills to France in 1533 through Catherine de Medici, and justifiably claim to have influenced French cooking. Italy is noted for its pastas, risottos, pizzas, cheeses and much more.

German and Austrian

The food of Germany and Austria is substantial with meat and sausages (*wursts*) of many varieties.

There is also a wide repertoire of regional dishes which reflect the type of produce available in those countries. Viennese pastry cooks and bakers have developed high quality skills and have a worldwide reputation.

Eastern European

Russia, Hungary, Poland and other Eastern European countries have a legacy of foods and cooking which have contributed to the international classic repertoire: Russian caviar served with blini, coulibiac, chicken Kiev. Goulash is a traditional Hungarian paprika-flavoured stew. Rum babas are a worldwide favourite.

Swiss

France, Italy and Germany border on Switzerland, influencing the cooking in a country already famous for its cheeses. The country is divided into over 20 regions known as Cantons and each Canton has a répertoire of local dishes.

Spanish and Portuguese (The Iberian Peninsula)

Food from Iberia is usually plain looking and hearty, appetising in a simple way and rarely over-decorated. One exception is the most famous Spanish dish, the paella. Spanish food in general is not heavily spiced or over-rich. Portuguese food tends to be spicier and richer because of more use of butter and cream. Fish dishes are very popular.

Scandinavian

Denmark, Norway and Sweden, due to their proximity to the sea, eat large quantities of fish, particularly herring. Butter, bacon and blue cheese is imported into Britain in large quantities. Rye, which grows in northern climates, is used for crispbreads which are popular, particularly for low-calorie diets.

Smörgäsbord (a buffet) is famous, where a wide variety of dishes including lots of fish is offered.

Smorrebrod are Danish open sandwiches.

Mediterranean and Middle Eastern

Cooking in this area is affected by religious, as well as by geographical and historical influences, sometimes making it unclear where certain dishes originated. Foods from the Mediterranean area include olives, aubergines, lemons, squid, octopus, yogurt and lamb; from the Middle East, wheat, rice, beans, chick peas, lentils, figs, dates and citrus fruits. Burghul, known as 'cracked wheat', is whole wheat grains partially cooked, dried and cracked, and used in many soups, stews and salads. Cous cous is popular, see page 59, African.

American

In a country as cosmopolitan as the United States the cooking is influenced by the many immigrants from all over the world and consequently the cookery repertoire is vast. America has developed an immense fast food industry which has been franchised worldwide. A versatile nation with a vast wealth of gastronomy, a country that anyone aspiring to a career in catering would be well advised to visit and work in for a period of time.

Mexican

For many years Mexican food has been the largest growing food industry in the United States and its popularity has spread to other countries including the UK. Over the years the influence of the Aztecs, the French and the Spanish have left their mark on Mexican cooking. Maize is the staple food and Mexican menus are designed to make meat go a long way. Carbohydrates from the maize, vitamins from vegetables (which are grown in abundance) and protein and fibre from beans make up a well-balanced diet.

Caribbean

The cooking of the Caribbean islands is spicy and hearty and based mainly on the products of their rich tropical soil – guavas, mango, paw paw, pineapple, coconut, okra, bread fruit, plantain and sweet potato. There are also endless varieties of tropical fish which include spiny lobster, prawns and conch.

Indian, Pakistani and Bangladeshi

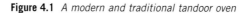

Figure 4.1 *A modern and traditional tandoor oven*

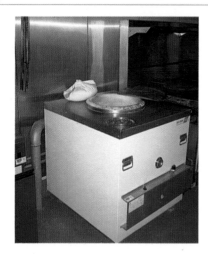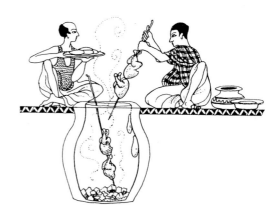

Indian cookery is noted for its use of spices, herbs and flavourings, but the subcontinent should not be associated only with curry. Northern India's speciality, tandoori cooking, is named after the unusual oven called the *tandoor* which produces slightly charred spiced chicken and lamb dishes. Southern India features vegetarian dishes and *vindaloo*. Bangladesh favours seafood. Pakistan uses yogurt extensively, and kebabs are common.

Chinese

China is a vast country with a wide climatic variation, and therefore many kinds of foods are available. Because of its size, four major styles of cooking have developed over the centuries, and foods produced in these areas predominate. The areas are divided into:

○ **Eastern:** Shanghai (wide variety of fruit, vegetables and fish; light and delicate seasoning; stir fry and steaming are favoured cooking methods; soy sauce from this area is considered the best in China).

○ **Northern:** Beijing or Peking (wheat and corn are produced in this area, not rice, so noodles, pancakes and dumplings are served; due to the climate many foods are preserved; less meat is available; garlic, leeks, onions and sesame seeds are used extensively).

○ **Western:** Sichuam or Szechuan (strong flavourings and hot spices predominate, e.g. red chillies, peppercorns, ginger, fruit, vegetables, meat and fish are plentiful).

○ **Southern:** Guangdong or Canton (foods are not overcooked, and less use is made of garlic; rice is the staple food; sweet and sour dishes and dim sums are renowned; stir fry and steaming are the most common methods of cooking).

Chinese cooking is based on five flavours which affect parts of the body:

FLAVOUR	ORGAN
sweet	spleen
acid	liver
sour	kidneys
bitter	heart
sharp	lungs

The Chinese diet is characterised by cooking methods which preserve vitamins, the absence of dairy produce, and little meat. Foods are divided into: *yin*, cooling food; *yang*, heating foods; *yin yang*, neutral foods. Yin foods include crab and duck, and yang foods beef, coffee and smoked fish; *yin yang* foods include rice, fruit and vegetables.

All parts of animals and birds, other than the fur and feathers, are used for food.

Japanese cookery

Japanese cookery is unique in its artistic presentation and the wide variety of small amounts of different dishes served to please the eye as well as the appetite. Fish, rice, noodles and vegetables as well as soy sauce predominate. Raw fish which is exceptionally fresh is used extensively.

South East Asian

South East Asia is influenced by both Chinese and Indian cooking. Singapore, Indonesia, Burma and Thailand use rice extensively as well as pineapples, pomelos, mandarins, bananas, coconut, mangoes and paw paws.

This area produces many spices such as nutmeg, cloves, and ginger. Coconuts, rice and other tropical fruits including pineapples and bananas are common.

African

The climate of Africa enables bananas, paw paws, mangoes, grapes, citrus fruits and sugar cane to grow well. From North Africa comes *couscous*, the national dish of Morocco, Tunisia and Algeria, which is a fine semolina made from wheat steamed over soup, stew or fish. East Africa, which includes Ethiopia, is where coffee originated. Both coffee and tea are grown here and maize is an important crop. In West Africa *cassava* is the staple food, and Ghana is the main cocoa-producing country in the world. Groundnut is grown in Nigeria. South Africa produces sugar cane and maize and cattle and sheep are raised.

Some references to cultures elsewhere in the book

Taste	420	Speciality restaurants	13
Hospitality industry	1	Recipe development	425
Resources	360, 45		

Topics for Discussion

1 The effects of religion on the eating habits of certain cultures.
2 The most popular British foods; why they are the most popular.
3 The benefits of having a wide variety of ethnic restaurants in the country.
4 The effects of people's eating habits other than cultural or religious.

5 Examine the origin why and how Welsh, Scottish, Irish and/or English styles of cooking have developed.

6 What has developed as 'American Food', explain why this has become worldwide.

7 Why have oriental and Asian foods become popular in Britain?

8 The American fast food industry and its effect on Britain.

PART 3

Food Commodities, Nutrition and Science

FOOD COMMODITIES

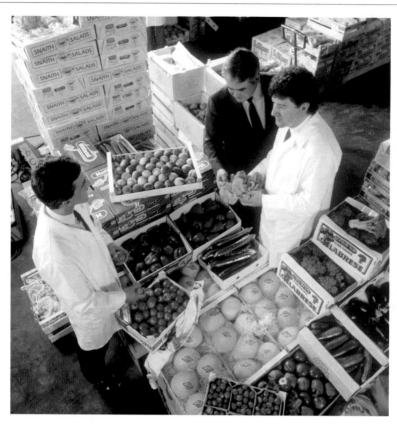

Figure 5.1 *Purchasing fruit and vegetables*

THE STUDY OF COMMODITIES

Further information about Meat, Poultry, Fish, Fruit and Vegetables can be found in *Practical Cookery* and *Advanced Practical Cookery*.

When studying commodities, students are recommended to explore the markets to get to know both fresh foods and all possible substitutes such as convenience or ready-prepared foods. Comparison should be made between various brands of foods, and between convenience and fresh unprepared foods. Factors to be considered when comparing should include quality, price, hygiene, labour, cost, time, space required and disposal of waste.

Students are advised to be cost conscious from the outset in all their studies and to form the habit of keeping up to date with current prices of all commodities, equipment, labour and overheads. An in-built awareness of costs is an important asset to any successful caterer. A list of food prices is printed weekly in *The Caterer and Hotelkeeper*.

Organic foods

Consumers are gradually becoming more organic and environmentally friendly. There are no nutritional reasons for using organic produce. Organic foods are said to contain fewer contaminants. They have a lower content of pesticides, or none at all, but global sources of contamination cannot be avoided by the organic farmer.

Food inspection particularly by the Department of Environment, Food and Rural Affairs keep a good check on the content of undesirable substances in conventional produce. The aspect of contamination, therefore, is not a good reason for using organically grown produce either. The main argument for using organic produce is that they support an environmentally sensible development in farming. Caterers may thus consider using organic produce as a social priority. Some caterers have started using organic produce as they become environmentally conscious.

Today's consumers, whether guests in a restaurant or staff in firms' restaurants or hospital patients, have a national expectation that insensitive use of the environment or resources should be avoided. Staff in catering have a natural expectation with regard to a sensible working environment.

One of the problems for the organic market is the lack of a good distribution network. It is difficult to establish a distribution network as long as there are only a few catering kitchens which use organic vegetables. The solution to the problem is to distribute organic produce through traditional distribution channels which is being developed. The quality of organic produce is variable. The majority of caterers and food manufacturers at present take organic produce seriously. The trend for the future is likely to be towards environmentally friendly food products rather than organic food products.

ENVIRONMENTALLY FRIENDLY FOOD PRODUCTS

These are foods that are produced under conditions which save on electricity and water as well as other environmental factors, or they can be products made with environmentally friendly technology. Products may be packed in environmentally friendly packaging and produce is grown with a limited use of fertilisers and crop sprays, but is not necessarily totally organic. In this way a trend may be expected in which industry slowly takes on the idea of organic production and increasingly begins to market environmentally friendly food products to the catering industry. Organic is a term defined by European law and all organic food production and processing is governed by strict legislative standards. Catering operations preparing and selling organic menus must be certified with a UK certification body such as Soil Association Certification Ltd.

MEAT

Cattle, sheep and pigs are reared for fresh meat and certain pigs are specifically produced for bacon. Tenderness, flavour and moistness are increased if beef is hung after slaughter. Pork and veal are hung for 3–7 days according to the temperature. Meat is generally hung at a temperature of 1°C (34°F).

Conversion of muscle to meat

Glycogen is a carbohydrate energy reserve stored in the muscle of animals. Glycogen is used to provide energy in the living animal and is broken down to water and carbon dioxide. In muscle after slaughter there is no supply of oxygen and therefore the glycogen is converted to lactic acid. The build up of lactic acid reduces the pH from about 7.0 to 5.6 (makes the meat more acidic). This natural acidity is important for keeping the quality of meat.

Under some conditions this process cannot follow the normal pattern. In particular, if there is insufficient glycogen present in the muscle at slaughter the pH does not fall to the same extent and dark, firm dry meat results. This is caused by insufficient feed prior to slaughter or a prolonged period of stress. Another condition, known as PSE (pale soft exudative) results if animals (especially pigs) are subjected to a period of acute stress prior to slaughter. This results in the pH fall occurring too rapidly which gives rise to denaturation of the muscle protein.

Carcase hanging

The method of carcase hanging can give rise to marked differences in eating quality. Hanging the carcase by the hip bone (aitch bone) instead of the traditional achilles tendon, puts tension on the important muscles of the hindquarter. This 'stretching' effect makes them more tender. Traditionally carcases were 'hung' (held as carcases) for a period of several days. In fact, boning can take place as soon as 12 hours (pigs), 24 hours (sheep) or 48 hours (cattle) after slaughter provided a period of ageing is allowed following butchery.

Ageing of meat

Like cheese and wine, meat benefits both from a period of ageing or maturation, before it is consumed. This gives an increase in both the tenderness and flavour. The increase in tenderness occurs as enzymes, naturally present within the meat, break down key proteins. The so called calpain enzymes are important for the development of tenderness. Flavour may be increased by the release of small protein fragments with strong flavour. Enzymes released from the lysosomes (cell bodies that store protein attacking enzymes) may also be involved. Minimum ageing periods of 7 days from slaughter to consumption are often recommended for beef, lamb and pork.

STORAGE

Meat should be stored at its appropriate temperature, usually between 1 and 5°C (34–41°F). Raw meat should be stored separately from cooked meat or meat products. Chilled meat must be used by the 'use-by date' unless written permission to use it later has been given by the supplier.

Temperatures of chillers and freezers should be measured regularly. Chilled cooked meat must generally be stored below 8°C (46.4°F) but if it has been prepared for consumption without further cooking or reheating the temperature must be at or below 5°C (41°F). Cut or sliced, smoked or cured meats must be stored at or below 5°C (41°F).

CUTS AND JOINTS

For economic reasons of saving on both labour and storage space, very many caterers purchase meat by joints or cuts rather than by the carcass.

The Meat Buyer's Guide to Caterers is a manual which has been designed to assist caterers who wish to simplify and facilitate their meat purchasing.

FOOD VALUE

Meat, having a high protein content, is valuable for the growth and repair of the body and as a source of energy. It is an important source of several vitamins, minerals and other nutrients e.g. vitamins B/z, A and D, zinc and iron.

PRESERVATION

- **Salting.** Meat can be pickled in brine, and this method of preservation may be applied to silverside, brisket and ox-tongues. Salting is also used in the production of bacon, before the sides of pork are smoked. This also applies to hams.
- **Chilling.** This means that meat is kept at a temperature just above freezing point in a controlled atmosphere.
- **Freezing.** Small carcasses, such as lamb and mutton, can be frozen and the quality is not affected by freezing. They can be kept frozen until required and then thawed out before being used. Some beef is frozen, but it is inferior in quality to chilled beef.
- **Canning.** Large quantities of meat are canned and corned beef is of importance since it has a very high protein content. Pork is used for tinned luncheon meat.

Further information

Institute of Meat, Third Floor, 50–60 St John St, London EC1M 4DT; Meat and Livestock Commission, PO Box 44, Winterhill House, Snowdon Drive, Milton Keynes, MK6 1AX www.britishmeat.org.uk. See also *Practical Cookery* and *Advanced Practical Cookery* and *The Meat Buyers Guide*.

Beef

The hanging or maturing of beef at a chill temperature of 1°C (34°F) for up to 14 days has the effect of increasing tenderness and flavour. This hanging process is essential as animals are generally slaughtered around the age of 18 months, and the beef can be tough. Also a short time after death an animal's muscles stiffen, a condition known as *rigor mortis*. After a time chemical actions caused by enzymes and increasing acidity relax the muscles and the meat becomes soft and pliable. As meat continues to hang in storage *rigor mortis* is lost and tenderness, flavour and moistness increase. (Pork, lamb and veal are obtained from young animals so that toughness is not a significant factor.)

Large quantities of beef are prepared as chilled boneless prime cuts, vacuum packed in film. This process has the following advantages: it extends the storage life of the cuts. The cuts are boned and fully trimmed thus reducing labour costs and storage space.

Figure 5.2 *Side of beef*

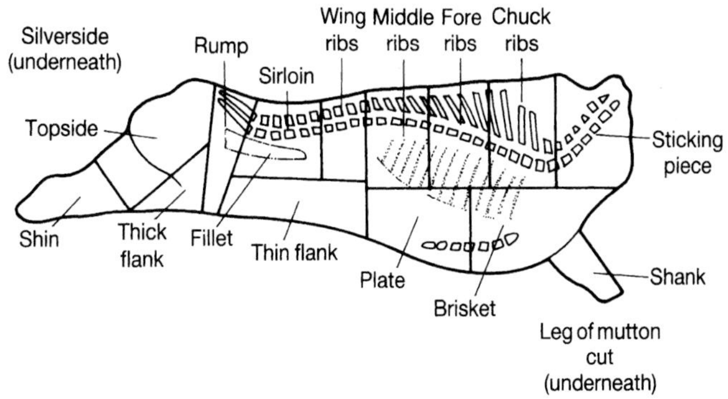

Silverside (underneath)
Rump
Wing ribs
Middle ribs
Fore ribs
Chuck ribs
Sirloin
Topside
Sticking piece
Shin
Thick flank
Fillet
Thin flank
Plate
Brisket
Shank
Leg of mutton cut (underneath)

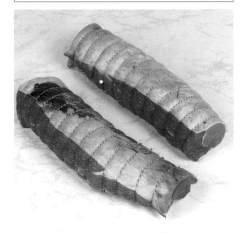

Figure 5.3 *Beef, silverside (rolled)*

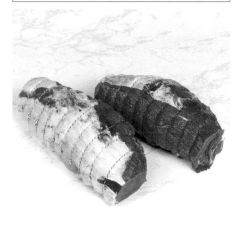

Figure 5.4 *Rolled topside of beef*

Figure 5.5 *Boned shin of beef*

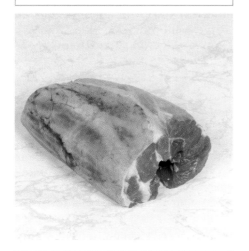

Figure 5.6 *Rump and loin of beef*

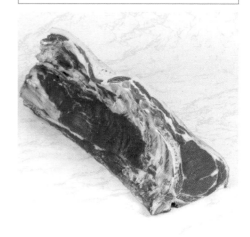

Figure 5.7 *Forerib of beef*

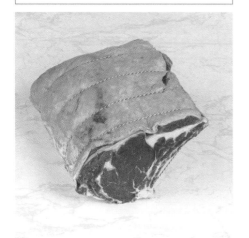

Figure 5.8 *Beef, chuck steak*

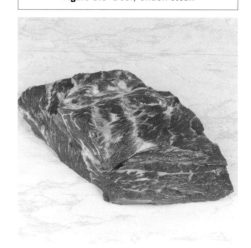

Figure 5.9 *T-Bone steaks*

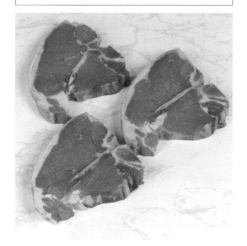

Figure 5.10 *Sirloin steaks*

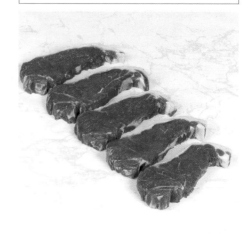

Figure 5.11 *Fillet steaks*

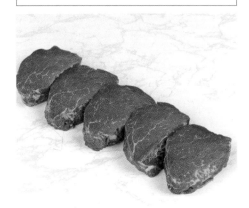

Figure 5.12 *Rib eye steaks*

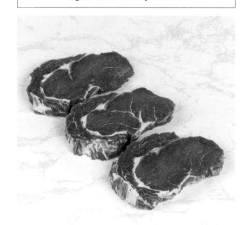

Figure 5.13 *Veal kidneys*

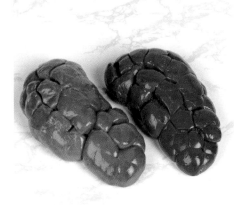

Figure 5.14 *Veal escalopes*

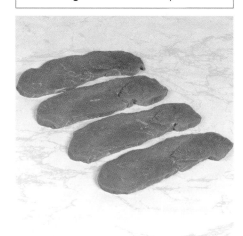

Figure 5.15 *Veal sweetbreads*

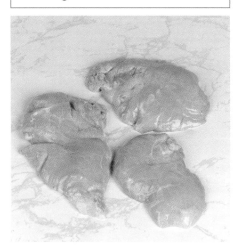

Figure 5.16 *Leg of pork*

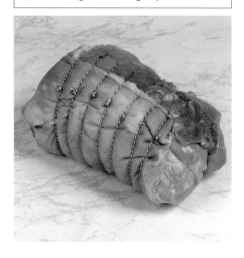

Figure 5.17 *Loin of pork*

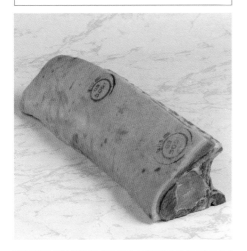

Figure 5.18 *Boned leg of pork*

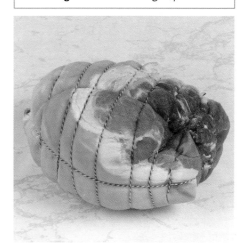

Figure 5.19 *Pork chops*

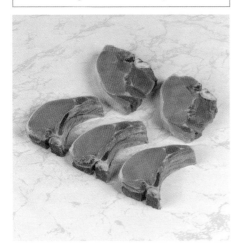

Figure 5.20 *Boned and rolled gammon*

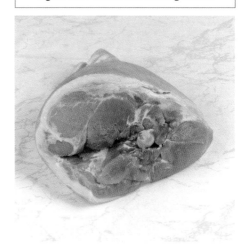

Figure 5.21 *Gammon steaks*

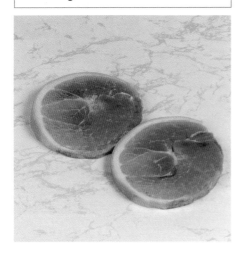

Figure 5.22 *Back bacon*

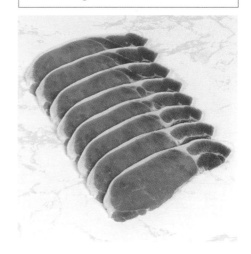

Figure 5.23 *Streaky bacon*

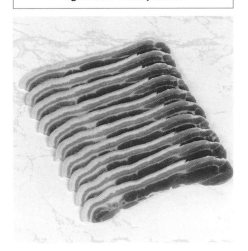

Figure 5.24 *Suckling pig*

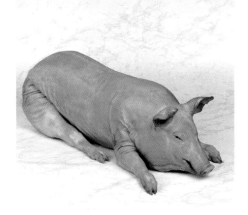

Figure 5.25 *Pigs trotters*

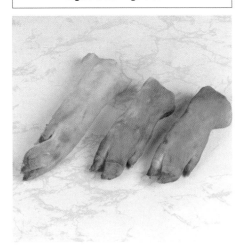

Figure 5.26 *Saddle of lamb*

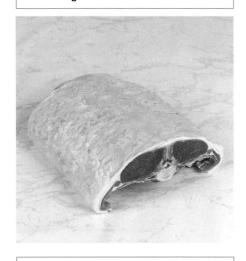

Figure 5.27 *Pair of best ends of lamb*

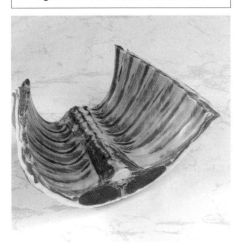

Figure 5.28 *Boned and rolled lamb shoulder*

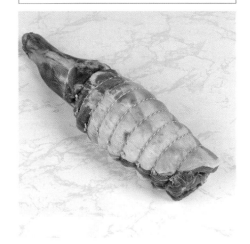

Figure 5.29 *Shoulder of lamb*

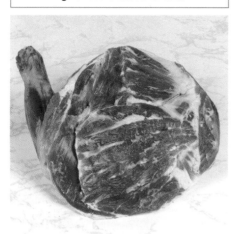

Figure 5.30 *Double loin chops of lamb*

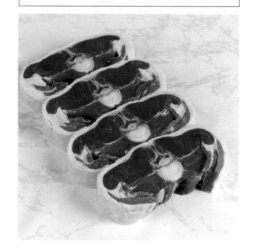

Figure 5.31 *Lamb loin chops*

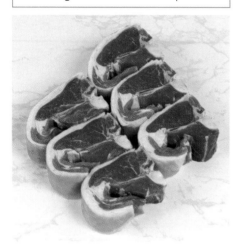

Figure 5.32 *Lamb cutlets*

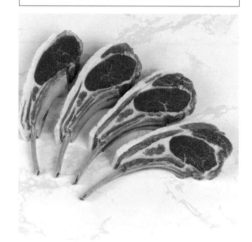

Figure 5.33 *Valentines of lamb*

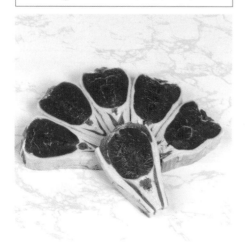

Figure 5.34 *Best ends of lamb (racks, french trimmed)*

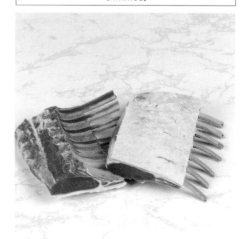

Figure 5.35 *Leg steaks of lamb*

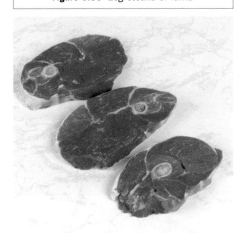

Figure 5.36 *Lamb rosettes*

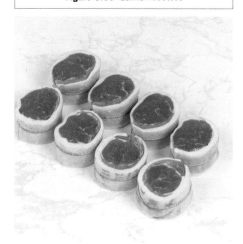

Figure 5.37 *Lamb kidneys*

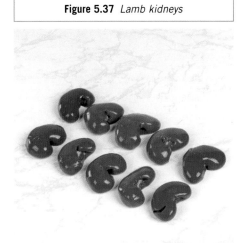

Figure 5.38 *Lamb hearts*

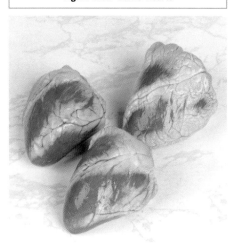

Figure 5.39 *Calves' liver*

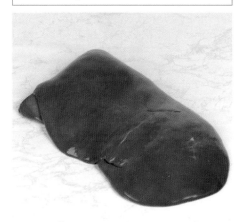

Figure 5.40 *Wholesale purchasing of meat*

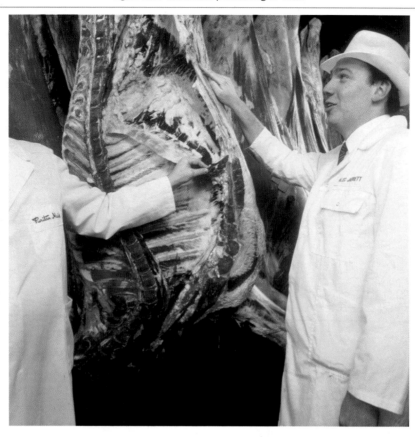

It is essential to store and handle vacuum packed meat correctly. Storage temperature should be 0°C (32°F) with the cartons the correct way up so that the drips cannot stain the fatty surface. A good circulation of air should be allowed between cartons.

When required for use, the vacuum film should be punctured in order to drain away any blood before the film is removed. On opening the film a slight odour is usually discernible, but this should quickly disappear on exposure to the air. The vacuum packed beef has a deep red colour, but when the film is broken the colour should change to its normal characteristic red within 20–30 minutes. Once the film is punctured the meat should be used as soon as possible.

QUALITY

○ Lean meat should be bright red, with small flecks of white fat (marbled).

○ The fat should be firm, brittle in texture, creamy white in colour and odourless.

Meat of traceable origin is best.

Veal

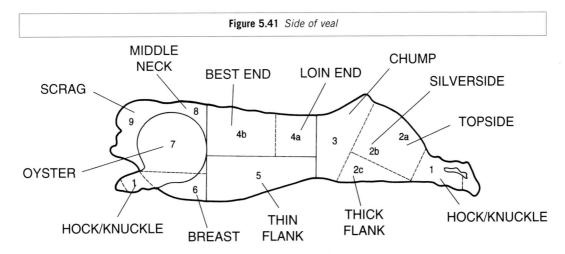

Figure 5.41 *Side of veal*

SCRAG — MIDDLE NECK — BEST END — LOIN END — CHUMP — SILVERSIDE — TOPSIDE — OYSTER — HOCK/KNUCKLE — BREAST — THIN FLANK — THICK FLANK — HOCK/KNUCKLE

Originally most top quality veal came from Holland, but as the Dutch methods of production are now used extensively in Britain, supplies of home-produced veal welfare are available all the year round. Good quality carcasses weighing around 100 kg (220 lb) can be produced from calves slaughtered at 12–24 weeks. This quality of veal is necessary for first-class cookery.

○ The flesh of veal should be pale pink, firm, not soft or flabby.
○ Cut surfaces must not be dry, but moist.
○ Bones in young animals should be pinkish white, porous and with a small amount of blood in their structure.
○ The fat should be firm and pinkish white.
○ The kidney ought to be firm and well covered with fat.
○ Welfare veal comes from calves that are loosely penned. The colour of the meat as a consequence is a deeper shade of pink.

Pork

Approximately 95% of pork used in Britain is home produced.

○ Lean flesh of pork should be pale pink.
○ The fat should be white, firm, smooth and not excessive.
○ Bones must be small, fine and pinkish.
○ The skin, or rind, ought to be smooth.

Suckling pigs weigh 5–9 kg (10–20 lb) dressed and are usually roasted whole. Boars are wild or uncastrated male pigs. The meat of boars is available from special farms.

Boars

Boars are wild or uncastrated male pigs. The meat of boars is available from special farms. It is better to obtain good quality animals from suppliers using as near as possible 100% pure breeding stock. Animals that are free to roam and forage for food have a much better flavour than farm reared ones that have been penned and fed. Animals are best between 12–18 months old weighing 70–75 kg on the hoof. Slaughtering is best done during late summer when the fat content is lower. Recommended hanging time is between 7–10 days at a temperature between 1 and 4°C. Marinading greatly improves the taste and texture of boar meat before cooking.

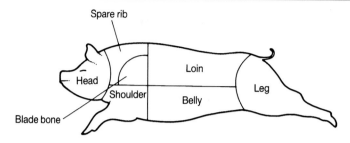

Figure 5.42 *Side of pork*

Bacon

Bacon is the cured flesh of a pig (60–75 kg (120–150 lb) dead weight) often specifically reared for bacon because its shape and size yield economic bacon joints.

The curing process consists of salting either by a dry method and smoking, or by soaking in brine followed by smoking.

Unsmoked bacon is brine cured but not smoked; it has a milder flavour but does not keep as long as smoked bacon.

○ There should be no sign of stickiness.

○ There must be no unpleasant smell.

○ The rind should be thin, smooth and free from wrinkles.

○ The fat ought to be white, smooth and not excessive in proportion to the lean.

○ The lean meat of bacon should be deep pink in colour and firm.

Bacon should be kept in a well-ventilated cold room. Joints of bacon should be wrapped in muslin and hung, preferably in a cold room. Sides of bacon are also hung on hooks. Cut bacon is kept on trays in the refrigerator or cold room. But bacon can also be vaccumed packed.

Pancetta are rolled slices of curled pork belly. Lardo is extremely fatty Italian bacon.

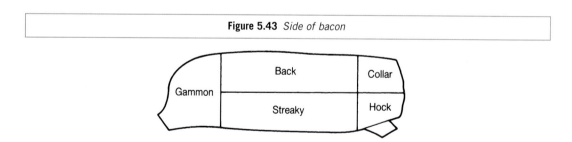

Figure 5.43 *Side of bacon*

Hams *(see page 158)*

Lamb and mutton

In Britain, more lamb and mutton is eaten than in any other European country.

○ Lamb is generally meat from animals under one year old – mutton is the term for older animals.

○ The carcass should be compact and evenly fleshed.

○ The lean flesh of lamb ought to be firm and of a pleasing dull red colour and of a fine texture or grain.
○ The fat should be evenly distributed, hard, brittle, flaky and clear white in colour.
○ The bones should be porous in young animals.

The factors influencing lamb composition, quality and value are essentially similar to those previously described for beef.

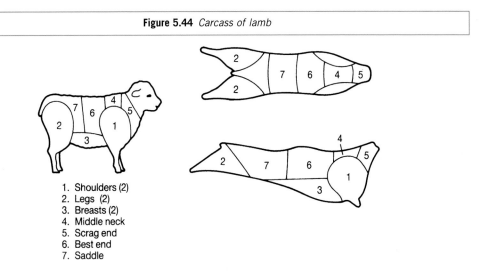

Figure 5.44 *Carcass of lamb*

1. Shoulders (2)
2. Legs (2)
3. Breasts (2)
4. Middle neck
5. Scrag end
6. Best end
7. Saddle

Offal and other edible parts of the carcass

Offal is the name given to the edible parts taken from the inside of the carcass: liver, kidney, heart and sweetbread. Tripe, brains, oxtail, tongue and head are sometimes included under this term. Fresh offal (unfrozen) should be purchased as required and can be refrigerated under hygienic conditions at a temperature of − 1°C (30°F), at relative humidity of 90% for up to seven days. Frozen offal should be kept frozen until required.

TRIPE

Tripe is the stomach lining or white muscle of beef cattle. Honeycomb tripe is from the second compartment of the stomach and considered the best. Smooth tripe is the first compartment of the stomach, and is not considered to be as good as honeycomb tripe. Sheep tripe, darker in colour, is obtainable in some areas. Tripe may be boiled or braised.

OXTAIL

Oxtails should be $1\frac{1}{2}$–$1\frac{3}{4}$ kg) (3–5 lb), lean and with no signs of stickiness. They are usually braised or used for soup.

SUET

Beef suet should be creamy white, brittle and dry. It is used for suet paste. Other fat should be fresh and not sticky. Suet and fat may be rendered down for dripping.

BONES

Bones must be fresh, not sticky; they are used for stock, which is the base for soups and sauces.

LIVER *(see Figure 5.39, page 71)*

Calves' liver is the most expensive and is considered the best in terms of tenderness and delicacy of flavour and colour.

Lamb's liver is mild in flavour, tender and light in colour.

Ox or beef liver is the cheapest and if taken from an older animal can be coarse in texture and strong in flavour.

Pig's liver is full flavoured and used in many pâté recipes.

QUALITY

○ Liver should appear fresh and have an attractive colour.
○ It must not be dry or contain tubers.
○ It should be smooth in texture.

FOOD VALUE

Liver is valuable as a protective food; it consists chiefly of protein and contains useful amounts of vitamin A and iron.

KIDNEY *(see Figures 5.13 and 5.37, pages 67 and 71)*

Lamb's kidney is light in colour, delicate in flavour and is ideal for grilling and frying.

Calf's kidney is light in colour, delicate in flavour and can be used in a wide variety of dishes.

Ox kidney is dark in colour, strong in flavour and is generally used mixed with beef, for steak and kidney pie or pudding.

Pig's kidney is smooth, long and flat by comparison with sheep's kidney; it has a strong flavour.

QUALITY

○ Ox kidney should be fresh and deep red in colour.
○ Lamb's kidney should be covered in fat which is removed just before use; the fat should be crisp and the kidney moist.

FOOD VALUE

The food value of kidney is similar to liver, i.e. containing vitamin A and iron.

HEARTS *(see Figure 5.38, page 71)*

Ox or beef hearts are the largest used for cooking. They are dark coloured, solid and tend to be dry and tough.

Calf's heart, coming from a younger animal, is lighter in colour and more tender.

Lamb's heart is smaller and lighter and is normally served whole. Larger hearts are normally sliced before serving.

QUALITY

Hearts should not be too fatty and should not contain too many tubes. When cut they should be moist.

FOOD VALUE

They have a high protein content and are valuable for growth and repair of the body.

TONGUE

- Tongues must be fresh.
- They should not have an excessive amount of waste at the root end.
- Ox tongues may be used fresh or salted.
- Sheep's tongues are used unsalted.

SWEETBREADS

Sweetbread is the name given to two glands, one is the pancreas and is undoubtedly the best as it is round flat and plump; the other is the elongated sausage-shaped thymus gland.

QUALITY

Sweetbread should be fleshy, large and creamy white in colour.

FOOD VALUE

Sweetbreads are valuable foods, particularly for hospital diets. They are very easily digested and useful for building body tissues.

FURTHER INFORMATION

Further information on meats and offal can be found in *Practical Cookery Advanced Practical Cookery* and *The Meat Buyers Guide*.

Meat substitutes

TEXTURED VEGETABLE PROTEIN (TVP)

This is a meat substitute manufactured from protein derived from wheat, oats, cotton-seed, soya bean and other sources. The main source of TVP is the soya bean, due to its high protein content.

TVP is used chiefly as a meat extender, varying from 10–60% replacement of fresh meat. Some caterers on very tight budgets make use of it, but its main use is in food manufacturing.

By partially replacing the meat in certain dishes, such as casseroles, stews, pies, pasties, sausage rolls, hamburgers, meat loaf and pâté, it is possible to reduce costs, provide nutrition and serve food acceptable in appearance.

MYCO-PROTEIN

A meat substitute is being produced from a plant which is a distant relative of the mushroom. This myco-protein contains protein and fibre and is the result of a fermentation process similar to the way yogurt is made. It may be used as an alternative to chicken or beef or in vegetarian dishes.

QUORN

Quorn is the brand name of Rank Hovis McDougall's myco-protein, produced by fermentation process from a plant which is a distant relative of the mushroom (fungi).

POULTRY (see Figures 5.45 and 5.46, pages 80 and 81)

Poultry is the name given to domestic birds specially bred to be eaten and for their eggs.

SEASON

Owing to present-day methods of poultry breeding and growing, poultry is available all the year round either chilled or frozen.

FOOD VALUE

The flesh of poultry is more easily digested than that of butchers' meat. It contains protein and is therefore useful for building and repairing body tissues and providing heat and energy. Fat content is low and contains a high percentage of unsaturated acids.

STORAGE

Fresh poultry must be hung by the legs under chilled conditions, otherwise it will not be tender; the innards are removed as soon as possible after slaughter.

Frozen birds must be kept in a deep-freeze cabinet below −5°C until required. To reduce the risk of food poisoning, it is essential that frozen birds be completely thawed, preferably in a refrigerator before being cooked. Chilled birds should be kept between 3 and 5°C.

For information on quality, types and use see *Practical Cookery* and *Advanced Practical Cookery*.

FURTHER INFORMATION

○ For further information contact: British Poultry Meat Federation Ltd. Europoint House, 5 Lavington St London SE1 0HZ http://www.britishpoussin.co.uk/about.htm

Duck/duckling and Goose/gosling (see Figure 5.46, page 81)

Goose is traditionally in season from Michaelmas, September 29 until Christmas.

QUALITY

○ The feet and bills should be bright yellow.
○ The upper bill should break easily.
○ The web feet must be easy to tear.

Ducks and geese may be roasted or braised.

Turkey

QUALITY

○ The breast should be large, the skin undamaged and with no signs of stickiness.
○ The legs of young birds are black and smooth, the feet supple with a short spur.
○ As the bird ages the legs turn reddish grey and become scaly. The feet become hard.

Turkeys are usually roasted and served hot or cold. Turkey meat is also used for a variety of other dishes.

Guinea fowl *(see Figure 5.46, page 81)*

When plucked these grey-and-white feathered birds resemble a chicken with darker flesh. The young birds are known as squabs.

The quality points relating to chicken apply to guinea fowl.

Pigeon *(see Figure 5.46, page 81)*

Pigeon should be plump, the flesh mauve-red in colour and the claws pinkish. Tame pigeons are smaller than wood pigeons. Squabs are young specially reared pigeons.

Peacock

Peacock has a light, gamey flavour, similar to guinea fowl and should be treated like a well exercised turkey.

Ostrich

Ostrich is usually sold as a fillet (taken from the thigh) or leg steak. The neck or offal is also available and is cheaper. It is often compared to beef, but it has a slightly coarser texture with less fat and cholesterol.

GAME *(Figures 5.49 and 5.50, pages 82, 83)*

Game is the name given to certain wild birds and animals which are eaten; there are two kinds of game:

○ feathered;   ○ furred.

FOOD VALUE

As it is less fatty than poultry or meat, game is easily digested, with the exception of water fowl, which has oily flesh. Game is useful for building and repairing body tissues and for energy.

STORAGE

○ Hanging is essential for all game. It drains the flesh of blood and begins the process of disintegration which is vital to make the flesh soft and edible, and also to develop flavour.

○ The hanging time is determined by the type, condition and age of the game and the storage temperature.

○ Old birds need to hang for a longer time than young birds.

○ Game birds are not plucked or drawn before hanging.

○ Venison and hare are hung with the skin on.

○ Game must be hung in a well-ventilated, dry, cold storeroom; this need not be refrigerated.

○ Game birds should be hung by the neck with the feet down.

GAME AVAILABILITY

Game is available fresh in season between the following dates and frozen for the remainder of the year:

- ○ Grouse   August 12–December 10
- ○ Snipe   August 12–January 31
- ○ Partridge   September 1–February 1
- ○ Wild duck   September 1–January 31
- ○ Pheasant   October 1–February 1
- ○ Woodcock   October 31–February 1
- ○ Venison, hares, rabbits and pigeons are available throughout the year.

Figure 5.45 Poultry (left to right, top to bottom): boiling fowl 2 kg (4 lb), turkey 5 kg (10 lb), chicken 1 kg (2 lb), French chicken (Bresse) 1 kg (2 lb), corn-fed chicken 1 kg (2 lb), chicken fermier 1 kg (2 lb), Poussin 400g (1 lb)

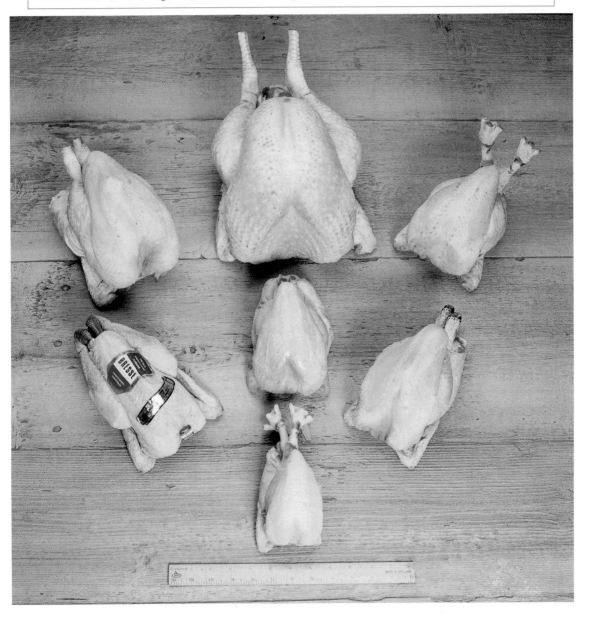

Venison *(see Figure 5.47, page 82)*

Venison is the flesh from any member of the deer family which includes elk, moose, reindeer, caribou and antelope. Red deer meat is a dark, blood-red colour; the flesh of the roe deer is paler and the fallow deer is considered to have the best flavour.

Meat from animals over 18 months in age tends to be touch and dry and is usually marinated to counteract this. Young animals up to 18 months produce delicate, tender meat which does not require marinating. Nowadays, venison is extensively farmed in the UK.

Venison contains 207 calories per 100 g and young venison has only about 6% fat (compared to beef, lamb and pork around 20% fat). It has the highest protein content of the major meats.

Continued on p 94

Figure 5.46 *Poultry (left to right, top row first): croise duck 1 kg (2 lb), duck 2 kg (4 lb), guinea fowl 1 kg (2 lb), squab 32 g, quail 13 g, woodpigeon 28 g*

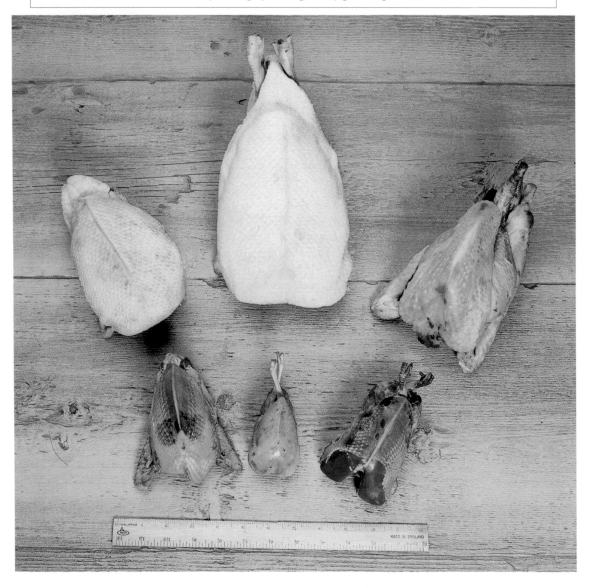

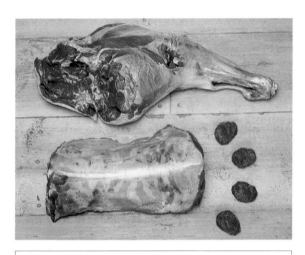

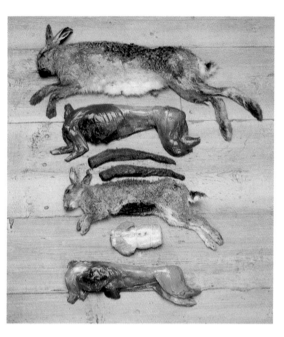

Figure 5.47 *Haunch of venison 23 kg (46 lb) (top), and saddle of venison 13 kg (26 lb)*

Figure 5.48 *hare 2½ kg (5 lb) (top), skinned hare and fillets of hare; tame rabbit 750 g (1½ lb), saddle of rabbit and skinned rabbit*

Figure 5.49 *Cock pheasant 1 kg (2 lb), prepared hen pheasant, prepared cock pheasant*

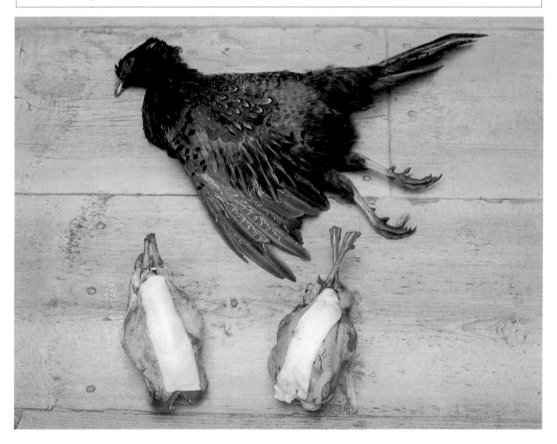

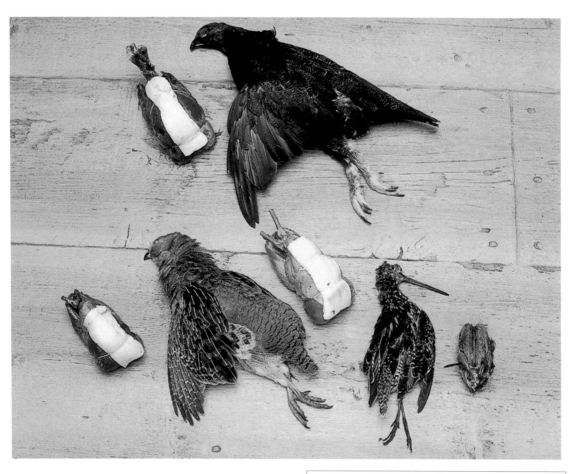

Figure 5.50 *Prepared grouse (top), grouse 750 g (1½ lb), prepared partridge, partridge 750 g (1½ lb), prepared red legged partridge, snipe 300 g (12 oz) and prepared snipe (note trussed with beak)*

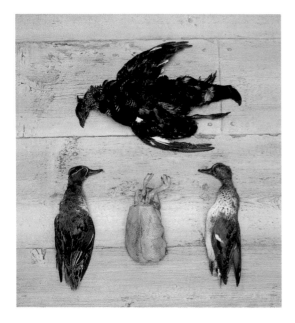

Figure 5.51 *Capercaillie 1 kg (2 lb) (top), wild duck 750 g (1½ lb), oven-ready wild duck, wild duck 750g (1½ lb)*

Figure 5.52 *Conger eel 1 kg (2 lb), octopus, squid*

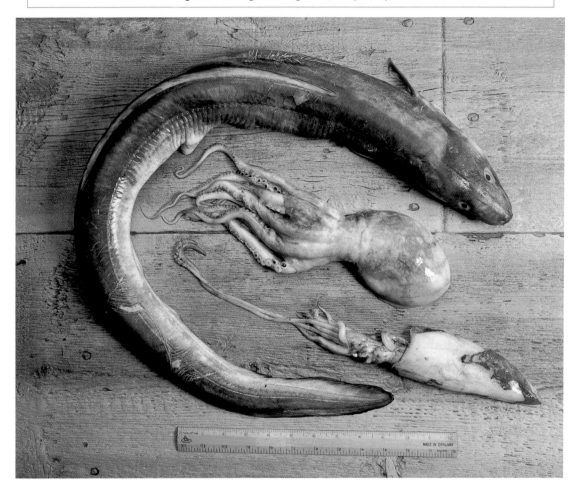

Figure 5.53 *Brill 4 kg (9 lb) on the left*

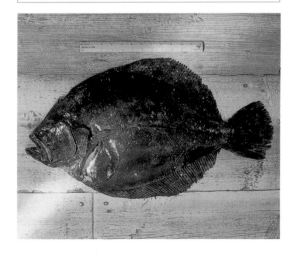

Figure 5.54 *Halibut 2.5 kg (5 lb)*

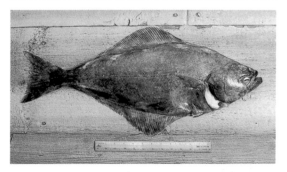

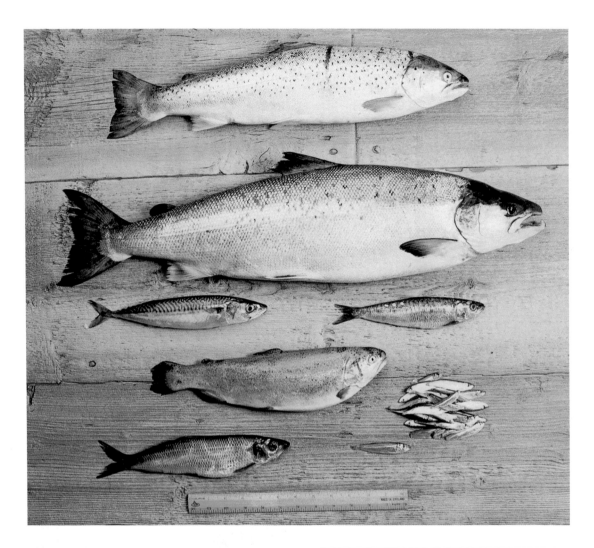

Figure 5.55 *Top to bottom: salmon trout 2 kg (4 lb), salmon 5 kg (10 lb), mackerel 400 g (1 lb), sardine 300 g (12 oz), trout 1 kg (2 lb), herring 400 g (1 lb), whitebait*

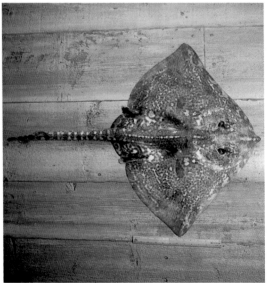

Figure 5.56 *Skate 5.5 kg (12 lb)*

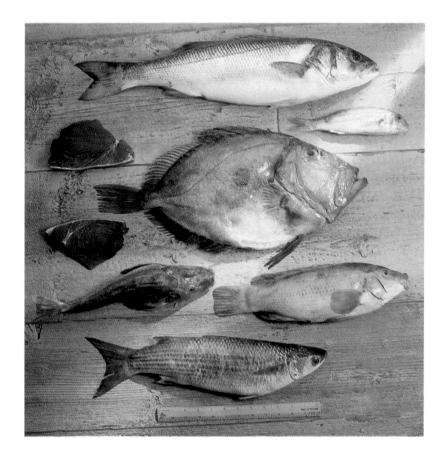

Figure 5.57 *Sea bream 2 kg (4 lb) (top), red mullet 200 g (8 oz), tuna steaks, John Dory 2 kg (4 lb), gurnard 550 g (1¼ lb), wrasse 1 kg (2 lb), grey mullet 1 kg (2 lb)*

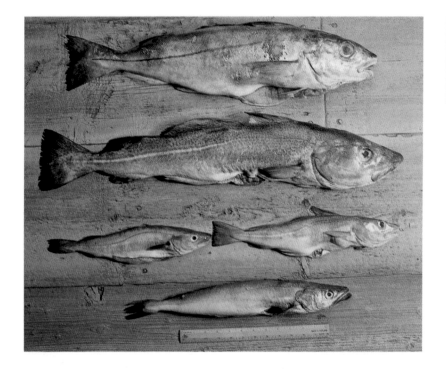

Figure 5.58 *Haddock 3 kg (6 lb) (top), cod 3 kg (6 lb), hake 1 kg (400 g 1 lb, (2 lb) (left), codling 500 g (1¼ lb), whiting 300 g 400 g 1 lb (12 oz)*

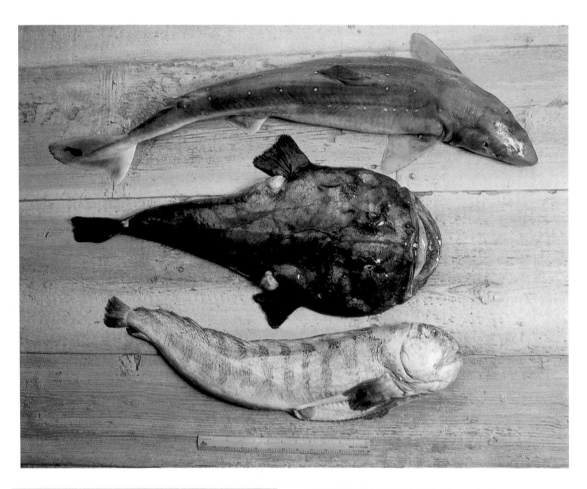

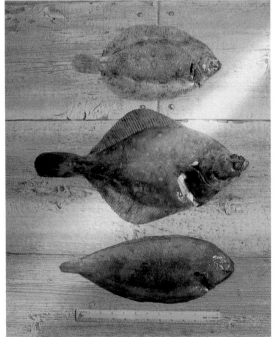

Figure 5.59 *Dogfish 4 kg (9 lb) (top), monkfish 4 kg (9 lb), catfish 2.5 kg (5 lb)*

Figure 5.60 *Lemon sole 500 g (1 lb) (top), plaice 1 kg (2 lb), Dover sole 500 g (1 lb)*

Figure 5.61 *Turbot 5 kg (10 lb)*

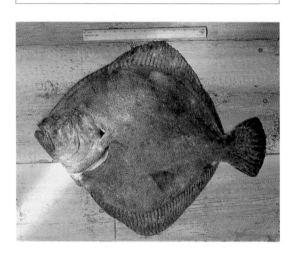

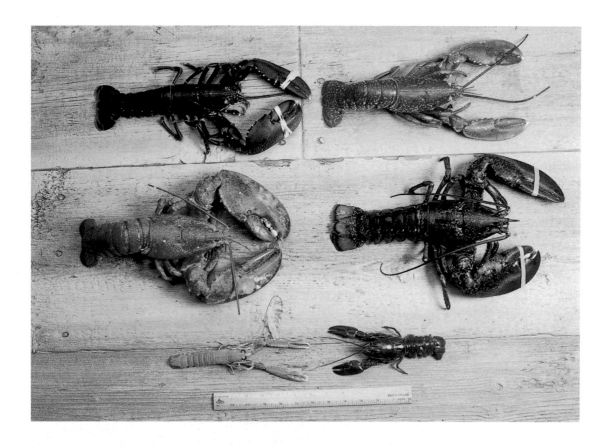

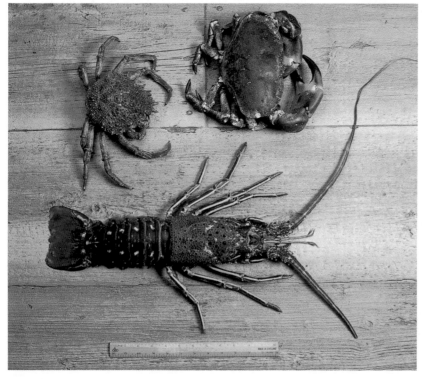

Figure 5.62 *Scottish lobster, raw and cooked (top), Canadian lobster, cooked and raw, crayfish, langoustine*

Figure 5.63 *Spidercrab (top left), crab, crawfish*

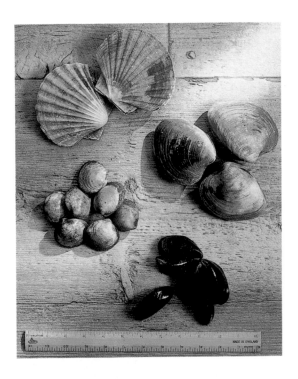

Figure 5.64 *Scallops (top), large clams, small clams, mussels*

Figure 5.65 *Smoked salmon (top), smoked haddock (natural), smoked haddock (coloured), kipper, cod's roe, smoked halibut, smoked trout, Arbroath smoky*

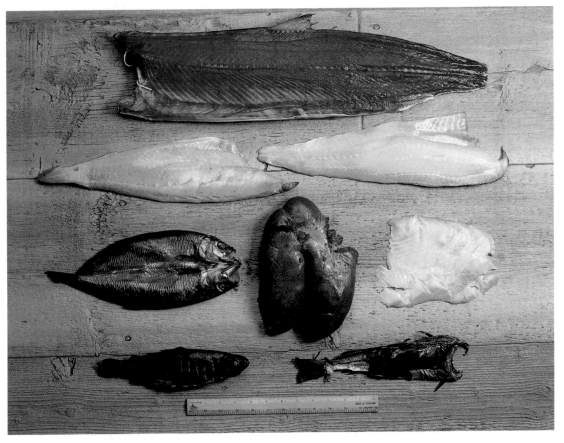

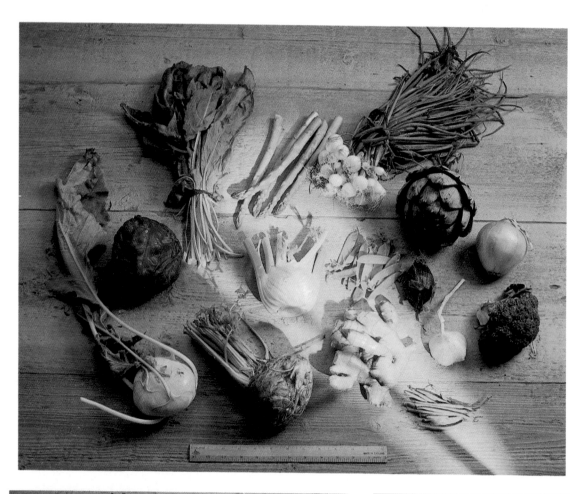

Figure 5.66 *Bulbs, leafy vegetables and pods (from top left), sorrel, asparagus, grelots, globe artichoke, red cabbage, fennel, mange-tout, red onion, onion, kohlrabi, celeriac, ginger, garlic, broccoli, haricots verts*

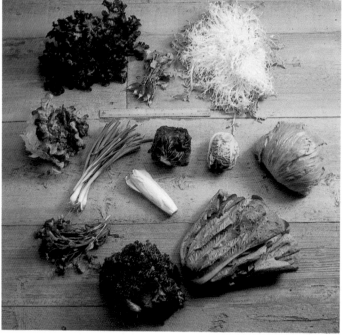

Figure 5.67 *Salad vegetables, (from top left), oakleaf, radishes, frisé endive, lettuce, spring onions, Belgian endive, radiccio, little gem, iceberg, watercress, lollo rosso, cos*

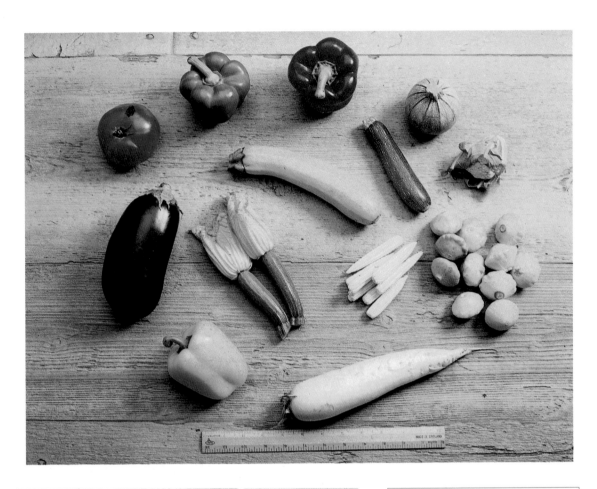

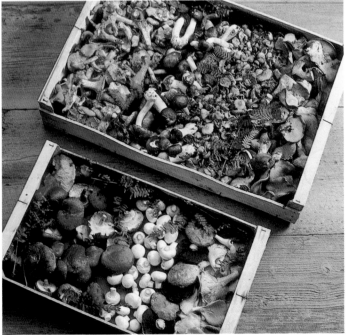

Figure 5.68 *Various vegetables (from top left), beef tomato, green pepper, red pepper, squash, aubergine, courgette flowers, yellow courgette, green corgette, baby cauliflower, yellow pepper, mooli, baby corn, squash*

Figure 5.69 *Mushrooms, wild and cultivated*

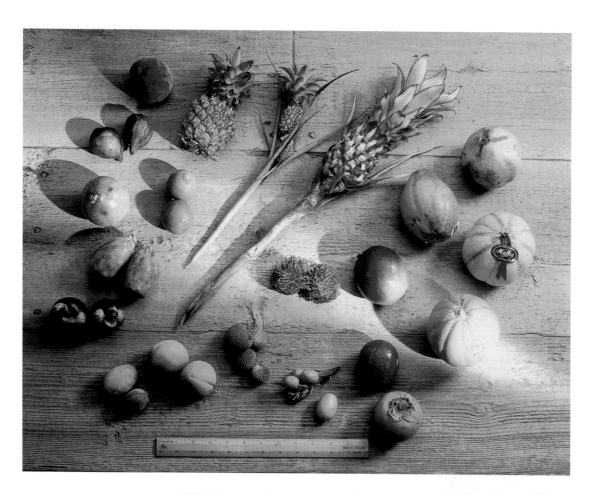

Figure 5.70 *Fruits: figs, peach, pineapple, pineapple flowers, pomegranate, granadillo, limes, paw=paw, charentis melon, prickly pear, rambukin, mango, ogen melon, mangostines, almonds, apricots, lychees, kumquat, blood orange, persimmon*

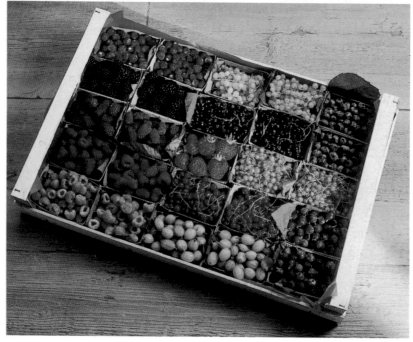

Figure 5.71 *Soft fruits: wild strawberries, white currants, blueberries, blackberries, blackcurrants, loganberries, strawberries, pink currants, raspberries, red currants, red gooseberries, golden raspberries, gooseberries*

Figure 5.72 *A selection of soft cheeses*

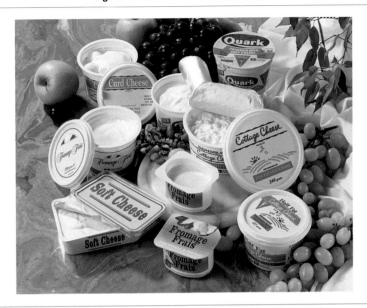

Figure 5.73 *Herbs (left to right, top to bottom) thyme, dill, sage, mint, tarragon, fennel, chives, corriander, rosemary, basil, flat leaf parsley*

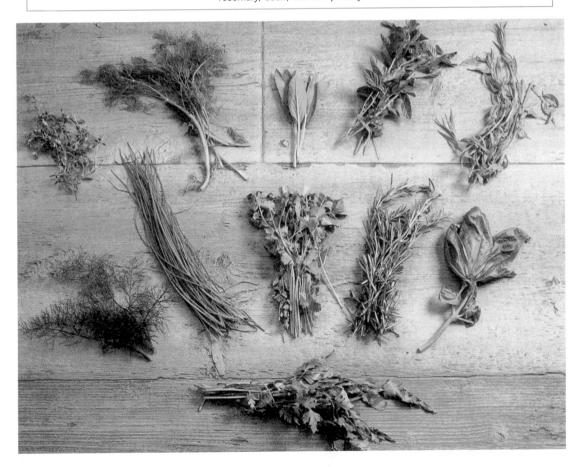

Venison is very suitable for a low-cholesterol diet because the fat is mainly polyunsaturated. The carcass has little intramuscular fat; the lean meat contains only low levels of marbling fat.

Both farmed and wild venison are available. Joints should be well fleshed and a dark brownish red colour. Venison is usually roasted or braised in joints, served hot or cold with a peppery/sweet type sauce. Small cuts may be fried and served in a variety of ways. Venison is available as shoulder, boned and rolled; haunch, boned and rolled; prepared saddles and steaks; also as pâté, in sausages, burgers; and smoked.

Other meats

Alligator has a white meat, with a veal-like texture and a shellfish-like flavour.

Bison should be treated like a gamey, well-hung version of beef. However, because it is so lean it needs to be cooked quickly and served rare or medium rare.

Camel is available as fillet, steak of diced. It comes in frozen from Africa.

Crocodile has a firm-textured, light-coloured meat with a delicate fishy taste, similar to monkfish, that absorbs other flavours well. It is surprisingly fatty.

European wild boar has been reintroduced to British farms. It produces rich, dark red meat with a dense texture.

Kangaroo is similar to venison in flavour. It has a fine-grained meat which, once cooked, is likened in texture to liver and is best served rare or medium rare.

Kid usually comes from goats bred for their milk. However, the South African Boer goat, which is bred for its meat, has recently been introduced into this country. It has a rich, yet delicate flavour with very little fat.

Kudu is a breed of wild African antelope that is culled in a controlled way. They are very large and the meat has a stronger flavour than wild venison. It needs to be tenderised by marinating and cooking.

HARE AND RABBIT (see Figure 5.48, page 82)

The ears of hares and rabbits should tear easily. In old hares the lip is more pronounced than in young animals. The rabbit is distinguished from the hare by shorter ears, feet and body.

Hare may be cooked as a red wine stew called jugged hare and the saddle can be roasted.

Birds

- ○ The beak should break easily.
- ○ The breast plumage should be soft.
- ○ The breast should be plump.
- ○ Quill feathers should be pointed, not rounded.
- ○ The legs should be smooth.

PHEASANT (see Figure 5.49, page 82)

This is one of the most common game birds. Average weight is $1\frac{1}{2}$–2 kg (2–4 lb). Young birds have a pliable breast bone and soft pliable feet. Hang for five to eight days. Used for roasting, braising or pot roasting.

PARTRIDGE (see Figure 5.50, page 83)

The most common varieties are the grey legged and the red legged. Average weight is 200–400 g ($\frac{1}{2}$–1 lb). Hang for three to five days. Used for roasting or braising.

GROUSE *(see Figure 5.50, page 83)*

A famous and popular game bird is the red grouse which is shot in Scotland and Yorkshire. Average weight is 300 g (12 oz). Young birds have pointed wings and rounded soft spurs. Hang for five to seven days. Used for roasting.

SNIPE *(see Figure 5.50, page 83)*

Weight is about 100 g (4 oz). Hang for three to four days. The heads and neck are skinned, the eyes removed; birds are then trussed with their own beaks. When drawing the birds only the gizzard, gallbladder and intestines are removed. The birds are then roasted with the liver and heart left inside.

WOODCOCK

Small birds with long thin beaks. Average weight is 200–300 g (8–12 oz). Prepare as for snipe. Usually roasted.

QUAIL

Small birds weighing 50–75 g (2–3 oz) produced on farms, usually packed in boxes of 12. Quails are not hung. They are usually roasted or braised.

WILD DUCK *(see Figure 5.51, page 83)*

Wild duck include mallard and widgeon. Average weight is $1–1\frac{1}{2}$ kg (2–3 lb). Hang for one or two days. Usually roasted or braised.

TEAL

The smallest duck, weighing 400–600 g ($1–1\frac{1}{2}$ lb). Hang for one to two days. Usually roasted or braised. Young birds have small pinkish legs and soft down under the wings. Teal and wild duck must be eaten in season otherwise the flesh is coarse and has a fishy flavour. Usually roasted or braised.

FISH *(see pages 84–87)*

Fish have formed a large proportion of our food because of their abundance and relative ease of harvesting.

Because the fish supply is not unlimited due to overfishing, fish farms (e.g. for trout and salmon) have been established to supplement the natural sources. This is not the only problem: due to contamination by man, the seas and rivers are increasingly polluted, thus affecting both the supply and the suitability of fish, particularly shellfish, for human consumption.

Fish are valuable, not only because they are a good source of protein, but because they are suitable for all types of menus and can be cooked and presented in a wide variety of ways. The range of different types of fish of varying textures, taste and appearance is indispensable to the creative chef.

TYPES OR VARIETIES *(see tables on pages 96, 97, and 105)*

○ Oily fish – round in shape (herring, mackerel, salmon).
○ White fish – round (cod, whiting, hake) or flat (plaice, sole, turbot).
○ Shellfish and cephalopods are discussed on pages 104–106.

KINDS OF FISH: SEASONS AND PURCHASING UNITS

FISH	SEASON	PURCHASING UNIT
Oily		
anchovy	imported occasionally June to December (home waters)	number and weight
common eel	all year, best in autumn	number and weight
conger eel	March to October	weight
herring	all year except spring	number and weight
kingfish – check with supplier – and weigh with fillets		
mackerel	September to July	number and weight or fillets
pilchard (mature sardines)	all year	number and weight
salmon (farmed)	all year	number and weight
salmon (wild)	February to August	number and weight
salmon trout	February to August	number and weight
salmon (Pacific)	July to November	number and weight
sprat	September to March	number and weight
sardines	all year	number and weight
trout	February to September	number and weight
trout (farmed)	all year	number and weight
tuna	all year	steaks or pieces
whitebait	when available	weight
White flat		
brill	June to February	number and weight
dab	March to December	number and weight
flounder	May to February, best in winter	number and weight
halibut	June to March	number and weight or steaks
megrim	April to February	number and weight
plaice	May to February	number and weight or fillets
skate	May to February	wings, number and weight
sole, Dover	May to March	number and weight or fillets
sole, lemon	all year, best in spring	number and weight or fillets
turbot	all year	number and weight or fillets
turbot (farmed)	when available	number and weight
witch	all year, best in spring	number and weight or fillets
Round		
barracuda – check with supplier number and weight of fillets		

KINDS OF FISH: SEASONS AND PURCHASING UNITS – continued

FISH	SEASON	PURCHASING UNIT
bass, wild/farmed	June to September	number and weight or fillets
bream, fresh water	August to April	number and weight or fillets
bream, sea	June to December	number and weight or fillets
carp (mostly farmed)	fluctuates throughout year	number and weight or fillets
cod	all year, not at best in spring	number and weight or fillets
dogfish (huss, flake, rigg)	all year, best autumn	steaks or fillets
grey mullet	May to February, best autumn and winter	number and weight
grouper – check with supplier number and weight of fillets		
haddock	all year, best autumn and winter	number and weight or fillets
hake	June to February	number and weight or fillets
John Dory	September to May	number and weight or fillets
ling	September to July	number and weight or fillets
monkfish (angler-fish)	all year, best in winter	number and weight or tails
pike	all year	number and weight
perch	May to February	number and weight
pollack (yellow, green)	May to December	number and weight
redfish	all year	number and weight or fillets
red gurnard	all year, best from July to April	number or weight
red mullet	imported best in summer, UK autumn	number and weight and fillets
sea bream	June to February	number and weight
smelt	occasionally	number and weight
shark (porbeagle)	occasionally	steaks or pieces
snapper, red snapper	check with supplier	
whiting	all year, best in winter	number and weight or fillets

PURCHASING UNIT

Fresh fish is bought by the kilogram, by the number of fillets or whole fish of the weight that is required. For example, 30 kg (66 lb) of salmon could be ordered as 2 × 15 kg (33 lb), 3 × 10 kg (22 lb) or 6 × 5 kg (11 lb). Frozen fish can be purchased in 15 kg (33 lb) blocks. Fish may be bought on the bone or filleted in steaks or supremes. (The approximate loss from boning and waste is 50% for flat fish, 60% for round fish.) Fillets of plaice and sole can be purchased according to weight. They are graded from 45 g ($1\frac{1}{2}$ oz) to 180 g (6 oz) per fillet and go up in weight by 15 g ($\frac{1}{2}$ oz).

STORAGE

- ○ Fresh fish are stored in a fish-box containing ice, in a separate refrigerator or part of a refrigerator used only for fish at a temperature of 1–2°C (34–36°F).
- ○ The temperature must be maintained just above freezing point.
- ○ Frozen fish must be stored in a deep-freeze cabinet or compartment at −18°C (0°F).
- ○ Smoked fish should be kept in a refrigerator.

FOOD VALUE

Fish is as useful a source of animal protein as meat. The oily fish, such as sardines, mackerel, herrings and salmon contain vitamins A and D in their flesh; in white fish, such as halibut and cod, these vitamins are present in the liver. Since all fish contains protein it is a good body-building food and oily fish is useful for energy and as a protective food because of its vitamins.

The bones of sardines, whitebait and tinned salmon, which can be eaten, provide calcium and phosphorus.

Owing to its fat content oily fish is not so digestible as white fish and is not suitable in cookery for invalids.

Oily fish

ANCHOVIES

Anchovies are small round fish used mainly tinned in this country; they are supplied in 60g and 390g tins. They are filleted and packed in oil.

They are used for making anchovy butter and anchovy sauce, for garnishing dishes and for savouries, snacks and salads.

COMMON EEL

Eels live in fresh water and are also farmed and can grow up to 1m (39in) in length. They are found in many British rivers and considerable quantities are imported from Holland. Eels must be kept alive until the last minute before cooking and they are generally used in fish stews.

CONGER EEL *(see Figure 5.52, page 84)*

The conger eel is a dark grey sea-fish with white flesh which grows up to 3m (10ft) in length. It may be used in the same way as eels, or it may be smoked.

HERRING *(see Figure 5.55, page 85)*

Fresh herrings are used for breakfast and lunch menus; they may be grilled, fried or soused. Kippers (which are split, salted, dried) and smoked herrings are served for breakfast and also as a savoury. Average weight is 250g (9oz).

King Fish come from the Spanish Mackerel family with orangey, pink coloured flesh

MACKEREL *(see Figure 5.55, page 85)*

Mackerel are grilled, shallow fried, smoked or soused, and may be used on breakfast and lunch menus. They must be used fresh because the flesh deteriorates very quickly. Average weight, 360g (12oz).

PILCHARDS

These are mature sardines and can grow up to 24 cm (10 in). They have a good distinctive flavour and are best grilled or baked.

SALMON *(see Figure 5.55, page 85)*

Salmon is perhaps the most famous river fish and is caught in British rivers like the Dee, Tay, Severn, Avon, Wye and Spey. It is also extensively farmed in Scotland and Norway. A considerable number are imported from Scandinavia, Canada, Germany and Japan. Apart from using it fresh, salmon is tinned or smoked. When fresh, it is used in a wide variety of dishes.

SALMON TROUT (SEA TROUT) *(see Figure 5.55, page 85)*

Salmon trout are a sea fish similar in appearance to salmon, but smaller, and they are used in a similar way. Average weight, $1\frac{1}{2}$–2 kg (3–4 lb).

SARDINES

Sardines are small fish of the pilchard family which are usually tinned and used for hors-d'œuvre, sandwiches and as a savoury. Fresh sardines are also available and may be cooked by grilling or frying.

SPRATS

Sprats are small fish fried whole and are also smoked and served as an hors-d'œuvre.

TROUT *(see Figure 5.55, page 85)*

Trout live in rivers and lakes and in the UK they are cultivated on trout farms. Trout may be poached and served grilled or shallow fried, and may also be smoked and served as an hors d'œuvre. Average weight, 200 g (7 oz).

TUNA

Tuna has dark reddish-brown flesh which when cooked turns to a lighter colour. Thin texture and a mild flavour. If overcooked it dries out and is best cooked medium rare. It is used fresh for a variety of dishes or tinned in oil and used mainly in hors-d'œuvre and salads.

WHITEBAIT *(see Figure 5.55, page 85)*

Whitebait are the fry or young of herring, 2–4 cm ($\frac{3}{4}$–$1\frac{1}{2}$ in) long, and they are usually deep fried.

White flat fish

BRILL *(see Figure 5.53, page 84)*

Brill is a large flat fish which is sometimes confused with turbot. Brill is oval in shape; the mottled brown skin is smooth with small scales. It can be distinguished from turbot by its lesser breadth in proportion to length; average weight, 3–4 kg (7–9 lb). It is usually served in the same way as turbot.

DAB

Dab is an oval-bodied fish with sandy brown upper skin and green freckles. Usual size is 20–30 cm (8–10 in). It has a pleasant flavour when fresh, and may be cooked by all methods.

FLOUNDER

This is oval, with dull brown upper skin (or sometimes dull green with orange freckles). Usual size is 30 cm (12 in). Flesh is rather watery and lacks flavour, needing good seasoning. It can be cooked by all methods.

HALIBUT *(see Figure 5.54, page 84)*

Halibut is a long and narrow fish, brown, with some darker mottling on the upper side; it can be 3m (10 ft) in length and weigh 150 kg (330 lb). Halibut is much valued for its flavour. It is poached, boiled, grilled or shallow fried. It is also smoked.

MEGRIM

Megrim has a very long slender body, sandy-brown coloured with dark blotches. Usual size is 20–30 cm (8–12 in). It has a softish flesh and an unexceptional flavour, so needs good flavouring. It is best breadcrumbed and shallow-fried.

PLAICE *(see Figure 5.60, page 87)*

Plaice are oval in shape, with dark brown colouring and orange spots on the upper side, used on all types of menus; they are usually deep fried or grilled. Average weight, 360–450 g (12 oz–1 lb).

SKATE *(see Figure 5.56, page 85)*

Skate, a member of the ray family, is a very large fish and only the wings are used. It is usually served on the bone and either poached shallow or deep fried or cooked in a court-bouillon and served with black butter.

SOLE *(see Figure 5.60, page 87)*

Sole is considered to be the best of the flat fish. The quality of the Dover sole is well known to be excellent. Soles are cooked by poaching, grilling or frying, both shallow and deep. They are served whole or filleted and garnished in a great many ways.

LEMON SOLE *(see Figure 5.60, page 87)*

This is related to Dover sole, but is broader in shape, and its upper skin is warm, yellowy brown and mottled with darker brown. It can weigh up to 600g (1 lb 5 oz), and may be cooked by all methods.

TURBOT *(see Figure 5.61, page 87)*

Turbot has no scales and is roughly diamond in shape; it has knobs known as tubercules on the dark skin. In proportion to its length it is wider than brill; $3\frac{1}{2}$–4 kg (8–9 lb) is the average weight.

Turbot may be cooked whole, filleted or cut into portions on the bone. It may be boiled, poached, grilled or shallow fried.

WITCH

This is similar in appearance and weight to lemon sole, with sandy-brown upper skin. It is best fried, poached, grilled or steamed.

Round fish

BARRACUDA

A game fish with reddish flesh which when cooked turns pastel white. A mild flavoured fish but cooked as a supreme with the skin left on to prevent drying out.

BASS

Bass have silvery grey backs and white bellies; small ones may have black spots. They have an excellent flavour, with white, lean, softish flesh (which must be very fresh). Bass can be steamed, poached, stuffed and baked, or grilled in steaks. Usual length is 30 cm (1 ft) but they can grow to 60 cm (2 ft).

Bass is usually farmed but sea bass is available (also called wild or nature) from the south coast of Britain. Farmed bass is also available from France and Greece.

BREAM *(see Figure 5.57, page 86)*

Sea bream is a short, oval-bodied, plump, reddish fish, with large scales and a dark patch behind the head. It is used on many less expensive menus; it is usually filleted and deep fried, or stuffed and baked, but other methods of cooking are employed. Average weight, $\frac{1}{2}$–1 kg (1–2 lb); size 28–30 cm (11–12 in). Bream are caught fresh or farmed.

CARP

This is a freshwater fish, usually farmed. The flesh is white with a good flavour, and is best poached in fillets or stuffed and baked. The usual size is 1–2 kg (2–4 lb).

COD *(see Figure 5.58, page 86)*

Cod varies in colour but is mostly greenish, brownish or olive grey. It can measure up to $1\frac{1}{2}$ m (5 ft) in length. Cod is cut into steaks or filleted and cut into portions; it can be deep or shallow fried or poached. Small cod are known as codling. Average weight of cod, $2\frac{1}{2}$–$3\frac{1}{2}$ kg (6–8 lb).

COLEY (SAITH, COALFISH, BLACKJACK)

Coley is dark greenish-brown or blackish in colour, but the flesh turns white when cooked. It has a coarse texture and a dry undistinctive flavour, so is best for mixed fish stews, soups or pies. Size is 40–80 cm (16–31 in).

DOGFISH (HUSS, FLAKE, RIGG) *(see Figure 5.59, page 87)*

These are slender, elongated small sharks. The non-bony white or pink flesh is versatile, and is usually shallow or deep fried. It has a good flavour when very fresh. Length is usually 60 cm (24 in) and weight is $1\frac{1}{4}$ kg ($2\frac{1}{2}$ lb).

GREY MULLET *(see Figure 5.57, page 86)*

This has a scaly streamlined body, which is grey-silver or blue-green. Deep-sea or off-shore mullet has a fine flavour, with firm, moist flesh. It may be stuffed and baked or grilled in steaks.

Some people believe that flavour is improved if the fish is kept in a refrigerator for two to three days, without being cleaned. Length is usually about 30 cm (1 ft); weight 500 g (1 lb 2 oz).

GROUPER

Types include brown, brown spotted, golden strawberry, red speckled. Grouper have a light pinkish flesh that cooks to a greyish-white with a pleasant mild flavour.

GUDGEON

Gudgeon are small fish found in Continental lakes and rivers. They may be deep fried whole. On menus in this country the French term *en goujon* refers to other fish such as sole or turbot, cut into pieces the size of gudgeon.

GURNARD *(see Figure 5.57, page 86)*

A large family of tasty fish with many culinary uses.

HADDOCK *(see Figure 5.58, page 86)*

Haddock is distinguished from cod by the thumb mark on the side and by the lighter colour. Every method of cooking is suitable for haddock, and it appears on all kinds of menus. Apart from fresh haddock, smoked haddock may be served for breakfast, lunch and for a savoury. Average weight, $\frac{1}{2}$–2 kg (1–4 lb).

HAKE *(see Figure 5.58, page 86)*

Owing to overfishing, hake is not plentiful. It is usually poached and is easy to digest. The flesh is very white and of a delicate flavour.

JOHN DORY *(see Figure 5.57, page 86)*

John Dory has a thin distinctive body, flattened from side to side, which is sandy beige in colour and tinged with yellow, with a blue silver grey belly. There is a blotch on each side referred to as 'thumbprint of St Peter'. It has very tough sharp spikes. The flavour is considered superb, and the fish may be cooked by all methods but is best poached, baked or steamed. The large bony head accounts for two-thirds of the weight. Usual size 36 cm (14 in).

LING

This is the largest member of the cod family, and is mottled brown or green with a bronze sheen; the fins have white edges. Size can be up to 90 cm (3 ft). Ling has a good flavour and texture and is generally used in fillets or cutlets, as for cod.

MONKFISH *(see Figure 5.59, page 87)*

Monkfish has a huge flattened head, with a normal fish-shaped tail. It is brown with dark blotches. The tail can be up to 180 cm (6 ft); weight 1–10 kg (2–22 lb). It may be cooked by all methods, and is a firm, close textured white fish with excellent flavour.

PIKE

Pike has a long body usually 60 cm (2 ft) which is greeny-brown, flecked with lighter green, with long toothy jaws. The traditional fish for quenelles, it may also be braised or steamed.

PERCH

Perch has a deep body, marked with about five shadowy vertical bars, and the fins are vivid orange or red. Usual size 15–30 cm (6–12 in). It is generally considered to have an excellent flavour, and may be shallow-fried, grilled, baked, braised or steamed.

POLLACK

This is a member of the cod family, and has a similar shape and variable colours. Its usual size is 45 cm (18 in). It is drier than cod, and can be poached, shallow fried or used for soups and stews.

REDFISH

This is bright red or orange-red, with a rosy belly and dusky gills. Usual size is 45 cm (18 in). It may be poached, baked or used in soups.

RED GURNARD (GREY AND YELLOW GURNARD MAY ALSO BE AVAILABLE) *(see Figure 5.57, page 86)*

This has a large 'mail-checked', tapering body with very spiky fins. Usual size is 20–30 cm (8–12 in). It is good for stews, braising and baking.

RED MULLET *(see Figure 5.57, page 86)*

Red mullet is on occasion cooked with the liver left in, as it is thought that they help to impart a better flavour to the fish. Mullet may be filletted or cooked whole, and the average weight is 360 g (12 oz).

ROCKFISH

Rockfish is the fishmonger's term applied to catfish, coalfish, dogfish, conger eel, etc., after cleaning and skinning. It is usually deep fried in batter.

SHARK

The porbeagle shark, mako or hammerhead, fished off the British coast, gives the best quality food. It is bluish-grey above with a white belly and matt skin. Size is up to 3m (10 ft). It may be cooked by all methods, but grilling in steaks or as kebabs are particularly suitable.

SMELT

Smelts are small fish found in river estuaries and imported from Holland; they are usually deep fried or grilled. When grilled they are split open. The weight of a smelt is from 60 to 90 g (2–3 oz).

SNAPPER

There are several kinds of snapper all of which are brightly coloured. Deep red or medium sized ones give the best flavour. Snapper may be steamed, fried, grilled, baked or smoked.

SWORDFISH

Swordfish is popular grilled, barbecued, roasted or shallow fried.

WHITING *(see Figure 5.58, page 86)*

Whiting are very easy to digest and they are therefore suitable for cookery for invalids. They may be poached, grilled or deep fried and used in the making of fish stuffing. Average weight, 360 g (12 oz).

WRASSE *(see Figure 5.57, page 86)*

Fish of variable colours but usually tinged with red and blue, covered in white and green spots. Wrasse has a variety of culinary uses and can be baked and steamed.

FURTHER INFORMATION

Further information can be obtained from Seafish Industry Authority, 18 Logie Mill, Logie Green Road, Edinburgh EH7 4HG www.seafish.co.uk

Shellfish *(see table, page 105)*

Shellfish are of two types: ○ Crustaceans (lobster, crabs)   ○ Molluscs (oysters, mussels)

Crabs are used for hors-d'œuvre, cocktails, salads, dressed crab, sandwiches and bouchées. Soft-shelled crabs are eaten in their entirety. They are considered to have an excellent flavour and may be deep or shallow fried or grilled.

Shellfish is a good body-building food. As the flesh is coarse and therefore indigestible a little vinegar may be used in cooking to soften the fibres.

CRAWFISH *(see Figure 5.63, page 88)*

Crawfish are like large lobsters without claws, but with long antennae. They are brick red in colour when cooked. Owing to their size and appearance they are used mostly on cold buffets but they can be served hot. The best size is $1\frac{1}{2}$–2 kg (3–4 lb). Menu example includes Langouste parisienne (Dressed crawfish Paris-style).

CRAYFISH *(see Figure 5.62, page 88)*

Crayfish are a type of small fresh-water lobster used for salads, garnishing cold buffet dishes and for recipes using lobster. They are dark brown or grey, turning pink when cooked. Average size is 8 cm (3 in).

LOBSTER *(see Figure 5.62, page 88)*

Lobsters are served cold in cocktails, hors-d'œuvre, salads, sandwiches and on buffets. They are used hot for soup, grilled and served in numerous dishes with various sauces.

PRAWNS

Prawns are larger than shrimps; they may be used for garnishing and decorating fish dishes, for cocktails, canapés, salad, hors-d'œuvre and for hot dishes, such as curried prawns. Prawns are also popular served cold with a mayonnaise type sauce.

SCAMPI, DUBLIN BAY PRAWN

Scampi are found in the Mediterranean. The Dublin Bay prawn, which is the same family, is caught around the Scottish coast. These shellfish resemble small lobster about 20 cm (8 in) long and only the tail flesh is used for a variety of fish dishes, garnishing and salads.

SHRIMPS

Shrimps are used for garnishes, decorating fish dishes, cocktails, sauces, salads, hors-d'œuvre, potted shrimps, omelettes and savouries.

Shellfish: seasons and purchasing units

SHELLFISH	SEASON	PURCHASING UNIT
clams	all year	number and weight
cockles	all year, best in summer	weight
common crab	all year, best April to December	number and weight
spider crab	all year	number and weight
swimming crab	all year	number and weight
king crab, red crab	check with supplier	imported frozen, shelled, prepared
soft-shelled crab	check with supplier	number and weight
crawfish	April to October	number and weight
Dublin Bay prawn	all year	number and weight
freshwater crayfish	mainly imported, some farmed in the UK, wild have short season	number, weight and by case
lobster	April to November	number and weight
mussels	September to March	weight
oysters	May to August	by the dozen
prawn and shrimp	all year	number and weight
scallop	best December to March	number and weight
sea urchin	all year	number and by case

Molluscs

CLAMS *(see Figure 5.64, page 89)*

There are many varieties; the soft or long neck clams such as razor, Ipswich and small hard-shell clams such as cherrystones, can be eaten raw. Large clams can be steamed, fried or grilled and used for soups (chowders) and sauces.

COCKLES

These are enclosed in pretty cream-coloured shells of 2–3 cm (1–1½ in). Cockles are soaked in salt water to purge and then steamed or boiled. They may be used in soups, salads and fish dishes, or served as a dish by themselves.

MUSSELS *(see Figure 5.64, page 89)*

Mussels are extensively cultivated on wooden hurdles in the sea, producing tender, delicately flavoured, plump fish. British mussels are considered good; French mussels are smaller; Dutch and Belgian mussels are plumper. All vary in quality from season to season.

Mussels are kept in boxes, covered with a damp sack and stored in a cold room. They may be served hot or cold or as a garnish.

OYSTERS

Oysters are produced from centres in England, Scotland, Ireland and Wales. Since the majority of oysters are eaten raw it is essential that they are thoroughly cleansed before the hotels and restaurants receive them.

○ Oysters must be alive; this is indicated by the firmly closed shells.
○ They are graded in sizes and the price varies accordingly.
○ Oysters should smell fresh.
○ They should be purchased daily.
○ Oysters are in season from September to April (when there is an r in the month).
○ During the summer months oysters are imported from France, Holland and Portugal.

Oysters are stored in barrels or boxes, covered with damp sacks and kept in a cold room to keep them moist and alive. The shells should be tightly closed; if they are open, tap them sharply, and if they do not shut at once, discard them.

The popular way of eating oysters is in the raw state. They may also be served in soups, hot cocktail savouries, fish garnishes, as a fish dish, in meat puddings and savouries.

SCALLOPS *(see Figure 5.64, page 89)*

Great scallops are up to 15 cm (6 in) in size; Bay scallops up to 8 cm (3 in); Queen scallops are small-cockle-sized, and are also known as 'Queenies'. Scallops may be steamed, poached, fried or grilled.

SEA-URCHIN OR SEA HEDGEHOG

They have spine-covered spherical shells. Only the orange and yellow roe is eaten, either raw out of the shell or removed with a teaspoon and used in soups, sauces, scrambled eggs, etc.: 10 to 20 urchins provide approximately 200 g (7 oz) roe.

WINKLES

Winkles are small sea snails with a delicious flavour. They may be boiled for 3 minutes and served with garlic butter or on a dish of assorted shellfish.

Cephalopods and fish offal

CUTTLEFISH

They are usually dark with attractive pale stripes and the size can be up to 24 cm (10 in). They are available all year by number and weight. Cuttlefish are prepared like squid and may be stewed or gently grilled.

OCTOPUS *(see Figure 5.52, page 84)*

Octopus are available all year by number and weight. Large species are tough and need to be tenderised; they are then prepared as for squid. Small octopus can be boiled, then cut up for grilling or frying. When stewing, a long cooking time is needed.

SQUID *(see Figure 5.52, page 84)*

The common squid has mottled skin and white flesh, two tentacles, eight arms and flap-like fins. Usual size is 15–30 cm (6–12 in). Careful, correct preparation is important if the fish is to be tender. It may be stir-fried, fried, baked, grilled or braised.

LIVER

An oil rich in vitamins A and D is obtained from the liver of cod and halibut. This is used medicinally.

ROE

Those used are the soft and hard roes of herring, cod, sturgeon and the coral from lobster. Soft herring roes are used to garnish fish dishes and as a savoury. Cod's roe is smoked and served as hors-d'œuvre. The roe of the sturgeon is salted and served raw as caviar and the coral of lobster is used for colouring lobster butter and lobster dishes, and also as a decoration for fish dishes.

VEGETABLES

Fresh vegetables and fruits are important foods both from an economic and nutritional point of view. On average, each person consumes 125–150 kg (275–330 lb) per year of fruit and vegetables.

The purchasing of these commodities is difficult because the products are highly perishable and supply and demand varies. The high perishability of fresh vegetables and fruits causes problems not encountered in other markets. Fresh vegetables and fruits are living organisms and will lose quality quickly if not properly stored and handled. Improved transportation and storage facilities can help prevent loss of quality. For organic vegetables see page 62.

Automation in harvesting and packaging speeds the handling process and helps retain quality.

Vacuum cooling, which is a process whereby fresh produce is moved into huge chambers, where, for about half an hour, a low vacuum is maintained, inducing rapid evaporation which quickly reduces field heat, has been highly successful in improving quality.

Types of vegetables

ROOTS	TUBERS	BULBS	LEAFY
beetroot	Jerusalem	garlic	chicory
carrots	artichokes	leeks	Chinese leaves
celeriac	potatoes	onions	corn salad
horseradish	sweet potatoes	shallots	lettuce
mooli	yams	spring onions	mustard and cress
parsnips			radiccio
radish			sorrel
salsify			spinach
scorzonera			Swiss chard
swedes			watercress
turnips			

BRASSICAS	PODS AND SEEDS	FRUITING	STEMS AND SHOOTS	MUSHROOMS AND FUNGI
broccoli	broad beans	aubergine	asparagus	ceps
Brussels sprouts	butter or lima	avocado	beans	chanterelles
cabbage	beans	courgette	cardoon	horn of plenty
calabrese	runner beans	cucumber	celery	morels
cauliflower	mange-tout	goulds	endive	mushrooms
curly kale	okra	marrow	globe artichokes	
spring greens	peas	peppers	kohlrabi	
	sweetcorn	pumpkin	sea kale	
		squash		
		tomatoes		

Experience and sound judgement are essential for the efficient buying and storage of all commodities, but none probably more so than fresh vegetables and fruit.

The grading of fresh fruit and vegetables within the EU

There are four main quality classes for produce:

○ Extra Class – for produce of top quality,
○ Class I – for produce of good quality,
○ Class II – for produce of reasonably good quality,
○ Class III – for produce of low marketable quality.

Food value

○ Root vegetables – useful in the diet because they contain starch or sugar for energy, a small but valuable amount of protein, some mineral salts and vitamins; also useful sources of cellulose and water.
○ Green vegetables – no food is stored in the leaves, it is only produced there; therefore little protein or carbohydrate is found in green vegetables; they are rich in mineral salts and vitamins, particularly vitamin C and carotene; the greener the leaf the larger the quantity of vitamin present; chief mineral salts are calcium and iron.

Preservation

○ Canning – certain vegetables are preserved in tins: artichokes, asparagus, carrots, celery, beans, peas (fins, garden, processed), tomatoes (whole, purée), mushrooms, truffles.
○ Dehydration – onions, carrots, potatoes and cabbage are shredded and quickly dried until they contain only 5% water.
○ Drying – the seeds of legumes (peas and beans) have the moisture content reduced to 10%.
○ Pickling – onions and red cabbage are examples of vegetables preserved in spiced vinegar.
○ Salting – French and runner beans may be sliced and preserved in dry salt.
○ Freezing – many vegetables such as peas, beans, sprouts, spinach and cauliflower are deep frozen.

Types of vegetables

ROOTS

○ Beetroot – two main types, round and long; used for soups, salads and as a vegetable.
○ Carrots – grown in numerous varieties and sizes; used extensively for soups, sauces, stocks, stews, salads, and as a vegetable.
○ Celeriac – large, light-brown, celery-flavoured root, used in soups, salads and as a vegetable.
○ Horseradish – long, light-brown, narrow root, grated and used for horseradish sauce.
○ Mooli – long, white, thick member of radish family, used for soups, salads or as a vegetable.
○ Parsnips – long, white root tapering to a point; unique nut-like flavour; used in soups, added to casseroles and as a vegetable (roasted, purée, etc.).
○ Radishes – small summer variety, round or oval, served with dips, in salads or as a vegetable in white or cheese sauce.
○ Salsify – also called oyster plant because of similarity of taste; long, narrow root used in soups, salads and as a vegetable.

○ Scorzonera – long, narrow root, slightly astringent in flavour; used in soups, salads and as a vegetable.

○ Swede – large root with yellow flesh; generally used as a vegetable, mashed or parboiled and roasted; may be added to stews.

○ Turnip – two main varieties, long and round; used in soups, stews and as a vegetable.

TUBERS

○ Artichokes, Jerusalem – potato-like tuber with a bitter-sweet flavour; used in soups, salads and as a vegetable.

○ Purple congo are a blue potato. Truffle de Chine are a deep purple potato grown in France.

○ Turo-Eddo are two basic varieties found in tropical areas. A large barrel shaped tuber and a smaller variety which is often called eddo of dashheen. They are all a dark mahogony brown with a shaggy skin, looking like a cross between a beetroot and a swede.

○ Potatoes – many varieties are grown but all potatoes should be sold by name (King Edward, Desirée, Maris Piper); this is important as the caterer needs to know which varieties are best suited for specific cooking purposes. The various varieties fall into four categories: floury, firm, waxy or salad potatoes; Jersey Royals are specially grown, highly regarded new potatoes.

○ Sweet potatoes – long tubers with purple or sand-coloured skins and orange flesh; flavour is sweet and aromatic; used as a vegetable (fried, puréed, creamed, candied) or made into a sweet pudding.

○ Yams – similar to sweet potatoes, usually cylindrical, often knobbly in shape; can be used in the same way as sweet potatoes.

BULBS *(see Figure 5.66, page 90)*

○ Fennel – the bulb is the swollen leaf base and has a pronounced flavour. Used raw in salads and cooked.

○ Garlic – an onion-like bulb with a papery skin inside of which are small individually wrapped cloves; used extensively in many forms of cookery; garlic has a pungent distinctive flavour and should be used sparingly.

○ Leeks – summer leeks have long white stems, bright green leaves and a milder flavour than winter leeks; these have a stockier stem and a stronger flavour; used extensively in stocks, soups, sauces, stews, hors-d'œuvre and as a vegetable.

○ Onions – there are numerous varieties with different coloured skins and varying strengths; after salt, the onion is probably the most-used flavouring in cookery; can be used in almost every type of food except sweet dishes.

○ Shallots – have a similar but more refined flavour than the onion and are therefore more often used in top class cookery.

○ Spring onions – are slim and tiny like miniature leeks; used in soups, salads and Chinese and Japanese cookery. Ramp looks like a spring onion but is stronger.

LEAFY *(see Figures 5.66 and 5.67, page 90)*

○ Chicory – a lettuce with coarse, crisp leaves and a sharp, bitter taste in the outside leaves; inner leaves are milder.

○ Chinese leaves – long white, densely packed leaves with a mild flavour resembling celery; makes a good substitute for lettuce and can be boiled, braised or stir-fried as a vegetable.

○ Corn salad – sometimes called lamb's lettuce; small, tender, dark leaves with a tangy nutty taste.

- Culaboo are leaves of the tero plant, poisonous if eaten raw, but widely used in Asian and Caribbean cookery.
- Lettuce – many varieties: cabbage, cos, little gem, iceberg, oakleaf, Webbs; used chiefly for salads, or used as a wrapping for other foods, e.g. fish fillets.
- Mustard and cress – embryonic leaves of mustard and garden cress with a sharp warm flavour; used mainly in, or as a garnish to, sandwiches and salads.
- Nettles brache – once cooked the sting disappears. Should be picked young, used in soups.
- Radiccio – round, deep red variety of chicory with white ribs and a distinctive bitter taste.
- Rocket – a type of cress with larger leaves and a peppery taste.
- Sorrel – bright-green sour leaves which can be overpowering if used on their own; best when tender and young; used in salad and soups.
- Spinach – tender dark green leaves with a mild musky flavour; used for soups, garnishing egg and fish dishes, as a vegetable and raw in salads.
- Swiss chard – has large, ribbed, slightly curly leaves with a flavour similar to but milder than spinach; used as for spinach.
- Watercress – long stems with round, dark, tender green leaves and a pungent peppery flavour; used for soups, salads, and for garnishing roasts and grills of meat and poultry.
- Vine leaves – all leaves from grape vines can be eaten when young.

BRASSICAS

- Broccoli – various types: calabrese white, green, purple-sprouting; delicate vegetable with a gentle flavour used in soups, salads, stir-fry dishes and cooked and served in many ways as a vegetable.
- Broccoflower – a cross between broccoli and cauliflower. Chinese broccoli is a leafy vegetable with slender heads of flowers.
- Brussels sprouts – small green buds growing on thick stems; can be used for soup but are mainly used as a vegetable, and can be cooked and served in a variety of ways.
- Cabbage – three main types: green, white and red; many varieties of green cabbage available at different seasons of the year; early green cabbage is deep green and loosely formed; later in the season they firm up with solid hearts; Savoy is considered the best of the winter green cabbage; white cabbage is used for coleslaw; green and red as a vegetable, boiled, braised or stir-fried.
- Chinese mustard greens, deep green mustard flavoured. Pok Choi – Chinese cabbage with many varieties.
- Cauliflower – heads of creamy-white florets with a distinctive flavour; used for soup and cooked and served in various ways as a vegetable.
- Kale and Curly Kale – thick green leaves. The curly variety is the most popular Romanescue – pretty green or white cross between broccoli and cauliflower.

PODS AND SEEDS

- Broad beans – pale-green, oval-shaped beans contained in a thick fleshy pod; young broad beans can be removed from the pods and cooked in their shells and served as a vegetable in various ways; old broad beans will toughen and when removed from the pods will have to be shelled before being served.
- Butter or lima beans – butter beans are white, large, flattish and oval-shaped; lima beans are smaller; both used as a vegetable or salad, stew or casserole ingredient.

○ Runner beans – popular vegetable that must be used when young; bright green colour and a pliable velvety feel; if coarse, wilted, or older beans are used they will be stringy and tough.

○ Mange-tout – also called snow-peas or sugar peas; flat peapod with immature seeds which after topping, tailing and stringing, may be eaten in their entirety; used as a vegetable, in salads and for stir-fry dishes.

○ Okra – curved and pointed seed pods with a flavour similar to aubergines; cooked as a vegetable or in creole-type stews.

○ Peas – garden peas are normal size, petits pois are a dwarf variety; marrow fat peas are dried; popular as a vegetable, peas are also used for soups, salads, stews and stir-fry dishes.

○ Sweetcorn – also known as maize or Sudan corn; available 'on the cob' fresh or frozen or in kernels, canned or frozen; a versatile commodity and used as a first course, in soups, salads, casseroles and as a vegetable.

ROOTS AND STEMS

○ Thai beans – similar to French beans

○ Fallow wax beans – similar to French beans

○ Fiddlecoke fern – also called ostrich fern. 5 cm long, a cross between asparagus and used in oriental dishes.

○ Palm hearts – buds of cabbage palm trees.

○ Water Chestnuts – common name for a number of quatic herbs and their nut like fruit. The best known type is the Chinese water chestnut, sometimes known as the Chinese sedge.

○ Samphire – two types : marsh samphire grows in estuaries and salt marshes. White rock samphire sometimes called sea fennel grows on rocky shores. Marsh samphire is also kown as glass wort and is sometimes called sea asparagus.

FRUITING *(see Figure 5.68, page 91)*

○ Aubergine – firm, elongated, varying in size with smooth shiny skins ranging in colour from purple-red to purple-black; inner flesh is white with tiny soft seeds; almost without flavour, it requires other seasonings, e.g. garlic, lemon juice, herbs, to enhance its taste; may be sliced and fried or baked, steamed or stuffed. Varieties include baby, Japanese, white, striped, Thai.

○ Avocado – fruit that is mainly used as a vegetable because of its bland, mild, nutty flavour; two main types: summer variety that is green when unripe and purple-black when ripe with golden-yellow flesh; winter ones are more pear-shaped with smooth green skin and pale green to yellow flesh; eaten as first courses and used in soups, salads, dips and garnishes to other dishes hot and cold.

○ Courgette – baby marrow, light to dark green in colour, with a delicate flavour becoming stronger when cooked with other ingredients, e.g. herbs, garlic, spices; may be boiled, steamed, fried, baked, stuffed and stir-fried.

○ Cucumber – a long, smooth-skinned fruiting vegetable, ridged and dark green in colour; used in salads, soups, sandwiches, garnishes and as a vegetable.

○ Gourds (exotic). Bottle gourds chayotes (chow-chow), Chinese butter lemons.

○ Marrow – long, oval-shaped edible gourds with ridged green skins and a bland flavour; may be cooked as for courgettes.

○ Peppers – available in three colours: green peppers are unripened and they turn yellow to orange and then red (they must remain on the plant to do this); used raw and cooked in salads, vegetable dishes, stuffed and baked, casseroles and stir-fried dishes.

Seasons for home-grown vegetables

SPRING

asparagus	cauliflower	broccoli – white and purple
new carrots	new turnips	new potatoes
greens		

SUMMER

artichokes, globe	turnips	asparagus
cauliflower	aubergine	cos lettuce
beans, broad	peas	radishes
BEANS, French	carrots	sea-kale
sweetcorn		

AUTUMN

artichokes, globe	parsnips	field mushrooms
artichokes, Jerusalem	aubergine	peppers
beans, runner	cauliflower	red cabbage
broccoli	celery	shallots
salsify	swedes	marrow
celeriac	turnips	

WINTER

Brussels sprouts	chicory	cabbage
kale	celery	parsnips
cauliflower	broccoli	red cabbage
Savoy cabbage	celeriac	swedes
turnips		

ALL THE YEAR ROUND

Although the following vegetables are available all the year round, nevertheless at certain times, owing to bad weather, a heavy demand or other circumstances, supplies may be temporarily curtailed. However, owing to air transport, most vegetables are available all year round.

beetroot	tomatoes	spinach	onions
mushrooms	leeks	watercress	lettuce
cucumber	carrots	cabbage	potatoes

○ Pumpkins – vary in size and can weigh up to 50 kg (110 lb); associated with Hallowe'en as a decoration but may be used in soups or pumpkin pie.

○ Squash – many varieties e.g. acorn, butternut, summer crookneck, delicate, hubbond, kuboche, onion. Flesh firm and glowy; can be boiled, baked, steamed or puree'd.

○ Tomatoes – along with onions, probably the most-used vegetable in cookery; several varieties including cherry, yellow, globe, large ridged (beef) and plum; used in soups, sauces, stews, salads, sandwiches and as a vegetable.

STEMS AND SHOOTS *(see Figure 5.66, page 90)*

- Asparagus – three main types: white, with creamy white stems and a mild flavour; French, with violet or bluish tips and a stronger more astringent flavour; and green, with what is considered a delicious aromatic flavour; used on every course of the menu, except the sweet course.
- Bean sprouts – slender young sprouts of the germinating soya or mung bean, used as a vegetable accompaniment, in stir-fry dishes and salads.
- Cardoon – longish plant with root and fleshy ribbed stalk similar to celery, but leaves are grey-green in colour; used cooked as a vegetable or raw in salads.
- Celery – long-stemmed bundles of fleshy, ribbed stalks, white to light green in colour; used in soups, stocks, sauces, cooked as a vegetable and raw in salads and dips.
- Chicory – also known as Belgian endive; conical heads of crisp white, faintly bitter leaves used cooked as a vegetable and raw in salads and dips.
- Globe artichokes – resemble fat pine cones with overlapping fleshy, green, inedible leaves, all connected to an edible fleshy base or bottom; used as a first course, hot or cold; as a vegetable, boiled, stuffed, baked, fried or in casseroles.
- Kohlrabi – stem which swells to turnip shape above the ground; those about the size of a large egg are best for cookery purposes (other than soup or purées); may be cooked as a vegetable, stuffed and baked and added to stews and casseroles.
- Sea-kale – delicate white leaves with yellow frills edged with purple; can be boiled or braised or served raw like celery.

Plantains

- Ackee – tropical fruit used in Caribbean style savoury dishes.
- Breadfruit – fruit from a tropical tree found in the Islands of the South Pacific Ocean.

MUSHROOMS AND FUNGI *(see Figure 5.69, page 91)*

- Ceps – wild mushrooms with short, stout stalks with slightly raised veins and tubes underneath the cap in which the brown spores are produced.
- Chanterelles or Girolles – wild, funnel-shaped, yellow-capped mushrooms with a slightly ribbed stalk which runs up under the edge of the cap.
- Horns of plenty – trumpet-shaped, shaggy, almost black wild mushrooms.
- Morels – delicate, wild mushrooms varying in colour from pale beige to dark brown-black with a flavour that suggests meat.
- Oyster mushrooms – creamy gills and firm flesh; delicate with shorter storage life than regular mushrooms.
- Shitake mushrooms – solid texture with a strong, slightly meaty flavour.
- Mushrooms – field mushrooms found in meadows from late summer to autumn; creamy white cap and stalk and a strong earthy flavour.
- Cultivated mushrooms – available in three types: button (small, succulent, weak in flavour); cap and open or flat mushrooms.

All mushrooms both wild and cultivated have a great many uses in cookery, in soups, stocks, salads, vegetables, savouries and garnishes.

FRUITS

For culinary purposes fruit can be divided into various groups.

FOOD VALUE

The nutritive value of fruit depends on its vitamin content, especially vitamin C; it is therefore valuable as a protective food. The cellulose in fruit is useful as roughage.

STORAGE

- Hard fruits, such as apples, are left in boxes and kept in a cool store.
- Soft fruits, such as raspberries and strawberries, should be left in their punnets or baskets in a cold room.
- Stone fruits are best placed in trays so that any damaged fruit can be seen and discarded.
- Peaches and citrus fruits are left in their delivery trays or boxes.
- Bananas should not be stored in too cold a place because the skins turn black.

QUALITY AND PURCHASING POINTS

- Soft fruits deteriorate quickly, especially if not sound. Care must be taken to see that they are not damaged or too ripe when bought.
- Soft fruits should appear fresh; there should be no shrinking, wilting or signs of mould.
- The colour of certain soft fruits is an indication of ripeness (strawberries, dessert gooseberries).
- Hard fruits should not be bruised. Pears should not be over-ripe.

PRESERVATION

- Drying – apples, pears, apricots, peaches, bananas and figs are dried; plums when dried are called prunes, and currants, sultanas and raisins are produced by drying grapes.
- Canning – almost all fruits may be canned; apples are packed in water and known as solid packed apples; other fruits are canned in syrup.
- Bottling – bottling is used domestically, but very little fruit is commercially preserved in this way; cherries are bottled in maraschino.
- Candied, glacé and crystallised fruits are mainly imported from France.
- Jam – some stone fruits and all soft fruits can be used.
- Jelly – jellies are produced from fruit juice.
- Quick freezing – strawberries, raspberries, loganberries, apples, blackberries, gooseberries, grapefruit and plums are frozen and they must be kept below 0°C/32°F.
- Cold storage – apples are stored at temperatures between 1–4°C (34–39°F), depending on the variety of apple.
- Gas storage – fruit can be kept in a sealed store room where the atmosphere is controlled; the amount of air is limited, the oxygen content of the air is decreased and the carbon dioxide increased, which controls the respiration rate of the fruit.

Different fruits and their seasons

FRUIT	SEASON	FRUIT	SEASON
apple	all year round	greengage	August
apricot	May to September	lemon	all year round
avocado pear	all year round	mandarin	November to June
banana	all year round	melon	all year round
blackberry	September to October	orange	all year round
blackcurrants	July to September	peach	September
cherry	June to August	pear	September to March
clementine	winter	pineapple	all year round
cranberries	November to January	plum	July to October
damson	September to October	raspberry	June to August
date	winter	red currants	July to September
fig	July to September	rhubarb	December to June
gooseberry	July to September	strawberry	June to August
grapefruit	all year round	tangerine	winter
grapes	all year round		

Because of modern storage methods and air transport the majority of these fruits may be available all year round.

Fruit juices, syrups and drinks

Fruit juices such as orange, lemon, blackcurrant are canned. Syrups such as rose hip and orange are bottled. Fruit drinks are also bottled; they include orange, lime and lemon.

USES

With the exception of certain fruits (lemon, rhubarb, cranberries) fruit can be eaten as a dessert or in its raw state. Some fruits have dessert and cooking varieties, e.g. apples, pears, cherries and gooseberries.

STONE FRUITS

Damsons, plums, greengages, cherries, apricots, peaches and nectarines are used as a dessert; stewed (compote) for jam, pies, puddings and in various sweet dishes and some meat and poultry dishes. Peaches are also used to garnish certain meat dishes. Varieties of Plums include Dessert, Victoria, Gamota, Mayoris, Burbank, Cooking: Angelina, Stanley, Beech Cherry, Reeves Seedling.

HARD FRUITS

The popular English dessert apple varieties include Beauty of Bath, Discovery, Spartan, Worcester Pearmain, Cox's Orange Pippin, Blenheim Orange, Laxton's Superb and James Grieve; imported apples include Golden Delicious, Braeburn and Gala. The Bramley is the most popular cooking apple. The William, Conference and Doyenne du Comice are among the best known pears. Other varieties of Pear include: Anjou, Beurre-Beth, Beure-Bose, Beurve-Hardi, Beurre-Supersin, Forelle, Morton Poirde, Onwaide, Rocha, Housi, Perry Tieatsin.

Apples and pears are used in many pastry dishes. Apples are also used for garnishing meat dishes and for sauce which is served with roast pork and duck.

SOFT FRUITS *(see Figure 5.71, page 92)*

Raspberries, strawberries, loganberries and gooseberries are used as a dessert. Gooseberries, black and red currants and blackberries are stewed, used in pies and puddings. They are used for jam and flavourings and in certain sauces for sweet, meat and poultry dishes. Other varieties of soft fruit include: Dewberries, Jam berries, Young berries, Boysenberries, Sunberries, Wineberries, blue berries, elderberries. Varieties of gooseberries include: leveller, London, golden drop.

CITRUS FRUITS

Oranges, lemons, limes and grapefruit are not usually cooked, except for marmalade. Lemons and limes are used for flavouring and garnishing, particularly fish dishes. Oranges are used mainly for flavouring, and in fruit salads, also to garnish certain poultry dishes. Grapefruit are served at breakfast and as a first course generally for luncheon. Mandarins, clementines and satsumas are eaten as a dessert or used in sweet dishes. Kumquats look and taste like tiny oranges and are eaten with the skin on. Tangelos are a cross between tangerines and grapefruit, and are sometimes called uglis. Pomelos are the largest of the citrus fruits, predominantly round but with a slightly flattened base and pointed top.

TROPICAL AND OTHER FRUITS *(see Figure 5.70, page 92)*

- Bananas – as well as being used as a dessert, bananas are grilled for a fish garnish, fried as fritters and served as a garnish to poultry (Maryland); they are used in fruit salad and other sweet dishes.
- Cape gooseberries – a sharp, pleasant-flavoured small round fruit sometimes dipped in fondant and served as a type of petit four.
- Carambola – also known as starfruit, it has a yellowish-green skin with a waxy sheen. The fruit is long and narrow and has a delicate lemon flavour.
- Cranberries – these hard red berries are used for cranberry sauce, which is served with roast turkey.
- Dates – whole dates are served as a dessert; stoned dates are used in various sweet dishes and petits fours.
- Figs – fresh figs may be served as a first course or dessert. Dried figs may be used for fig puddings, and other sweet dishes.
- Granadillas – these are like an orange in shape and colour, are light in weight and similar to a passion fruit in flavour.
- Grapes – black and white grapes are used as a dessert, in fruit salad, as a sweet meat and also as a fish garnish.
- Guavas – varies size between that of a walnut to that of an apple; ripe guavas have a sweet pink flesh and they can be eaten with cream or mixed with other fruits.
- Kiwi fruit – have a brown furry skin; the flesh is green with edible black seeds which when thinly sliced gives a pleasant decorative appearance.
- Lychees – a Chinese fruit with a delicate flavour, obtainable tinned in syrup and also fresh.
- Mangoes – can be as large as a melon or as small as an apple; ripe mangoes have smooth pinky-golden flesh with a pleasing flavour; they may be served in halves sprinkled with lemon juice, sugar, rum or ginger; mangoes can also be used in fruit salads and for sorbets.
- Mangostines – are apple-shaped with tough reddish-brown skin which turns purple as the fruit ripens; they have juicy creamy flesh.
- Bubacos – hybrid of the papaya.

○ Custard apples – heart-shaped or oval light tan or greenish quilted skin. Soursops (prickly custard apples) have dark green skins covered in short spines.

○ Curuba – also known as banana passion fruit. Soft yellowish skin.

○ Dragon fruit – yellow or pink. Pink are large, about 10 cm long and covered with pointed green-tipped scales.

○ Durians – large fruit that can weigh up to 4.5 kg. Round or oval, have a woolly olive green outer layer covered with stubby, sharp pikes, which turn yellow as they ripen. Contains creamy white flesh with the texture of rich custard.

○ Feijons – member of the guava family, feijons resemble small slightly pear-shaped passion fruit, with a dark green skin which yellows as the fruit ripens.

○ Granadillas – largest members of the passion fruit family.

○ Jackfruit – related to breadfruit. The large irregularly shaped oval fruits can weigh up to 20 kg. They have a rough spiny skin which ripens from green to brown.

○ Jujubes – also known as Chinese jujubes, apples or dates. Small greeny brown fruit.

○ Kiwanos – also known as horned melon, horned cucumber or jelly melon. The oval fruits have thick, bright golden-orange skin covered with sharp spikes. The skin conceals a bright green, jelly-like flesh, encasing edible seeds, rather like a passion fruit.

○ Loquats – native to China and South Japan, also known as Japanese medlar. They have a sweet scent and a delicate mango-like flavour.

○ Maracoyas – also known as yellow passion fruit. Vibrant green with a thick shiny skin, which turns yellow as it ripens. Inside orange pulp enclosing hard grey seeds.

○ Pepinos – smooth golden skin heavily streaked with purple, sometimes called a tree melon. Native to Peru.

○ Pomegranates – apple-shaped fruit with leathery reddish-brown skin, and a large calyx or crown. Inside is a mass of creamy-white edible seeds, each encased in a translucent sac of deep pink or crimson pulp and held together by segments of bitter, inedible yellow membrane.

○ Prickly pears – also kown as 'indian figs'. Fruit of the cactus. Skin is covered in prickles. Greenish-orange skin and orangey-pink flesh with a melon-like texture.

○ Rambutans – related to lychees, sometimes kown as hairy lychees.

○ Sapodillas – oval fruit from central America. Light brown skin, the flesh is sweet, with inedible hard black pips.

○ Snake fruit – large member of the lychees family, the creamy flesh is divided into four segments each encasing a very large inedible brown stone.

○ Tamarillos – known as 'tree tomatoes', large egg-shaped tomatoes with thick, smooth wine-red skins. Each fruit has two lobes containing a multitude of black seeds.

○ Passion fruit – the name comes from the flower of the plant which is meant to represent the Passion of Christ; size and shape of an egg with crinkled purple-brown skin when ripe; flesh and seeds are all edible. Has many uses in pastry work.

○ Paw paw (papaya) – green to golden skin, orangey flesh with a sweet subtle flavour and black seeds; eaten raw sprinkled with lime or lemon juice. Served with crab or prawns and mayonnaise as a first course.

○ Persimmon – a round orange-red fruit with a tough skin which can be cut when the fruit is ripe; when under-ripe they have an unpleasant acid-like taste of tannin.

○ Pineapple – served as a dessert; it is also used in many sweet dishes and as a garnish to certain meat dishes.

○ Rhubarb – forced or early rhubarb is obtainable from January; natural rhubarb from April–June; used for pies, puddings, fool and compote.
○ Sharon fruit – a seedless persimmon tasting like a sweet exotic peach.
○ Tamarind – red, egg shaped, flavour a mix of tomato, apricot and coconut, used in sweet dishes and salads.

MELONS

There are several types of melon. The most popular are:
○ Honeydew – long, oval-shaped melons with dark green skins; the flesh is white with a greenish tinge.
○ Charentais – small and round with a mottled green and yellow skin; the flesh is orange coloured.
○ Cantaloup – large round melons with regular indentations; the rough skin is mottled orange and yellow and the flesh is light orange in colour.
○ Ogen – small round mottled green skins suitable for one portion (depending on size); mainly used as a dessert, hors-d'œuvre and sweet dishes.

Care must be taken when buying as melons should not be over- or under-ripe. This can be assessed by carefully pressing the top or bottom of the fruit and smelling the outside skin for sweetness. There should be a slight degree of softness to the cantaloup and charentais melons. The stalk should be attached, otherwise the melon deteriorates quickly.

Further information: Fresh fruit and vegetable information bureau, Bury House, 126–8, Cromwell Rd, London SW7 4ET www.ffvib.co.uk

Fresh produce consortium, Minerva House, Minerva Business Park, Lynch Wood, Peterborough PE2 6FT www.freshproduce.org.uk

NUTS

Nuts are the reproductive kernel (seed) of the plant or tree from which they come. Nuts are perishable and may easily become rancid or infested with insects. Some people have an allergy to nuts which can cause severe illness and possibly death.
SEASON
Dessert nuts are in season during the autumn and winter.

Food value

Nuts are highly nutritious because of their protein, fat and mineral salts. They are of considerable importance to vegetarians, who may use nuts in place of meat; they are therefore a food which builds, repairs and provides energy. Nuts are difficult to digest.

Storage

Dessert nuts, those with the shell on, are kept in a dry, ventilated store. Nuts without shells, whether ground, nibbed, flaked or whole, are kept in airtight containers.

Quality and purchasing points

○ Nuts should be of good size.
○ They should be heavy for their size.
○ There must be no sign of mildew.

Use

Nuts are used extensively in pastry and confectionery work and vegetarian cookery, and also for decorating and flavouring. They are used whole, or halves, and almonds are used ground, nibbed and flaked.

ALMONDS

Salted almonds are served at cocktail parties and bars. Ground, flaked or nibbed almonds are used in sweet dishes and for decorating cakes.

Marzipan (almond paste) has many uses in pastry work.

BRAZIL NUTS

Brazil nuts are served with fresh fruit as dessert and are also used in confectionery.

CHESTNUTS

Chestnuts are used as stuffing for turkeys; chestnut flour is used for soup, and as a garnish for ice cream. Chestnut purée is used in pastries and gâteaux.

COCONUT

Coconut is used in desiccated form for curry preparations, and in many types of cakes and confectionery.

HAZEL NUTS

These nuts are used as a dessert and for praline.

MACADAMIA NUTS

These expensive nuts have a rich, delicate, sweetish flavour. They can be used in pasta dishes, savoury sauces for meat, game and poultry and in ice-cream, sorbets and puddings.

PECANS

Pecan nuts are used salted for dessert, various sweets and ice-cream.

PEANUTS AND CASHEW NUTS

These are salted and used as bar snacks. Also used in some stir fry dishes.

PISTACHIO NUTS

These small green nuts, grown mainly in France and Italy, are used for decorating galantines, small and large cakes and petits fours. They are also used in ice-cream.

WALNUTS

Walnuts, imported mainly from France and Italy, are used as a dessert, in salads and for decorating cakes and sweet dishes. They are also pickled, while green and unripe.

EGGS

The term egg applies not only to those of the hen, but also to the edible eggs of other birds, such as turkeys, geese, ducks, guinea fowl, quails and gulls. Around 28 million hens eggs are consumed each day in the UK and approximately 95% of these are produced in the UK.

The British Egg Products Association (BEPA) introduced a strict Code of Practice in 1993 which covers all stages of production, from sourcing of raw materials to packaging and finished production standards. Members of BEPA can qualify to show a Date Stamp on their products which signifies that the products have been produced to standards higher than those demanded by UK and European law. The aim of the Date Stamp is to reduce the risk of infection in hens, to monitor and take remedial action where necessary and to ensure that eggs are held and distributed under the best conditions.

Food value

Eggs contain most nutrients and are low in calories: two eggs contain 180 calories. Egg protein is complete and easily digestible, therefore it is useful for balancing meals. Eggs may also be used as the main dish; they are a protective food and provide energy and material for growth and repair of the body.

Production

Hens' eggs are graded in four sizes:

- ○ small 48 g
- ○ medium 58 g
- ○ large 68 g
- ○ very large 76 g

The size of an egg does not affect the quality but does affect the price. The eggs are tested for quality, then weighed and graded under European law.

- ○ Grade A – naturally clean, fresh eggs, internally perfect with intact shells and an air cell not exceeding 6 mm ($\frac{1}{4}$ in) in depth.
- ○ Grade B – eggs which have been down-graded because they have been cleaned or preserved, or because they are internally imperfect, cracked or have an air cell exceeding 6mm ($\frac{1}{4}$ in) but not more than 9 mm ($\frac{3}{8}$ in) in depth.
- ○ Grade C – are eggs which are fit for breaking for manufacturing purposes but cannot be sold in their shells to the public.

Figure 5.74 *Quality of eggs*

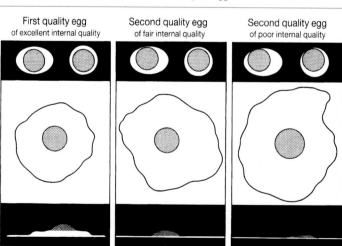

First quality egg
of excellent internal quality

Second quality egg
of fair internal quality

Second quality egg
of poor internal quality

They are then packed into boxes containing, 360 (or 180). The wholesale price of eggs is quoted per long hundred (120). All egg-boxes leaving the packing station are dated.

The lion quality mark on eggs and egg boxes means that the eggs have been produced to the highest standards of food safety in the world.

Raw eggs and Salmonella

In a number of Salmonella food poisoning cases, raw eggs have been suspected as being the cause. Most infections cause only mild stomach upsets but the effects can be serious in vulnerable people such as the elderly, the infirm, pregnant women and young children. Consumers, particularly the more vulnerable, are advised to avoid eating raw and lightly cooked eggs, uncooked foods made from raw eggs and products such as mayonnaise, mousses and ice creams. Caterers are advised to use pasteurised eggs. Dishes with an obvious risk of passing on contamination also include soft boiled eggs, scrambled eggs and omelettes. The Department of Health has issued the following guidelines which apply to raw eggs.

There does not appear to be a similar risk with eggs that are cooked thoroughly.

- Eggs should be stored in a cool dry place, preferably under refrigeration.
- Eggs should be stored away from possible contaminants such as raw meat.
- Stocks should be rotated: first in, first out.
- Hands should be washed before and after handling eggs.
- Cracked eggs should not be used.
- Preparation surfaces, utensils and containers should be regularly cleaned and always cleaned between the preparation of different dishes.
- Egg dishes should be consumed as soon as possible after preparation or, if not for immediate use, refrigerated.

Egg products

Most egg products are available in liquid, frozen or spray dried foam. Whole egg is used primarily for cake production where its foaming and coagulation properties are required. Egg whites are used for meringues and light sponges where their foaming property is crucial.

Usage of Egg Products	FROZEN			LIQUID			DRIED		
	Whole Egg	Yolk	Whites	Whole Egg	Yolk	Whites	Whole Egg	Yolk	Whites
Ready Meals	*	*	*	*	*	*	*	*	*
Pies/Flans	*	*	*	*	*	*	*	*	*
Baked Goods	*	*	*	*	*	*	*	*	*
Cakes	*	*	*	*	*	*	*	*	*
Dairy Products	*	*		*	*		*	*	
Desserts	*	*	*	*	*	*			*
Biscuits	*	*	*	*	*	*	*	*	*
Drinks	*	*	*	*	*	*			
Baby Food	*	*		*	*		*		
Soup		*			*			*	
Salad Dressing		*			*		*	*	
Noodles	*	*		*	*		*	*	
Meat Binder			*	*					*
Pet Foods	*	*		*	*		*	*	

Composition of eggs (approximate percentages)

	WHOLE EGG	WHITE	YOLK
water	73	87	47
protein	12	10	15
fat	11		33
minerals	1	0.5	2
vitamins			

Uses of fresh eggs

Eggs are used extensively in:

- hors-d'œuvre;
- soups;
- egg dishes;
- fish dishes;
- sauces;
- meat and poultry;
- pasta;
- salads;
- sweets and pastries;
- savouries.

USES OF EGG PRODUCTS

pasteurised whole egg*†‡ salted whole egg*† sugared whole egg*†‡ pasteurised yolk*†‡ salted yolk*† sugared yolk*†‡ pasteurised albumen*†‡ sugared albumen* egg granules†	hard-boiled eggs* pickled eggs chopped hard-boiled egg with mayonnaise* scrambled egg*† omelettes† egg custard blend*‡ quiche blend*† egg/milk blends*†‡

*Chilled †Frozen ‡Dried

Other types of eggs

- Turkeys' and guinea fowls' eggs may be used in place of hens' eggs.
- The eggs of the goose or duck may be used only if they are thoroughly cooked.
- Quails eggs are used in some establishments as a garnish, or as an hors-d'œuvre.

Availability

The table above, titled Uses of Egg Products shows the many egg products carrying the Date Stamp that are currently available. If you would like something a little different, it's worth talking to your supplier as he may be able to tailor the product to meet your specific needs.

Further information

British Egg Information, 2nd Floor, 89 Charterhouse Street, London EC1M 6HR
http://www.britegg.co.uk.

DAIRY PRODUCTS

Milk

Milk is a white nutritious liquid produced by female mammals for feeding their young. The milk most used in this country is that obtained from cows. Goats' milk and ewes' milk can also be used.

Food value

Milk can make a valuable contribution to our daily eating pattern and can help to meet our nutritional needs as part of a balanced, varied diet. Milk is one of the most nutritionally complete foods available, containing a wide range of nutrients which are essential for the proper functioning of the body. In particular, milk is a good source of protein, calcium and B group vitamins, and whole milk is a good source of vitamin A.

Storage

Milk is a perishable product and therefore must be stored with care. It will keep for 4–5 days in refrigerated conditions. Milk can be easily contaminated and therefore stringent precautions are taken to ensure a safe and good quality product for the consumer.

○ Fresh milk should be kept in the container in which it is delivered.

○ Milk must be stored in the refrigerator (4–5 days).

○ Milk should be kept covered as it easily absorbs smells from other foods, such as onion and fish.

○ Fresh milk should be ordered daily.

○ Tinned milk should be stored in cool, dry ventilated rooms.

○ Dried milk is packaged in airtight tins and should be kept in a dry store.

○ Sterilised milk will keep for 2–3 months if *unopened*, but once opened must be treated in the same way as pasteurised milk.

○ UHT (ultra-heat-treated) milk will keep unrefrigerated for several months. Before using, always check the date stamp which expires 6 months after processing and make sure to rotate stocks. Once opened it must be refrigerated and will keep for 4–5 days.

Packaging

Bulk fresh milk can be supplied in a variety of types of packaging. These come in the form of a plastic bag-in-box which holds a capacity of between 12–20 litres (3–5 gallons). They should be placed in the appropriate refrigerated unit and the contents can be drawn off as required by fitting the correct tap device.

All packs contain fresh pasteurised homogenised milk and can be obtained in either whole, semiskimmed or skimmed varieties.

Other types of packaging include

○ Polybottles (large plastic bottles) of fresh milk available in 1 litre/2 pint, 2 litre/4 pint and 3 litre/6 pint size.

○ Bottles of fresh milk available in $\frac{1}{2}$ litre/1 pint size.

○ Cartons of fresh milk available in $\frac{1}{2}$ litre/1 pint and 1 litre/2 pint sizes.

All the above milks are pasteurised and come in whole, homogenised whole, semiskimmed, and skimmed varieties; in addition milk in cartons is available as UHT (ultra-heat-treated) and milk in bottles is available in UHT and sterilised varieties.

Milk heat treatment and types of milk

Milk is heat treated in one of several ways to kill any harmful bacteria that may be present:

○ Approximately 99% of milk sold in the UK is heat treated.

○ Pasteurised milk – the milk is heated to a temperature of at least 71.7°C (161°F) for 15 seconds and then cooled quickly to less than 10°C (50°F).

○ UHT (ultra-heat-treated) milk – milk is homogenised (see below) and then heated to a temperature of at least 135°C for 1 second, the milk is then packed under sterile conditions.

○ Sterilised milk – milk is pre-heated to 50°C, separated and standardised to produce whole, semi-skimmed or skimmed milk. Filled bottles are then passed through a steam pressure chamber at temperatures between 110°C and 130°C for 10–30 minutes and then cooled in a cold water tank.

○ Homogenised milk – milk is forced through a fine aperture which breaks up the fat globules to an even size so that they stay evenly distributed throughout the milk and therefore do not form a cream line.

○ Whole milk (blue cap) – comes as pasteurised or pasteurised homogenised and has a fat content of an average 3.9%.

○ Semi-skimmed milk (green cap) – comes as pasteurised and has a fat content of between 1.5 and 1.8%.

○ Skimmed milk (red cap) – comes as pasteurised and UHT and contains just 0.1% fat.

○ Channel Islands milk – milk which comes from the Jersey and Guernsey breeds of cow and has a particularly rich and creamy taste and distinct cream line; it contains, on average 5.1% fat.

○ Evaporated milk – a concentrated sterilised product with a final concentration about twice that of the original milk.

○ Condensed milk – concentrated in the same way as evaporated milk but with addition of sugar; this product is not sterilised but is preserved by the high concentration of sugar it contains.

○ Dried milk powder – milk produced by the evaporation of water from the milk by heat, or other means, to produce solids containing 5% or less moisture; available as a whole, or skimmed product; dried filled milk powder is skimmed milk powder to which vegetable fat has been added.

○ Soya milk – can be offered as an alternative for people with an intolerance to cows milk.

○ Goats milk – nutritionally similar to cows milk and can be useful for people with a lactose intolerance.

○ Rice milk – an alternative to dairy milk for vegans and those with an intolerance to lactose. It is heat stable which makes it a good replacement for cows milk in corking although it tends to have a sweeter taste.

○ Coconut milk – is high in saturated fat but low in calories. It can be served as a drink but is more often used as a marinade and in cooking.

Uses of milk

Milk is used in:

○ soups and sauces;
○ cooking of fish, vegetables;
○ making of puddings, cakes, sweet dishes;
○ hot and cold drinks.

Cream

Cream is the lighter weight portion of milk which still contains all the main constituents of milk but in different proportions. The fat content of cream is higher than that of milk and the water content and other constituents are lower. Cream is separated from the milk and heat treated.

Cream is that part of cows' milk rich in fat which has been separated from the milk.

Types of cream and their fat content:

DESCRIPTION	MINIMUM BUTTERFAT CONTENT % BY WEIGHT
Clotted Cream	55
Double Cream	48
Whipping Cream	35
Whipped Cream	35
Sterilised Cream	23
Cream or Single Cream	18
Sterilised Half Cream	12
Half Cream	12

Other creams available include:
Extra thick double cream (48%) homogenised and pasteurised – will not whip.
Spooning cream or extra thick textured cream (30%).
Frozen cream (single, whipping or double).
Aerosol cream – heat treated by UHT method to give a whipped cream.
Soured cream (18%) cream soured by addition of a 'starter'.
Crème fraîche – is a similar product with a higher fat content.

Whipping of cream – for cream to be whipped it must have fat content of 38–42%. If the fat content is too low there will not be enough fat to enclose the air bubbles and form the foam. Conversely if the fat content is too high, the fat globules come into contact too easily, move against each other and form butter granules before the air can be incorporated to form the foam.

The addition of stabilisers to cream prevents seepage (particularly important when cream is used in flour confectionery).

Cream substitutes – are in the main based on vegetable fats or oils which are emulsified in water with other permitted substances.

Storage points

- Fresh cream should be kept in the container in which it is delivered.
- Fresh cream must be stored in the refrigeration until required.
- Cream should be kept covered as it easily absorbs smells from other foods, such as onion and fish.
- Fresh cream should be ordered daily.
- Tinned cream should be stored in cool, dry ventilated rooms.
- Frozen cream should only be thawed as required and not refrozen.
- Artificial cream should be kept in the refrigerator.

Yogurt

Yogurt is a cultured milk product made from cows, ewes', goats' or buffaloes' milk. Differences in the taste and texture of the product depends on the type of milk used and the activity of the micro-organisms involved. A bacterial 'starter culture' is added to the milk which causes the natural sugar 'lactose' to ferment and produce lactic acid. There are two types of yogurt:

○ stirred yogurt, which has a smooth fluid consistency;

○ set yogurt, which is more solid and has a firmer texture.

All yogurt is 'live' and contains live bacteria which remain dormant when kept at low temperatures, unless it clearly states on the packaging that it has been 'pasteurised, sterilised or ultra-heat-treated'. If stored at room temperature or above, the dormant bacteria become active again and produce more acid. Too high an acidity kills the bacteria, impairs the flavour and causes the yogurt to separate.

Yoghurt is available plain (Natural) or in a wide variety of flavours; it often has pieces of fruit added during manufacture.

Food value – yoghurt is rich in nutrients containing protein and a range of vitamins and minerals. It is particularly useful as a source of calcium.

YOGHURT

TYPE	% FAT CONTENTS PER 150 g POT	STORAGE AND CHARACTERISTICS
Very low fat – plain (natural)/fruit	0.3	14 days if refrigerated
Low fat – plain (natural)/fruit	1.1–1.2	14 days if refrigerated
Whole milk/creamy	4.2	14 days if refrigerated
Greek, Greek style	13.7	14 days if refrigerated
Bio or BA	percentage fat content as for very low fat, low fat and whole milk yoghurts	14 days if refrigerated. Has a less tart flavour and is said to aid digestion

Other fermented milk products

○ **Cultured buttermilk** – this product is made from skimmed milk with a culture added to give it a slightly thickened consistency and a sharp taste; it contains less than 0.5% fat and should be kept refrigerated.

○ **Smetana** – this is a cultured product containing 10% fat; it has a slightly sharp flavour and can be served chilled as a drink or used as an alternative to soured cream in recipes.

Further information

National Dairy Council, 5–7 John Princes Street, London W1M 0AP
http://www.dairytraining.org.uk.
Dairy Industry Federation Ltd, 19 Cornwall Terrace, London NW1 4QP.

CHEESE FATS AND OILS

Cheese

Cheese in made from milk protein coagulated by an enzyme e.g. rennet (an animal product). For vegetarian cheese a non-animal enzyme is used

Cheese is made worldwide from cows', ewes' or goats' milk and it takes approximately 5 litres (9 pints) of milk to produce $\frac{1}{2}$ kg (1 lb) of cheese.

There are many hundreds of varieties; most countries manufacture their own special cheeses.

Quality

- The skin or rind of cheese should not show spots of mildew, as this is a sign of damp storage.
- Cheese when cut should not give off an overstrong smell or any indication of ammonia.
- Hard, semi-hard and blue-vein cheese when cut should not be dry.
- Soft cheese when cut should not appear runny, but should have a delicate creamy consistency.

Hygiene

Cheese is a living product and should be handled carefully. It should always be wrapped in greaseproof or waxed paper or foil, or put in a closed container. Cheese stored in a refrigerator should have plenty of air circulating around it.

Natural rind can be exposed to air, so it can breathe, but cut surfaces should be covered with film to prevent drying out. Mould ripened cheeses should be separated from other cheeses. Remove cheese from the refrigerator about one hour before serving to allow it to return to room temperature.

Recent scares about food poisoning included soft unpasteurised cheeses – this is because listeria can grow and multiply at a lower temperature than most bacteria; at 10°C (50°F) or warmer, growth is rapid.

Storage

All cheese should be kept in a cool, dry, well-ventilated store and whole cheeses should be turned occasionally if being kept for any length of time. Cheese should be kept away from other foods which may be spoilt by the smell.

Food value

Cheese is a highly concentrated form of food. Fat, protein, mineral salts and vitamins are all present. Therefore it is an excellent body-building, energy-producing, protective food.

Preservation

Certain cheeses may be further preserved by processing. A hard cheese is usually employed, ground to a fine powder, melted, mixed with pasteurised milk, poured into moulds then wrapped in lacquered tinfoil, e.g. processed Gruyère, Kraft, Primula.

Uses

Soups, pasta, egg, fish and vegetable dishes, savouries.

Types
BRITISH CHEESE, SOME EXAMPLES

- Cheddar – golden colour with a close texture and a fresh mellow, nutty flavour.
- Cheshire – orange-red or white, loose crumbly texture and a mild mellow slightly salty flavour.
- Double Gloucester – orange-red, a buttery open texture with a delicate creamy flavour.
- Dunlop – a Scottish equivalent of Cheddar, milder and lighter in colour and texture.

○ Leicester – red in colour with a buttery open texture; a mellow medium-strength.
○ Caerphilly – white in colour and flaky, with a fresh, mild, slightly salty flavour.
○ Lancashire – white in colour, soft and crumbly with a fresh mild flavour.
○ Wensleydale – white in colour, moderately close texture with a fresh, mild, slightly salty flavour; excellent with crisp apples or apple pie.
○ Stilton – white with blue veins, soft and close texture and a strong flavour.

FRENCH CHEESE, SOME EXAMPLES

○ Brie – white, round cheese with close, soft, creamy texture and delicate flavour.
○ Camembert – white, round with soft, close, creamy texture and full flavour.
○ Chevre – a generic name for a wide range of goats' cheeses.
○ Fourme d'Ambert – sometimes called a French stilton; salty, full flavour.
○ Roquefort – blue cheese made from ewe's milk; rich, sharp flavour with salty aftertaste.

ITALIAN CHEESE, SOME EXAMPLES

○ Bel Paese – round, firm, pearly-white texture and a fresh, creamy taste.
○ Gorgonzola – blue vein with a rich, sharp flavour; Dolcelatte is a milder version.
○ Mozzarella – traditionally made from buffalo milk; pale and plastic looking, sweet flavour with a little bite.
○ Parmesan – hard, low-fat cheese; grated and used extensively in cooking.
○ Ricotta – fresh, white, crumbly and slightly sweet, similar to cottage cheese.

OTHER CHEESES, SOME EXAMPLES

○ Germany – Cambazola: creamy-white round blue vein cheese.
○ Netherlands – Edam: round, full-flavoured with low-fat content; covered in red skin.
○ Switzerland – Gruyere: firm, creamy-white with a full fruity flavour.
○ Greece – Fetta: white, moist, crumbly with a refreshing salty-sour taste.

SOFT CURD CHEESES *(see Figure 5.72, page 93)*

○ Curd cheese – made from pasteurised milk soured by the addition of a milk-souring culture and rennet; produce a soft, milk-flavoured, low fat (11%) cheese; made from either skimmed or medium-fat milk.
○ Cottage cheese – a low-fat, high protein product made from pasteurised skimmed milk; also available are very low-fat, sweet and savoury varieties.
○ Fromage frais – (fresh cheese) or fromage blanc is a fat-free soft curd cheese to which cream can be added to give richer varieties; also available, low-fat, medium-fat, savoury and fruit flavours.
○ Quark – a salt-free, fat-free soft cheese made from skimmed milk.

LOW-FAT HARD CHEESE

There is a range of hard cheese with half the fat of traditional cheese.

VEGETARIAN CHEESE

Traditional hard cheeses made using a non-animal rennet are also available.

FURTHER INFORMATION

National Dairy Council, 5–7 John Prince's Street, London W1M0AP.

www.dairytraining.org.uk

Storage of all fats

Fats should be kept in a cold store, and in a refrigerator in warm weather.

Butter

Butter is a natural dairy product made by churning fresh cream. During the churning process, the butterfat globules in the cream coalesce to form butter, and the excess liquid – known as buttermilk – is drained off. A little salt is added, between 1 and 2.5% depending on the type of butter, to enhance its flavour and keeping qualities.

Food value

Butter contains 80–82% fat and is therefore a high energy food. The remaining constituents are water (approximately 16%) and milk proteins. The fat soluble vitamins A and D are present in butter, and there is a small amount of calcium. Each 100g of butter supplies 733 kilocalories (3014 kilojoules).

Quality

- The flavour of butter is rich, creamy and mellow.
- The colour of butter varies from a delicate pale yellow to a rich, bright colour; both are entirely natural, as explained below.
- Butter's texture is smooth and creamy, and remains firm when chilled. It should be kept refrigerated, below 5°C (41°F) for optimum quality, where it can be kept for up to 6 weeks. Butter kept at room temperature soon deteriorates and exposure to light causes rancidity. As a recommendation, butter should be kept covered in a cool, dark place, away from strong flavours or smells which could taint its delicate taste.

Production

Essentially, there are two types of butter: lactic and sweetcream.

In lactic or 'continental taste' butter, the pasteurised cream is ripened before churning with a lactobacillus culture to produce a mildly acidic flavour. This mild acidity enhances the keeping properties, meaning that this type of butter can be purchased as unsalted or slightly salted, where 1–1.5% salt is added.

In sweetcream butter – traditionally produced in the UK and the Republic of Ireland, and imported from New Zealand – the cream is not ripened before churning and therefore the salt content needs to be a little higher to assist keeping qualities, between 1.5 and 2.5%.

Apart from the salt, there are no additives in butter. The colour of butter is entirely natural, and varies slightly according to the type of butter, the breed of cow and the pastures on which they feed. Seasonal variations affect the colour of the butter slightly, as the cow's diet changes during the year.

Use

The unique taste and texture of butter means that it is ideal for spreading and using in all types of cooking, both professionally and in the domestic kitchen. It is the foundation of many classic recipes, as it improves the flavour and appearance of a great many foods.

Butter is used as a base for making soups, sauces, compound butters and for hard butter sauces like brandy butter.

It is also used for making cakes and pastries, butter icings and frostings. Sometimes unsalted butter is chosen for these recipes.

Butter is ideal for shallow frying foods, but it is not suitable for stir-frying or deep frying where higher temperatures would cause the butter to burn. Melted butter makes an ideal baste for brushing grilled foods, and can be combined with chopped fresh herbs, spices, grated citrus rind, etc., to vary the flavour.

For finishing cooked foods, butter can be used as a glaze.

In sandwiches, butter acts as a protective layer, preventing moist foods from permeating the bread. The butter also gives the finished sandwich a delicious flavour.

Clarified butter can be made by gently heating butter until it has melted and separated. The milk solids can then be strained off. The resultant clarified butter can be used at higher temperatures. **Ghee** is a type of clarified butter, widely used as the basis of Indian cooking. A type of clarified butter known as **concentrated butter** is made by removing most of the water and milk solids. It is suitable for cooking and baking, but not for spreading or finishing foods.

Margarine

Margarine is produced from milk and a blend of vegetable oils emulsified with lecithin, flavouring, salt, colouring and vitamins A and D.

FOOD VALUE

Margarine is an energy and protective food. With the exception of palm oil, the oils used in the manufacture of margarine do not contain vitamins A and D; these are added during production. Margarine is not inferior to butter from the nutritional point of view.

QUALITY

There are several grades of margarine: block (hard or semi-hard); soft (butter substitute); semi-hard for making pastry; and cake margarine which creams easily and absorbs egg. Some margarines are blended with butter. Taste is the best guide to quality.

USE

Margarine can be used in place of butter, the difference being that the smell is not so pleasant, and nut brown (beurre noisette) or black butter (beurre noir) cannot satisfactorily be produced from margarine. The flavour of margarine when used in the kitchen is inferior to butter – it is therefore not so suitable for finishing sauces and dishes.

It should be remembered that it is equally nutritious and may be cheaper than butter.

Vegetable shortening and high-ratio fat are available. They are used extensively in bakery products.

Animal fats
LARD

Lard is the rendered fat from pigs. Lard has almost 100% fat content. It may be used in hot water paste and with margarine to make short paste. It can also be used for deep or shallow frying.

SUET

Suet is the hard solid fat deposits in the kidney region of animals. Beef suet is the best and it is used for suet paste and mincemeat.

DRIPPING

Dripping is obtained from clarified animal fats (usually beef) and it is used for deep or shallow frying.

FURTHER INFORMATION

Unilever Ltd, Unilever House, Blackfriars, London EC4.

OILS
CHOICE OF OIL

The choice of an oil as a food ingredient or for cooking will usually involve a compromise. The factors that will need to be taken into account may include:

Price – variations will occur according to supply and demand.

Intended use – some oils are versatile others are a limited use.

Durability – in use and in storage.

Nutritional – and health concerns.

Flash point – for frying purposes an oil must, when heated, reach a high temperature without smoking. Food being fried will absorb the oil if the oil smokes at a low temperature. As oils are combustibles they can catch fire (known as flash point). In some cases the margin between smoking and flash point may be narrow. See Practical Cookery for further information.

Food Value – as oil has a very high fat content it is useful as an energy food.

Storage:
○ oil should be kept in a cool place;
○ if refrigerated some oils congeal but will return to a fluid state when removed from the refrigerator;
○ oils keep for a fairly long time but may go rancid if not kept cool.

Types of Oils:

peanut (groundnut);	cotton seed;	palm;
rapeseed;	olive;	coconut;
soya bean;	sunflower;	speciality e.g. almond,
palm;	corn;	grapeseed, hazelnut, walnut.

Herbal oils are available or can be made by adding chopped fresh herbs (e.g. tarragon, thyme, basil etc) to olive oil and keeping refrigerated in screw top jars for about three weeks, then strained and rebottled. If fresh green herbs are used, blanching and refreshing them will enhance the colour of the oil.

Uses:

Mayonnaise, vinaigrette and hors d'oeuvre dishes.

Pasta, certain doughs and breads use olive oil.

Deep frying, lubrication of utensils and slabs.

Further information: National Edible Oils Distribution Association, 6 Catherine Street, London WC2B 5JJ

http://www.cybgroup.co.uk

CEREALS

Cereals are cultivated grasses, but the term is broadened to include sago, rice and arrowroot. All cereal products contain starch. The following are the important cereals used in catering: wheat, oats, rye, barley, maize, rice, tapioca, sago and arrowroot. A wide variety of cereals is processed into breakfast foods (barley, wheat, rice, bran and corn).

Wheat
Source

Wheat is the most common cereal produced in the Western world and is grown in most temperate regions. Large quantities are home-grown and a great deal, particularly in the form of strong flour, is imported from Canada.

Food value

Cereals are one of the best energy foods. Whole grain cereals provide vitamin B and are therefore protective foods.

Wheat and Flour quality

Flours vary in their composition and broadly speaking are defined by the quality of wheats used in the grist prior to milling and by their rate of extraction. The extraction is the percentage of whole cleaned wheatgrain that is present in the flour. A typical mill will produce hundreds of different types of flour using a wide range of home grown and imported wheats.

STORAGE OF FLOUR

○ The store room must be dry and well ventilated.
○ Flour should be removed from the sacks and kept in wheeled bins with lids.
○ Flour bins should be of a type that can be easily cleaned.

Flour is probably the most common commodity in daily use. It forms the foundation of bread, pastry and cakes and is also used in soups, sauces, batters and other foods.

○ White flour contains 72 to 85% of the whole grain (the endosperm only).
○ Wholemeal flour contains 100% of the whole grain.
○ Brown flour contains 85–95% of the whole grain.
○ High ratio or patent flour contains 40% of the whole grain.
○ 'Self-raising flour' is white flour with the addition of baking powder.
○ Semolina is granulated hard flour prepared from the central part of the wheat grain. White or wholemeal semolina is available. Semolina is used for cous-cous.
○ Burghul (cracked wheat) is used in Tabbouleh.

Uses of wheat products

○ Soft flour – cakes, biscuits, all pastes except puff and flaky, thickening soups and sauces, batters and coating various foods.
○ Strong flour – bread, puff and flaky pastry, and pasta.
○ Wholemeal flour – wholemeal bread and rolls.
○ Gnocchi, milk puddings.

FURTHER INFORMATION

Flour Advisory Bureau, 21 Arlington Street, London SW1 1RN www.fabflour.co.uk.

Rye

Rye flour is obtained from the cereal rye and is the most important European cereal after wheat.

Rye is the only cereal apart from wheat which contains gluten proteins. However these gluten proteins are not of the same quality or quantity as flour produced from wheat. Dough produced from rye flour has a sticky dense consistency. The baked product has a low volume. Rye flour is available as light, medium and dark rye. Likewise the colour and flavour of rye bread can range from light and mild to dark and strong, depending on the type of rye flour used.

Rye flour must be weighed accurately to ensure that:

The recipe remains balanced.	The correct yield is obtained.
A uniform product is obtained.	Faults are prevented

Store in dry conditions 10–16°C 50–61°F.

Oats

Oats are either rolled into flakes or ground into three grades of oatmeal: coarse, medium and fine.

SOURCE

Oats are one of the hardiest cereals, and are grown in large quantities in Scotland and the north of England.

FOOD VALUE

Oats have the highest food value of any of the cereals. They contain a good proportion of protein and fat.

STORAGE

Because of the fat content, the keeping quality of oat products needs extra care. They should be kept in containers with tight-fitting lids, and stored in a cool, well-ventilated store room.

USES

○ Rolled oats – porridge.
○ Oatmeal – porridge, thickening soups, coating foods, cakes and biscuits, haggis.
○ Patent rolled oats nowadays largely displace oatmeal and have the advantage of being already heat treated and consequently more quickly and easily cooked.

Barley

The whole grain of barley is known as pot or Scotch barley and requires soaking overnight. Pearl barley has most of the bran and germ removed, and it is then polished. These products are used for making barley water for thickening soups and certain stews.

Barley when roasted, is changed into malt and as such is used extensively in the brewing and distilling of vinegar.

Barley needs the same care in storage as oats.

Buckwheat is the seed of the plant 'bran buckwheat'. The grain is usually roasted before cooking, and is also ground into a strong savoury flour for pancakes and baking.

Maize

Maize is also known as corn, sweetcorn or corn-on-the-cob, and besides being served as a vegetable it is processed into cornflakes and cornflour. Maize yields a good oil suitable for cooking.

Cornflour

Cornflour is produced from maize and is the crushed endosperm of the grain which has the fat and protein washed out so that it is practically pure starch.

Cornflour is used for making custard and blancmange powders, because it thickens very easily with a liquid, and sets when cold into a smooth paste that cannot be made from other starches.

Custard powder consists of cornflour, colouring and flavouring.

Cornflour is used for thickening soups, sauces, custards and also in the making of certain small and large cakes.

Rice

Rice is the staple food for half the world's population, and is second only to wheat as the world's most important food grain.

There are three main types used in this country:

- Long grain – a narrow, pointed grain, best suited for savoury dishes and plain boiled rice because of its firm structure, which helps to keep the rice grains separate, e.g. basmati, patna.
- Medium grain – an all-purpose rice suitable for sweet and savoury dishes, e.g. carolina, arborio.
- Short grain – a short, rounded grain, best suited for milk puddings and sweet dishes because of its soft texture, e.g. arborio.

TYPES

- Brown rice – any rice that has had the outer covering removed but retains its bran and as a result is more nutritious.
- Whole grain rice – whole and unprocessed rice.
- Wild rice – seed of an aquatic plant related to the rice family. It has a nutty flavour and a checky texture.
- Ground rice – used for milk puddings.
- Rice flour – used for thickening certain soups, e.g. cream soups.
- Rice paper – a thin edible paper produced from rice, used in the preparations of macaroons and nougat.
- Precooked instant rice, par-boiled, ready cooked and boil in the bag is also available.

Storage

Rice should be kept in tight-fitting containers in a cool, well-ventilated store.

Tapioca

Tapioca is obtained from the roots of a tropical plant called cassava. Flake (rough) and seed (fine) are available. Tapioca may be used for garnishing soups and milk puddings.

Sago

Sago is produced in small pellets from the pith of the sago palm. It may be used for garnishing soups and for making milk puddings.

Arrowroot

Arrowroot is obtained from the roots of a West Indian plant called maranta.

It is used for thickening sauces and is particularly suitable when a clear sauce is required as it becomes transparent when boiled. Arrowroot is also used in certain cakes and puddings, and is particularly useful for invalids as it is easily digested.

Arrowroot is easily contaminated by strong-smelling foods; therefore it must be stored in air-tight tins.

Potato flour

Potato flour is a preparation from potatoes, suitable for thickening certain soups and sauces.

RAISING AGENTS

The method of making mixtures light or aerated may be effected in several ways.

Baking powder

Baking powder may be made from one part sodium bicarbonate to two parts of cream of tartar. In commercial baking the powdered cream of tartar may be replaced by another acid product, e.g. acidulated calcium phosphate.

When used under the right conditions it produces carbon dioxide gas; to produce gas, a liquid and heat are needed. As the acid has a delayed action, only a small amount being given off when the liquid is added, the majority of the gas is released when the mixture is heated. Therefore cakes and puddings when mixed do not lose the property of the baking powder if they are not cooked right away.

USE

Baking powder is used in sponge puddings, cakes and scones and in suet puddings and dumplings.

Yeast

Yeast is a fungus form of plant life available as a fresh or dried product.

Storage and quality points

- Yeast should be wrapped and stored in a cold place
- It is ordered only as required.
- It must be perfectly fresh and moist.
- It should have a pleasant smell.
- Yeast should crumble easily.
- Yeast should crumble easily.

Food value

Yeast is rich in protein and vitamin B. It is therefore a help towards building and repairing the body and provides protection.

Uses

Yeast is used in bread and bun doughs, cakes and batters.

SUGAR

Sugar is produced from sugar cane grown in a number of tropical and subtropical countries and from sugar beet which is grown in parts of Europe, including the UK.

Food value

As sugar contains 99.9% pure sugar, it is invaluable for producing energy.

Types

○ Refined white sugars: granulated, castor; cube; icing.
○ Unrefined sugar: brown sugar.
○ Partially refined sugar: demerara.

Storage

Sugar should be stored in a dry, cool place. When purchased by the sack, the sugar is stored in covered bins.

Further information

British Sugar PLC, Oundle Rd, Peterborough PE2 9QU www.britishsugar.co.uk.

BEVERAGES (DRINKS)

The simplest, cheapest drink of all is water which varies from place to place in taste and character according to the substances dissolved or suspended in it. Soft water has a low content of lime. Hard water has an abundance of lime (if the flavour of lime is too strong, the water may have to be softened to remove the excess of lime).

Water which has been artificially softened should not be used for coffee or tea making. The mineral content of water used for brewing can significantly affect the final taste of the coffee or tea. A blend of coffee or tea brewed in the very hard water of London has a completely different taste to the same blend brewed in Edinburgh, where the water is very soft. Water can also have varying degrees of other substances, e.g. iron and sulphur, which in some instances are considered to be beneficial to health and are known as mineral waters (see page 140).

Drink can be broadly classified into two categories, alcoholic and non-alcoholic (beverage or soft drink). Although the word beverage means a drink the generally accepted definition is a non-alcoholic liquid, e.g. chocolate, coffee, tea, cocoa, fruit drinks, mineral waters, milk.

Alcoholic drinks include cocktails, aperitifs, fancy drinks, wines, fortified wines, spirits, beers, cider, perry.

Low alcohol drinks are also available.

Non-alcoholic drinks
Coffee

Coffee is produced from the beans of the coffee tree, and is grown and exported from South America, Arabia, India, West Indies, Africa, Jarva and Sumatra. The varieties of coffee are named after the areas where they are grown, such as Mysore, Kenya, Brazil, Mocha and Java.

Purchasing unit

Coffee beans either unroasted, roasted or ground, are sold by the pound (500 g) and in 7 lb (3 kg) or 28 lb (14 kg) parcels or tins. Coffee essence is obtained in $5\frac{1}{2}$ fl oz (125 ml), 10 fl oz (250 ml), 25 fl oz (625 ml) and 1 gal ($4\frac{1}{2}$ l) bottles.

Food value

It is the milk and sugar served with coffee that have food value. Coffee has no value as a food by itself.

Types of Coffee

- Expresso – steam under pressure is forced through powdered coffee.
- Cappuchino – strong filtered coffee with whisked hot milk added.
- French coffee usually contains chicory; the root is washed, dried, roasted and ground. The addition of chicory gives a particular flavour and appearance to the coffee.
- Coffee essence is a concentrated form of liquid coffee which may contain chicory.
- Instant coffee is liquid coffee which has been dried into powder form.
- Decaffeinated coffee has most of the caffeine removed, and is, therefore, less of a stimulant.

Composition

The composition of coffee is complex with a large range of compounds including flavanoids, chlorogenic acids, nicotinic acids and caffeine.

Uses

Coffee is mainly used as a beverage which may be served with milk, cream or as a flavouring for cakes, icings, mousse and ice-cream.

It can be brewed to suit individual tastes. The many different pure blended and instant (soluble) coffees which can be brewed in a wide selection of different coffee makers, or by various special brewing methods, make it possible to provide a brew to suit everyone. Whatever type of coffee is drunk, and regardless of roasting time, fineness of grind or brewing method, there are basic rules to observe for making a good cup of coffee.

Rules for making coffee

- Use good coffee which is freshly roasted and ground.
- Use ground or vacuum-packed coffee within 10 days or the quality will deteriorate. Store in airtight containers in a cool place.
- Use freshly drawn, freshly boiled water cooled to 92–96°C (198–205°F) (to preserve the flavour and aroma of the coffee). Do **not** use boiling water.
- Measure the quantity of coffee carefully, 300–360 g (11–13 oz) per 5 litres (9 pints).
- After the coffee has been made it should be strained off, otherwise it will acquire a bitter taste if kept hot for more than 30 minutes. Do not reheat brewed coffee.
- Milk, if served with coffee, should be hot but not boiled.
- All coffee-making equipment must be kept scrupulously clean, washed thoroughly after each use and rinsed with clean hot water (never use soda).
- Make coffee in pots which have been thoroughly dried and warmed.

Figure 5.75 *Cafetière and filter coffee brewing machine*

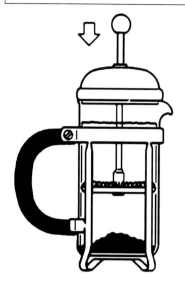
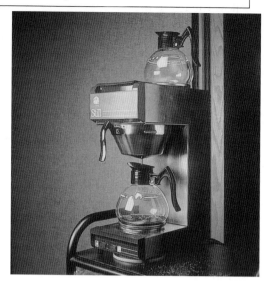

Instant coffee

The majority of people in the United Kingdom drink 'instant' coffee. After the seal is broken on the container of instant or soluble coffee it should be stored in an airtight container and kept in a cool place.

The flavour of instant coffee is improved if it is made in a pot using approximately one heaped teaspoon for each cup, and according to taste. Fresh water which is below boiling point should be added.

Instant coffee is convenient because it can be made into individual cups by adding water to the coffee and stirring.

Ways of making coffee

Jug method, cafetière, automatic drip, glass cone, Turkish or Greek, Expresso.

Further Information

The Roast Coffee Company, 84 High St, Tonbridge, Kent TN9 1AP. Email: sales@realcoffee.co.uk www.realcoffee.co.uk.

Tea

Tea is an evergreen plant of the Camellia family which is kept to bush size for easy plucking and only the two top leaves and bud are plucked.

There are more than 1500 blends of tea and tea grows in more than 31 countries.

○ Use a good quality loose leaf or bagged tea.
○ This must be stored in an air-tight container at room temperature.
○ Always use freshly drawn boiling water.
○ In order to draw the best flavour out of the tea the weater must contain oxygen, this is reduced if the water is boiled more than once.
○ Measure the tea carefully.

○ Use 1 tea bag or 1 rounded teaspoon of loose tea for each cup to be served.

○ Allow the tea to brew for the recommended time before pouring.

RECOMMENDED BREWING TIMES

	TYPE	COUNTRY OF ORIGIN	BREWING TIME	MILK/BLACK/ LEMON	CHARACTERISTICS
DARJEELING	BLACK	INDIA	3–5 minutes	BLACK or MILK	Delicate, slightly astringent flavour
ASSAM	BLACK	INDIA	3–5 minutes	BLACK or MILK	Full-bodied with a rich, smooth, malty flavour
CEYLON BLEND	BLACK	SRI LANKA	3–5 minutes	BLACK or MILK	Brisk, full flavour with a bright colour
KENYA	BLACK	KENYA (AFRICA)	2–4 minutes	BLACK or MILK	A strong tea with a brisk flavour
EARL GREY	BLACK	CHINA OR CHINA/ DARJEELING	3–5 minutes	BLACK or LEMON	Flavoured with the natural oil of citrus bergamot fruit
LAPSANG SOUCHONG	BLACK	CHINA	3–5 minutes	BLACK	Smoky aroma and flavour
CHINA OOLONG	OOLONG	CHINA	5–7 minutes	BLACK	Subtle, delicate, lightly flavoured tea

Blends

Blends of tea provide the widest possible choice of tea with many different characteristics and flavours. A popular brand leading blend can contain as many as 35 different teas.

Speciality teas take their name from the area or country in which they are grown; a blend of tea for a particular time of day; a blend of teas known after a person; a blend of teas to which fruit oil, flower petals or blossoms have been added or a 'made' processed tea.

Flavoured teas are real tea blended with fruit, herbs or spices. These should not be confused with tisanes and fruit infusions made from herbs, hibiscus leaves and fruits, but which do not contain any real tea. Several varieties of green tea are also available.

Buying

Tea comes in either tea bag or loose leaf packs which cover a wide variety of catering needs.

Storage

Packs of tea should be stored in a clean, dry and well ventilated storeroom, away from strong smelling products. Once a pack is opened tea should be kept in a dry, clean air-tight caddy because tea will pick up any aroma or flavour and become tainted.

Food value

Tea is a natural product. It contains no artificial colourings, preservations or flavourings, is virtually calorie free and has no fat content, if taken without milk or sugar.

Teas contains caffeine, 40 mg per cup which acts as a gentle stimulant and helps give tea its diuretic effect. Also manganese, potassium, fluoride and vitamins A, B1, B2 and C.

The main producers are India, Sri Lanka, Kenya, Malawi, Indonesia and China.

Further information

The Tea Council Limited, 9 The Courtyard, Gowan Avenue, London SW6 6RH www.tea.co.uk.

Cocoa

Cocoa is a powder produced from the beans of the cacao tree. It is imported mainly from West Africa.

Food value

As cocoa contains some protein and a large proportion of starch it helps to provide the body with energy. Iron is also present in cocoa.

Storage

Cocoa should be kept in airtight containers in a well-ventilated store.

Uses

For hot drinks, cocoa is mixed with milk, milk and water, or water. Hot liquid is needed to cook the starch and make it more digestible. Cocoa can be used to flavour puddings, cakes, sauces, icing and ice-cream.

Chocolate

Cocoa beans are used to produce chocolate, and over half of the cocoa bean consists of cocoa butter. To produce chocolate, cocoa butter is mixed with crushed cocoa beans and syrup. With baker's chocolate, the cocoa fat (butter) is replaced by vegetable fat thus giving a cheaper product which does not need tempering. For commercial purposes, chocolate is sold in blocks known as *couverture*. Pure chocolate couverture is made from cocoa mass, highly refined sugar and extracted cocoa butter. It is the additional cocoa butter which gives couverture its qualities for moulding, its flavour and therefore its higher price.

Uses

Chocolate or couverture is used for icings, butter creams, sauces, dipping chocolates and moulding into shapes.

Drinking chocolate

This is ground cocoa from which less fat has been extracted and to which sugar has been added. It can be obtained in flake or powder form.

Mineral waters and soft drinks

A wide range of mineral waters are available, both home produced and from overseas, and either natural (still) in character or treated with gas (carbon dioxide) to give a light sparkle or fizz. Examples of natural mineral waters are Buxton and Malvern. Manufactured soft drinks include grapefruit, lime juice (still) and tonic water, Coca-Cola, ginger beer (sparkling) etc.

Squashes and cordials are all concentrated fruit extracts, meant to be broken down with fresh or aerated water into a long drink, and to be served hot or iced. Fruit juices are the unfermented juice of fresh fruits such as apple, grape, orange, tomato.

Fruit syrups are concentrated fruit juices preserved with sugar or manufactured from compound colourings and flavours (orange, lime, cherry). A large range of compound flavourings is available.

Milk drinks

Milk can be offered plain either hot or cold. Other milk drinks include:

○ Milkshakes – a mixture of fresh milk, ice-cream and a flavouring syrup, rapidly whisked and served in a tall glass.

○ Ice-cream sodas – combination of fruit syrup and fresh cream in a long glass filled with soda water and topped with ice-cream.

○ Egg noggs – beaten eggs (preferably pasteurised) with fruit syrup and sugar added, mixed with hot or cold milk in a tall glass and topped with grated nutmeg.

○ Other products from which beverages are made either by the addition of hot water or milk include Bournvita, Bovril, Horlicks, Ovaltine.

Alcoholic drinks

WINE

Wine has been made for over 6000 years and is produced in most parts of the world. It is the fermented juice of the grape and is available in many styles: red, white, rose, sparkling, organic, alcohol-free, de-alcoholised and low alcohol. Wines may be dry, medium dry or sweet in character and according to the type and character they may be drunk while young (within a short time of bottling) or allowed to age (in some cases for many years).

Bottled wines should always be stored on their sides so that the wine remains in contact with the cork. This keeps the cork expanded and prevents air from entering the wine which, if allowed to happen, will turn the wine to vinegar.

FORTIFIED WINES

Fortified wines are those which have been strengthened by the addition of alcohol usually produced from grape juice; the best known are port, sherry and Madeira.

AROMATISED WINES

Aromatised wines are produced by flavouring a simple basic wine with a blend of ingredients (fruit, roots, bark, peel, flowers, quinine, herbs). Vermouth and Dubonnet are two examples of aromatised wines popular as aperitifs.

SPIRITS

Spirits are distillations of fermented liquids which are converted into liquid spirit; they include whisky, gin, vodka, brandy and rum.

LIQUEURS

Liqueurs are flavoured and sweetened spirits. A wide range of flavouring agents are employed (e.g.: aniseed, caraway, peaches, raspberries, violets, rose petals, cinnamon, sage, honey, coffee beans). Many different liqueurs are available (Cointreau, cherry brandy, etc.).

COCKTAILS AND MIXED DRINKS

Cocktails are usually a mixture of a spirit with one or more ingredients from liqueurs, fruit juices, fortified wines, eggs, cream, etc. Cocktails may be garnished with mint, borage, fresh fruit, olives, etc.

Mixed drinks have an assortment of names that include flips, fizzes, noggs, sours, cups. Cocktails and mixed drinks can also be made from non-alcoholic ingredients.

BEER

Beer is a term that covers all beer-like drinks such as ale, stouts and lagers. It is made from a combination of water, grain (e.g. barley), hops, sugar and yeast. Types of beer include: bitter, mild, Burton, strong ale, barley wine, porter, lager.

Reduced alcohol beers are also available.

Beers are good sources of energy, they contain high levels of carbohydrates and protein. Beers are richer in minerals than wines, but lower in alcohol at only 3–5%.

CIDER

Cider is fermented apple juice. Also in this category are:
○ Pomagne – a sparkling cider.
○ Scrumpy – strong, homemade, rough cider.

PERRY

Perry is fermented pear juice.

FURTHER INFORMATION

The Beverage Book, Durkan and Cousins, Hodder and Stoughton, 1995.

PULSES

Pulses are the dried seeds of plants which form pods.

Types

○ Aduki beans – small, round, deep red, shiny beans.
○ Black beans – glistening black skins and creamy flesh.
○ Black-eyed beans – white beans with a black blotch.
○ Borlotti beans – pink blotched mottled colour.
○ Broad beans – strongly flavoured beans, sometimes known as fava beans.
○ Butter beans – available large or small, also known as Lima beans.
○ Cannellini – Italian haricots, slightly fatter than the English.
○ Chick-peas – look like the kernel of a small hazel-nut.
○ Dhal – is the Hindi word for dried peas and beans.
○ Dutch brown beans – light brown in colour.
○ Flageolets – pale-green, kidney-shaped beans.
○ Ful medames or Egyptian brown beans – small, brown, knobbly beans, also known as the field bean in England.
○ Haricot beans – white, smooth oval beans.
○ Lentils – available in bright orange, brown or green.
○ Mung beans – chiefly used for bean sprouts.

- Pinto beans – pink blotched mottled colour.
- Puy lentils – grey coloured beans; do not require soaking and they hold their shape when cooked. Considered the finest of lentils.
- Red kidney beans – used in Chilli con carne.
- Soissons – the finest haricot beans.
- Soya beans – the most nutritious of all beans.
- Split peas – available in bright green or golden yellow.

Food value

Pulses are good sources of protein and carbohydrate and therefore help to provide the body with energy. With the exception of the soya bean, they are completely deficient in fat.

Storage

All pulses should be kept in clean containers in a dry, well-ventilated store.

Use

Pulses are used extensively for soups, stews, vegetables, salads and accompaniments to meat dishes and vegetarian cookery.

HERBS *(see Figure 5.73, page 93)*

Of the thirty well known types of herbs, approximately twelve are generally used in cookery. Herbs may be used fresh, but the majority are dried, so as to ensure a continuous supply throughout the year. The leaves of herbs contain an oil which gives the characteristic smell and flavour.

Herbs have no food value but are important from a nutritive point of view in aiding digestion because they stimulate the flow of gastric juices. These are the most commonly used herbs:

Basil

Basil is a small leaf with a pungent flavour and sweet aroma. Used in raw or cooked tomato dishes or sauces, salads and lamb dishes.

Bay leaves

Bay leaves are the leaves of the bay laurel or sweet bay trees or shrubs. They may be fresh or dried and are used for flavouring many soups, sauces, stews, fish and vegetable dishes, in which case they are usually included in a faggot of herbs (bouquet garni).

Borage

This is a plant with furry leaves and blue flowers that produces a flavour similar to cucumber when added to vegetables and salads.

Chervil

Chervil has small, neatly shaped leaves with a delicate aromatic flavour. It is best used fresh, but may also be obtained in dried form. Because of its neat shape it is employed a great deal for decorating chaud-froid work. It is also one of the *fines herbes*, the mixture of herbs used in many culinary preparations.

Chive

Chive is a bright green member of the onion family resembling a coarse grass. It has a delicate onion flavour. It is invaluable for flavouring salads, hors-d'œuvre, fish, poultry and meat dishes, and chopped as a garnish for soups and cooked vegetables. It should be used fresh.

Coriander

A member of the parsley family, coriander is one of the oldest flavourings used by man. It is both a herb and a spice. The leaves have a distinctive pungent flavour.

Dill

Dill has feathery green-grey leaves and is used in fish recipes and pickles.

Fennel

Fennel has feathery bright green leaves, and a slight aniseed flavour and is used for fish sauces, meat dishes and salads.

Lemon grass

Lemon grass is a tall plant with long spear-shaped grass-like leaves with a strong lemon flavour.

Lovage

Lovage leaves have a strong celery-like flavour; when finely chopped they can be used in soups, stews, sauces and salads.

Marjoram

Marjoram is a sweet herb which may be used fresh in salads and pork, fish, poultry, cheese, egg and vegetable dishes, and when dried can be used for flavouring soups, sauces, stews and certain stuffings.

Mint

There are many varieties of mint. Fresh sprigs of mint are used to flavour peas and new potatoes. Fresh or dried mint may be used to make mint sauce or mint jelly for serving with roast lamb. Another lesser known but excellent mint for the kitchen is apple mint. Chopped mint can be used in salads.

Oregano

Oregano has a flavour and aroma similar to marjoram but stronger. It is used in Italian and Greek-style cooking in meats, salads, soups, stuffings, pasta, sauces, vegetable and egg dishes.

Parsley

Parsley is probably the most common herb in Britain and has numerous uses for flavouring, garnishing and decorating a large variety of dishes.

Rosemary

Rosemary is a strong fragrant herb which should be used sparingly and may be used fresh or dried for flavouring sauces, stews, salads and for stuffings. Rosemary can also be sprinkled on roasts or grills of meat, poultry and fish during cooking and on roast potatoes.

Sage

Sage is a strong, bitter, pungent herb which aids the stomach to digest rich fatty meat and is therefore used in stuffings for duck, goose and pork.

Tarragon

This plant has a bright green attractive leaf. It is best used fresh, particularly when decorating chaud-froid dishes. Tarragon has a pleasant flavour and is used in sauces, one well-known example being sauce béarnaise. It is one of the *fines herbes* and as such is used for omelettes, salads, fish and meat dishes.

Thyme

Thyme is a popular herb in the UK and is used fresh or dried for flavouring soups, sauces, stews, stuffings, salads and vegetables.

Fine herbs *(fines herbes)*

This is a mixture of fresh herbs, usually chervil, tarragon and parsley, which is referred to in many classical cookery recipes.

Balm, Bergamot, Fennel, Savory, Sorrel, Tansy, Lemon Thyme

These and other herbs are used in cookery, but on a much smaller scale.

SPICES

Spices are natural products obtained from the fruits, seeds, roots, flowers or the bark of a number of different trees or shrubs. They contain oils which aid digestion by stimulating the gastric juices. They also enhance the appearance of food and add a variety of flavours. As spices are concentrated in flavour, they should be used sparingly, otherwise they can make foods unpalatable. Most spices are grown in India, Africa, the West Indies and the Far East.

Allspice or Pimento

This is so called because the flavour is like a blend of cloves, cinnamon and nutmeg. It is the unripe fruit of the pimento tree which grows in the West Indies. Allspice is picked when still green, and dried when the colour turns to reddish brown. Allspice is ground and used as a flavouring in sauces, sausages, cakes, fruit pies and milk puddings. It is one of the spices blended for mixed spice.

Anise

This is also known as sweet cumin, and has a sweet aniseed flavour. It is used for fish, sweets, creams and cakes.

Anise (Pepper)

A strong, hot-flavoured red pepper.

Anise (Star)

Stronger than anise, this has a slight liquorice flavour. Used in Chinese cookery with pork and duck.

Asafoetida

This is used in Indian cookery to add flavour to vegetarian dishes. Available in block or powder form.

Cardamom

Cardamom is frequently used in curry, and has a warm, oily sharp taste.

Caraway

Caraway seeds come from a plant grown in Holland. The seeds are about $\frac{1}{2}$ cm ($\frac{1}{4}$ in) long, shaped like a new moon and brown in colour. Caraway seeds are used in seed-cake and certain breads, sauerkraut, cheese and confectionery. Also for flavouring certain liqueurs such as Kümmel.

Cassia

This comes in thicker sticks than cinnamon, and is less delicate and more expensive. Used in spiced meats and curries.

Celery seed

Slightly bitter, this should be used sparingly if celery or celery salt is not available.

Chillies and Capsicums

These are both from the same family and grow on shrubs. The large bright red type are capsicums and these are ground and known as paprika. There are many types of chillies and they vary in taste, colour, piquancy and heat (always test the heat by cutting off a small piece and taste with the tip of the tongue). The seeds are one of the hottest parts of the chilli and they can be removed by splitting the chilli in half then scooping them out with the point of the knife. Hands should always be thoroughly washed after preparing chillies because the oils are exceptionally strong and will burn the eyes, mouth and other delicate areas of the body. Chillies are used in many dishes: pizzas, pasta and in Indian, Thai and Mexican cookery.

Chinese Five spice powder

Usually consists of: powdered anise, fennel, cloves, cinnamon and anise pepper. Used extensively in Chinese cookery.

Cinnamon

Cinnamon is the bark of the small branches of the cinnamon shrub which grows in China and Sri Lanka. The inner pulp and the outer layer of the bark are removed and the remaining pieces dried. It is a pale brown colour and is obtained and used in stick or powdered form, mainly by bakeries and for pastry work.

Cloves

Cloves are the unopened flower-buds of a tree which grows in Zanzibar, Penang and Madagascar. The buds are picked when green, and dried in the sun until they turn to a rich brown colour. They are used for flavouring stocks, sauces, studding roast ham joints and in mulled wine.

Coriander

Coriander is a pleasant spice obtained from the seed of an annual plant grown chiefly in Morocco. It is a yellowish brown colour and tastes like a mixture of sage and lemon peel. It is used in sauces, curry powder and mixed spice.

Cumin

This is frequently used in curry and is powerful, warm, sweet and has a slightly oily taste.

Dill seeds

These are used for flavouring fish soups, stews and cakes.

Fennel seeds

Fennel seeds have a sweet aniseed flavour, used in fish dishes and soups.

Fenugreek

Fenugreek is roasted, ground and frequently used in curry; slightly bitter, with a smell of fresh hay.

Garam Masala

This literally means 'hot spices' and is not a standardised recipe, but a typical mixture which could include: cardamom seeds, stick cinnamon, cumin seeds, cloves, black peppercorns, nutmeg.

Ginger

Ginger is the rhizome or root of a reed-like plant grown in the Far East. The root is boiled in water and sugar syrup until soft. Ground ginger is used mainly for pastry and bakery work and for mixed spice. Whole root is used for curries, pickles, stir-fry dishes and sauces.

Krachai

is a type of ginger with a slightly strange flavour.

Juniper berries

If these are added to game, red cabbage, pork, rabbit and beef dishes, they give an unusual background flavour.

Nutmegs and Mace

The tropical nutmeg bears a large fruit like an apricot which, when ripe, splits. Inside is a dark brown nut with a bright red net-like covering which is the part that becomes mace. Inside the nut is the kernel or seed which is the nutmeg. Although the two spices come from the same fruit, the flavour is different. Mace is more delicate and is used for flavouring sauces and certain meat and fish dishes. Nutmeg is used in sweet dishes (particularly milk puddings), sauces, soups, vegetable and cheese dishes. It is also used for mixed spice.

Poppy seeds

Poppy seeds are used as a topping for bread and cakes, etc.

Saffron

The stigmas from a crocus known as the saffron crocus (grown chiefly in Spain) are dried and form saffron, which is a flavouring and colouring spice. It is used in soups, sauces and particularly in rice dishes, giving them a bright yellow colour and distinctive flavour. Saffron is very expensive as it takes the stigmas from approximately 4000 crocus flowers to yield 30 g (1 oz).

Sesame seeds

These are used as a topping for bread, cakes and in Chinese and vegetarian cookery.

Surmac seeds

These are used in Middle Eastern cooking for their acidic lemon peppery flavour. Deep red-maroon colour.

Turmeric

Turmeric grows in the same way as ginger and it is the rhizome which is used. It is without any pronounced flavour and its main use is for colouring curry powder. It is ground into a fine powder, which turns it yellow. Tumeric is also used in pickles, relishes and as a colouring in cakes and rice.

Some additional ingredients used in Asian and Fusion Cuisine (a mixture of food styles and ingredients from the cookery styles of the East and West)

AJOWAN

A native Indian plant used in Indian recipes. An ingredient of Bombay mix and breads such as parathas, bean and pulse recipes.

ANNATTO

Shrub indigenous to both the Caribbean and tropical America, has heart-shaped glossy leaves, pink flowers. The seeds are washed and dried separately for culinary use. An orange food colour is made from the husk.

ASAFOETIDA

Indigenous to Iran and Afghanistan and in the North of India. Used in vegetable, fish, pulse and pickle ingredients.

BAMBOO SHOOTS

Mild flavoured, tender shoots of the young bamboo. Widely available fresh, or sliced or halved in cans.

BENGALI FIVE SPICES

Bengal origin, also known as panch phoron. Cumin seeds, fennel seeds, mustard seeds, fenngreek seeds, nigella seeds.

BERBERA

An Ethiopian blend of spices. Dried red chillies, white cardamons, allspice berries, black peppercorns, cumin seeds, coriander seeds, ajowan seeds, ground ginger, fenngreek seeds, cloves, ground nutmeg, salt.

BLACKBEAN SAUCE

Made from salted black beans crushed and mixed with flour and spices (such as ginger, garlic or chilli) to form a paste. Sold in jars and cans.

CARDAMON PODS

Available both as small green pods and larger black pods containing seeds. They have a strong aromatic quality.

CAJUN SPICE MIX

Spice mixture used for fish, chicken and meat. Garlic, dried oregano, white mustard seeds, salt, black peppercorns, chilli powder, cumin seeds, paprika, dried thyme.

CHILLIES

There are over 24 different types of chillies, for example, small green or red, garlic etc.

CHILLI BEAN SAUCE

Made from fermented bean paste mixed with hot chilli and other seasonings.

CHILLI OIL

Made from fermented bean paste mixed with hot chilli and other seasonings.

CHILLI POWDER

Milder than cayenne pepper and more coarsely ground; prepared from a variety of mild and hot chillies.

CHILLI SAUCE

A very hot sauce made from chillies, vinegar, sugar and salt. Sold in bottles.

CHINESE RICE WINE

Made from glutinous rice, also known as yellow wine huang jin or chiew because of its colour. The best variety is called shuo hsing or shuoxing and comes from South-East China. Dry sherry may be used as a substitute.

CHINESE CHIVES

Also known as garlic chives.

COCONUT MILK AND CREAM

Not to be confused with the 'milk' or juice found inside the fresh coconut. The coconut milk used for cooking is produced from the white flesh of the coconut. If left to stand, the thick part of the milk will rise to the surface like cream.

CURRY LEAVES

Comes from the tropical tree of the citrus-rue family, native of Southern India, Sri Lanka. Strong, curry aroma.

A classical way of using curry leaves is by frying mustard seeds in hot ghee, then adding a little asafoetida and several curry leaves for a few seconds, before stirring them into a plain dhal dish or dhal based Indian soup.

DASHI

Light Japanese stock, available in powder form. The flavour derives from kelp seaweed.

DRIED SHRIMPS AND SHRIMP PASTE

Dried shrimps are tiny shrimps that are salted and dried. They are used as a seasoning for stir-fry dishes. Shrimp paste, also known as terasi, is a dark, odorous paste made from fermented shrimps.

GALANGAL

Fresh galangal, also known as lengkuas, tastes and looks a little like ginger with a pinkish tinge to its skin.

GRAM FLOUR

Made from ground chick peas, this flour has a unique flavour.

HARISSA

Spice mix used in Moroccan, Tunisian and Algerian cooking. Used as a dip or accompaniment. Dried red chillies, olive oil, coriander seeds, garlic, cumin seeds, salt.

HOI SIN SAUCE

A thick, dark brownish-red sauce which is sweet and spicy.

KAFFIR LIME LEAVES

These are used like bay leaves, to give an aromatic lime flavour to dishes.

JUNIPER

Grown in Hungary, southern Europe. An evergreen coniferous tree of the cypress family. The berries taste of gin, used in the production of gin. A seasoning for some birds, venison, duck, rabbit, pork, ham and lamb.

LA KAMA

Moroccan spice mix. Black peppercorns, ground ginger, ground turmeric, ground nutmeg, cinnamon stick.

LIQUORICE

Native of the Middle East and South-East Europe. The root is the most important part, sends out a deep and extensive network of rhizomes, which are grown for 3–5 years before they are harvested. The roots and rhizomes are cleaned, pulped, then boiled and the liquorice extract is then concentrated by evaporation.

Liquorice is best known as an ingredient in confectionery, also used in the making of Guinness and the flavour of Italian liquor Sambucco.

MAHLEBI

Tree found only in Middle East and Turkey. The ground spice is used in breads and pastries.

MANGO POWDER

The unriped mangoes are sliced, sun-dried and ground to a powder, then mixed with a little ground turmeric. Used in vegetarian dishes, curries, chutneys.

MIRIN

A mild sweet, Japanese rice wine used in cooking.

MISO

A fermented bean paste that adds richness and flavour to Japanese soups.

NIGELLA

Grown in India. The seeds are held in a seed head similar to a poppy head. Sometimes used as a substitute for pepper. Nigella is one of the five spices in Bengali five Spices (panch phoron). It is widely used in Indian cooking, in dhal and vegetable dishes, pickles and chutneys. The seeds are often scattered on naan bread.

NOODLES

Cellophane noodles – also known as bean thread, transparent or glass noodles. Made from ground mung beans.

Egg noodles – are made from wheat flour, egg and water.

Rice noodles – are made from ground rice and water.

Rice vermicelli – are thin brittle noodles that look like white hair.

Somen noodles – are delicate thin white Japanese noodles made from wheat flour.

Udon noodles – Japanese noodles made of wheat flour and water.

NORI

Paper thin sheets of Japanese seaweed.

OYSTER SAUCE

Made from oyster extract.

PAK CHOI

Also known as bok choi this is a leaf vegetable with long, smooth milky white stems and dark green foliage.

PALM SUGAR

Strongly flavoured, hard brown sugar made from the sap of the coconut palm tree.

PAPAYA SEEDS

Seeds of the papaya fruit. Can be used fresh or dried. Rich in enzyme papain which is an efficient meat tenderiser of commercial value.

POMEGRANATE SEEDS

Grown in Mediterranean countries, South America, the USA and parts of Africa.

Grenadine is a syrup made from the juice of the pomegranate. Fresh pomegranate seeds are sprinkled on hummus.

RAS EL HANOUT

Moroccan spice mixture. Black peppercorns, coriander seeds, cumin seeds, cloves, green cardamons, ground turmeric, cinnamon stick, ground ginger, salt nutmeg, dried red chillies, dried flowers.

RED BEAN PASTE

A reddish-brown paste made from pureèd red beans and crystallised sugar.

RICE VINEGAR

There are two basic types:

Red vinegar – made from fermented rice and has a distinctive dark colour

White vinegar – stronger in flavour, distilled from rice.

SAKE

A strong powerful fortified rice wine from Japan.

SAMBALS

Sambals is an accompaniment that is spooned directly on to the plate. Made from seeded red chillies pureèd with salt.

SAMBAL KEEAP

Indonesian sauce used as an accompaniment on a dip. Dark soy sauce, lemon juice, garlic, red chilli, deep fried onion slices.

SAMBAAR POWDER

Also known as sambar used in South Indian dishes, made from red chillies, coriander seeds, black peppercorns, fenngreek seeds, urad dhal, channu dhal, mung dhal, ground turmeric and cumin seeds.

SOY SAUCE

A major seasoning ingredient in Chinese cooking, made from fermented soya beans, combined with yeast, salt and sugar. Chinese soy sauce falls into two main categories:

Light and dark. Light has more flavour than the sweeter dark sauce, which gives food a rich, reddish colour.

SPRING ROLL WRAPPERS

Paper thin wrappers made from wheat or rice flour and water.

SUMAC

Bush grown in Italy, Sicily and the Middle East. Red berries are dried. Widely used in Lebanese, Syrian, Turkish and Iranian cuisines.

SZECHUAN PEPPERCORNS

Also known as tarchiew, aromatic, best used roasted and ground. Not so hot as white or black peppercorns.

TAMARIND

The brown, sticky pulp of the bean-like seed pod of the tamarind tree. Used in Indian, Thai and Indonesian cooking.

THAI FISH SAUCE – NAM PLA

The most common flavouring in Thai food, in the same way soy sauce is used in Chinese dishes. It is made from salted anchovies and has a strong, salty flavour.

THAI NAM PRIK SAUCE

This is the most famous of the Thai sauces, it can be served on its own or used as a dip. Brown sugar, lemon juice, fish sauce, fresh red chillies, dried prawns, blanchan, cooked prawns, garlic, fresh coriander.

THAI PARSLEY

Similar in appearance to spring onion but without the bulb.

THAI RED CURRY PASTE

Krueng gueng phed is the Thai name. Used for meat, poultry and vegetable dishes. Red chillies, groundnut oil, red onion, blanchan, lemon grass, salt, cumin seeds, citrus peel, garlic, galangal, green chillies, white onion, fresh coriander, coriander seeds.

TOEY LEAVES

Also known as pandanus leaves, these are long, flat blades bright green in colour.

TOFU

Pureèd, pressed soya beans. Also known as bean curd, rich in protein.

WASABI

Edible root used in Japanese cooking, to make a condiment with a sharp, pungent and fiery flavour. Similar to horseradish.

WATER CHESTNUTS

Walnut-sized bulbs from an Asian water plant that looks like sweet chestnuts.

WONTON WRAPPERS

Small, paper-thin squares of wheat flour and egg dough.

YARD LONG BEANS

Long thin beans similar to French beans but three or four times longer.

YELLOW BEAN SAUCE

A thick paste made from salted, fermented yellow soya beans crushed with flour and sugar.

ZEDOURY

A member of the ginger and turmeric family, bright yellow in colour. Has a musky aroma with a hint of camphor.

CONDIMENTS

Salt

FOOD VALUE

Salt (sodium chloride) is essential for stabilising body fluids and preventing muscular cramp.

STORAGE

Salt must be stored in a cool, dry store as it readily absorbs moisture. It should be kept in airtight packets, drums or bins.

USE

Salt is used for curing fish such as herrings and haddocks and for cheese and butter making. Salt is also used for the pickling of foods, in the cooking of many dishes and as a condiment on the table.

Pepper

Pepper is obtained from black peppercorns, which are the berries of a tropical shrub.

White peppercorns are obtained by removing the skin from the black peppercorn. White pepper is less pungent than black, and both may be obtained in ground form.

Green peppercorns are fresh unripe pepper berries, milder than dried peppercorns, available frozen or in tins. Pink peppercorns are softer and milder than green peppercorns, available preserved in vinegar.

Ground pepper is used for seasoning many dishes and as a condiment at the table.

CAYENNE PEPPER

Cayenne is a red pepper used on savoury dishes and cheese straws. It is a hot pepper which is obtained from grinding chillies and capsicums.

PAPRIKA

Paprika is a bright red mild pepper used in goulash.

Mustard

Mustard is obtained from the seed of the mustard plant. It is sold in powder form and is diluted with water, milk or vinegar for table use or sold ready mixed in jars.

A large variety of continental mustards are sold as a paste in jars, having been mixed with herbs and wine vinegar.

Vinegar

Malt vinegar is made from malt, which is produced from barley.

Artificial, non-brewed, pure or imitation vinegars are chemically produced solutions of acetic acid in water. They are cheaper and inferior to malt vinegar, having a pungent odour and a sharp flavour.

Spirit vinegars are produced from potatoes, grain or starchy vegetables, but they do not have the same flavour as malt vinegar.

Red or white vinegars are made from grapes and are more expensive and have a more delicate flavour than the other vinegars.

All vinegars can be distilled; this removes the colour. The colour of vinegar is no indication of its strength as burnt sugar is added to give colour.

Balsamic vinegar is a specially matured vinegar from Italy with a distinctive flavour which varies in strength according to the age of the vinegar which can be up to 30 years.

Other vinegars include chilli, sherry, cider, rice, herb (especially tarragon) thyme, oregano, sage, rosemary and fruit such as raspberry and strawberry.

USES

Vinegar is used as a preservative for pickles, rollmops and cocktail onions; and as a condiment on its own or with oil as a salad dressing; it is used for flavouring sauces such as mayonnaise and in reductions for sharp sauces (sauce piquante, sauce diable).

COLOURINGS, FLAVOURINGS, ESSENCES

Colourings

A number of food colourings are obtained in either powder or liquid form. Natural colours include:

COCHINEAL

Cochineal is a red colour, produced from the cochineal beetle, used in pastry and confectionery work.

GREEN COLOURING

This can be made by mixing indigo and saffron, but chlorophyll, the natural green colouring of plants, such as in spinach, may also be used.

INDIGO

Indigo is the blue colour seldom used on its own, but which, when mixed with red, produces shades of mauve.

YELLOW COLOURING

A deep yellow colour can be obtained from turmeric roots and is prepared in the form of a powder mainly used in curry and mustard pickles.

Yellow is also obtained by using egg yolks or saffron.

BROWN

Brown sugar is used to give a deep brown colour in rich fruit cakes; it also adds to the flavour.

BLACKJACK OR BROWNING

Blackjack or commercial caramel is a dark brown, almost black liquid, and is used for colouring soups, sauces, gravies, aspics and in pastry and confectionery.

CHOCOLATE COLOUR

This can be obtained in liquid or powder form, and is used in pastry and confectionery.

COFFEE COLOUR

This is usually made from coffee beans with the addition of chicory.

A large range of artificial colours are also obtainable; they are produced from coal tar and are harmless. Some mineral colours are also used in foodstuffs. All colourings must be pure and there is a list of those permitted for cookery and confectionery use.

Essences

Essences are generally produced from a solution of essential oils with alcohol, and are prepared for the use of cooks, bakers and confectioners.

Among the many types of essence obtainable are:

- almond;
- lemon;
- orange;
- peppermint;
- pineapple;
- raspberry;
- strawberry;
- vanilla.

Essences are available in three categories: natural, artificial and compound.

NATURAL ESSENCES

- Fruit juices pressed out of soft fruits (raspberries or strawberries).
- Citrus fruit peel (lemon, orange).
- Spices, beans, herbs, roots, nuts (caraway seeds, cinnamon, celery, mint, sage, thyme, clove, ginger, coffee beans, nutmeg and vanilla pod).

ARTIFICIAL ESSENCES

Artificial essences such as vanilla, pineapple, rum, banana, coconut, are produced from various chemicals blended to give a close imitation of the natural flavour.

COMPOUND ESSENCES

Compound essences are made by blending natural products with artificial products.

The relative costs vary considerably and it is advisable to try all types of flavouring essence before deciding on which to use for specific purposes.

GROCERY, DELICATESSEN

Delicatessen literally means 'provision store', but the name is commonly used to cover the place where a wide range of table delicacies may be bought.

Agar Agar

This is obtained from the dried purified stems of a seaweed; also known as vegetable gelatine, and is used in vegetarian cookery.

Anchovy essence

This is a strong, highly seasoned commodity used for flavouring certain fish sauces and fish preparations such as anchovy sauce or fish cakes.

Aspic

Aspic jelly is a clear savoury jelly which may be the flavour of meat, game or fish. It may be produced from fresh ingredients (see *Advanced Practical Cookery*) or obtained in a dried form.

It is used for cold larder work, mainly for coating chaud-froid dishes, and may also be chopped or cut into neat shapes to decorate finished dishes.

Bresaola

A cured beef speciality of Valtellina, in Lombardy, Italy.

Coppa

Salted and dried sausage made from the neck and shoulder of pork.

Caviar

Caviar is the uncooked roe of the sturgeon which is prepared by carefully separating the eggs from the membranes of the roe and gently rubbing them through sieves of coarse hemp. It is then soaked in a brine solution, sieved and packed.

Sturgeon fishing takes place in the estuaries of rivers which run into the Caspian or Black Sea, therefore caviar is Russian or Iranian in origin. The types normally obtainable in Britain are Beluga, Osetrova and Sevruga. These names refer to the type of sturgeons from which the caviar is taken.

Caviar is extremely expensive and needs to be handled with great care and understanding. Caviar should be kept at a temperature of 0°C (32°F) but no lower otherwise the extreme cold will break the eggs down. Caviar must never be deep frozen.

A red caviar (keta) is obtained from the roe of salmon. From the lumpfish a mock caviar is obtained. These are considerably cheaper than genuine caviar.

Continental sausages

A large variety of these are imported from European countries, e.g. Salami, Cervelat, Chorizo, Mortadella, Luganege, Zampone etc.

Extracts (meat and vegetable)

Extracts are highly concentrated forms of flavouring used in some kitchens to strengthen stocks and sauces (Bovril, Marmite, Maggi, Jardox).

Foie Gras

This expensive delicacy is obtained from the livers of specially fattened geese and is produced mainly in Strasbourg.

Galantine

This is a cooked meat preparation made from well-seasoned finely minced chicken, veal or other white meat.

Gelatine

Gelatine is obtained from the bones and connective tissue, collagen, of certain animals; it is manufactured in leaf or powdered form and used in varying sweets such as bavarois. (See also 'Agar agar' on page 157.)

Haggis

This traditional Scottish dish is made from the heart, lungs (lights) and liver of the sheep, mixed with suet, onion and oatmeal and sewn up in a stomach bag. It is boiled and served with mashed potatoes.

Hams

A ham is the hind leg of a pig cured by a special process which varies according to the type of ham. One of the most famous English hams is the York ham weighing 6–7 kg (13–15 lb) which is cured by salting, drying and sometimes smoking. The Bradenham ham is of coal-black colour and is a sweet-cured ham from Chippenham in Wiltshire. Hams are also imported from Northern Ireland and Denmark.

Continental raw hams, Bayonne and Ardenne from France, Parma from Italy and Serrano from Spain, are cut in thin slices and served raw.

Horseradish

Horseradish is a plant of which only the root is used. The root is washed, peeled, grated and used for horseradish sauce and horseradish cream.

Pâté maison

Pâté is a well seasoned cooked mixture of various combinations of meat, poultry, game, fish or vegetables, usually served cold as a first course. There are numerous recipes, one of which can be found in *Practical Cookery*.

Panettone

An Italian light textured yeast bread containing sultanas and candied fruit.

Pickles

These are vegetables and/or fruits preserved in vinegar or sauce and include:
○ Red cabbage, gherkins, olives, onions, walnuts, capers.
○ Mango chutney is a sweet chutney which is served as an accompaniment to curried dishes.

Smoked herring fillets and Anchovy

These are preserved in oil and used as hors-d'œuvre.

Smoked salmon

British, Scandinavian or Canadian salmon weighing between 6–8 kg (13–18 lb) are used for smoking. A good quality side of smoked salmon should have a bright deep colour and be moist when lightly pressed with the finger tip at the thickest part of the flesh. A perfectly smoked side of salmon will remain in good condition for not more than seven days when stored at a temperature of 18°C (64°F). This versatile food is used for canapés, hors-d'œuvre, sandwiches, and as a fish course for lunch, dinner or supper.

Snails

These edible snails are raised on the foliage of the vine. They are obtainable in boxes which include the tinned snails and the cleaned shells. The snails are replaced in the shells with a mixture of butter, garlic, lemon juice and parsley, then heated in the oven and served in special dishes as a fish course. Snails are now farmed in Britain.

CONFECTIONERY AND BAKERY GOODS

Cake covering

This is produced from hardened vegetable fat with the addition of chocolate flavouring and colour.

Cape gooseberries

A tasty, yellow-berried fruit resembling a large cherry. Cape gooseberries are often dipped into fondant and served as a petit four.

Chocolate vermicelli

A ready-made preparation of small fine chocolate pieces used in the decorating of small and large cakes and some chocolate-flavoured sweets.

Cocktail cherries

Bright red cherries preserved in a syrup often flavoured with a liqueur known as maraschino. In addition to being used for cocktails they are also used to give colour to grapefruit and grapefruit cocktails.

Fondant

A soft, white preparation of sugar which has many uses in pastry and confectionery work, chiefly for coating petit fours, pastries and gâteaux.

Gum tragacanth

A soluble gum used for stiffening pastillage; only a very clear white type of gum tragacanth should be used. It is obtained from the shrubs of the genus *Astragalus*.

Honey

A natural sugar produced by bees working upon the nectar of flowers. It is generally used in the form of a preserve and in pastry work.

Ice-cream

A frozen preparation of a well-flavoured, sweetened mixture which can be made in many ways and in many flavours. Ice-cream may be bought ready prepared, usually in 5 litre (9 pint) containers which are suitable for deep-freeze storage. The storage temperature for ice-cream should not exceed −19°C (−32°F). All caterers must comply with the Ice-Cream Regulations which govern the production and labelling of ice-cream; if in doubt, contact the local Environmental Health Officer.

Jam

A preserve of fruit and sugar which is obtainable in 28 g (1 oz), $\frac{1}{2}$ kg (1 lb) and 1 kg (2 lb) jars and 3 kg (7 lb) tins. Raspberry and apricot jams are those mostly used in the pastry.

Marmalade

A preserve of citrus fruits and sugar, which is used mainly for breakfast menus and for certain sweets.

Marrons glacés

Peeled and cooked chestnuts preserved in syrup. They are used in certain large and small cakes, sweet dishes and as a variety of petit fours.

Marzipan

A preparation of ground almonds, sugar and egg yolks used in the making of petits fours, pastries and large cakes. Marzipan may be freshly made and is also obtained as a ready-prepared commodity.

Mincemeat

A mixture of dried fruit, fresh fruit, sugar, spices, nuts, etc., chiefly used for mince-pies. It can also be obtained in $\frac{1}{2}$ kg (1 lb) and 1 kg (2 lb) jars and 3 kg (7 lb) tins.

Pastillage (gum paste)

A mixture of icing sugar and gum tragacanth which may be moulded into shapes for set pieces for cold buffets and also for making baskets, caskets, etc., for the serving of petits fours.

Piping jelly

A thick jelly of piping consistency obtainable in different colours and flavours. It is used for decorating pastries and gâteaux and cold sweets. Piping jelly is obtainable in large tins.

Redcurrant jelly

A clear preserve of redcurrants used as a jam as an accompaniment and also in the preparation of savoury sweet sauces.

Rennet

A substance originally obtained from the stomach of calves, pigs and lambs, and can now be obtained in synthetic form. Rennet is prepared in powder, extract or essence form and is used in the production of cheese and for making junket. Vegetable rennet, for vegetarians, is also available.

Vanilla

This is the dried pod of an orchid used for infusing mild sweet flavour into dishes. After use rinse the vanilla stick, dry and store in a sealed jar of castor sugar ready for reuse.

Wafers

Thin crisp biscuits of various shapes and sizes usually served with ice-cream. They are obtainable in large tins of approximately 1000 and half-tins of approximately 500 wafers.

Some references to commodities elsewhere in the book

Topics for Discussion

1. Factors that affect the quality of meat.
2. Fors and againsts of using meat substitute such as TVP, Quorn.
3. Purchasing of meat (by carcass, joints or portion controlled cuts).
4. Much of today's poultry lacks flavour. How can this be remedied?
5. The popularity of fish compared to meat and poultry.
6. The best ways to purchase fish.
7. Buying policy for vegetables and fruit.
8. The importance of vegetables and fruit in the diet.
9. Eggs and the caterer.
10. Compare the uses of butter, margarine or oil in cooking.
11. What is a sensible policy for selling cheese in a restaurant?
12. Is the average caterer sufficiently knowledgeable about the different types of flour and their suitability for specific purposes?
13. Should the caterer be offering a wider range of choice of teas and coffees?
14. The values of using pulses.
15. The values of using herbs and spices.

CHAPTER 6

ELEMENTARY NUTRITION, FOOD SCIENCE, DIET AND HEALTH

FOOD AND NUTRIENTS

A food is any substance, liquid or solid, which provides the body with materials:

○ for heat and energy;
○ for growth and repair;
○ for regulating the body processes.

The materials are known as *nutrients*. They are:

○ proteins;　　　　　○ vitamins;
○ fats;　　　　　　　○ minerals;
○ carbohydrates;　　○ water.

The study of these nutrients is termed nutrition. Only those substances containing nutrients are foods (alcohol is an energy-provider but it also has the effects of a drug, so it is not listed under the nutrients). Most foods contain several nutrients; a few foods contain only one nutrient, such as sugar.

For the body to obtain the maximum benefit from food it is essential that everyone concerned with the buying, storage, cooking and serving of food and the compiling of menus should have some knowledge of nutrition.

The main function of nutrients

ENERGY	GROWTH AND REPAIR	REGULATION OF BODY PROCESSES
carbohydrates fats proteins	proteins minerals water	vitamins minerals water

Digestion *(see Figure 6.1, below)*

This is the breaking down of the food with the help of enzymes. Enzymes are proteins which speed up (catalyse) the break down processes. Digestion takes place

- in the mouth, where food is mixed with saliva, and starch is broken down by the action of an enzyme in saliva;
- in the stomach, where the food is mixed and gastric juices are added, and proteins are broken down;
- in the small intestine, where proteins, fats and carbohydrates are broken down further and additional juices are added.

Absorption

To enable the body to benefit from food it must be absorbed into the bloodstream; this absorption occurs after the food has been broken down; the product then passes through the walls of the digestive tract into the bloodstream.

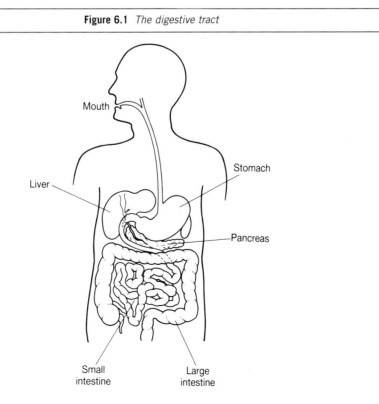

Figure 6.1 *The digestive tract*

This occurs in:

○ the stomach where simple substances, such as alcohol and glucose, are passed through the stomach lining into the bloodstream;

○ the small intestine where more of the absorption of nutrients takes place due to a further breakdown of the food;

○ the large intestine, where water is reabsorbed from the waste.

Food should smell, look and taste attractive in order to stimulate the flow of saliva and digestive juices. This will help the digestive process and ensure that most food is broken down and absorbed.

If digestion and absorption is not efficient this could lead to a deficiency of one or more nutrients and a state of malnutrition.

Proteins

Protein is an essential part of all living matter; it is therefore needed for the growth of the body and for the repair of body tissues.

There are two kinds of protein:

○ Animal protein, found in meat, game, poultry, fish, eggs, milk, cheese: myosin, collagen (meat, poultry and fish); albumin, ovovitellin (eggs); casein (milk and cheese).

THE PROTEIN CONTENT (%) PER 100G OF SOME ANIMAL AND VEGETABLE FOODS

braised beef	30.0
roast pork	30.0
roast lamb	28.0
roast chicken	25.0
roasted peanuts	24.0
baked cod	20.0
eggs	12.0
white bread	8.0
milk	3.0

○ Vegetable protein, found mainly in the seeds of vegetables. The proportion of protein in green and root vegetables is small. Peas, beans and nuts contain most protein and the grain of cereals, such as wheat, has a useful amount because of the large quantity eaten; for example gliadin and glutenin forming gluten with water (wheat and rye).

The table above shows the proportion of protein in some common foods and Figure 6.3 represents the main sources of protein and the contribution made by different protein foods in the typical Western diet. The proportion of animal foods contributing to the total would be very much reduced in developing countries.

It follows that, because protein is needed for growth, growing children and expectant and nursing mothers will need more protein than other adults, whose requirements are mainly for repair. Any spare protein is used for producing heat and energy. In diets where the protein intake is minimal, it is important that there is plenty of carbohydrate available so that protein is used for growth and repair, rather than for energy purposes.

WHAT IS PROTEIN?

Protein is composed of different amino acids; so the protein of cheese is different from the protein of meat because the number and arrangement of the acids are not the same. A certain number of these amino acids is essential to the body and must be provided by food. Proteins containing all the essential amino acids in the correct proportion are said to be of high biological value. The human body is capable of converting the other kinds of amino acids to suit its needs.

It is preferable that the body has both animal and vegetable protein, so that a complete variety of the necessary amino acids is available.

During digestion protein is split into amino acids; these are absorbed into the bloodstream and used for building body tissues and to provide some heat and energy.

Fats

There are two main groups of fats: animal and vegetable. The function of fat is to protect vital organs of the body, to provide heat and energy, and certain fats also provide vitamins.

Fats can be divided into:

○ solid fat;

○ oils (fat which is liquid at room temperature).

Fats are obtained from the following foods (see below).

○ animal origin: dripping, butter, suet, lard, cheese, cream, bacon, meat fat, oily fish;

○ vegetable origin: margarine, cooking fat, nuts, soya-beans.

Oils are obtained from the following foods:

○ animal origin: halibut and cod-liver oil;

○ vegetable origin: from seeds or nuts.

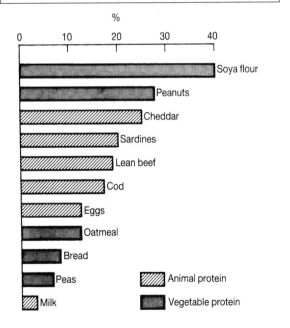

Figure 6.2 *Proportion of protein in some foods*

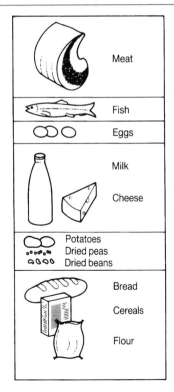

Figure 6.3 *Main sources of protein in the average diet*

COMPOSITION OF FATS

Fats are composed of glycerol to which are attached three fatty acids (hence the name triglyceride). Fats differ because of the fatty acids from which they are derived. These may be, for example, butyric acid in butter, stearic acid in solid fat, such as beef suet, oleic acid in most oils. These fatty acids affect the texture and flavour of the fat. The fatty acids found in animal foods (meat and dairy products) are of a different type from those found in other foods (fish, seed and nut oils). The former are termed 'saturated' fatty acids and produce saturated fats whereas the other types of fatty acids are 'unsaturated' and produce unsaturated fats or oils.

To be useful to the body, fats have to be broken down into glycerol and fatty acids so that they can be absorbed; they can then provide heat and energy.

The food value of the various kinds of fat is similar, although some animal fats contain vitamins A and D.

PERCENTAGE OF SATURATED* FAT IN AN AVERAGE DIET

milk, cheese, cream	16.0
meat and meat products	25.2
other oils and fats	30.0
other sources	
including eggs, fish, poultry	7.4
biscuits and cakes	11.4
The 25.2% for meat and meat	
products split down into:	
other meat products	9.1
beef	4.1
lamb	3.5
pork, bacon and ham	5.8
sausage	2.7

The contribution of animal fat in the Western diet is gradually changing as healthy eating policies encourage a reduction in the total fat intake, particularly animal fats. There has been a swing towards skimmed milk, leaner cuts of meat, cooking with vegetable oils and a reduced market for eggs, high fat cheeses and butter.

Figure 6.4 *Proportion of fat in some foods*

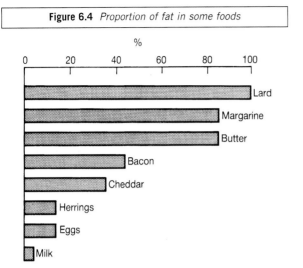

Figure 6.5 *Main sources of fat in the average diet*

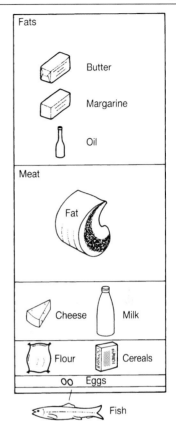

Fats should be eaten with other foods such as bread, potatoes, etc., as they can then be more easily digested and utilised in the body.

Certain fish, such as herrings, mackerel, salmon and sardines, contain oil (fat) in the flesh. Other fish, such as cod and halibut, contain the oil in the liver.

Vegetables and fruit contain very little fat, but nuts have a considerable amount.

EFFECTS OF COOKING ON FAT

Cooking has little effect on fat except to make it more digestible.

Carbohydrates

Figure 6.6 *Main sources of carbohydrates in the average diet*

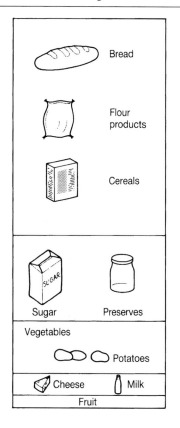

Figure 6.7 *Proportion of carbohydrate in some foods*

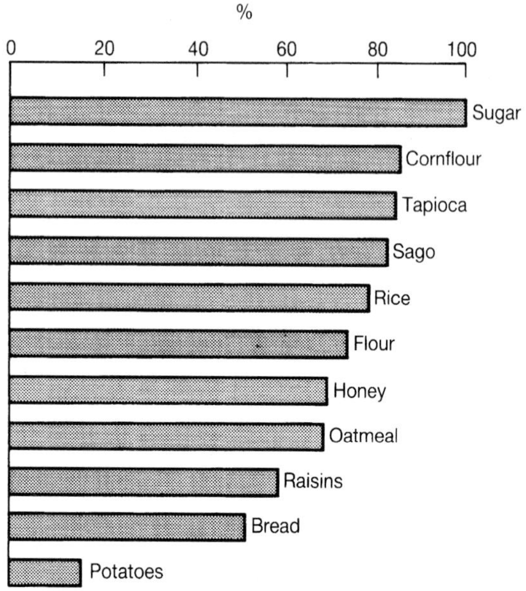

There are three main types of carbohydrates:
○ sugar (saccharide);
○ starch (polysaccharide);
○ cellulose.

The function of carbohydrates is to provide the body with most of its energy. Starch is composed of a number of glucose molecules (particles), and during digestion starch is broken down into glucose. It is often now referred to as dietary fibre or NSP (non-starch polysaccharide).

SUGAR

There are several kinds of sugar:
○ glucose: found in the blood of animals and in fruit and honey;
○ fructose: found in fruit, honey and cane sugar;
○ sucrose: found in beet and cane sugar;
○ lactose: found in milk;
○ maltose: produced naturally during the germination of grain.

Sugars are the simplest form of carbohydrate and the end-products of the digestion of carbohydrates. They are absorbed in the form of glucose and simple sugars and used to provide heat and energy.

STARCH

Starch is present in the diet through the following foods:

○ whole grains: rice, barley, tapioca;

○ powdered grains: flour, cornflour, ground rice, arrowroot;

○ vegetables: potatoes, parsnips, peas, beans;

○ unripe fruit: bananas, apples, cooking pears;

○ cereals: cornflakes, shredded wheat, etc.;

○ cooked starch: cakes, biscuits;

○ pastas: macaroni, spaghetti, vermicelli, etc.

Cooking effects on starch

Uncooked starch is not digestible. Foods containing starch have cells with starch granules, covered with a cellulose wall which breaks down when heated or made moist. When browned, as with the crust of bread, toast, roast potatoes, skin on rice pudding, etc., the starch forms dextrins and these taste sweeter. On heating with water or milk, starch granules swell and absorb liquid, thus thickening the product, (thickened gravy or cornflour sauce). This thickening process is known as gelatinisation of starch.

CELLULOSE

Cellulose is the coarser structure of vegetables and cereals which is not digested but is used as roughage in the intestine. It is often now referred to as dietary fibre.

Vitamins

Vitamins are chemical substances which are vital for life, and if the diet is deficient in any vitamin, ill-health results. As they are chemical substances they can be produced synthetically.

GENERAL FUNCTION OF VITAMINS

Vitamins assist the regulation of the body processes:

○ to help the growth of children;

○ to protect against disease.

VITAMIN A (see page 170)

Function

Vitamin A:

○ assists in children's growth;

○ helps the body to resist infection;

○ enables people to see better in the dark.

Vitamin A is fat soluble; therefore it is to be found in fatty foods. It can be made in the body from carotene, the yellow substance found in many fruits and vegetables.

Dark green vegetables are a good source of vitamin A, the green colour masking the yellow of the carotene. Carotene is gradually destroyed by light (hence the fading of orange coloured spices and vegetables on prolonged storage).

Sources of vitamin A

○ halibut-liver oil
○ cod-liver oil
○ kidney
○ liver
○ butter
○ margarine (to which vitamin A is added)
○ cheese
○ eggs

○ milk
○ herrings
○ carrots
○ spinach
○ watercress
○ tomatoes
○ apricots

Fish-liver oils have the most vitamin A. The amount of vitamin A in dairy produce varies. Because cattle eat fresh grass in summer and stored feeding-stuffs in winter, the dairy produce contains the highest amount of vitamin A in the summer. Kidney and liver are also useful sources of vitamin A.

VITAMIN D

Function

Vitamin D controls the use the body makes of calcium. It is therefore necessary for healthy bones and teeth. Like vitamin A it is fat soluble.

Sources of vitamin D

An important source of vitamin D is from the action of sunlight on the deeper layers of the skin (approximately 75% of our vitamin D comes from this source). Others include:

○ fish-liver oils;
○ oily fish;
○ egg yolk;
○ margarine (to which vitamin D is added);
○ dairy produce.

VITAMIN B

When first discovered vitamin B was thought to be one substance only; it is now known to consist of at least 11 substances, the two main ones being:

○ thiamin (B_1);
○ riboflavin (B_2);

Others include folic acid and pyridoxine (B_6).

Sources of vitamin B

THIAMIN (B_1)	RIBOFLAVIN (B_2)	NICOTINIC ACID
○ yeast	○ yeast	○ meat extract
○ bacon	○ liver	○ brewers' yeast
○ oatmeal	○ meat extract	○ liver
○ peas	○ cheese	○ kidney
○ wholemeal bread	○ egg	○ beef

Function

Vitamin B which is water soluble and can be lost during cooking is required to:

○ keep the nervous system in good condition;

○ enable the body to obtain energy from the carbohydrates;

○ encourage the growth of the body.

VITAMIN C (ASCORBIC ACID)

Function

Vitamin C:

○ is necessary for the growth of children;

○ assists in the healing of cuts and uniting of broken bones;

○ prevents gums and mouth infection.

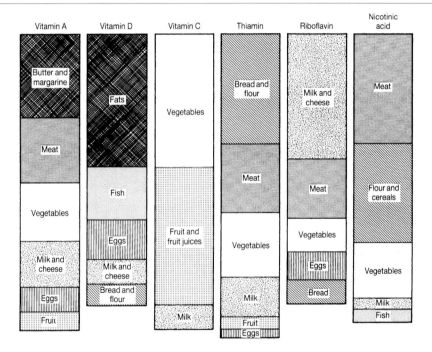

Figure 6.8 *Main sources of vitamins in the average diet*

Vitamin C is water soluble and can be lost during cooking or soaking in water. It is also lost by bad storage (keeping foods for too long, bruising, or storing in a badly ventilated place) and by cutting vegetables into small pieces.

Sources of vitamin C

○ blackcurrants   ○ potatoes   ○ Brussels sprouts and other greens

○ strawberries   ○ lemons   ○ oranges

○ grapefruit   ○ tomatoes   ○ bananas

○ fruit juices

The major sources in the British diet are potatoes and green vegetables.

MINERAL ELEMENTS

There are 19 mineral elements, most of which are required by the body in very small quantities. The body has at certain times a greater demand for certain mineral elements and there is a danger then of a deficiency in the diet. Calcium, iron and iodine are those most likely to be deficient.

Calcium

Calcium is required for:
- building bones and teeth;
- clotting of the blood;
- the working of the muscles.

The use the body makes of calcium is dependent on the presence of vitamin D.

SOURCES OF CALCIUM

Calcium can be found in:
- milk and milk products;
- bones of tinned oily fish;
- wholemeal bread and white bread (to which calcium is added). *Note* It is still the practice to add calcium, iron, thiamin and nicotinic acid to flour despite the DHSS report No. 23 (1981) which recommended that it should be discontinued.
- vegetables (greens);
- Drinking water.

Although calcium is present in certain foods (spinach, cereals) the body is unable to make use of it as it is not in a soluble form and therefore cannot be absorbed.

Because of the need for growth of bones and teeth, infants, adolescents, expectant and nursing mothers have a greater demand for calcium.

Phosphorus

Phosphorus is required for:
- building the bones and teeth (in conjunction with calcium and vitamin D);
- the control of the structure of the brain cells.

SOURCES OF PHOSPHORUS

- liver
- cheese
- kidney
- bread
- eggs
- fish

Iron

Iron is required for building the haemoglobin in blood and is therefore necessary for transporting oxygen and carbon dioxide round the body.

SOURCES OF IRON

- lean meat
- offal
- egg yolk
- wholemeal flour
- green vegetables
- fish

Iron is most easily absorbed from meat and offal, and its absorption is helped by the presence of vitamin C.

Iron may also be present in drinking water and obtained from iron utensils in which food is prepared.

As the haemoglobin in the blood should be maintained at a constant level, the body requires more iron at certain times than others (after loss of blood).

Sodium

Sodium is required in all body fluids, and is found in salt (sodium chloride). Excess salt is continually lost from the body in urine. The kidneys control this loss. We also lose sodium in sweating, a loss over which we have no control.

SOURCES OF SODIUM

Many foods are cooked with salt or have salt added (bacon and cheese) or contain salt (meat, eggs, fish). Excess sodium can cause hypertension (high blood pressure) in middle age.

Iodine

Iodine is required for the functioning of the thyroid gland which regulates basal metabolism (see page 175).

SOURCES OF IODINE

○ sea foods
○ iodised salt
○ drinking water obtained near the sea
○ vegetables grown near the sea

Other minerals

Potassium, magnesium, sulphur and copper are some of the other minerals required by the body.

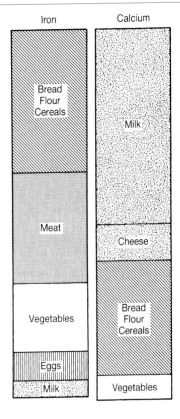

Figure 6.9 *Main sources of iron and calcium in the average die*

Water

Water is required for:

○ regulation of body temperatures by evaporation of perspiration;
○ all body fluids;   ○ metabolism;
○ digestion;   ○ excretion;
○ absorption;   ○ secretion.

SOURCES OF WATER

○ drinks of all kinds;
○ foods, such as fruits and vegetables, meat, eggs;
○ combustion or oxidation: when fats, carbohydrates and protein are used for energy a certain amount of water (metabolic water) is produced within the body.

THE EFFECTS OF COOKING ON NUTRIENTS

Protein

When protein is heated it coagulates and shrinks. Too much cooking can spoil the appearance of the food, such as scrambled eggs, as well as causing destruction of certain vitamins. On being heated, the different proteins in foods set or coagulate at different temperatures; above these temperatures shrinkage occurs, and this is particularly noticeable in grilling or roasting meat. Moderately cooked protein is the most easy to digest: a lightly cooked egg is more easily digested than a raw egg or a hard-boiled egg.

Carbohydrate

Unless starch is thoroughly cooked it cannot be digested properly (insufficiently cooked pastry or bread). When cooked, the starch granules swell, burst and then the starch can be digested. (This is called gelatinisation of starch.)

When sugar is heated it melts and with further heating loses water, gradually turning brown, dark brown and then black. This is known as the caramelisation of sugar.

Fat

The nutritive value of fat is not affected by cooking. During cooking processes a certain amount of fat may be lost from food when the fat melts, such as in the grilling of meat.

Mineral elements

There is a possibility of some minerals being lost in the cooking liquor, so diminishing the amount available in the food. This applies to soluble minerals, such as salt, but not to calcium or iron compounds which do not dissolve in the cooking liquor.

Iron

Iron may be acquired from foods cooked in iron utensils. The iron in foods is not affected by the cooking.

Calcium

Cooking foods in hard water may very slightly increase the amount of calcium in food.

Vitamins

- Vitamins A and D withstand cooking temperatures, and they are not lost in the cooking.
- Vitamin B_1 (thiamin) can be destroyed by high temperatures and by the use of bicarbonate of soda. It is soluble in water and can be lost in the cooking.
- Vitamin B_2 (riboflavin) is not destroyed easily by heat but bright sunlight can break it down.
- Vitamin C is lost by cooking and by keeping food warm in a hot place. It is also soluble in water (the soaking of foods for a long time and bruising are the causes of losing vitamin C). It is unstable and therefore easily destroyed in alkaline conditions (bicarbonate of soda must not be used when cooking green vegetables).

FOOD REQUIREMENTS

Energy is required to enable the heart to beat, for the blood to circulate, the lungs and other organs of the body to function, for every activity such as talking, eating, standing, sitting and for strenuous exercise and muscular activity.

Young and active people require a different amount of food from elderly, inactive people because they expend more energy, and this energy is obtained from food during chemical changes taking place in the body.

The energy value of a food is measured by a term called a kilocalorie or Calorie (this term should be written with a capital C although popularly is often written with a small c). This is the amount of heat required to raise the temperature of 1000 grammes of water from 15 to 16°C.

A new unit is now gradually replacing the Calorie. This is the joule. Since the joule is too small for practical nutrition, the kilojoule (kJ) is used.

1 Calorie=4.18 kJ

(Both units will be given here and for ease of conversion 1 Calorie will be taken to equal 4.0 kJ.)

Foods contain certain amounts of the various nutrients, which are measured in grammes.

The energy value of nutrients is as follows:

1 g carbohydrate produces 4 Calories   (16 kJ);

1 g protein produces 4 Calories   (16 kJ);

1 g fat produces 9 Calories   (36 kJ).

The energy value of a food, diet or menu is calculated from the nutrients it contains; 28 g of food containing:

10 g carbohydrate	will produce 10 × 4 =	40 Calories (160 kJ)
2 g protein	will produce 2 × 4 =	8 Calories (32 kJ)
5 g fat	will produce 5 × 9 =	<u>45</u> Calories (180 kJ)
	Total	<u>93</u> Calories (372 kJ)

Foods having a high fat content will have a high energy value; those containing a lot of water, a low energy value. All fats, cheese, bacon and other foods with a high fat content have a high energy value.

Men require more Calories (kJ) than women, big men and women require more than small men and women, and people engaged in energetic work require more Calories (kJ) than those with sedentary occupations.

BASAL METABOLISM

Basal metabolism is the term given to the amount of energy required to maintain the functions of the body and to keep the body warm when it is still and without food. The number of Calories (kJ) required for basal metabolism is affected by the size, sex and general condition of the body. The number of Calories (kJ) required for basal metabolism is approximately 1700 per day.

In addition to the energy required for basal metabolism, energy is also required for everyday activities, such as getting up, dressing, walking, and the amount required will be closely related to a person's occupation.

The approximate energy requirements per day for the following examples are:

○ Clerk   2000 Calories (8000 kJ)
○ Carpenter   3000 Calories (12000 kJ)
○ Labourer   4000 Calories (16000 kJ)

VALUE OF FOODS IN THE DIET

Milk and milk products

Cows' milk is almost the perfect food for human beings; it contains protein, carbohydrate, fat, minerals, vitamins and water.

When milk is taken into the body it coagulates in the same way as in the making of junket. This occurs in the stomach when digestive juices (containing the enzyme rennin) are added. Souring of milk is due to the bacteria feeding on the milk sugar (lactose) and producing lactic acid from it, which brings about curdling.

COMPOSITION OF MILK

The approximate composition is as follows:

○ 87% water
○ 3–4% proteins (mostly casein)
○ 3–4% fat
○ 4–5% sugar
○ 0.7% minerals (particularly calcium)
○ Vitamins A, B and D

In Channel Island milk (Jersey and Guernsey) the percentage of fat must be 4%; in all other milk the minimum is 3%.

Milk, therefore, is a body-building food because of its protein, an energy food because of the fat and sugar, and a protective food as it contains vitamins and minerals. Because of its high water content, while it is a suitable food for infants, it is too bulky to be the main source of protein and other nutrients after the first few months of life. It is also deficient in iron and vitamin C.

However, it may be included in everyone's diet as a drink and it can be used in a variety of ways.

Skimmed milk, which has had the cream layer removed, is increasing in popularity. Not only does it provide a lower calorie intake for those watching their weight, but also the potentially harmful animal fat has been removed.

CREAM

Cream is the fat of milk and the minimum fat content of single cream is approximately 18%, for double cream 48% and clotted cream 60%.

Cream is therefore an energy-producing food which also supplies vitamins A and D. It is easily digested because the fat is in a highly emulsified form (i.e. the fat globules are very small).

Butter

Butter is made from the fat of milk and contains vitamins A and D, the amount depending on the season. Like cream it is easily digested.

COMPOSITION OF BUTTER

The approximate composition is:

- 84% fat;
- 15% water;
- 1% salt;
- vitamins A and D.

Butter is also an energy-producing food and a protective food in so far as it provides vitamins A and D.

Cheese

Cheese is made from milk; its composition varies according to whether the cheese has been made from whole milk, skimmed milk or milk to which extra cream has been added.

The composition of cheddar cheese is approximately:

- 40% fat;
- 30% water;
- 25% protein.
- calcium;
- vitamins A and D;

The food value of cheese is exceptional because of the concentration of the various nutrients it contains. The minerals in cheese are useful, particularly the calcium and phosphorus. Cheese is also a source of vitamins A and D.

It is a body-building, energy-producing and protective food because of its protein, fat and mineral elements and vitamin content.

Cheese is easily digested, provided it is eaten with starchy foods and eaten in small pieces as when grated.

Margarine

Margarine, which is made from animal and/or vegetable oils, and skimmed milk, has vitamins A and D added to it. The composition and food value of margarine are similar to butter.

Meat, poultry and game

Meat consists of fibres which may be short, as in a fillet of beef, or long, as in the silverside of beef. The shorter the fibre the more tender and easily digested the meat. Meat is carved across the grain to assist mastication and digestion of the fibres.

Hanging the meat helps to make the flesh of meat more tender; this is because acids develop and soften the muscle fibres. Marinading in wine or vinegar prior to cooking also helps to tenderise meat so that it is more digestible. Expensive cuts of meat are not necessarily more nourishing than the cheaper cuts.

Meat contains proteins, variable amounts of fat, water, also iron and thiamin. (Bacon is particularly valuable because of its thiamin, and pork and pork products are especially rich in thiamin.) Tripe, in addition to its protein, is a good source of calcium as it is treated with lime during its preparation. It is also easily digested. Meat of all kinds is therefore important as a body-building food.

Fish

Fish is as useful a source of animal protein as meat.

The amount of fat in different fish varies: oily fish contain 5–18%, white fish less than 2%.

When the bones are eaten, calcium is obtained from fish (tinned sardines or salmon).

Oily fish is not so easily digested as white fish because of the fat; shellfish is not easily digested because of the coarseness of the fibres.

Fish is important for body building, and certain types of fish (oily fish) supply more energy and are protective because of the fat and vitamins A and D contained in the fish.

Eggs

Egg white contains protein known as egg albumin and the amount of white is approximately twice the amount of the yolk.

The yolk is more complex; it contains more protein than the white, also fat, vitamins A and D, thiamin, riboflavin, calcium, iron, sulphur and phosphorus. Lecithin (an emulsifying agent) and cholesterol are also present.

Because of the protein, vitamins, mineral elements and fat, eggs are a body-building, protective and energy-producing food.

Fruit

The composition of different fruit varies considerably: avocado pears contain about 20% fat, whereas most other fruits contain none. In unripe fruit the carbohydrate is in the form of starch which changes to sugar as the fruit ripens.

The cellulose in fruits acts as a source of dietary fibre.

Fruit is valuable because of the vitamins and minerals it contains. Vitamin C is present in certain fruits, particularly citrus varieties (oranges, grapefruit) and blackcurrants and other summer fruits. Dried fruits such as raisins and sultanas are a useful source of energy because of their sugar content, but they contain no vitamin C.

COMPOSITION OF FRUIT

The approximate composition is:

- water 85%;
- carbohydrate 5–10%;
- cellulose 2–5%;
- minerals 0.5%;
- vitamin C varying amounts.

Very small amounts of fat and protein are found in most fruits. Fruit is a protective food because of its minerals and vitamins.

Nuts

Nuts are highly nutritious because of the protein, fat and minerals they contain. Vegetarians may rely on nuts to provide the protein in their diet.

Nuts are not easily digested because of their fat content and cellulose.

Vegetables

GREEN VEGETABLES

Green vegetables are particularly valuable because of their vitamin and mineral content; they are therefore protective foods. The most important minerals they contain are iron and calcium. Green vegetables are rich in carotene, which is made into vitamin A in the body.

The greener the vegetable the greater its nutritional value. Vegetables which are stored for long periods, or are damaged or bruised, quickly lose their vitamin C value, therefore they should be used as quickly as possible.

Green vegetables also act as a source of dietary fibre in the intestines.

ROOT VEGETABLES

Compared with green vegetables most root vegetables contain starch and sugar; they are therefore a source of energy. Swedes and turnips contain a little vitamin C and carrots and other yellow-coloured vegetables contain carotene, which is changed into vitamin A in the body.

POTATOES

Potatoes contain a large amount of starch (approximately 20%) and a small amount of protein just under the skin. Because of the large quantities eaten, the small amount of vitamin C they contain is of value in the diet.

ONIONS

The onion is used extensively and contains some sugar, but its main value is to provide flavour.

PEAS AND BROAD BEANS

These vegetables contain carbohydrate, protein and carotene.

Cereals

Cereals contain from 60 to 80% carbohydrate in the form of starch and are therefore energy foods. They also contain 7–13% protein, depending on the type of cereal, and 1–8% fat.

The vitamin B content is considerable in stoneground and wholemeal flour, and B vitamins are added to other wheat flours, as are calcium and iron salts.

Oats contain good quantities of fat and protein.

Sugar

There are several kinds of sugar, such as those found in fruit (glucose), milk (lactose), cane and beet sugar (sucrose).

Sugar, with fat, provides the most important part of the body's energy requirements.

Saccharin, although sweet, is chemically produced and has no food value.

Liquids

WATER

Certain waters contain mineral salts; hard waters contain soluble salts of calcium. Some spas are known for the mineral salts contained in the local water. Bottled natural mineral waters are sold in many places (particularly supermarkets), and are being used more widely in the catering industry and in the home. Fluoride may be present naturally in some waters, and makes children's teeth more resistant to decay.

FRUIT JUICES

In recent years there has been a tremendous increase in the consumption of fruit juices sold in cartons as a chilled drink or in a 'long-life' form which will keep almost indefinitely before being opened. In addition, freshly squeezed orange juice is a popular alternative drink in many places, including airport and rail terminal restaurants.

BEVERAGES

Tea and coffee have no food value in themselves, but they do act on the nervous system as a stimulant.

Cocoa contains some fat, starch and protein, also some vitamin B and mineral elements.

When tea, coffee and cocoa are served with milk and sugar they do have some food value.

Catering for health

NEW PRACTICAL GUIDANCE TO HEALTHIER CATERING

Concern that many catering courses include little information about nutrition, led to the publication of new guidance by the Food Standards Agency and Department of Health: *Catering for Health, A guide for teaching healthier catering practices.*

ENCOURAGE A BALANCED DIET

A food intake to provide the vitamins, minerals, protein and fibre the body requires, without too much fat, sugar and salt.

Following the widely accepted model of five good groups, *The Balance of Good Health* developed in 1994 by the Health Education Authority, the Department of Health and the Department of Environment, Food and Rural Affairs means, for most people:

1 starchy foods – a third of total food intake;

2 fruit and vegetables – a further third of total food intake: five portions of a variety of fruit and vegetables each day – a portion would be any of the following: half a large grapefruit, a whole apple, orange or banana, two plums, small bunch of grapes, half to one tablespoon of dried fruit, two to three tablespoons of cooked or canned fruit, two tablespoons raw, cooked, frozen or canned vegetables, a bowl of salad, a glass of fruit juice (not more than one per day);

3 meat, fish and other non-dairy sources of protein – moderate amounts only;

4 milk and dairy foods – moderate amounts only;

5 foods containing fat and foods containing sugar – relatively small amounts only. Fats which contain a small proportion of saturates and a high proportion of unsaturates (polyunsaturates or monounsaturates) are better for health.

To follow these guidelines, most people need to increase by half their intake of starchy food, double the amount of fruit and vegetables, and reduce substantially on fat and sugar.

Most people also need to cut down on the amount of salt in their diet.

Caterers can assist customers achieve a more balanced diet, within the parameters of their eating out experience. When the customer-base is all or mostly captive in a home for the elderly, hospital, boarding school, the armed forces, workers on an oil rig, etc there are three meals a day, and a menu cycle that can be viewed over a week or fortnight. So, for example, the number of red meat main courses can be limited to two or three days a week, while fish is offered on one or two days a week. A variety of fruit can be included in all meals, with perhaps fruit juice or grapefruit segments at breakfast. So can starchy foods, with cereals and/or porridge at breakfast and bread rolls. Vegetables and salads can feature more prominently for mid-day and evening meals. Dishes relatively high in fat and sugar can be limited to treats, perhaps once a week.

When the customer base is transient as in most restaurants, pubs, wine bars, hotels, cafés, etc the menu choice can be varied to offer for example a pasta dish, white meat and fish as well as red meat, dishes which are low in fat, interesting vegetables and salads, and imaginative, appealing dishes based on these. Alternatives might be offered to all-time favourites: a baked jacket potato with a salad garnish as an option to french fries with the main course.

Healthy catering by stealth has more chance of success than any attempt to corral customers into a better lifestyle unless you are confident of reaching that quite narrow market segment which wants only healthy dishes. Just as high street retailers do with sandwiches and snacks aimed at the lunchtime market, it may work well to brand one or two dishes as healthy choices. But this description could deter sales where the customers are eating out for a celebration, leisure or entertainment. Fashion and peer pressure play a powerful role in influencing what is acceptable.

'Bear in mind your customers' approach to food...'

The customers' approach to food is through experience, education, background, sophistication, travel etc. Some people enjoy experimenting, others not. Some enjoy wholegrain pastas, rice and bread, for example, others won't touch them. Healthy catering should not be introduced in such a way that it alienates people.

Even where there is quite strong customer resistance, subtle changes can be introduced over time if necessary to the content, presentation and service of favourite dishes.

ADAPT RECIPES, PREPARATION AND COOKING METHODS

With thought and skill, a substantial contribution can be made to a balanced diet, without loss of flavour or texture, or restricting customer choice. Nor should it jeopardise operating margins. Indeed the process, by encouraging creativity, could lead to improved profits, with high added value yet less expensive ingredients.

There are many practical changes that can be made to the way food is prepared and cooked, which will lead to a healthier choice for your customers. To get the best results, some trialing and experimentation is recommended!

Possibilities include...

Adapt recipes – use alternative flavourings to salt and proprietary products high in salt; reduce quantity of fat/oil; replace butter with olive oil or a mixture of butter and olive oil; thicken with purées of vegetables/fruit/pulses, or potatoes in place of a roux; enrich with lower/reduced fat products; use natural fruit juice to sweeten; use wholemeal with white flour for pastry.

Adjust preparation methods – trim visible fat, remove poultry skin; leave skin on potatoes, vegetables and fruit (to increase fibre content and reduce vitamin loss); use chunky/thick cuts (to reduce fat absorption/vitamin loss).

Selected ingredients – lean cuts and joint of meat; skinless poultry; fish rich in oils beneficial to health (eg salmon, mackerel, herring, trout); white fish (very little fat); prepared dishes that can be oven baked or grilled instead of fried; unsugared breakfast cereals; fruit juices and products in their natural juices/unsweetened; oils, fats and spreads which are high in monounsaturates or polyunsaturates; pre-prepared and convenience products which are low in salt/sugar/fat.

Change to low-fat cooking methods – grill, bake, poach, microwave, stir-fry (quick cooking, minimum oil), shallow fry in non-stick pans (to use less oil), steam chips to blanch.

For vegetables, favour cooking methods which reduce vitamin loss – steam or microwave or stir-fry, cook in small batches (to reduce hot holding time).

MARKETING AND PRESENTATION

Describe dishes and menu choices in ways which will appeal to your customers. Avoid terms like 'health', 'low in fat', 'low in saturates', especially if your customers are eating out for enjoyment. Emphasise the positive: unusual flavours and combinations, freshly cooked, tasty, satisfying, interesting textures, colourful garnishes, exotic ingredients, associations with foreign travel, ethnic cuisines, etc.

Feature as dishes of the day, special promotions, house specialities, and in counter and buffet display those dishes which have been prepared and cooked according to healthy catering guidelines. Expand the choice of accompaniments and sauces to give appealing, healthier alternatives to those which are high in fat or sugar. Choose garnishes which increase the starch, fibre, vegetable and/or fruit content.

Package healthy additions in the price, such as a granary or wholemeal roll with soup, fresh fruit with a sandwich or lunch-time snack, rice or Naan bread with a curry. Select healthy choices for promotional offers.

Involve your staff: brief them on the dish content so that descriptions are appealing and accurate, and questions can be answered helpfully.

Take care not to use misleading or false descriptions, or terms which have a specific legal meaning under the food labelling regulations, such as 'low fat', 'reduced fat', 'low salt'.

FURTHER REFERENCE

Catering for Health – A guide to teaching healthier catering practices is available through the Food Standards Agency publications, PO Box 367, Hayes, Middlesex, UB3 1UT.

The national diet and nutrition survey, 1st June 2000

This survey conducted by the Department of Health, sampled over 1700 young people, representative of the UK population as a whole. Their physical measurement patterns of food consumption and levels of physical activity over a period of a week were measured. The main findings were that young people were eating insufficient amounts of fruit and vegetables to maintain a balanced diet, resulting in serious shortages of bone strengthening minerals in both males and females which could result in osteoporosis in later life. Lack of iron in the oldest girls suggests anaemia is a major problem; lack of zinc contributes to an overall deterioration of health and the immune system.

SALT

Intake of salt, excluding additions during cooking and at the table, were on average twice the government recommendations.

Salt consumption is known to be a risk factor for increased levels of blood pressure.

The most popular foods – white bread, savoury snacks, chips, biscuits, boiled, mashed and jacket potatoes and chocolate confectionery. The most commonly consumed meats were chicken and turkey.

The government guidelines are to consume at least five portions of fruit or vegetables a day. Not only are these sources of a range of vitamins and minerals, they also provide fibre and naturally occurring energy in the form of glucose. High fruit and vegetable consumption is recognised as a significant protective factor against the development of heart disease and some cancers. It also assists in weight maintenance. It is essential that all children develop the habit of consuming a wide range of fruits and vegetables on a daily basis in order to maintain good health in adult life.

VEGETARIANS

10% of 15–18 years old girls claimed to be vegetarian or vegan.

Vegetarians, especially vegans, need to carefully balance their menus to ensure that they do not go short of iron, vitamin B12, zinc, vitamin D and calcium. The less restricted the diet the better. Vegetarians have a lower risk of heart disease, stroke, diabetes, gallstones, kidney stones and colon cancer, they are also less likely to become overweight or to have raised cholesterol levels.

Figure 6.10 *Which foods in this bun are healthy and which are unhealthy?*

YOU ARE WHAT YOU EAT

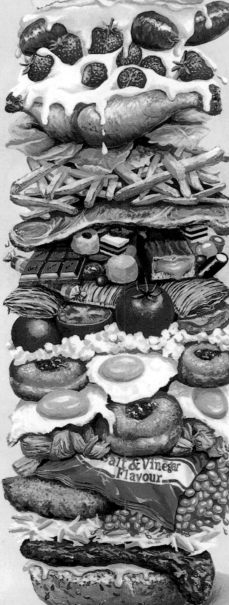
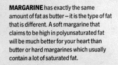

WHITE BREAD ROLLS. It's a good idea to include bread in your daily diet, but choose wholemeal bread whenever possible because it contains more vitamins, minerals and fibre than white bread.

STRAWBERRIES with a yoghurt topping would be far better than with cream because cream contains a lot of saturated fat. Fresh fruit has lots of vitamins and fibre and we should all eat at least one portion a day.

GRILLED OR ROAST CHICKEN with the skin removed is low in fat and therefore good for your heart. Try using chicken as a sandwich filling instead of luncheon meat or cheddar cheese.

FRIED, CRISPY BACON tastes great but so does grilled crispy bacon and this would be much better for your heart. Frying simply coats the bacon with an extra layer of fat. The fat on bacon, like all meat fat, is high in saturated fat and it is best to avoid eating it.

SWEETS AND CHOCOLATES are high in sugar and fat and therefore are not good for your teeth, your appearance or your heart. A piece of fresh fruit such as an apple or tangerine would be a good substitute!

DOUGHNUTS are high in calories and therefore fattening. Deep-fried in oil and then coated in sugar, doughnuts contain very little goodness for all those calories.

TUNA SALAD makes a wonderful filling for a roll or sandwich. Fish is one of the best foods you can eat because it is low in saturated fats and high in protein which helps build healthy growing bodies.

POTATO CRISPS are potatoes with a lot of fat and salt added to them, which is bad for your heart.

COLESLAW is a tasty way of eating vegetables. Try using a low fat mayonnaise or a yoghurt-based dressing on this and other salads.

The British Heart Foundation spends more on heart research than any other charity in Britain. Its aim is to find out what causes heart disease and how it can be prevented.

BRITISH
HEART
FOUNDATION

MARGARINE has exactly the same amount of fat as butter – it is the type of fat that is different. A soft margarine that claims to be high in polyunsaturated fat will be much better for your heart than butter or hard margarines which usually contain a lot of saturated fat.

SAUSAGES AND PIES contain a lot of fat, especially saturated fat, so it's best not to have them too often. A five ounce pork pie contains nearly eight teaspoons of fat, a large sausage almost four teaspoons of fat.

CHEDDAR CHEESE, like many hard cheeses, is high in calcium (essential for the development of strong bones and teeth). It is, however, also rather high in saturated fat, so try to choose a medium or low fat cheese whenever you can.

FRIED CHIPS contain lots of fat, but large chips have less surface area to absorb fat and so contain less fat than french fries. Oven chips usually have less fat than deep fried chips, but a potato baked in its jacket is the best choice of all.

WHOLEWHEAT BREAKFAST CEREALS contain lots of fibre, vitamins and minerals such as iron. Oats, either as porridge or muesli (preferably unsweetened) are also very nutritious.

COTTAGE CHEESE is one of the best cheeses for your heart because it is low in fat, yet still contains lots of calcium as well as protein.

EGGS contain a lot of essential vitamins, minerals and protein but they are also high in cholesterol so it is probably wise to restrict the number you eat to three or four a week.

BAKED BEANS ON TOAST is a healthy nutritious meal. Beans contain lots of fibre and protein and very little fat which makes them a good heart food.

BEEFBURGERS are best when made of lean meat and grilled rather than fried.

BUTTER is high in saturated fat which tends to increase the cholesterol in your blood. This is bad for your heart.

Figure 6.11 *A basic preparation area*

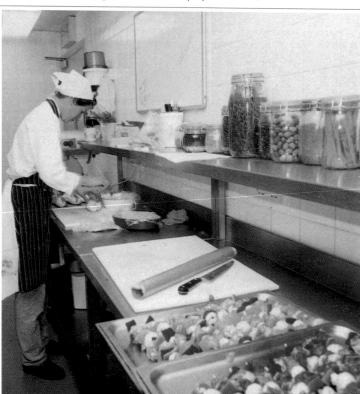

Figure 6.12 *Vacuum Packing*

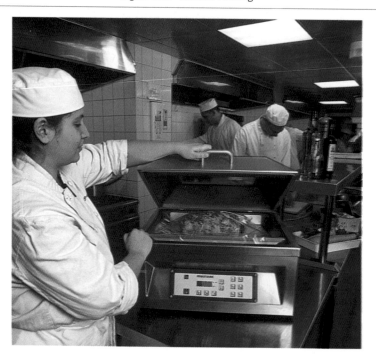

SPECIAL DIETS

DIET	FOODS TO AVOID
Vegetarian and other ethical diets	Meat or fish or any type, or dishes made with or containing the products of animals. *Check for vegetarians who:* – occasionally eat fish and/or meat: *semi-vegetarian or demi-vegetarian* – do not eat milk and dairy products: *ovo-vegetarian* – do not eat eggs: *lacto-vegetarian* – do not eat any food of animal origin (including honey, dairy products, egg): *vegan* (note: vegetables, fruits, grains, legumes, pasta made without eggs, soya products and other products of plans *are* acceptable) – only eat far fruit, nuts and berries: *frutarian or fructarian*
Religious diets	*Muslim:* pork, meat which is not Halal (slaughtered according to custom), shellfish and alcohol (even when used in cooking). *Hindu:* meat, fish or eggs (orthodox Hindus are usually strict vegetarians); less strict Hindus may eat lamb, poultry and fish but definitely not beef as cattle have a deep religious meaning (milk, however, is highly regarded) *Sikh:* beef, pork, lamb, poultry and fish may be acceptable to Sikh men, Sikh women tend to avoid all meat. *Jewish:* pork, pork products, shellfish and eels, meat and milk served at the same time or cooked together; strict Jews eat only Kosher meat; milk and milk products are usually avoided at lunch and dinner (but acceptable at breakfast) *Rastafarian:* all processed foods, pork, fish without fins (eels), alcohol, coffee, tea
Medical diets	*Diabetes:* dishes which are high in sugar and/or fat (low-calorie sweeteners can be used to sweeten desserts) *Low cholesterol and saturated fat:* liver, egg yolks and shellfish (which are high in cholesterol), beef, pork and lamb (which contain saturated fats), butter, cream, groundnut oil, margarine (use oils and margarines labelled high in polyunsaturated fats) *Low fat:* any food which contains fat or has been fried or roasted *Low salt:* foods and dishes which have had salt added in cooking or processing (including smoked and cured fishes and meats and hard cheeses), or contain monosodium glutamate *Low residue:* wholemeal bread, brown rice and pasta, fried and fatty foods. *Milk-free:* milk, butter, cheese, yoghurt and any pre-prepared foods which include milk products (check label) *Nut allergy:* nuts, blended cooking oils and margarine (since these may include nut oil; use pure oils or butter), and any dishes containing these (check label) *Gluten-free:* wheat, wholemeal, wholewheat and wheatmeal flour, wheat bran, rye, barley and oats (some doctors say oats are permitted, the Coeliac Society advises against), and any dishes made with these including pasta, noodles, semolina, bread, pastries, some yoghurts (e.g. museli), some cheese spreads, barley-based drinks, malted drinks, beer, some brands of mustard proprietary sauces made with flour, (use cornflour to thicken; rice, potato, corn and sage are also acceptable).

FURTHER INFORMATION

Health Development Authority, Trevelynan House, 30 Great Peter St, London SW1P 2HW.

Foods containing the various nutrients and their use in the body

NUTRIENT	FOOD IN WHICH IT IS FOUND	USE IN BODY
protein	meat, fish, poultry, game, milk, cheese, eggs, pulses, cereals	for building and repairing body tissues; some heat and energy
fat	butter, margarine, cooking-fat, oils, cheese, fat meat, oily fish	provides heat and energy
carbohydrate	flour, flour products and cereals, sugar, syrup, jam, joney, fruit, vegetables	provides heat and energy
vitamin A	oily fish, fish-liver oil, dairy foods carrots, tomatoes, greens	helps growth; resistance to disease
vitamin B_1 – thiamin	yeast, pulses, liver, whole grain, cereals meat and yeast extracts	helps growth; strengthens nervous system
vitamin B_2 – riboflavin	yeast, liver, meat, meat extracts, whole grain cereals	helps growth, and helps in the production of energy
nicotinic acid (niacin)	yeast, meat, liver, meat extracts, whole grain cereals	helps growth
vitamin C – ascorbic acid	fruits such as strawberries, citrus fruits, green vegetables, root vegetables, salad	helps growth, promotes health
vitamin D (sunshine vitamin)	fish-liver oils, oily fish, dairy foods	helps growth; builds bones and teeth
iron	lean meat, offal, egg yolk, wholemeal flour, green vegetables, fish	building up the blood
calcium (lime)	milk and milk products, bones of fish, wholemeal bread	building bones and teeth, clotting the blood, the working of the muscles
phosphorus	liver and kidney, eggs, cheese, bread	building bones and teeth, regulating body processes
sodium (salt)	meat, eggs, fish, bacon, cheese	prevention of muscular cramp

Special diets

There will be occasions when caterers will be asked to provide some special diets or to cater for a guest with special dietary needs.

The tables on pages 185 and 190 are examples of some of the special diets that a caterer may have to produce.

Today there is a body of opinion amongst the medical profession that suggests that a regular diet of fresh fruit and vegetables can help to eliminate a number of diseases and certain types of cancers. Also it is advisable to reduce fat intake, eat more fish, wholegrain breads, pulses and rice.

It is advisable for the caterer to prepare the meal in close consultation with the individuals concerned. It is also advisable to ensure that all members of the restaurant and kitchen staff are aware of the need to have a sound knowledge of the commodities and raw materials that they are using and the products they are serving to the customer. If in any doubt the restaurant staff should consult the chef. Not only is this good practice but failure to do this could well be life-threatening.

Further information

○ British Nutrition Foundation, High Holborn House, 52–54 High Holborn, London WC1V 6RQ www.nutrition.org.uk

○ Nutrition Society, 10 Cambridge Court, 210 Shepherd's Bush Rd, London W6 7NJ www.nutsoc.org.uk.

FOOD ADDITIVES

These can be divided into 12 categories, and except for purely 'natural' substances, their use is subject to certain legislation.

○ Preservatives: natural ones include salt, sugar, alcohol and vinegar; synthetic ones are also widely used.

○ Colouring agents: natural, including cochineal, caramel and saffron, and many synthetic ones.

○ Flavouring agents: synthetic chemicals to mimic natural flavours (monosodium glutamate to give a meaty flavour to foods).

○ Sweetening: saccharin, sorbitol and aspartame.

○ Emulsifying agents (to stop separation of salad creams, ice-cream, etc.); examples are lecithin and glyceryl monostearate (GMS).

○ Antioxidants: to delay the onset of rancidity in fats due to exposure to air, such as vitamin E and Butylated Hydroxy Toluene (BHT).

○ Flour improvers: to strengthen the gluten in flour, such as vitamin C.

○ Thickeners: animal (gelatine); marine (agar-agar); vegetable (gum tragacanth (used for pastillage), pectin; synthetic products.

○ Humectants: to prevent food drying out, such as glycerine (used in some icings).

○ Polyphosphate: injected into poultry before rigor mortis develops; it binds water to the muscle and thus prevents 'drip', giving a firmer structure to the meat.

○ Nutrients: vitamins and minerals added to breakfast cereals, vitamins A and D added to margarine.

○ Miscellaneous: anticaking agents added to icing sugar and salt; firming agents (calcium chloride) added to tinned fruit and vegetables to prevent too much softening in the processing; mineral oils added to dried fruit to prevent stickiness.

Further information

Food Standards Agency, Room No 213 Whitehall Place (East Block), London SW1A 2HH.

FOOD SPOILAGE

Unless foods are preserved they deteriorate; therefore, to keep them in an edible condition it is necessary to know what causes food spoilage. In the air there are certain micro-organisms called moulds, yeasts and bacteria which cause foods to go bad.

Moulds

These are simple plants which appear like whiskers on foods, particularly sweet foods, meat and cheese. To grow, they require warmth, air, moisture, darkness and food; they are killed by heat and sunlight. Moulds can grow where there is too little moisture for yeasts and bacteria to grow, and will be found on jams and pickles.

Although not harmful they do cause foods to taste musty and to be wasted – the top layer of a jar of jam should be removed if it has mould on it.

Correct storage in a dry cold store prevents moulds from forming.

Not all moulds are destructive. Some are used to flavour cheese (stilton, roquefort) or to produce antibiotics (penicillin, streptomycin).

Yeasts

These are single-cell plants or organisms larger than bacteria, which grow on foods containing moisture and sugar. Foods containing only a small percentage of sugar and a large percentage of liquid, such as fruit juices and syrups, are liable to ferment because of yeasts. Although they seldom cause disease, yeasts do increase food spoilage; foodstuffs should be kept under refrigeration or they may be spoiled by yeasts. Yeasts are also destroyed by heat. The ability of yeast to feed on sugar and produce alcohol is the basis of the beer and wine-making industry.

Bacteria

Bacteria are minute plants, or organisms, which require moist, warm conditions and a suitable food to multiply. They spoil food by attacking it, leaving waste products, or by producing poisons in the food.

Their growth is checked by refrigeration and they are killed by heat. Certain bacterial forms (spores) are more resistant to heat than others and require higher temperatures to kill them.

Pressure cooking destroys heat-resistant bacterial spores provided the food is cooked for a sufficient length of time, because increased pressure increases the temperature; therefore heat-resistant bacterial spores do not affect canned foods as the foods are cooked under pressure in the cans. Acids are generally capable of destroying bacteria, such as vinegar in pickles.

Dehydrated foods and dry foods do not contain much moisture and, provided they are kept dry, spoilage from bacteria will not occur. If they become moist then bacteria can multiply: if dried peas are soaked and not cooked the bacteria present can begin to multiply.

Other causes

Food spoilage can occur due to other causes, such as by chemical substances called enzymes, which are produced by living cells. Fruits are ripened by the action of enzymes; they do not remain edible indefinitely because other enzymes cause the fruit to become over-ripe and spoil.

When meat and game are hung they become tender; this is caused by the enzymes. To prevent enzyme activity going too far, foods must be refrigerated or heated to a temperature high enough to destroy the enzymes. Acid retards the enzyme action – lemon juice prevents the browning of bananas or apples when they are cut into slices.

The acidity and alkalinity of foods

The level of acidity or alkalinity of a food is measured by its pH value. The pH can range from 1 to 14, with pH7 denoting neutral (neither acid nor alkaline).

Most micro-organisms grow best at near neutral pH. Bacteria (particularly harmful ones) are less acid tolerant than fungi, and no bacteria will grow at pH less than 3.5. Spoilage of high acid foods such as fruit is usually caused by yeasts and moulds. Meat and fish are more susceptible to bacterial spoilage, since their pH is nearer neutral.

The pH may be lowered so that the food becomes too acidic (less than pH1.5) for any micro-organisms to grow, such as the use of vinegar in pickling. In the manufacture of yogurt and cheese, bacteria produce lactic acid; this lowers the pH, and retards the growth of food poisoning and spoilage organisms.

Figure 6.13 *The pH range in some foods*

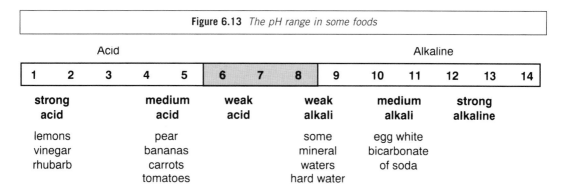

FOOD ALLERGIES

Some people are allergic to some foods which, when handled or eaten, cause an allergic reaction which may prevent employment because they cannot handle the item (tomatoes which may cause a rash), or they become ill and in a small number of cases they die. Only in rare cases is it fatal.

Foods which may cause an allergic reaction to a very small number of people include milk and dairy products, fish, shellfish, eggs and nuts (particularly peanuts but also cashew, pecan, Brazil and walnuts). Peanuts are often commonly used in Bombay mix, peanut butter, satay sauce, nut-coated cereals, groundnut and arachide oils, salted peanuts, chopped nuts, vegetarian dishes and salads containing nuts etc and fresh fruit.

The Anaphylaxis Campaign has warned caterers to be on the alert for foods containing flour made from lupin seeds as this can cause an allergic reaction similar to that of peanuts. Lupin flour is widely used as an ingredient in France, Holland and Italy because of its nutty taste, attractive yellow colour and because it is guaranteed GM free.

Persons suffering an allergy to nuts need to know if and where they are used.

Food allergies are on the increase and can cause death, warns the Food Standards Agency. It has launched a major campaign warning caterers to tell customers exactly what is in their food.

Further information

British Allergy Foundation, St Bart's Hospital, London EC1A 7BE.

Some special diets

TYPE OF DIET	PROBLEMS	FOODS TO AVOID	PERMITTED FOODS
Coeliac	An allergy to gluten. Results in severe inflammation of the gastro-intestinal tract, pain and diarrhoea, and malnutrition due to inability to absorb nutrients.	All products made from wheat, barley or rye, this includes bread. Always check the label on all commercial products.	Potatoes, rice and flours made from potatoes and rice. Also cornflour, fresh fruit and vegetables.
Food allergies	Individuals can suffer severe and rapid reactions to any food which can be fatal. Common allergies are to peanuts and their derivatives, sesame seeds, cashew nuts, pecan nuts, walnuts, hazel nuts, milk, fish, shellfish and eggs.	Peanuts, chopped nuts, groundnut oil, satay sauce, arachide oil, peanut products and other nut products.	
Low cholesterol	High levels of cholesterol circulating in the bloodstream are associated with an increased risk of cardiovascular disease.	Liver, kidney, egg yolks, fatty meats, bacon, ham, pâté, fried foods, pastry, cream, full fat milk, full fat yoghurt, cheeses, salad dressings, biscuits, cakes.	Lean meat and fish grilled or poached, fresh fruit and vegetables, low fat milk, low fat yogurt, porridge, muesli.
Diabetic	The body is unable to control the level of glucose in the blood. This can lead to comas and long-term problems such as increased risk of cardiovascular disease, blindness and kidney problems.	As above plus high sugar dishes.	As above plus wholemeal bread, pasta, rice, potatoes, pulses.

Further information

HCIMA Technical brief No 43.

http://zingsolutions.com/food/hiddenz.htm

http://www.hiaid.nih.gov/factsheets/food.htm

http://www.foodallergy.org/questions.html

Keeping up-to-date

Changes are occurring constantly regarding food production and manufacture which may affect the use of foods in the kitchen. Consumers' reaction to reports of changes published in the press or seen or heard on the TV or radio may affect demand. Similarly information about nutritional values can affect customers' preferences and thus cause trends and affect menu selection.

It is therefore essential to be aware of these reports and when necessary to act according to government recommendations. An example of research which has affected kitchen practice has been the use of eggs. In recent years, the rise in fatalities from bacteria such as BSE and E. coli has led to renewed concern and scrutiny of food production techniques.

Recommendations and contradictions produced by dietetic research can cause trends and affect consumer habits. The use of butter and margarine is such an example.

It is essential to keep up to date through the media and adopt a commonsense attitude to the comments made but to take action when serious recommendations are made by valid research bodies.

METHODS OF PRESERVATION

Foods may be preserved by:
○ removing the moisture from the food – drying, dehydration;
○ making the food cold – chilling, freezing;
○ applying heat – canning, bottling;
○ radiation, using X- or gamma-rays;
○ chemical means – salting, pickling, crystallising;
○ vacuum packing;
○ smoking;
○ chemical;
○ gas storage.

Drying or dehydration

This method of preserving is achieved by extracting the moisture from the food, thus preventing moulds, yeasts and bacteria from growing. In the past this was done by drying foods, such as fruits, in the sun; today many types of equipment are used, and the food is dried by the use of air at a regulated temperature and humidity.

FREEZE DRYING

This is a process of dehydration whereby food requires no preservation or refrigeration yet, when soaked in water, regains its original size and flavour. It can be applied to every kind of food. The food is frozen in a cabinet, the air is pumped out and the ice vaporised. This is called freeze drying and it is the drying of frozen foods by sublimation under conditions of very low pressure. Sublimation is the action of turning from solid to gas without passing through a liquid stage; in this case it is ice to steam without first turning to water.

When processed in this way the food does not lose a great deal of its bulk, but it is very much lighter in weight. When water is added the food gives off its natural smell.

ADVANTAGES OF DRYING

○ If kept dry, food keeps indefinitely.
○ Food preserved by this method occupies less space than food preserved by other methods. Some dried foods occupy only 10% of the space that would be required when fresh.
○ Dried foods are easily transported and stored.
○ The cost of drying and the expenses incurred in storing are not as high as other methods of preservation.
○ There is no waste after purchase, therefore portion control and costing are simplified.

FOODS PRESERVED BY DRYING

○ Vegetables: peas, onions, beetroot, beans, carrots, lentils, cabbage, mixed vegetables, potatoes;
○ Herbs; eggs; milk; coffee;
○ Fruits: apples, pears, plums (prunes), apricots, figs, grapes (sultanas, raisins, currants);
○ Meat; fish.

VEGETABLES

Many vegetables are dried; those most used are the pulse vegetables (beans, peas and lentils) which are used for soups, vegetable purées and many vegetarian dishes. Usually potatoes are cooked, mashed and then dried. The other dried vegetables are used as a vegetable (cabbage, onions).

Pulse vegetables may be soaked in water before use, then washed before being cooked. Vegetables which are dehydrated (having a lower content of water as more moisture has been extracted) are soaked in water.

Dehydrated potatoes are in powder form and are reconstituted with water, milk, or milk and water. They often have manufactured vitamin C added as dehydration results in loss of vitamin C.

HERBS

Fresh herbs are tied into bundles and allowed to dry out in a dry place.

FRUITS

Sultanas, currants and raisins are dried grapes which have been dried in the sun or by hot air. Figs, plums, apricots, apples and pears are also dried by hot air. Apples are usually peeled and cut in rings or diced and then dried.

All dried fruits must be washed before use, and fruits such as prunes, figs, apricots, apples and pears are cooked in the water in which they are soaked.

Little flavour or food value is lost when drying fruits, with the exception of loss of vitamin C.

MILK

Milk is dried either by the roller or spray process. With the roller method the milk is poured onto heated rollers which cause the water to evaporate; the resulting powder is then scraped off. This method is not widely used now as it damages the milk proteins and results in a less soluble dried product, which is more difficult to reconstitute. With the spray process the milk is sent through a fine jet as a spray into hot air, the water evaporates and the powder drops down. The temperature is controlled so that the protein in the milk is not cooked.

Milk powder may be used in place of fresh milk mainly for economic purposes (especially skimmed milk powder) and is used for making custard and white sauce.

EGGS

Eggs are dried in the same way as milk, and although they have a food value similar to fresh eggs, dried eggs do not have the same aerating quality. When reconstituted the eggs should be used at once; if they are left in this state in the warm atmosphere of a kitchen, bacteria can multiply and food poisoning may result; although pasteurised before drying, the mixture may be contaminated in the kitchen and it is a very suitable food for the growth of bacteria. Dried eggs are mainly used in the bakery trade.

Chilling and freezing *(see also pages 271 and 283)*

Refrigeration is a method of preservation where the micro-organisms in food are not killed; they are only prevented from multiplying. The lower the temperature the longer foods will keep. Refrigerators kept at a temperature between 0–7°C (32–45°F) prevent foods from spoiling for only a short time; most frozen foods can be kept at −17°C (1°F) for a year and at −28°C (–18°F) for two years. Foods must be kept in a deep freeze until required for use.

Cold chilled storage of fresh foods merely retards the decay of the food; it does not prevent it from eventually going bad. The aim of chilling is to slow down the rate of spoilage; the lower the chill temperature within the range −1°C (30°F) and +8°C (46°F) the slower the growth of micro-organisms and the biochemical changes which spoil the flavour, colour, texture and nutritional value of foods. Lowering the temperature to this range also reduces food poisoning hazards although it is important to remember that the food must not be contaminated before chilling.

If food is frozen slowly, large uneven crystals are formed in the cells. The water in each cell contains the minerals which give flavour and goodness to food; if food is frozen slowly, the minerals are separated from the ice crystals which break through the cells; on thawing, the goodness and flavour drain away. Quick-freezing is satisfactory because small ice crystals are formed in the cells of food; on thawing, the goodness and flavour are retained in the cells.

MEAT

○ Chilling – meat which is chilled is kept at a temperature just above freezing-point and will keep for up to 1 month, if the atmosphere is controlled with carbon dioxide the time can be extended to 10 weeks.

○ Freezing – imported lamb carcasses are frozen; beef carcasses are not usually frozen because owing to the size of the carcass it takes a long time to freeze and this causes ice crystals to form which, when thawed, affect the texture of the meat; frozen meat must be thawed before it is cooked.

QUICK-FREEZING OF RAW FOODS AND COOKED FOODS

During the cooking and freezing process, foods undergo physical and/or chemical changes. If it is found that these changes are detrimental to the product, then recipe modification is required. The following products require some modification: sauces, casseroles, stews, cold desserts, batters, vegetables, egg dishes.

Conventional recipes normally use wheat flour for thickening, but in the cook-freeze system this will not give an acceptable final product because separation of the solids from the liquids in the sauce will occur if the product is kept in frozen storage for more than a period of several weeks. To overcome this problem it is necessary to use wheat flour in conjunction with any of a number of classically modified starches, such as tapioca starch, waxy maize starch. Many recipes prove successful with a ratio of 50% wheat flour with 50% modified starch.

Rapid freezing of foodstuffs can be achieved by a variety of methods using different types of equipment, for example:

○ plate freezer;

○ blast freezer;

○ low-temperature immersion freezer;

○ still-air cold room;

○ spray freezer (using liquid nitrogen or carbon dioxide) – known as cryogenic freezing this is a method of freezing food by very low temperature; it also freezes food more quickly than any other method; the food to be frozen is placed on a conveyor belt and passed into an insulated freezing tunnel; the liquefied nitrogen or carbon dioxide is injected into the tunnel through a spray, and vaporises, resulting in a very rapid freezing process;

○ freeze flow – this is a system which freezes food without hardening it.

FOODS WHICH ARE FROZEN

A very wide variety of foods are frozen, either cooked or in an uncooked state.

○ Cooked foods: whole cooked meals; braised meat; vol-au-vents; éclairs; cream sponges; puff pastry items.

○ Raw foods: fillets of fish; fish fingers; poultry; peas; French beans; broad beans; spinach; sprouts; broccoli; strawberries; raspberries; blackcurrants.

With most frozen foods, cooking instructions are given; these should be followed to obtain the best results.

Fillets of fish may be thawed out before cooking; vegetables are cooked in their frozen state. Fruit is thawed before use and as it is usually frozen with sugar the fruit is served with the liquor.

ADVANTAGES OF USING FROZEN FOODS

○ Frozen foods are ready-prepared, therefore saving time and labour.

○ Portion control and costing are easily assessed.

○ Foods are always 'in season'.

○ Storage is compact.

○ Additional stocks are to hand.

○ Quality is guaranteed.

○ Very little vitamin C is lost from fruits and vegetables even after several months in a deep freeze.

Canning and bottling

Bottled and canned foods are sealed in airtight bottles or tins and heated at a high enough temperature for a sufficient period of time to destroy harmful organisms.

Dented cans which do not leak are safe to use, but blown cans, that is those with bulges at either end, must not be used.

Tinned hams are canned at a low temperature in order to retain their flavour and avoid excessive shrinkage in the can and therefore should be stored in a refrigerator and consumed soon after purchase. Other tinned foods are kept in a dry, cool place and the table below indicates the advised storage time.

Foods are canned in tins of various sizes (see the table over).

Storage of tinned foods

TYPE OF TINNED FOOD	ADVISED STORAGE TIME
fruit	up to 12 months
milk	up to 12 months
vegetables	up to 2 years
meat	up to 5 years
fish in oil	up to 5 years
fish in tomato sauce	up to 1 year

Tin sizes

SIZE	APPROX. WEIGHT	USE
	142 g	baked beans, peas
	227 g	fruits, meats, vegetables
A1	284 g	baked beans, soups, vegetables, meats, pilchards
14Z	397 g	fruits, vegetables
A2	567 g	fruits, vegetables, fruit and vegetable juices
A2$\frac{1}{2}$	795 g	fruits, vegetables
A10	3079 g	fruits, vegetables, tongues

The advantages of canned foods are similar to those of frozen foods, but a disadvantage is that due to the heat processing a proportion of the vitamin C and B_1 (thiamin) may be lost.

Preservation by salting and smoking

SALTING

Micro-organisms cannot grow in high concentrations of salt. This method of preservation is used mainly to preserve meat and fish, and the advantage lies chiefly in the fact that a wider variety of dishes with different flavours can be put on the menu.

The salt added to butter and margarine and also to cheese acts as a preservative.

MEATS

Meats which are salted or 'pickled' in a salt solution (brine) are brisket, silverside of beef, ox tongues, legs of pork.

FISH

Fish are usually smoked as well as being salted and include: salmon, trout, haddock, herrings.

The amount of salting varies. Bloaters are salted more than kippers and red herrings more than bloaters.

SMOKING

The difference between smoke cooking and curing

Smoke cooking is done at higher temperatures in order to cook the meat. Smoke curing is really just smoking cured meat or sausage. Although smoking meat does provide some preservative effect, it alone is not sufficient to allow long term storage.

Smoke is a very complex material, with upward of 200 components that include alcohols, acids, phenolic compounds, and various toxic, sometimes carcinogenic substances. The toxic substances inhibit the growth of microbes, and the phenolics retard fat oxidation, and the whole complex imparts the characteristic flavour of burning wood to the meat or fish or vegetables.

The temperature of smoke cooking meat

The temperature is very important, there are a variety of different smokes on the market all with temperature guides, some recommend 93°C–104°C, 200–220°F.

Temperature control is very important, excess heat will melt the fat and leave a dry product.

Examples of woods used for smoking

Alder

The traditional wood for smoking salmon in the Pacific Northwest, alder also works well with other fish. It has a light delicate flavour.

Apple and Cherry

Both woods produce a slightly sweet, fruity smoke that is mild enough for chicken or turkey, but capable of favouring a ham.

Hickory

Hickory is the king of the woods. The strong, hearty taste is perfect for pork shoulder and ribs, but it also enhances any red meat or poultry.

Maple

Mildly smoky and sweet, maple mates well with poultry, ham and vegetables.

Mesquite

It's great for grilling because it burns very hot, but below average for barbecuing for the same reason. Also, the smoke taste turns from tangy to bitter over an extended cooking time.

Oak

If hickory is the king of barbecue woods, oak is the queen. The most versatile of hardwoods, blending well with a wide range of flavours.

Pecan

Pecan burns cool and offers a subtle richness of character.

Grapevines

Very distinctive aroma, ideal for grilling food.

The smoking process

Before smoking commences, the raw meat or fish is either dry salted or soaked in brine. In hot countries the salting is still used for the purpose of preservation, but in more temperate climates the salt is used only as a seasoning.

During smoking, weight loss occurs in the product, due to evaporation of water content from within the flesh of the meat or fish. This weight loss is essential to successful smoking. It follows that the greater the weight loss the greater the keeping qualities. Today flavour tends to be more important than keeping qualities so it is better to create humid conditions to produce a succulent product.

Hot and cold smoking

Cold smoking flavours but does not cook the product. It is usually carried out at a temperature between 10°C–29°C, 50°F–85°F. Some cold smoked products are eaten without further cooking e.g. salmon, beef fillet, halibut and cods' roes, whereas others such as haddock, herring (kippers) and cod fillets require a further period of cooking, although obviously not such as a completely raw product as the cooking process has already been started.

Hot smoked products after salting or brining are first cold smoked to partially dry them out and to impart a smoked flavour. In the case of fish the temperature is then raised to 93°C–104°C, 200–240°F and the fish are then cooked. Care must be taken during the initial cold smoking to see that the temperature does not exceed 26°C, 85°F, as this will harden the outside and stop further smoke penetration. Again, during hot smoking, temperatures must be monitored to see that the fish do not become overcooked. Herbs and spices may be incorporated into the smoking process.

Preservation by sugar

A high concentration of sugar prevents the growth of moulds, yeasts and bacteria. This method of preservation is applied to fruits in a variety of forms: jams, marmalades, jellies, candied, glacé and crystallised.

○ Jams are prepared by cooking fruit and sugar together in the correct quantities to prevent the jam from spoiling. Too little sugar means the jam will not keep.

○ Jellies, such as redcurrant jelly, are prepared by cooking the juice of the fruit with the sugar.

○ Marmalade is similar to jam in preparation and preservation, citrus fruits being used in place of other fruits.

○ Candied fruit is made when the peel of such fruit as orange, lemon, grapefruit and lime, and also the flesh of pineapple, are covered with hot syrup; the syrup's sugar content is increased each day until the fruit is saturated in a very heavy syrup, then it is allowed to dry slowly.

○ Crystallised fruit is made following candying. It is left in fresh syrup for 24 hours and then allowed to dry slowly until crystals form on the fruit. Angelica, ginger, violet and rose petals are prepared in this way.

○ Glacé fruit, usually cherries, is first candied, then dipped in fresh syrup to give a clear finish.

Preservation by acids *(see page 189 for explanation of pH)*

Foods may be preserved in vinegar, which is acetic acid (ethanoic acid) diluted with water. In the UK, malt vinegar is most frequently used, although distilled or white wine vinegar is used for pickling white vegetables such as cocktail onions and also for rollmops (herrings).

Foods usually pickled in vinegar are: gherkins, capers, onions, shallots, walnuts, red cabbage, mixed pickles and chutneys.

Preservation by chemicals

A number of chemicals are permitted by law to be used to preserve certain foods such as sausages, fruit pulp, jam. For domestic fruit bottling, Campden preserving tablets can be used.

Preservation by gas storage

Gas storage is used in conjunction with refrigerators to preserve meat, eggs and fruit. Extra carbon dioxide added to the atmosphere surrounding the foods increases the length of time they can be stored. Without the addition of gas these foods would dry out more quickly.

Preservation by radiation
WHAT IS IRRADIATION?

Foods are exposed to ionising radiation which transfers some of its energy as it passes through the food, killing the pathogenic bacteria, which would otherwise make the food unsafe to eat, or at lower doses the spoilage bacteria, which cause food to rot. Ionising radiation is electromagnetic like radio waves, infrared light or ultraviolet light. It is similar to ultraviolet radiation but has a higher frequency and much greater energy. This is sufficient to protect food effectively, but not enough to make it radioactive.

Irradiation methods have other key advantages over heating, chilling and chemical preservation methods.

○ Irradiation works well with frozen or heat-sensitive products, as it does not cause any significant increase in temperature.

○ Packaged products can be sterilised in the final pack, thus preventing contamination.

○ Irradiation has a minimal impact on the nutritional value of the food. Proteins and carbohydrates are unaffected.

○ Irradiation processing is a clean technology. No chemical additives are used or residues left behind in the food and the process does not contaminate or damage the environment.

The chemical changes caused in the food by the ionising radiation are in general much less severe than those arising from other food processing methods such as cooling and heating.

At present 36 countries allow irradiation of about thirty individually specified foods. In 21 of these countries there are active commercial food irradiative plants.

The Food Labelling (Amendment) (Irradiated Food) Regulations 1990 came into force on 1 January 1991 in parallel with those regulations setting out the controls on irradiation. The regulations require all foods which have been irradiated to carry an indication of treatment using the specified words 'irradiated' or 'treated with ionising radiation'.

Vacuum packing

There are two distinct methods in which vacuum packaging can be incorporated into kitchen procedures.

The first process relates to preparation and preservation.

The second is a process of cooking sous vide and is a process of preparation, sealing inside a pouch or bag, cooking at low temperatures followed by rapid chilling and storage at no more than 2°C.

BENEFITS TO THE CATERER

Reduced dehydration and drip loss

Weight loss can be considerably reduced when meat is vacuum packed and when this also cuts out the need to trim, financial benefits are significant.

Increased storage life

Use by times can be extended on chill items (5°C maximum) as follows:

Fresh meat	14 days
Cheese	14 days
Fruit and vegetables	7 days
Fish	7 days

Increased hygiene and reduced cross contamination

Vacuum pouches provide external barriers and will ensure food is protected in a hygienic condition, unaffected by any cross contamination after packaging.

Improved workflow

In any restaurant, there will inevitably be periods of time which are quiet. To spend that time vacuum packaging is not only an excellent use of your staff but also helps to relieve the workload when staff are busy. Vacuum packaging will make optimum use of all available time by helping to even out the workload.

Pre-packaging

Food may be pre-portioned and vacuum packed without the pressure of time, accurate weights and a reduction of waste should be obtained. The food can be kept chilled until wanted. This also allows planning to take place for banquets and can help overcome labour shortages at weekends and through holidays.

Wastage

Vacuum packaging in advance can help minimise waste.

Satellite kitchens

These can readily be supplied with vacuum packed portions, eliminating the need for preparation in several areas.

Bulk buying

Many foods like meat and fish are affected by burn or dehydration in the freezer. The protective qualities of a vacuum pouch ensures this problem is eliminated.

PRECAUTIONS

There are certain precautions that the chef has to be aware of when using vacuum packaging. The shelf-life of cooked foods should be kept to a minimum under chilled conditions. Cooked meats and fish should not be packed unless sous vide techniques are used. Stock rotation must be strictly observed. All packs must be clearly labelled with the description of the contents weight, date and use-by date. In the event of any pack becoming blown or leaking, the contents should be immediately opened, examined and repacked only if satisfactory. Strict hygiene, the immediate packing of foodstuffs, and accurate chill conditions are vital parts of the process.

Modified atmosphere packaging (MAP) *(see page 200)*

This is a flexible way of extending the shelf-life of many kinds of fresh foods up to two to three times the normal levels. The method involves replacing the normal surrounding or dead space atmosphere within food packages with specific mixtures of gases or single gases. Its objectives are to inhibit the growth of pathogenic bacteria and moulds and to extend the shelf-lives of chilled and certain ambient food products.

Originally the system was known as Controlled Atmosphere Packaging and was used for retail portioning and packaging of red meat. The method was based on what is now known as the date of packaging+5 days' system using an 80% oxygen/20% carbon dioxide gas mixture. The inert gases used are carbon dioxide, nitrogen and oxygen. They are natural gases like those present in the air but for MAP they are supplied purified and free of bacteria.

○ Carbon dioxide (CO_2) inhibits the growth of pathogenic bacteria at temperatures not exceeding 8°C (46.4°F) for a restricted period. CO_2 does not kill the bacteria but will restrict mould growth over long periods.

○ Nitrogen has a neutral effect on food stuffs and is used in 100% strength for dried and roasted foods, dairy cakes, cream and milk powders. The gas is also used in conjunction with CO_2 as a support gas.

○ Oxygen sustains basic metabolism and prevents spoilage caused by anaerobic bacteria. It is also used in MAP gas mixtures for packaging red meats where it preserves the red colour of the meat.

MAP effectively increases the length of time certain foods can be stored in the refrigerator. The gas mixtures used vary according to the product being packaged. MAP is particularly successful with bakery products where elevated CO_2 content permits high relative humidities with negligible mould growth.

Chefs employed in large food production operations and those employed as development chefs use MAP to aid food preparation and quality. Over the next few years we are likely to see further developments in this area as the catering industry becomes more involved in using gases to aid preservation of ingredients.

FURTHER INFORMATION

McCance and Widdowson, *The Composition of Foods* (HMSO).

Manual of Nutrition (HMSO).

Eating for Health (HMSO).

Kilgour, *Science for Catering Students* (Heinemann).

Gaman and Sherrington, *Science of Food* (Pergamon).

Guidelines on Pre-cooked Chilled Foods (HMSO).

Food (Control of Irradiation) Regulation 1990 (HMSO).

Education Department, Unilever Ltd, Unilever House, Blackfriars, London EC4.

RECOMMENDED GAS MIXTURE PERCENTAGES (%) FOR MAP
(based on refrigeration storage)

PRODUCT	OXYGEN (%)	NITROGEN (%)	CARBON DIOXIDE (%)	SHELF-LIFE
red meat	80	–	20	5–8 days
white fish	30	30	40	5–6 days
fatty fish	–	40	60	5–6 days
salmon	20	20	60	5–6 days
poultry	–	75	25	17–18 days
hard cheese	–	–	100	3 weeks
bacon, cooked meats	–	65–80	20–35	3–4 days
bread	–	30–40	60–70	3 weeks
dairy cakes	–	100	–	3 weeks

Health Education Authority, Trevelyan House, 30 Great Peter Street, London SW1P 2HW.

Nutrition Society, 10 Cambridge Court, 210 Shepherd's Bush Rd, London W6 7NJ

Some references to nutrition and food science elsewhere in the book

Topics for Discussion

1   Why is a balanced diet desirable? What do you consider to be necessary to provide a balanced diet?

2   Why do you think trends, fads and fashions occur in our eating? Discuss how you could encourage a positive approach to having healthy eating habits.

3   How has presentation of foods changed and why have these changes come about?

4   What problems are associated with certain people's diets? What specific considerations are there for the diets of children, the elderly, nursing mothers and teenagers?

5   For what reasons may the nutritional value of foods be affected? Discuss examples of how this may occur and how such effects be prevented.

6   Why do food habits, fads, styles etc occur?

7   What are the main source sof nutritional information?

8   Do you consider TV adverts and/or programmes affect peoples diets?

PART 4

Planning, production and service

CHAPTER 7

KITCHEN PLANNING, EQUIPMENT, SERVICES AND ENERGY CONSERVATION

INFLUENCING FACTORS ON DESIGN

Factors which influence kitchen planning and design include

- the size and extent of the menu and the market it serves;
- services – gas, electricity and water;
- labour, skill level of staff;
- amount of capital expenditure, costs;
- use of prepared convenience foods;
- types of equipment available;
- Hygiene and the Food Safety Act of 1990/01–05;
- design and decor;
- multi-usage requirements.

The size and extent of the menu

Before a kitchen is planned, the management must know its goals and objectives in relationship to market strategy. In other words what markets are you aiming at and what style of operation are you going to operate? The menu will then determine the type of equipment you will require in order to produce the products that you know from the market research that the customer is going to buy. You also need to know target numbers that you intend to service.

Services

The designer must know where the services are located and how efficient use can be made of them.

Labour and skill level

What kind of people does the company intend to employ? This will have an effect on the technology and equipment to be installed. The more prepared food used, the more this will effect the overall kitchen design.

Amount of capital expenditure

Most design has to work with a detailed capital budget. Often it is not always possible to design, then worry about the cost afterwards. Finance will very often determine the overall design and acceptability.

Because space is at a premium, kitchens are generally smaller. Equipment is therefore being designed to cater for this trend, becoming more modular and streamlined and generally able to fit into less space. This is seen as a cost-reduction exercise. Labour is a significant cost factor so equipment is being designed for ease of operation, maintenance and cleaning.

Use of prepared convenience foods

A fast-food menu using prepared convenience food will influence the planning and equipping very differently from à la carte or cook-chill kitchen. Certain factors will have to be determined:

- Will sweets and pastries be made on the premises?
- Will there be a need for larder or butcher?
- Will fresh or frozen food or a combination of both be used?

Types of equipment available

The type, amount and size of the equipment will depend on the type of menu being provided. The equipment must be suitably sited. When planning a kitchen, standard symbols are used which can be produced on squared paper to provide a scale design. Computer-aided design (CAD) is now often used.

Hygiene and the Food Safety Act 1990/91/95

Design and construction of the kitchen must comply with the Hygiene and Food Safety Act 1990/91/95. The basic layout and construction should enable adequate space to be provided in all food handling and associated areas for equipment as well as working practices and frequent cleaning to be carried out.

Design and decor

The trend towards provision of more attractive eating places, carried to its utmost perhaps by the chain and franchise operators, has not been without its effect on kitchen planning and design. One trend has been that of bringing the kitchen area totally or partially into view, with the development of back bar type of equipment; for example, where grills or griddles are in full public view and food is prepared on them to order.

While there will be a continuing demand for the traditional heavy duty type of equipment found in larger hotels and restaurant kitchens, the constant need to change and update the design and decor of modern restaurants means that the equipment life is generally shorter, reduced perhaps from ten years to seven or five or even less, to cope with the demand for change and redevelopment.

This has resulted in the generally improved design of catering equipment with the introduction of modular units.

Multi-usage requirements

Round the clock requirements such as in hospitals, factories doing shift work, the police and armed forces, have also forced kitchen planners to consider design of kitchens with a view to their partial use outside peak times. To this end kitchen equipment is being made more adaptable and flexible, so that whole sections can be closed down when not in use, in order to maximise savings on heating, lighting and maintenance.

KITCHEN DESIGN

Kitchens must be designed so that they can be easily managed. The management must have easy access to the areas under their control and have good visibility in the areas which have to be supervised. Large operations should work on separate work floors, for reasons of efficiency and hygiene:

○ Product – raw materials to finished product.
○ Personnel – how people move within the kitchen; for example, staff working in dirty areas (areas of contamination) should not enter areas of finished product, or where blast chilling is taking place.
○ Containers/Equipment/Utensils – equipment should, where possible, be separated out, into specific process areas.
○ Refuse – refuse must be kept separated and should not pass into other areas in order to get to its storage destination.

Product flows

Each section should be subdivided into high risk and contaminated sections. High risk food is that which during the process is likely to be easily contaminated.

Contaminated food is that which is contaminated on arrival before processing: unprepared vegetables, raw meat.

Back tracking or cross-over of materials and product must be avoided.

Work flow

Food preparation rooms should be planned to allow a 'work flow' whereby food is processed through the premises from the point of delivery to the point of sale or service with the minimum of obstruction. The various processes should be separated as far as possible and food intended for sales should not cross paths with waste food or refuse. Staff time is valuable and a design which reduces wasteful journeys is both efficient and cost-effective.

The overall sequence of receiving, storing, preparing, holding, serving and clearing is achieved by:

○ minimum movement;
○ minimal back tracking;
○ maximum use of space;
○ maximum use of equipment with minimum expenditure or time and effort.

Work space

Approximately 4.2 m (15 sq. ft) is required per person; too little space can cause staff to work in close proximity to stoves, steamers, cutting blades, mixers, etc., thus causing accidents. A space of 1.37 m ($4\frac{1}{2}$ ft) from equipment is desirable and aisles must be adequate to enable staff to move safely. The working area must be suitably lit and ventilated with extractor fans to remove heat, fumes and smells.

Working sections

The size and style of the menu and the ability of the staff will determine the number of sections and layout that is necessary. A straight line layout would be suitable for a snack bar whilst an island layout would be more suitable for a hotel restaurant.

Access to ancillary areas

A good receiving area needs to be designed for easy receipt of supplies with nearby storage facilities suitably sited for distribution of foods to preparation and production areas.

Hygiene must be considered so that kitchen equipment can be cleaned and all used equipment from the dining area can be cleared, cleaned and stored. Still room facilities may also be required.

Equipment

The type, amount and size of equipment will depend on the type of menu being provided. Not only should the equipment be suitably situated but the working weight is very important to enable the equipment to be used without excess fatigue. When a kitchen is being planned, standard symbols are used which can be produced on squared paper to provide a scale design. Wash hand facilities and storage of cleaning equipment should not be omitted.

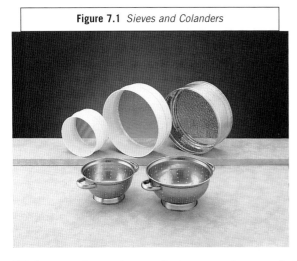

Figure 7.1 *Sieves and Colanders*

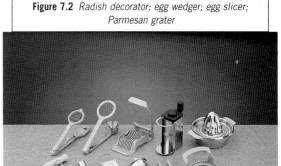

Figure 7.2 *Radish decorator; egg wedger; egg slicer; Parmesan grater*

Kitchen equipment manufacturers and gas and electricity suppliers can provide details of equipment relating to output and size.

The various preparation processes require different areas depending on what food is involved. A vegetable preparation area means that water from the sinks and dirt from the vegetables are going to accumulate and therefore adequate facilities for drainage should be provided. Pastry preparation on the other hand entails mainly dry processes.

Whatever the processes, there are certain basic rules that can be applied which not only make for easier working conditions but which help to ensure that the food hygiene regulations are complied with.

Food preparation areas

Proper design and layout of the preparation area can make a major contribution to good food hygiene. Staff generally respond to good working conditions by taking more of a pride in themselves, in their work and in their working environment.

Adequate work space must be provided for each process and every effort must be made to separate dirty and clean processes. Vegetable preparation and wash up areas should be separate from the actual food preparation and service areas. The layout must ensure a continuous work flow in one direction in order that cross-over of foods and any cross-contamination is avoided. The staff should not hamper each other by having to cross each others' paths more than is absolutely necessary.

Actual work-top areas should be adequate in size for the preparation process and should be so designed that the food handler has all equipment and utensils close to hand.

Accommodation must be based on operational need. The layout of the kitchen must focus on the working and stores area, and the equipment to be employed. These areas must be designed and based on the specification of the operation.

Kitchens can be divided into sections; these must be based on the process:

○ Dry areas: for storage.
○ Wet areas: for fish preparation, vegetable preparation, butchery, cold preparation.
○ Hot wet areas: for boiling, poaching, steaming; equipment needed will include:
  ○ atmospheric steamers;   ○ bratt pans;
  ○ pressure steamers;   ○ steam jacketed boilers.
  ○ combination oven;

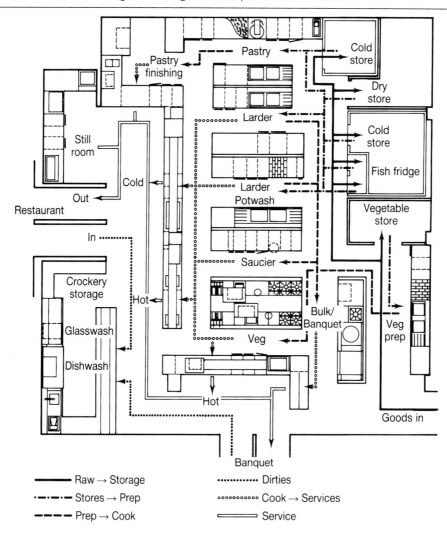

Figure 7.3 *Design for a well-planned basic kitchen*

○ Hot dry areas: for frying, roasting, grilling; equipment needed will include:

○ cool zone fryers;   ○ salamanders;

○ pressure fryers;   ○ induction cookers;

○ bratt pans;   ○ halogen cookers;

○ roasting ovens;   ○ microwave;

○ charcoal grills;   ○ cook and hold ovens.

○ Dirty areas: for refuse, pot wash areas, plate wash; equipment needed will include:

○ compactors;   ○ dishwashers;

○ refuse storage units;   ○ glass washers.

○ pot wash machines;

Size of kitchen and food preparation areas

Size is determined also by purpose and function.

○ The operation is based on the menu and the market it is to service.

○ The design and equipment is based on the market.

○ Consideration must be given to the management policy on buying raw materials. Choice will determine kitchen plans on handling raw materials.

Prepared food will require different types of equipment and labour requirements compared to part-prepared food or raw state ingredients.

Prepared food examples are sous vide products, cook/chill, cook/freeze, prepared sweets. Part-prepared food examples are peeled and cut vegetables, convenience sauces and soups, portioned fish/meat. Raw state food examples are unprepared vegetables, meat which requires butchering, fish requiring filleting and portioning.

Consideration must also be given to the service policy on using all plate service or a mixture of plate and silver service or self-service, and how all this will affect the volume and type of dishwashing.

Planning and layout of the cooking area

Because 'raw materials' enter the cooking section from the main preparation areas (vegetables, meat and fish, dry goods), this section will be designed with a view to continuing the flow movement through to the servery. To this end, roasting ovens for example, are best sited close to the meat preparation area, the steamers adjacent to the vegetable preparation area.

Layout is not, however, just a question of equipment siting and selection, much depends on the type of management policy on the use of prepared foods and the operating cycle. Clearly the cooking section should contain no through traffic lanes, used by other staff to travel from one section to another. The layout should be so planned that raw foodstuffs arrive at one point, are processed in the cooking section and are then despatched to the servery. There should be a distinctive progression in one direction.

As with other areas, the cooking section should be designed with a view to making maximum use of the available area and to provide economy of effort in use.

ISLAND GROUPINGS

In an island arrangement, equipment is placed back-to-back in the centre of the cooking area. There will need to be sufficient space to allow for this, including adequate gangways around the equipment and space to place other items along the walls.

WALL SITING

An alternative arrangement involves siting equipment along walls. This arrangement is possible where travel distances are reduced and normally occurs in smaller premises (or sections thereof).

L- OR U-SHAPED LAYOUTS

L- or U-shaped arrangements create self-contained sections that discourage entry by non-authorised staff and can promote efficient working, with distances reduced between work centres.

When planning the layout of the cooking section the need to allow sufficient space for access to equipment such as ovens should be borne in mind. Opening doors creates an arc that cannot be reduced and the operator must have sufficient room for comfortable and safe access. It is likely also that trolleys will be used for loading and unloading ovens, or rolling tables drawn into position in front of the oven.

THE CHOICE OF LAYOUT

A selection of equipment will be made after detailed consideration of the functions that will be carried out within the cooking area of the kitchen. The amount of equipment will depend upon the complexity of the menus offered, the quantity of meals served, and the policy of use of materials, from the traditional kitchen organisation using only fresh vegetables and totally unprepared items, to the use of prepared foods, chilled items, frozen foods, where the kitchen consists of a regeneration unit only.

Given, however, that a certain amount of equipment is required, the planner has the choice of a number of possible layouts, within the constraints of the building shape and size, and the location of services. The most common are the island groupings, wall siting and the use of an L- or U-shaped layout and variations upon these basic themes.

Siting of equipment

The kitchen operation must work as a system. It is advisable to site items of equipment used for specific functions together. This will help increase efficiency and avoid shortcuts.

Wash hand basins must be sited strategically to encourage frequent hand washing in all food preparation areas. One should be in evidence at each work station.

The kitchen environment

SPACE

The Office, Shop and Railway Premises Act 1963, stipulates 11.32 cu metres (400 cu ft) per person, discounting height in excess of 3 m (10 ft).

HUMIDITY

A humid atmosphere creates side effects such as food deterioration, infestation risk, condensation on walls and slippery floors. Anything higher than 60% humidity lowers productivity. Provision for replacement of extracted air with fresh air is essential.

TEMPERATURE

No higher than 20–26°C (68–79°F) is desirable for maximum working efficiency and comfort with 16–18°C (61–64°F) in preparation areas.

NOISE

Conversation should be possible within 4 m (13 ft).

LIGHT

Minimum legal level in preparation areas is 20 lumens per sq ft with up to 38 lumens preferable in all areas.

VENTILATION

It is estimated by the Health & Safety Executive (HSE) that 65% of commercial kitchens have poor ventilation resulting in health hazards.

Commercial kitchens are a working environment where cooking processes emit large amounts of vapours, impurities and excess heat. These include potential carcinogens such as exhaust gases from live fuel appliances including gas, charcoal and mesquite. The provision of good ventilation in the kitchen areas reduces the risks to health and should enhance the effectiveness and productivity of the kitchen.

Legislation requires that "adequate" ventilation must be provided in commercial kitchens but this cannot be precisely defined in law.

Air should be extracted from kitchen and subsidiary areas at a constant rate. The fresh air which replaces the extracted air should be provided through a separate air intake system. The air intake system should aim to replace all the air extracted from the kitchen, so that only minimal amounts of air are drawn from areas surrounding the kitchen. The amount of air which is extracted from the kitchen should slightly exceed the amount of air which is pumped into the kitchen, maintaining a negative pressure. The way in which a kitchen is ventilated depends on the type of cooking equipment, the cooking processes used and the layout of the kitchen.

AIRFLOW RATES

The rates of extraction recommended for each type of appliance from the manufacturers. This information can then be used to calculate how much air should be extracted from and introduced to the kitchen per minute. Generally the aim should be a complete change of air in the kitchen 20–30 times an hour depending on the type of cooking processes being carried out in the kitchen. It is possible to find recommended air change rates of 120 per hour in small, low ceilinged basement kitchens.

VENTILATION CANOPIES

Canopies over equipment must be of the correct size to effectively capture dirty air from kitchen equipment. The canopy must overhang the cooking appliance on all sides with an overhang within the range of 150–600 mm. The underside of the canopy should be positioned about 2 m above the floor. Canopies are usually made of stainless steel. Filters should be installed within the canopy to remove grease from the air stream. Canopies must be designed to pull fumes away from the cooking oven towards the rear of the cooking unit. For any ventilation system to be effective the correct size of ductwork and fans must be used. The system must also be accessible and easy to clean and maintain.

FURTHER INFORMATION

Technical brief No 30. Kitchen Ventilation HCIMA.

MAINTENANCE

Planning and equipping a kitchen is an expensive investment, therefore to avoid any action by the Environmental Health Officer, efficient, regular cleaning and maintenance is essential. (The Dorchester kitchens are swept during the day, given soap/detergent and water treatment after service and any spillages cleaned up immediately. At night, contractors clean the ceilings, floors and walls.)

Kitchen design industry trends

In most cases throughout the industry, companies are looking to reduce labour costs while maintaining or enhancing the meal experience for the customer. Trends in various situations are given below:

○ Hotels: greater use of buffet and self-assisted service units.
○ Banqueting: move towards plated service, less traditional silver service.
○ Fast food: new concepts coming onto the market, more specialised chicken and seafood courts, more choices in ethnic food.
○ Roadside provision: increase in number of operations, partnerships with oil companies, basic grill menus now enhanced via factory-produced à la carte items.

- Food courts: development has slowed down; minor changes all the time; most food courts offer an 'all day' menu. Restaurant Associates (COMPASS) are introducing food courts into hotels.
- Restaurants/hotels: less emphasis on luxury end, 5-star experience.
- Theme restaurants: will continue to improve and multiply.
- Hospitals: greater emphasis on bought-in freezer and chilled foods; reduced amount of on-site preparation and cooking.
- Industrial: more zero-subsidy staff restaurants, increased self-service for all items; introduction of cashless systems will enable multi-tenant office buildings to offer varying subsidy levels.
- Prisons, institutions: little if any change; may follow hospitals by buying in more preprepared food; may receive foods from multi-outlet central production units, tied in with schools, meals on wheels provision, etc.
- University/colleges: greater move towards providing food courts; more snack bars and coffee shops.

Kitchen equipment trends

- Refrigeration: more concentration on providing CFC-free equipment.
- Environmental: with an environmentally conscious society, energy conservation will feature higher in the development agenda; these will include heat recovery systems, recirculated air systems, improved working conditions and lighting systems.
- Cooking: more use of induction units, combination ovens, microwave and tunnel ovens.
- Servery counters: more decorative units being used.
- Dishwasher/potwash: greater economy of water, more mechanised and automated use of combination machines.
- Ventilation: moves towards integrated wash systems, recirculated air systems, integral air supply, integral fire suppression.

General trend will be towards self-diagnostic equipment and automated service call out. With the use of replacement components, there is less emphasis on repairs.

Consultants

There are a number of specialist consultants involved in kitchen design. Consultants are often used by companies to provide independent advice and specialist knowledge. Their expertise should cover:

- equipment;
- food service systems and methods;
- architectural elements;
- statutory legislation (Food Act, Health and Safety Act, fire regulations);
- green issues/legislation (waste management);
- refrigeration;
- mechanical and electrical services;
- drainage;
- ventilation/air conditioning;
- energy conservation;
- recycling.

Consultants should provide the client with unbiased opinions and expertise not available in their company. Their aim should be to raise the standards of provision, equipment installation, while providing an efficient and effective food production operation which also takes into account staff welfare.

WATER MANAGMENT
LEGISLATION

Each country has its own laws governing the use of water. In the United Kingdom these include Water Industry Act 1991, Health & Safety at Work Act 1974 and Water Supply Bylaw 1989.

The purpose of water law is to:

a discourage undue consumption of water;

b prevent contamination of the water supply.

Substantial savings in water can be made through the renewal and replacement of wasteful older water using equipment.

Self-closing taps reduce water consumption by as much as 55%.

In many countries it is an offence for owners or occupiers of buildings to intentionally or negligently allow any "fitting to waste" or to unduly consume water.

Examples:

○ Taps constantly dripping or left running.

○ Overflows from storage and WC cisterns dripping.

○ Water leaks not repaired.

There is evidence to show that the undertaking of a water management audit can save money. The audit examines and quantifies possible savings.

IMMEDIATE PRACTICAL ACTION

○ Water metering.

○ Tap flow regulator – flow control.

○ Urinals using less water.

○ Shut off device and self closing taps.

○ Automatic or programmed mains shut off device when buildings are not in use.

○ Low flow shower heads.

FURTHER INFORMATION

Water Training International
Burn Hall
Tollerton Road
Huby
Yorkshire
YO6 1JB.

EQUIPMENT DESIGN

The Food Safety (General Food Hygiene) Regulations, 1995, requires all articles, fittings and equipment with which food comes into contact, to be kept clean and be so constructed, of such materials and maintained in such condition and repair as to minimise risk of contamination and enable thorough cleaning and, where necessary, disinfected. Equipment must also be installed in such a way that the surrounding area is able to be cleaned.

Recommendations for equipment

Equipment is preferable with:

○ tubular machinery frames;

○ stainless steel table legs;

○ drain cocks and holes instead of pockets and crevices which could trap liquid;

○ dials fitted to machines having adequate clearance to facilitate cleaning.

Preparation surfaces

The choice of surfaces on which food is to be prepared is vitally important. Failure to ensure a suitable material may provide a dangerous breeding ground for bacteria. Stainless steel tables are the best as they do not rust and their welded seams eliminate unwanted cracks and open joints. Sealed tubular legs are preferable to angular ones because again they eliminate corners in which dirt collects. Tubular legs have often been found to provide a harbourage for pests.

Preparation surfaces should be jointless, durable, impervious, correct height and firm based.

Surfaces must withstand repeated cleaning at the required temperature without premature deterioration through pitting and corrosion.

Choosing cutting boards

Look at the following aspects when choosing cutting boards:

○ Water absorbency: soft woods draw fluids into them and with the fluids, bacteria is also drawn in.

○ Wooden cutting boards made of hard wood if cleaned and sterilised are perfectly acceptable in catering premises.

○ Resistance to stains, cleaning chemicals, heat and food acids.

○ Toxicity: the cutting board must not give off toxic substances.

○ Durability: the cutting board must withstand wear and tear.

○ Cutting boards must not split or warp.

Appearance can be deceptive. Dean Cliver and Afese AK, two researchers at the University of Wisconsin, Madison, USA set out ways of decontaminating wooden kitchen surfaces and ended up finding that such surfaces are pretty good at decontaminating themselves.

When working with wood from nine different species of tree, four sorts of plastic, the results were always the same. They spread salmonella, listeria and *Escherichia coli* over the various samples and left them there for three minutes. The level of bacteria on the plastic remained the same, while the level on the wood plummeted often by as much as 99.9%. Left overnight at room temperature the bacteria on the plastic actually multiplied, while the wooden surfaces cleaned themselves so thoroughly that De Cliver and Ms AK could not record anything from them.

This is because the porous structure of the wood, previously thought to be a disadvantage in soaking up the fluid with the bacteria in it. Once inside the bacteria sticks to the wood's fibres and they are 'strangled' by one of the many noxious anti-microbial chemicals with which living trees protect themselves.

Colour coding

To avoid cross contamination, it is important that the same equipment is not used for handling raw and high risk products without being disinfected. To prevent the inadvertent use of equipment for raw and high risk foods, it is recommended that where possible, different colours and shapes are used to identify products or raw materials used.

Fixing and siting of equipment

Where practicable, equipment should be mobile to facilitate its removal for cleaning, that is castor mounted with brakes on all the wheels.

A guide for stationary equipment

To allow for the cleaning of wall and floor surfaces stationary equipment must be:

○ 500 mm from the walls;
○ 250 mm clearance between the floor and underside of the equipment.

KITCHEN ORGANISATION

The purpose of kitchen organisation is to produce the right quantity of food of the highest standard, for the required number of people, on time, by the most effective use of staff, equipment and materials. Regardless of whether the organisation is simple or complex, the factors which have the greatest effect on the organisation will be the menu and the system used to prepare and present the menu items. For example, a very extensive menu can be offered if much of the *mise-en-place* (preparation prior to service) is prepared throughout the day and kept refrigerated until required at service time. If an establishment has a finishing kitchen for the final preparation and presentation by a small number of skilled cooks, then, with adequate *mise-en-place*, fish, meat, vegetables, potatoes, pastas and eggs, cooked by sautéing, grilling, deep frying and so on, can be completed quickly and efficiently to the benefit of the customer. This system, which has been operated very effectively in some establishments for many years, means that all staff are fully used. The design of the finishing kitchen is important here and needs to include refrigerated cabinets for holding perishable foods, adequate cooking facilities and bain-marie space for holding sauces, etc.

Restaurants which provide a limited menu, such as steak houses, are able to organise very few staff to cope with large numbers of customers to quite a high degree of skill. The required standard can be produced because few skills are needed. Nevertheless an employee producing grilled steaks, pancakes or whatever has to be organised in a systematic way and the flow of the work should be smooth.

Other kinds of establishments which are required to produce large amounts of food to be served at the same time include schools, hospitals, industrial establishments, airlines and departmental stores. Staff have to be well organised and supplied with large-scale preparation and production equipment and the means of finishing dishes quickly. To enable this to happen satisfactorily the preparation-production-freezing or chilling-reheat cycle has been developed, enabling staff to be involved in simply reheating or finishing the foods. It is essential that very high standards of hygiene must be practised in situations using a system of deep freezing or chilling and reheating.

As costs of space, equipment, fuel, maintenance and labour are continually increasing, considerable time, thought and planning have had to be given to the organisation and layout systems of kitchens. The requirements of the kitchen have to be clearly identified with regard to the type of food that is to be prepared, cooked and served. All areas of space and the different types of equipment available must be fully justified and the organisation of the kitchen personnel must also be planned at the same time.

In the late nineteenth century, when labour was relatively cheap, skilled and plentiful, public demand was for elaborate and extensive menus; and in response to this, Auguste Escoffier, one of the most respected chefs of the past era, devised what is known as the *partie* system. The number of parties required and the number of staff in each will depend on the size of the establishment.

With a sound knowledge of fresh, part-prepared and ready prepared foods, together with an understanding of kitchen equipment and planning (see Figure 7.3, page 208), the organisation of a kitchen can be economically and efficiently implemented. Even with two similar kitchens the internal organisation is liable to vary as each person in charge will have their own way of running the kitchen. However, everyone working in the system should know what he or she has to do, and how and when to do it.

The kitchen organisation will vary mainly due to the size and type of establishment. Obviously where a kitchen has 100 chefs preparing banquets for up to 1000 people, a lunch and dinner service for 300 customers with an à la carte menu, and floor service, the organisation will be quite different to a small restaurant serving 30 table d'hôte lunches, or a full-view coffee shop, a speciality restaurant with a busy turnover, or a hospital kitchen.

Figure 7.4 *Example of correct sequence for working methods*

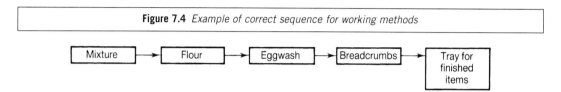

WORKING METHODS

A skilled craftsman or craftswoman is one who, among other things, completes the skill in the minimal time, to the highest standard and with the *least* effort. Effort requires expenditure of energy, and energy is the commodity which needs to be conserved, not wasted, in the kitchen. Any person working in a hot environment, with the stress of working against the clock, needs to get into the habit of working in such a way that energy is not wasted. To achieve this it is necessary to use commonsense and to know how to save energy so that the habit of working methodically and economically becomes second nature (Figure 7.4). This state of mind can be developed by students producing 12 items even though the real effects will only be evident when producing, say, 100 or 500 items.

Simplifying an operation

The objective is to make work easier and this can be achieved by simplifying the operation, eliminating unnecessary movements, combining two operations into one or improving old methods. For example, if you are peeling potatoes and you allow the peelings to drop into the container in the first place, the action of moving the peelings into the bowl and the need to clean the table could have been eliminated. This operation is simplified if, instead of a blunt knife, a good hand potato peeler is used, because it is simple and safe to use, requires less effort, can be used more quickly and requires less skill to produce a better result. If the quantity of potatoes is sufficient, then a mechanical peeler could be used, but it would be necessary to remember that the electricity used would add to the cost and that the time needed to clean a mechanical aid may lessen its work-saving value. If it takes 25 minutes to clean a potato mashing machine which has been used to mash potatoes for 500 meals, it could be time well spent in view of the time and energy saved mashing the potatoes. It may not be considered worthwhile using the machine to mash potatoes for 20 meals. Factors such as this need to be taken into account.

Overcoming fatigue

Working methods may be observed in catering at many different levels, from the experienced methodical chef wiping the knife after cutting a lemon, to the complexity of the Ganymede system in a large hospital or the carefully planned call-order unit in a fast-food operation where, because of careful thought and study, wastage of time, money and materials is reduced to a minimum. But even with the aid of mechanical devices, labour-saving equipment and the extensive use of foods which have been partially or totally prepared, people at work still become fatigued. It is most important to stand correctly, well balanced with the weight of the body divided on to both legs with the feet sensibly spaced and the back reasonably straight when working for long periods in one place. Particular care is needed when lifting: stand with legs apart and bend the knees (not the back) and use the leg muscles to assist lifting. The object to be raised should be held close to the body.

Figure 7.5 *Work flow, incorporating delivery, storage, preparation, cooking and service*

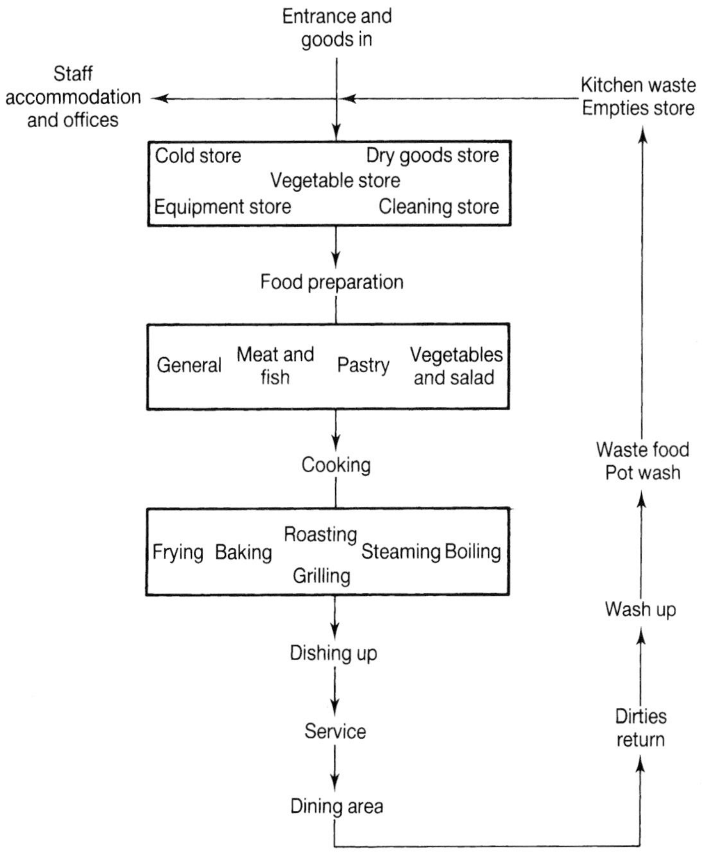

It is possible to cultivate the right attitude to work as well as good working habits. Certain jobs are repetitive, some require considerable concentration, while others cause physical strain; not all work provides equal job satisfaction. If 500 fish cakes have to be shaped it is worthwhile setting targets to complete a certain number in a certain time. Such simple things as not counting the completed items but counting those still to be done motivates some people to greater effort. Some circumstances do not lend themselves to overcoming the physical pressures: for example if 150 people require 150 omelettes then, provided the eggs are broken and seasoned and kept in bulk with the correct size ladle for portioning, the attitude to adopt may be to try to do each omelette better and quicker than the last. If careful thought and study are given to all practical jobs wastage of time, labour and materials can often be eliminated.

Equipment and layout *(Figure 7.3, page 208)*

Properly planned layouts with adequate equipment, tools and materials to do the job are essential if practical work is to be carried out efficiently. If equipment is correctly placed then work will proceed smoothly in proper sequence without backtracking or criss-crossing. Work tables, sinks and stores and refrigerators should be within easy reach in order to eliminate unnecessary walking. Equipment should be easily available during all working times.

The storage, handling of foods, tools and utensils and the movement of food in various stages of production needs careful study. Many people carry out practical work by instinct and often evolve the most efficient method instinctively (Figure 7.4, page 216). Nevertheless careful observation of numerous practical workers will show a great deal of time and effort wasted through bad working methods. It is necessary to arrange work so that the shortest possible distance exists between storage and the place where the items are to be used.

When arranging storage see that the most frequently used items are nearest to hand. Place heavy items where the minimum of body strain is required to move them. Keep all items in established places so that time is not lost in hunting and searching. Adjustable shelving can be a help in organising different storage requirements. Only after all the preplanning of the job is complete comes the actual work itself.

Careful preparation of foods and equipment (a good mise-en-place) is essential if a busy service is to follow and is to be operated efficiently so that orders move out methodically without confusion.

The work to be done must be carefully planned so that the items requiring long preparation or cooking are started first. Where a fast production is required lining up will assist efficiency. Work carried out haphazardly, without plan or organisation, obviously takes longer to do than work done according to plan. There is a sequence to work that leads to high productivity and an efficient worker should learn this sequence quickly.

When French beans are prepared they should all be topped and tailed, then cut – not topping, tailing then cutting each bean separately. When food is cut, articles to be cut should be on the left of the chopping board (for right-handed people), drawn with the left hand to the centre of the board, cut and pushed to the right. This should be a continuous, smoothly flowing process.

Food is often wasted by the use of bad working methods. For example, when spinach is prepared, to tip a whole box of spinach into the sink of water, then pick off the stalks so that they drop back on to the unpicked spinach will always result in waste. This is a bad practice used by careless cooks because three-quarters of the way through the job the contents of the sink (including an amount of good spinach) are thrown away. This can happen in the preparation of other vegetables such as sprouts, potatoes, carrots.

These are just a few examples of how planning and working methodically can save time, energy and materials.

KITCHEN SUPERVISION/MANAGEMENT

The organisation under different industries varies according to their specific requirements and the names given to people doing similar jobs may also vary. Some companies or organisations will require operatives, technicians, technologists, others need crafts people, supervisors and managers. The supervisory function of the technicians, chef de partie or supervisor may be similar.

The hospitality and catering industry is made up of people with craft skills. The crafts person is involved with food production, the chef de partie may be the supervisor, supervising a section or sections of the food production system. The head chef will have both managerial and supervisory skills and he/she will determine the kitchen policies.

Supervisors are involved with the successful deployment of money, material and people.

The primary role of the supervisor is to ensure that a group of people work together to achieve the goals set by the business. Managing physical and human resources to achieve customer service goals requires planning, organising, staffing, directing and controlling.

Supervisors and head chefs need to motivate people, to persuade them to act in certain ways. In the kitchen/restaurant as in any other department staff must first be motivated to follow procedures. This can be done in a positive way by offering rewards, or in a negative way in the catering staff who do not comply with requirements. Both methods can be effective and can be used by supervisors to achieve their goals. One of the mot effective ways is for a supervisor to build a team and offer incentives for good performance. However, staff can become indifferent to repeated schemes such as 'employee of the month'. A good supervisor will attempt to introduce novelty and fun into the reward system.

Supervisory function

Certain leadership qualities are needed to enable the supervisor to carry out his or her role effectively. These qualities include the ability to:

- communicate;
- co-ordinate;
- motivate;
- organise.
- initiate;
- mediate;
- inspire;
- make decisions;

Those under supervision should expect from the supervisor:

- consideration;
- respect;
- understanding;
- consistency;

and in return the supervisor can expect:

- loyalty;
- respect;
- co-operation.

The good supervisor is able to obtain the best from those for whom he or she has responsibility and can also completely satisfy the management of the establishment that a good job is being done.

The job of the supervisor is essentially to be an overseer. In the catering industry the name given to the supervisor may vary – sous-chef, chef de partie, kitchen supervisor or section chef. In hospital catering the name would be sous-chef, chef de partie or kitchen supervisor. The kitchen supervisor will be responsible to the catering manager, while in hotels and restaurants the chef de parties will be responsible to the head chef. The exact details of the job will vary according to the different areas of the industry and the size of the various units, but generally the supervisory role involves three functions: technical; administrative; social.

TECHNICAL FUNCTION

Culinary skills and the ability to use kitchen equipment are essential for the kitchen supervisor. Most kitchen supervisors will have worked their way up through the section or sections before reaching supervisory responsibility. The supervisor needs to be able 'to do' as well as knowing 'what to do' and 'how to do it'. It is also necessary to be able to do it well and to be able to impart some of these skills to others.

ADMINISTRATIVE FUNCTION

The supervisor or chef de partie will, in many kitchens, be involved with the menu planning, sometimes with complete responsibility for the whole menu but more usually for part of the menu, as happens with the larder chef and pastry chef. This includes the ordering of foodstuffs (which is an important aspect of the supervisor's job in a catering establishment) and, of course, accounting for and recording materials used. The administrative function includes the allocation of duties and, in all instances, basic work-study knowledge is needed to enable the supervisor to operate effectively. The supervisor's job may also include the writing of reports, particularly in situations where it is necessary to make comparisons and when new developments are being tried.

SOCIAL FUNCTION

The role of the supervisor is perhaps most clearly seen in staff relationships because the supervisor has to motivate the staff under his or her responsibility. 'To motivate' could be described as the initiation of movement and action; and having got the staff moving the supervisor needs to exert control. Then in order to achieve the required result the staff need to be organised.

Thus the supervisor has a threefold function regarding the handling of staff, namely: to organise, to motivate, to control; this is the essence of staff supervision.

Elements of supervision

The accepted areas of supervision include:

○ forecasting and planning;
○ organising;
○ commanding;
○ co-ordinating;
○ controlling.

Each of these will be considered within the sphere of catering.

FORECASTING

Before making plans it is necessary to look ahead, to foresee possible and probable outcomes and to allow for them. For example, the chef de partie knows that the following day is their assistant's day off, so looks ahead and plans accordingly; when the catering supervisor in the hospital knows that there is a 'flu epidemic and two cooks are feeling below par he or she plans for their possible absence; if there is a spell of fine hot weather and the cook in charge of the larder foresees a continued demand for cold foods, or when an end to the hot spell is anticipated, then the plans are modified. For the supervisor forecasting is the good use of judgement acquired from previous knowledge and experience. For example, because many people are on holiday in August fewer meals will be needed in the office restaurant; no students are in residence at the college hostel, but a conference is being held and 60 meals are required. The Motor Show, bank holidays, the effects of a rail strike or a wet day, as well as less predictable situations, such as the number of customers anticipated on the opening day of a new restaurant, all need to be anticipated and planned for.

PLANNING

From the forecasting comes the planning: how many meals to prepare; how much to have in stock (should the forecast not have been completely accurate); how many staff will be needed; which staff and when. Are the staff capable of what is required of them? If not, the supervisor needs to plan some training. This, of course, is particularly important if new equipment is installed. Imagine an expensive item, such as a new type of oven, ruined on the day it is installed because the staff have not been instructed in its proper use; or, more likely, equipment lying idle because the supervisor may not like it, may consider it is sited wrongly, does not train staff to use it, or for some similar reason.

As can be seen from these examples it is necessary for forecasting to precede planning, and from planning we now move to organising.

ORGANISING

In the catering industry organisational skills are applied to food, to equipment and to staff. Organising in this context consists of ensuring that what is wanted is where it is wanted, when it is wanted, in the right amount and at the right time.

Such organisation involves the supervisor in the production of duty rotas, maybe training programmes and also cleaning schedules. Consider the supervisor's part in organising an outdoor function where a wedding reception is to be held in a church hall: 250 guests require a hot meal to be served at 2pm and in the evening a dance will be held for the guests, during which a buffet will be provided at 9pm. The supervisor would need to organise the staff to be available when required, to have their own meals and maybe to see that they have got their transport home. Calor gas stoves may be needed, and the supervisor would have to arrange for the stoves to be serviced and for the equipment used to be cleaned after the function. The food would need to be ordered so that it arrived in time to be prepared. If decorated hams were to be used on the buffet then they would need to be ordered in time so that they could be prepared, cooked and decorated over the required period of time. If the staff have never carved hams before, instruction would need to be given; this entails organising training. Needless to say, the correct quantities of food, equipment and cleaning materials would also have to be at the right place when wanted; and if all the details of the situation were not organised properly problems could occur.

COMMANDING

The supervisor has to give instructions to staff on how, what, when and where; this means that orders have to be given and a certain degree of order and discipline maintained. The successful supervisor is able to do this effectively, having made certain decisions and, usually, having established the basic priorities. Explanations of why a food is prepared in a certain manner, why this amount of time is needed to dress up food, say for a buffet, why this decision is taken and not that decision, and how these explanations and orders are given, determine the effectiveness of the supervisor.

CO-ORDINATING

Co-ordinating is the skill required to get staff to co-operate and work together. To achieve this, the supervisor has to be interested in the staff, to deal with their queries, to listen to their problems and to be helpful. Particular attention should be paid to new staff, easing them into the work situation so that they quickly become part of the team or *partie*. The other area of co-ordination for which the supervisor has particular responsibility is in maintaining good relations with other departments. However, the important persons to consider will always be the customers, the patients, the school children, who are to receive the service, and good service is dependent on co-operation between waiters and cooks, nurses and catering staff, stores staff, caretakers, teachers, suppliers and so on. The supervisor has a crucial role to play here.

CONTROLLING

This includes the controlling of people and products, preventing pilfering as well as improving performance; checking that staff arrive on time, do not leave before time and do not misuse time in between; checking that the product, in this case the food, is of the right standard, that is to say, the correct quantity and quality; checking to prevent waste, and also to ensure that staff operate the portion control system correctly.

This aspect of the supervisor's function involves inspecting and requires tact; controlling may include the inspecting of the swill-bin to observe the amount of waste, checking the disappearance of a quantity of food, supervising the cooking of the meat so that shrinkage is minimised and reprimanding an unpunctual member of the team.

The standards of any catering establishment are dependent on the supervisor doing his or her job efficiently, and standards are set and maintained by effective control, which is the function of the supervisor.

Responsibilities of the supervisor

DELEGATION

It is recognised that delegation is the root of successful supervision; in other words, by giving a certain amount of responsibility to others the supervisor can be more effective.

The supervisor needs to be able to judge the person capable of responsibility before any delegation can take place. But then, having recognised the abilities of an employee, the supervisor who wants to develop the potential of those under his or her control must allow the person entrusted with the job to get on with it.

MOTIVATION

Since not everyone is capable of, or wants, responsibility, the supervisor still needs to motivate those who are less ambitious. Most people are prepared to work so as to improve their standard of living, but there is also another very important motivating factor: most people desire to get *satisfaction* from the work they do. The supervisor must be aware of why people work and how different people achieve job satisfaction and then be able to act upon this knowledge. A supervisor should have been on a training course to attempt to understand what motivates people as there are a number of theories a supervisor can use to stimulate ideas.

SYMPTOMS OF POOR MOTIVATION

There are many symptoms of poor motivation, in general terms they reveal themselves as a lack of interest in getting the job done correctly and within the required time. Although they may be indicators of poor motivation, the lack of efficiency and effectiveness could also be a result of the staff overworking, personal problems, poor work design, repetitive work, lack of discipline, inter-personal conflict, lack of training, failure of the organisation to value its staff. An employee may be highly motivated but may find the work physically impossible to do.

WELFARE

People always work best in good working conditions and these include freedom from fear: fear of becoming unemployed, fear of failure at work, fear of discrimination. Job security and incentives, such as opportunities for promotion, bonuses, profit sharing and time for further study, encourage a good attitude to work; but as well as these tangible factors people need to feel wanted and to feel that what they do is important. The supervisor is in an excellent position to ensure that this happens. Personal worries affect individuals' performance and can have a very strong influence on how well or how badly they work. The physical environment will naturally cause problems if, for example, the atmosphere is humid, the working situation ill-lit, too hot or too noisy, and there is constant rush and tear, and frequent major problems to be overcome. In these circumstances staff are more liable to be quick-tempered, angry and aggressive, and the supervisor needs to consider how these factors might be dealt with.

UNDERSTANDING

The supervisor needs to try to understand both men and women (and to deal with both sexes fairly), to anticipate problems and build up a team spirit so as to overcome the problems. This entails always being fair when dealing with staff and giving them encouragement. It also means that work needs to be allocated according to each individual's ability; everyone should be kept fully occupied and the working environment must be conducive to producing their best work.

COMMUNICATION

Finally, and most important of all, the supervisor must be able to communicate effectively. To convey orders, instructions, information and manual skills requires the supervisor to possess the right attitude to those with whom he or she needs to communicate. The ability to convey orders and instructions in a manner which is acceptable to the one receiving the orders is dependent not only on the words but on the emphasis given to the words, the tone of voice, the time selected to give them and on who is present when they are given. This is a skill which supervisors need to develop. Instructions and orders can be given with authority *without* being authoritative.

Thus the supervisor needs technical knowledge and the ability to direct staff and to carry responsibility so as to achieve the specified targets and standards required by the organisation; this he or she is able to do by organising, co-ordinating, controlling and planning but, most of all, through effective communication.

Skills for effective supervision

Robert L Katz (1974) has suggested that there are three types of skills required for effective management:

- technical;
- people;
- conceptual.

TECHNICAL SKILLS

These are the skills chefs, restaurant managers etc need to do the job. The supervisor must be skilled in the area they are supervising because they will be required in most cases to train other staff under them. Supervisors who do not have the required skills will find it hard to gain credibility with the staff.

PEOPLE SKILLS

Supervisors are team leaders therefore they must be sensitive to the needs of others. They must be able to communicate effectively, be able to build a team to achieve the agreed goals. Listening, questioning, communicating clearly, handling conflicts and providing support and praise when praise is due.

CONCEPTUAL SKILLS

A supervisor must be able to think things through, especially when planning or analysing why things are not going as expected. A supervisor must be able to solve problems and make decisions. For supervisors, conceptual skills are necessary for reasonably short-term planning. Head chefs and hospitality managers require conceptual skills for long-term strategic planning.

Henry Mintzberg (1973) suggested that the supervisor has three broad roles:

- Inter-personal   –   people skills
- Informational   –   people and technical skills
- Decision making   –   conceptual skills

SUPERVISORS AND ETHICAL ISSUES

A supervisor must be consistent when handling staff avoiding favouritism and perceived inequity. Such inequity can rise from the amount of training or performance counselling given, from the promotion of certain employees, and from the way in which rostering of shifts are allocated. Supervisors should engaged in conversation with all staff not just a selected few and also do not single out some staff for special attention.

Ethical treatment of staff is fair treatment of staff. A good supervisor will gain respect if they are ethical.

Confidentiality is an important issue for the supervisor. Employees or customers may wish to take the supervisor into their confidence and the supervisor must not betray this confidence.

Identifying recruitment needs

A supervisor must be able to identify what staff are required and where they are required in order to cope with the level of business. At the same time labour costs must be kept to a minimum. The supervisor must therefore ensure adequate staffing at the lowest possible cost.

An important aspect is to be able to carefully analyse projected business in order to adopt the best staffing mix.

Job design and the allocation of duties also have to be considered where jobs are simple and require little training, employment of casual labour can be justified. For more skilled staff full time employment has to be considered with investment in staff development and training.

Often the supervisor has to write job descriptions. These documents are used for a number of purposes, which include:

○ deciding on the knowledge, experience and skills required to carry out the duties specified;
○ allowing new staff to understand the requirements of their jobs;
○ allowing new staff to develop accurate expectation of the jobs;
○ identifying training needs;
○ assist in the development of recruitment strategies.

Job descriptions allow supervisors and managers to monitor performance and to manage discipline and discipline when performance is below standard. Job descriptions assist in allowing everyone to focus on the precise requirements of the job that everyone is clear about their expectations.

AN EXAMPLE OF A JOB DESCRIPTION

Senior Sous Chef

Reporting to Head Chef.

The Senior Sous Chef position reports to the Head Chef and is responsible for the day to day kitchen operation, overseeing the stores preparation and production areas. The position involves supervising and managing the kitchen staff with direct responsibility for rostering and scheduling production. In the absence of the Head Chef, the Senior Sous Chef will be required to take on the duties of the Head Chef and to attend Senior Management meetings in his/her absence.

Duties

○ Monitoring and checking stores operation.
○ Training new staff and existing staff in Health & Safety, HACCP etc.
○ Chair of the Kitchen Health and Safety Committee.
○ Developing new menus and concepts together with the Senior Management.
○ Scheduling and rostering all kitchen staff.
○ Maintain accurate records of staff absences.
○ Maintain accurate kitchen records.
○ Responsible for the overall cleanliness of the kitchen operation.
○ Assist in the production of management reports.

- ○ Establish an effective and efficient team.
- ○ Assist with the overall establishment and monitoring of budgets.

Conditions
- ○ Grade 3 Management Spine.
- ○ Private Health Insurance.
- ○ 5 day week.
- ○ 20 days holiday.
- ○ Profit Share Scheme after one year's service.

PERSONAL SPECIFICATION

Senior Sous Chef

Qualifications	○ BSc in International Culinary Arts Management or equivalent.
Experience	○ 5 years experience in 4 and 5 star hotel kitchens
	○ Restaurant and banqueting experience.
Skills	○ Proficiency in Culinary Arts
	○ Microsoft Excel, Access, Word
	○ Operation of inventory control software
	○ Written and oral communication skills
	○ Team building skills.
Knowledge	○ Current legislation in Health & Safety
	○ Food Hygiene
	○ HACCP
	○ Risk Assessment
	○ Production systems
	○ Current technology.
Other attributes	○ Honesty
	○ Reliability
	○ Attention to detail
	○ Initiative
	○ Accuracy.
Essential	○ Basic computer skills
	○ High degree of culinary skills
	○ Good communication skills
	○ Supervisory and leadership skills.
Desirable	○ Knowledge of employment law
	○ Public relations profile.

Induction programmes
WHY INDUCTION

Every establishment should have a detailed induction system. The induction process settles the new employees into their new position. It is important for the company to make a good impression as this will influence the person's attitude to the job. The new employee needs to be aware of their responsibilities. This will include not just their day to day procedures but also their role in legislation, food hygiene, health and safety.

TOPICS FOR INDUCTION

- ○ Company procedures, policies.
- ○ Tour of establishment and facilities.
- ○ Fire drill procedures, Health & Safety procedures.
- ○ Reporting procedures.
- ○ Job description explained.
- ○ condition of employment.
- ○ Emergency procedures.
- ○ Where to go for advice or assistance.
- ○ Equal opportunities.
- ○ Accident reporting.
- ○ Dismissal procedures.

During the first few weeks of employment the following topics need to be explained to the new employee.

- ○ Organisational aims and objectives.
- ○ Occupational health and safety.
- ○ Performance appraisal.
- ○ Job description explained.
- ○ Grievance procedures.
- ○ Quality standards.
- ○ Staff development.

Where possible new employees should be issued with an employee handbook with information on the company. The supervisor should take time to explain the contents of the handbook. Staff retention is an important issue in the hospitality and catering industry. Supervisors have a key role in developing teams to achieve effective working relationships which value people. These can help to reduce turnover. Staff turnover is extremely costly and every attempt should be made to reduce unnecessary turnover.

THE COST OF STAFF TURNOVER TO AN ESTABLISHMENT

- ○ Replacement costs – advertising, training etc.
- ○ Overtime to existing staff.
- ○ Extra pressure on existing staff.
- ○ Time taken to recruit staff.
- ○ Agency costs.
- ○ Payroll and administration costs.
- ○ Loss of business due to insufficient staff on duty to supply the required level of service.
- ○ Loss of business through damage of reputation.

The supervisor and performance appraisal

Supervisors manage performance informally through instructions and advice and by providing constructive feedback. The supervisor should give praise when it is due and reprimand an employee if necessary. Informal feedback takes place on a day-to-day basis but most large organisations operate a formal appraisal system. This involves the supervisor or the manager conducting a formal interview with the employee, examining past performance and assessing the opportunities for the future. Overall performance may be ranked on a performance scale. During the interview, training needs and career development are analysed to establish the employee's performance objectives and plans for achievement.

Performance appraisal forms may cover efficiency, reliability, teamwork and working relationships. In service organisations this may also include customer relations. To be more specific the job description criteria may also be included in the form. Focusing on the job description promotes discussion about what is happening in the workplace and how hurdles to ineffective performance can be overcome.

Performance objectives and training plans should also relate to the job requirements.

When a supervisor conducts a performance appraisal they should advise the employee in advance, explaining the purpose of the appraisal.

In addition, sufficient time must be allocated to the process. The following should also be taken into account:

○ creating an appropriate climate for the interview;
○ reviewing specific job performances against specific job targets;
○ openly discussing issues which may have an impact on performance;
○ agreeing on new performance targets;
○ giving positive constructive feedback.

Topics for Discussion

1 Who should be responsible for planning a kitchen?
2 Discuss the worst organised kitchen that you have seen and how it could be improved.
3 Give good and bad examples of working methods.
4 Discuss advantages and disadvantages of the straight shift and split-shift systems from the point of view of the staff and the employer.
5 Compile a list of all the factors which affect the good design of a kitchen. Discuss why they are necessary to enable efficiency.
6 Poor design may cause accidents in the kitchen. Discuss the ways in which accidents can be prevented.
7 Discuss the reasons why organisation of staff needs to be considered in relation to a specific menu and the factors which influence the composition of the menu.
8 Discuss the qualities which go towards being a good a) head chef; b) chef de partie.
9 Organising ability is a quality which is often quoted as an essential element to being successful in the kitchen. Discuss, with examples if possible, of your understanding of organising ability regarding a) the resources; b) staff; c) yourself.
10 Discuss the role of supervision and relate if possible to an establishment you know.
11 As an employee how do you like to be supervised?
12 What are the characteristics of a good supervisor?

EQUIPMENT

Cooking equipment provides the backbone of any busy catering operation. It is the key to catering success and quality. In terms of food safety it controls the most critical step in the food production process. A mistake at the cooking stage by undercooking of raw food is likely to result in a mass food poisoning incident.

Kitchen equipment is expensive so initial selection is important, and the following points should be considered before each item is purchased or hired:

- Overall dimensions (in relation to available space).
- Weight – can the floor support the weight?
- Fuel supply – is the existing fuel supply sufficient to take the increase?
- Drainage – where necessary, are there adequate facilities?
- Water – where necessary, is it to hand?
- Use – does the food to be produced justify good use?
- Capacity – can it cook the quantities of food required efficiently?
- Time – can it cook the given quantities of food in the time available?
- Ease – is it easy for staff to handle, control and use properly?
- Maintenance – is it easy for staff to clean and maintain?
- Attachments – is it necessary to use additional equipment or attachments?
- Extraction – does it require extraction facilities for fumes or steam?
- Noise – does it have an acceptable noise level?
- Construction – is it well made, safe, hygienic and energy efficient, and are all handles, knobs and switches sturdy and heat resistant?
- Appearance – if equipment is to be on view to customers does it look good and fit in with the overall design?
- Spare parts – are they and replacement parts easily obtainable?

Further information

Technical brief No 28, Purchasing Catering Equipment – HCIMA.

Kitchen equipment may be divided into three categories:

- Large equipment – ranges, steamers, boiling pans, fish-fryers, sinks, tables.
- Mechanical equipment – peelers, mincers, mixers, refrigerators, dish-washers.
- Utensils and small equipment – pots, pans, whisks, bowls, spoons.

Manufacturers of all kitchen equipment issue instructions on how to clean and keep their apparatus in efficient working order, and it is the responsibility of everyone using the equipment to follow these instructions (which should be displayed in a prominent place near the machines).

Arrangements should be made with the local gas board for regular checks and servicing of gas-operated equipment; similar arrangements should be made with the electricity supplier. It is a good plan to keep a log-book of all equipment, showing where each item is located when servicing takes place, noting any defects that arise, and instructing the fitter to sign the log-book and to indicate exactly what has been done.

LARGE EQUIPMENT
Ranges and ovens

A large variety of ranges are available operated by gas, electricity, solid fuel, oil, microwave or microwave plus convection.

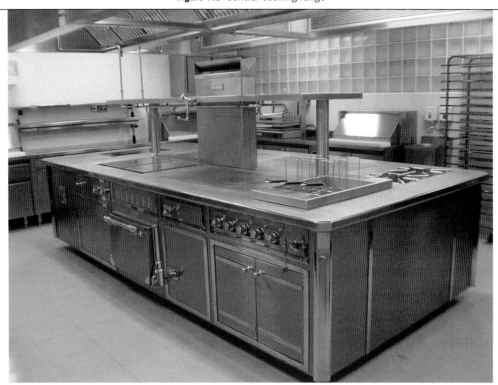

Figure 7.6 *Central cooking range*

Oven doors should not be slammed as this is liable to cause damage.

The unnecessary or premature lighting of ovens can cause wastage of fuel, which is needless expense. This is a bad habit common in many kitchens.

When a solid-top gas range is lit, the centre ring should be removed to reduce the risk of blow back, but it should be replaced after approximately five minutes, otherwise unnecessary heat is lost.

CONVECTION OVENS

These are ovens in which a circulating current of hot air is rapidly forced around the inside of the oven by a motorised fan or blower. As a result, a more even and constant temperature is created which allows food to be cooked successfully in any part of the oven. This means that the

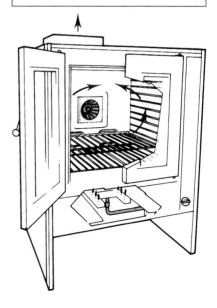

Figure 7.7 *Forced air convection oven*

heat is used more efficiently, cooking temperatures can be lower, cooking times shortened and overall fuel economy achieved.

Forced air convection can be described as fast conventional cooking; conventional in that heat is applied to the surface of the food, but fast since moving air transfers its heat more rapidly than does static air. In a sealed oven, fast hot air circulation reduces evaporation loss, keeping shrinkage to a minimum, and gives the rapid change of surface texture and colour which are traditionally associated with certain cooking processes.

Figure 7.8 *Hot air convection oven*

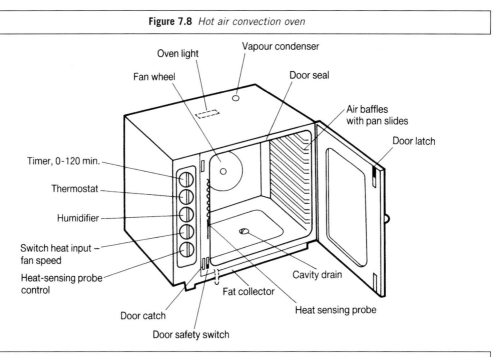

Figure 7.9 *Hot air steamer oven*

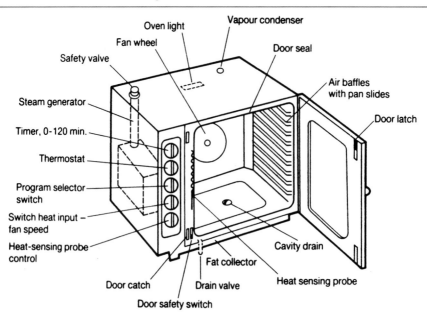

There are four types of convection oven.

○ Where forced air circulation within the oven is accomplished by means of a motor-driven fan, the rapid air circulation ensures even temperature distribution to all parts of the oven.

○ Where low velocity, high volume air movement is provided by a power blower and duct system.

○ A combination of a standard oven and a forced convection oven designed to operate as either by the flick of a switch.

○ A single roll-in rack convection oven with heating element and fan housed outside the cooking area. An 18-shelf mobile oven rack makes it possible to roll the filled rack directly from the preparation area into the oven.

COMBINATION OVENS

Combination ovens have brought about a revolution in baking, roasting and steaming. There are now many varieties of combination ovens available on the market. These ovens are now widely used in most sectors of the catering industry, fuelled by gas or electricity. They are especially used in large banqueting operations.

Ovens can be easily programmed to produce exact cooking times and the regeneration of chilled food, allowing chefs to produce consistent products every time.

The special features of combination ovens are:

○ reduce cooking times;

○ fully automatic – enable desired browning levels and exact core temperatures to be achieved;

○ self cleaning;

○ a combination oven system will allow more food to be produced in less space;

○ energy efficiency;

○ increased productivity.

A new type of combination oven of a different kind has been manufactured, it is a hybrid of fridge and oven. Designed for use in cook-chill food systems for banqueting or industrial catering. The chilled food is held in chill until the predetermined moment when the chilling unit switches off and the oven facility kicks in, bringing the food safely up to eating temperature.

The Cooking Process Management System

This links the combi-oven to a PC which monitors the cooking process to help with HACCP.

The computer software monitors not just the combi-ovens, but other items of cooking equipment in the kitchen, such as pressure bratt pans, steamers and boiling kettles. The chef inputs into the software what the day's food production is to be, and the computer will work out the order in which the food should be cooked, and in what pieces of equipment, to deliver the food just in time for freshness.

The HACCP management part of this system can track food from the goods delivery to the plate by using probes – for example, a chilled or frozen chicken can be probed to monitor and record temperatures before the cooking process so that if a problem occurs in the food cycle, the kitchen manager can check to see if there were any discrepancies in the goods storage procedures.

During the cooking the probes will record any variations to the pre-set cooking programme. This means the software system can alert the kitchen management team not just that a problem has occurred during the cooking procedure, but where it occurred.

More Information

EIM – Swiss equipment

COMBINATION OVENS – COOKING PROFILE

Example – Rationale

These are pre-programmed, ideal procedures for cooking different meats in particular for roasts such as leg of lamb, roast pork etc.

The special feature of these intelligent profiles is that they detect automatically the size of the meat and the volume of the food in the cooking cabinet. In addition, with the assistance of the IQT sensor, they also determine the exact core temperature of the food, the remaining cooking time and the current level of browning. The profiles are self-regulating – i.e. they adjust the cooking processes to the size of the meat and the load of food in the cooking cabinet.

IQT Sensor – (Rationale)

The sensor is inserted into the food to facilitate the detection of the core temperature. This prevents overcooking of joints and less weight loss.

Alto-Shaam Cook and Hold Ovens

These ovens reduce labour, product shrinkage, provides product consistency and increases holding life for banqueting service. Two items are available, one for holding and serve, the other for regeneration and serve.

SMOKING OVENS

Smoking certain foods is a means of cooking, injecting different flavours and preserving. Smoking ovens or cabinets are well insulated with controlled heating elements on which wood chips are placed (different types of wood chips give differing flavours). As the wood chips burn, the heated smoke permeates the food (fish, chicken, sausages, etc.), which is suspended in the cabinet.

MICROWAVE OVENS *(Figure 7.11, page 236)*

Microwave is a method of cooking and heating food by using high frequency power. The energy used is the same as that which carries the television signal from the transmitter to the receiver, but is at a higher frequency.

The waves disturb the molecules or particles of food and agitate them, thus causing friction which has the effect of heating the food. In the conventional method of cooking, heat penetrates the food only by conduction from the outside. Food being cooked by microwave needs no fat or water, and is placed in a glass, earthenware, plastic or paper container before being put in the oven. Metal is not used as the microwaves are reflected by it.

All microwave ovens consist of a basic unit of various sizes with varying levels of power. Some feature additions to the standard model, such as automatic defrosting systems, browning elements, 'stay-hot' controls and revolving turntables.

The oven cavity has metallic walls, ceiling and floor which reflect the microwaves. The oven door is fitted with special seals to ensure that there is minimum microwave leakage. A cut-out device automatically switches off the microwave energy when the door is opened.

FURTHER INFORMATION

Further information can be obtained from The Microwave Association, 3 Popham Gardens, Lower Richmond Rd, Surrey TW9 4LJ

COMBINATION CONVECTION AND MICROWAVE COOKER

This cooker combines forced air convection and microwave, either of which can be used separately but which are normally used simultaneously, thereby giving the advantages of both systems: speed, coloration and texture of food. Traditional metal cooking pans may also be used without fear of damage to the cooker.

AN INTRODUCTION TO INDUCTION COOKING

The History

The principle of induction heating was discovered by Michael Faraday towards the end of the 19th century when he noticed a heating effect in iron cored transformers. This later became known as Faraday's iron loss laws for transformers.

The effect was recognised but was of pure academic interest until the 1930s when the British steel industry needing a fast way of heating steel, successfully exploited Faraday's iron loss laws by wrapping a copper coil around the steel rod and energising the coil with alternating current. This produced a strong magnetic field that in turn instantly heated the steel rod. Induction heating was born. Induction became popular for fast heating of large objects containing iron, but the equipment used to do this was expensive, bulky and by today's standards was fairly crude.

In the early 80s the advent of solid state power electronics persuaded a few companies to look at the principle for induction cooking, using a flat coil to react with the iron in the base of a pan and produce heat directly in the pan. Crude systems began to emerge which showed the promise of induction cooking but most were withdrawn from the market as it became apparent that neither the technology nor the electronic power devices were sufficiently developed to provide the market with the product it required; special pans were needed and chefs were forced to adapt their cooking techniques. Some companies persevered with the original technology but it is only in the 1990s that electronic power technology advanced sufficiently to enable Induced Energy Limited to develop a comprehensive range of cooking hobs with the reliability, control and design flexibility to fully meet market needs.

Advantages of Induction Cooking Hobs

○ **Power Savings.** The induction hob has a very high energy efficiency and only draws power when a pan is on the ring. Energy costs are substantially reduced.

○ **Safety.** Only the pan gets hot therefore you cannot burn yourself on this type of hob.

○ **Cool Working Environment.** As virtually all the energy is developed as heat directly in the pan very little heat escapes to the atmosphere therefore providing a cool working environment.

○ **Less Extraction.** Because of the cool working environment the kitchen needs much less extraction, further reducing energy bills.

○ **Hygiene.** The flat ceramic top provides a wipe clean hygienic surface which remains cool and therefore spillage will not burn onto the cooking surface.

○ **No Combustion Gases.** Unlike gas hobs, induction hobs do not emit any combustion gases and are environmentally friendly.

○ **Speed of Cooking.** Modern induction hob designs are faster than gas hobs.

WHAT YOU NEED TO KNOW WHEN PURCHASING AN INDUCTION HOB

Pans

Try to find an induction hob which works using normal pans. Beware of induction hobs which need special pans or do not give constant performance pan to pan.

Power Supply

The best hobs feature a near unity power factor which gives the ideal loading on the main supply and is preferred by the electricity suppliers. You will need to check if a particular induction hob will require the upgrading of the power supply.

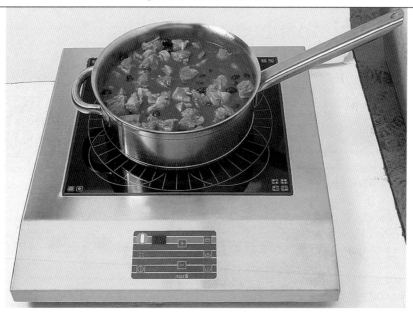

Figure 7.10 *An induction hob*

Power Control

Most chefs are trained on gas hobs which have infinite power control i.e. heat which can be continuously varied from low to high without steps. Choose a hob with infinitely variable power control (0 to full power) and preferably one that has its power control set to mimic the power profile of the gas tap.

Repeatability

Choose a hob that is designed to take a range of pans without power variations pan to pan. In this way precise cooking to power settings can be achieved irrespective of pan type. This is particularly helpful to the chef who can quickly 'eyeball' a power setting and achieve consistent results.

Cooking Zone

Choose a hob with a high depth of field. This allows the pan to be moved about naturally during cooking, just like cooking over a gas flame.

Warranty

Check the warranty cover for the induction hob and the service backup. Plug in Plug out designs usually mean fast service units.

Energy Efficiency

This forms part of the commercial decision for a particular hob. The more energy efficient the hob the ore you will save on running costs.

SAFETY FEATURES

Excess Temperature Control

It is important that the induction hob has an excess temperature control which will protect the hob, if for example the hob cooling air was blocked.

Boil Dry Protection

If a pan is inadvertently left to boil dry on the hob there must be an automatic cut out which safely switches off – saving the pan, hob and the kitchen from damage.

CONVENIENCE

Digital Display

Unlike a gas hob, the induction hob does not have a physical indication of the power being developed (a flame), so some form of digital display is required to show, for example, the power.

Totally Flat Top

It is very convenient to have a flat unobstructed cooking surface. Not only is it easily cleaned but it allows the hob to be used front of house with the customer served directly from the back of the hob. Similarly hobs can be placed back to back on an island site giving access from all sides.

One Pan Over 2 Rings or 2 Pans over 1 Ring

Often it is necessary to put a large pan over 2 rings. Make sure that your prospective hob provides this feature. Additionally check that you can cook using two or more smaller pans from a single ring.

Griddle

For steaks etc. some hobs convert to a griddle using a cast iron or ferritic stainless steel griddle top.

Portable Trolley

Some chefs prefer to have their boiling table portable and use various sockets around the kitchen.

Further information

Induced Energy Limited
Westminster Road
Northamptonshire
NN13.

HALOGEN HOB

This runs on electricity, and comprises five individually controlled heat zones, each of which has four tungsten halogen lamps located under a smooth ceramic glass surface. The heat source glows red, when switched on, getting brighter as the temperature increases.

When the hob is switched on, 70% of the heat is transmitted as infrared light directly into the base of the cooking pan, the rest is from conducted heat via the ceramic glass. Ordinary pots and pans may be used on the halogen hob, but those with a flat, dark or black base absorb the heat most efficiently.

The halogen range includes a convection oven, and the halogen hob unit is also available mounted on a stand.

STEAMERS

There are basically three types of steaming ovens:

○ atmospheric;
○ pressure;
○ pressureless (see Figure 7.12, page 236).

There are also combination steaming ovens: pressure/convection steam; pressureless/fully

Figure 7.11 *(a) Microwave energy being reflected off cooking cavity walls; (b) microwave energy being absorbed by food; (c) microwave energy passing through cooking container material*

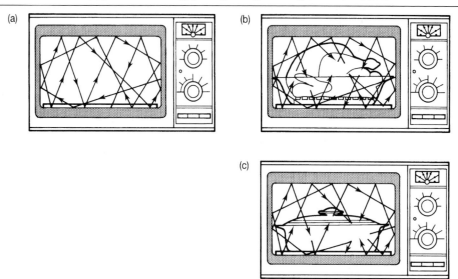

pressurised; steaming/hot air cooking; combination of hot air and steam; combination of hot air and steam with two settings (Figure 7.13 on page 237).

In addition, dual pressure steamers, switchable between low pressure and high pressure, and two pressure settings plus zero are available. Steaming ovens continue to develop, improve and become more versatile. The modern combination steamers which can be used for steaming, stewing, poaching, braising, roasting, baking, vacuum cooking, gratinating, reconstituting, blanching and defrosting, have electronic controls for easier setting and more precise time/temperature control. The advantage of the electronic controls is that they assist in fuel efficiency. They are available in several sizes and there are many examples of their efficiency. For example, one large hotel quotes: 'using five electrically heated combi-steamers we served 500 English breakfasts straight from the oven – no messing about with hot plates and cupboards'.

With such a wide range of models available it is increasingly important to consider carefully which model is best suited to a particular kitchen's requirements.

Figure 7.12 *Pressureless steamer*

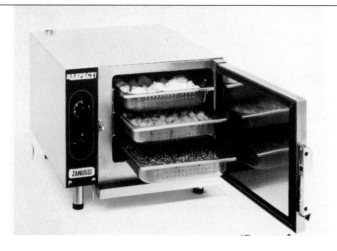

Figure 7.13 *Combination oven*

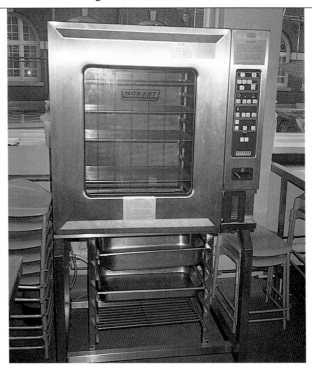

FURTHER INFORMATION

Further information can be obtained from Catering Equipment Manufacturers Association of Great Britain (CEMA), Carlyle House, 235–237 Vauxhall Bridge Road, London SW1V 1EJ.

Large pans, boilers and fryers
BRATT PAN

The bratt pan is one of the most versatile pieces of cooking equipment in the kitchen because it is possible to use it for shallow frying, deep frying, stewing, braising and boiling. A bratt pan can cook many items of food at one time because of its large surface area. A further advantage is that it can be tilted so that the contents can be quickly and efficiently poured out on completion of the cooking process. Bratt pans are heated by gas or electricity and several models are available incorporating various features to meet differing catering requirements.

BOILING PANS

Many types are available in different metals – aluminium, stainless steel, etc. – in various sizes (10, 15, 20, 30 and 40 litre capacity) and they may be heated by gas or electricity. As they are used for boiling or stewing large quantities of food, it is important that they do not allow the food to burn; for this reason the steam-jacket type boiler is the most suitable. Many of these are fitted with a tilting device to facilitate the emptying of the contents.

After use, the boiling pan and lid should be thoroughly washed with mild detergent solution and then well rinsed. The tilting apparatus should be greased occasionally and checked to see that it tilts easily. If gas fired, the gas jets and pilot should be inspected to ensure correct working. If a pressure gauge and safety valve are fitted these should also be checked.

PASTA COOKER

This equipment is fitted with water delivery and drain taps and can be used for the cooking of several types of pasta simultaneously. It is electrically operated.

DEEP FAT-FRYERS

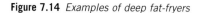
Figure 7.14 *Examples of deep fat-fryers*

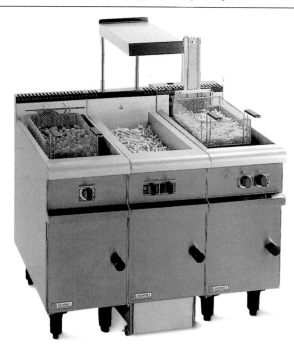

A deep fat-fryer is one of the most extensively used items of equipment in many catering establishments. The careless worker who misuses a deep fat-fryer and spills food or fat can cause accidents and waste money.

Fryers are heated by gas or electricity and incorporate a thermostatic control in order to save fuel and prevent overheating. There is a cool zone below the source of heat into which food particles can sink without burning, thus preventing spoiling of other foods being cooked. This form of heating also saves fat.

PRESSURE FRYERS

Food is cooked in an air-tight frying vat thus enabling food to be fried a lot faster and at a lower oil temperature.

HOT AIR ROTARY FRYERS

These are designed to cook batches of frozen blanched chips or battered foods without any oil in 4–6 minutes.

Computerised fryers are available which may be programmed to control automatically cooking temperatures and times, on and off switches, basket lifting and product holding times. Operational information is fed from a super-sensitive probe, which is immersed in the frying medium and passes information about temperature and rates of temperature change which may be caused by: the initial fat temperature, amount of food being fried, fryer efficiency and capacity, fryer recovery rate, quantity and condition of fat, product temperature and water content.

With all the above information the fryer computes exact cooking times and an automatic signalling device indicates the end of a cooking period.

Deep fat-fryers should be cleaned daily after use by following the manufacturers instructions:

○ turning off the heat and allow the fat or oil to cool;

○ draining off and straining the fat or oil;

○ closing the stopcock, filling the fryer with hot water containing detergent and boiling for 10–15 minutes;

○ draining off the detergent water, refilling with clean water plus litre of vinegar per 5 litres of water and reboiling for 10–15 minutes;

○ draining off the water, drying the fryer, closing the stopcock and refilling with clean fat or oil.

HOT-CUPBOARDS (COMMONLY REFERRED TO IN THE TRADE AS THE HOTPLATE)

Hot-cupboards are used for heating plates and serving dishes and for keeping food hot. Care should be taken to see that the amount of heat fed into the hot-cupboard is controlled at a reasonable temperature. This is important, otherwise the plates and food will either be too hot or too cold and this could obviously affect the efficiency of the service. A temperature of 60–76°C (140–169°F) is suitable for hot-cupboards and a thermostat is a help in maintaining this.

Hot-cupboards may be heated by steam, gas or electricity. The doors should slide easily, and occasional greasing may be necessary. The tops of most hot-cupboards are used as serving counters and should be heated to a higher temperature than the inside. These tops are usually made of stainless steel and should be cleaned thoroughly after each service.

BAINS-MARIE

Bains-marie are open wells of water used for keeping foods hot, and are available in many designs, some of which are incorporated into hot-cupboards, some in serving counters, and there is a type which is fitted at the end of a cooking range. They may be heated by steam, gas or electricity and sufficient heat to boil the water in the bain-marie should be available. Care should be taken to see that a bain-marie is never allowed to burn dry when the heat is turned on. After use the heat should be turned off, the water drained and the bain-marie cleaned inside and outside with hot detergent water, rinsed and dried. Any drain-off tap should then be closed.

FOOD DISTRIBUTION EQUIPMENT

In situations requiring mobile equipment e.g. hospitals, banqueting, etc wheeled items are essential to facilitate service particularly of hot foods.

Grills and salamanders

The salamander or grill heated from above by gas or electricity probably causes more wastage of fuel than any other item of kitchen equipment through being allowed to burn unnecessarily for long unused periods. Most salamanders have more than one set of heating elements or jets and it is not always necessary to have them all turned on full.

Salamander bars and draining trays should be cleaned regularly with hot water containing a grease solvent such as soda. After rinsing they should be replaced and the salamander lit for a few minutes to dry the bars.

For under-fired grills (Figure 7.15) to work efficiently they must be capable of cooking food quickly and should reach a high temperature 15–20 minutes after lighting, and the heat should be turned off immediately after use. When the bars are cool they should be removed and washed in hot water containing a grease solvent, rinsed, dried and replaced on the grill. Care should be taken with the fire bricks if they are used for lining the grill as they are easily broken.

CONTACT GRILLS

These are sometimes referred to as double-sided or infragrills and have two heating surfaces arranged facing each other. The food to be cooked is placed on one surface and is then covered by the second. These grills are electrically heated and are capable of cooking certain foods very quickly, so extra care is needed, particularly when cooks are using this type of grill for the first time.

FRY PLATES, GRIDDLE PLATES *(Figure 7.16)*

These are solid metal plates heated from below, and are used for cooking individual portions of meat, hamburgers, eggs, bacon, etc. They can be heated quickly to a high temperature and are suitable for rapid and continuous cooking. Before cooking on griddle plates a light film of oil should be applied to the food and the griddle plate to prevent sticking. To clean griddle plates, warm them and scrape off loose food particles; rub the metal with pumice stone or griddle stone, following the grain of the metal; clean with hot detergent water, rinse with clean hot water and wipe dry. Finally reseason (prove) the surface by lightly oiling with vegetable oil.

Griddles with zone heating are useful when demand varies during the day. These reduce energy consumption in quiet periods while still allowing the service to be maintained.

Figure 7.15 *An under-fired grill*	**Figure 7.16** *Griddle*

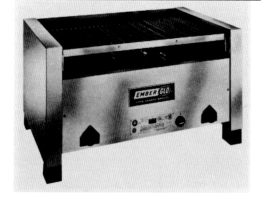
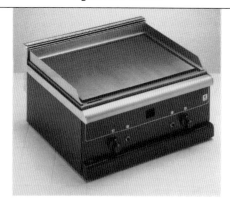

Mirror chromed griddles have a polished surface which gives off less radiated heat which saves energy and makes for a more pleasant working environment.

Barbecues

Barbecues are becoming increasingly popular because it is easy to cook and serve quick tasty food on them and the outdoor location, smell and sizzle develop an atmosphere which many customers enjoy.

There are three main types of barbecue: traditional charcoal, gas (propane or butane) and electric. Remember that the charcoal-fired type takes about an hour before the surface is ready. With gas and electricity the barbecue is ready to cook almost immediately.

Gas is the more flexible and controllable. Propane gas is recommended because it can be used at any time of the year. Butane, does not work when it is cold. Propane is, however, highly flammable and safety precautions are essential. Anyone connecting the gas container must be competent in the use of bottle gas. The supply pipe must be guarded to avoid accidental interference, and the cylinder must be placed away from the barbecue. The cylinder must be upright and stable with the valve uppermost and securely held in position. Connections must be checked for leaks.

Sinks

Stainless steel is generally used for all purposes

Tables

- Formica or stainless steel topped tables should be washed with hot detergent water then rinsed with hot water containing a sterilising agent – alternatively, some modern chemicals act as both detergent and sterilising agents. Wooden tables should not be used.
- Marble slabs should be scrubbed with hot water and rinsed. All excess moisture should be removed with a clean, dry cloth.

No cutting or chopping should be allowed on table tops; cutting boards should be used.

Hot pans should not be put on tables; triangles must be used to protect the table surface.

The legs and racks or shelves of tables are cleaned with hot detergent water and then dried. Wooden table legs require scrubbing.

BUTCHER'S OR CHOPPING BLOCK

A scraper should be used to keep the block clean. After scraping, the block should be sprinkled with a few handfuls of common salt in order to absorb any moisture which may have penetrated during the day.

Do not use water or liquids for cleaning unless absolutely necessary as water will be absorbed into the wood and cause swelling.

Storage racks

All type of racks should be emptied and scrubbed or washed periodically.

FURTHER INFORMATION

British Meat Foodservice. Tel: 01908 844114 email: foodservice@m/c.org.uk. www.britishmeatfoodservice.com

MECHANICAL EQUIPMENT

The Health and Safety Executive have two publications on catering machinery, both obtainable from HMSO. If a piece of mechanical equipment can save time and physical effort and still produce a good end result then it should be considered for purchase or hire. The performance of most machines can be closely controlled and is not subject to human variations, so it should be easier to obtain uniformity of production over a period of time.

The caterer is faced with two considerations:

- the cost of the machine: installation, maintenance, depreciation and running cost;
- the possibility of increased production and a saving of labour cost.

The mechanical performance must be carefully assessed and all the manufacturer's claims as to the machine's efficiency thoroughly checked. The design should be fool-proof, easy to clean and operated with minimum effort.

When a new item of equipment is installed it should be tested by a qualified fitter before being used by catering staff. The manufacturer's instructions must be displayed in a prominent place near the machine. The manufacturer's advice regarding servicing should be followed and a record book kept showing what kind of maintenance the machine is receiving, and when. The following list includes machines typically found in catering premises which are classified as dangerous under the Prescribed Dangerous Machines Order, 1964.

Warning: before cleaning, all machines should be switched off and the plug removed from the socket.

○ Power-driven machines
  – Worm-type mincing machines.
  – Rotary knife bowl-type chopping machines.
  – Dough mixers.
  – Food mixing machines when used with attachments for mincing, slicing, chipping and any other cutting operation, or for crumbling.
  – Pie and tart making machines.
  – Vegetable slicing machines.
○ Potato-peelers
  – Potatoes should be free of earth and stones before loading into the machine.
  – Before any potatoes are loaded the water spray should be turned on and the abrasive plate set in motion.
  – The interior should be cleaned out daily and the abrasive plate removed to ensure that small particles are not lodged below.
  – The peel trap should be emptied as frequently as required.
  – The waste outlet should be kept free from obstruction.
○ Machines whether power-driven or not
  – Circular knife slicing machines used for cutting bacon and other foods (whether similar to bacon or not).
  – Potato chipping machines.

FOOD PROCESSING EQUIPMENT
Food mixer *(Figure 7.21, page 245)*

This is an important labour-saving, electrically operated piece of equipment used for many purposes: mixing pastry, cakes, mashing potatoes, beating egg whites, mayonnaise, cream, mincing or chopping meat and vegetables.

○ It should be lubricated frequently in accordance with manufacturer's instructions.
○ The motor should not be overloaded, which can be caused by obstruction to the rotary components. For example, if dried bread is being passed through the mincer attachment without sufficient care the rotary cog can become so clogged with bread that it is unable to move. If the motor is allowed to run, damage can be caused to the machine.
○ All components as well as the main machine should be thoroughly washed and dried. Care should be taken to see that no rust occurs on any part. The mincer attachment knife and plates will rust if not given sufficient care.

Food processing machines *(see Figures 7.20, 7.21 and 7.22, pages 245 and 246)*

Food processors are generally similar to vertical, high-speed cutters except that they tend to be smaller and to have a larger range of attachments. They can be used for a large number of mixing and chopping jobs but they cannot whisk or incorporate air to mixes.

LIQUIDISER OR BLENDER

Figure 7.17 *A portable liquidiser*

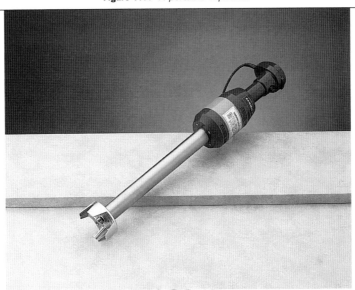

This is a versatile, labour-saving piece of kitchen machinery which uses a high-speed motor to drive specially designed stainless steel blades to chop, purée or blend foods efficiently and very quickly. They are also useful for making breadcrumbs. As a safety precaution food must be cooled before being liquidised.

FOOD-SLICERS

Food-slicers are obtainable both manually and electrically operated. They are labour-saving devices, but can be dangerous if not used with care so working instructions should be placed in a prominent position near the machine.

- ○ Care should be taken that no material likely to damage the blades is included in the food to be sliced. It is easy for a careless worker to overlook a piece of bone which, if allowed to come into contact with the cutting blade, could cause severe damage.
- ○ Each section in contact with food should be cleaned and carefully dried after use.
- ○ The blade or blades should be sharpened regularly.
- ○ Moving parts should be lubricated, but oil must not come into contact with the food.
- ○ Extra care must be taken when blades are exposed.

Figure 7.18 *Gastronorm counter*

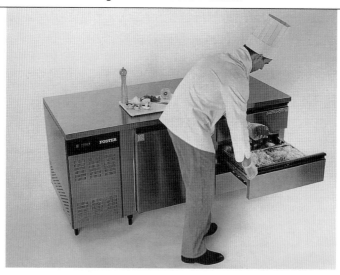

Figure 7.19 *Automatic pastry roller (dough brake)*

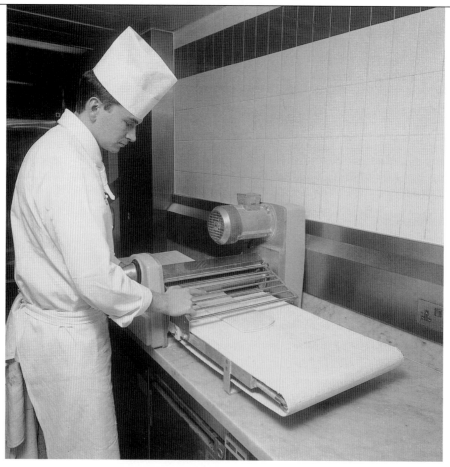

Figure 7.20 *Vertical, variable speed mixers*

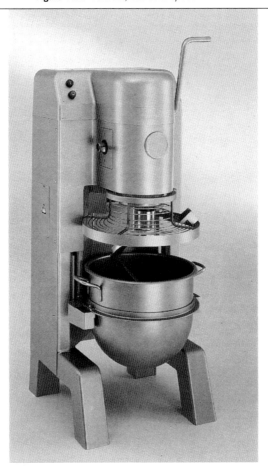

Figure 7.21 *Belt-driven food processor*

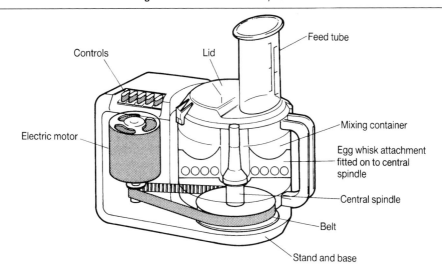

Controls

Lid

Feed tube

Electric motor

Mixing container

Egg whisk attachment fitted on to central spindle

Central spindle

Belt

Stand and base

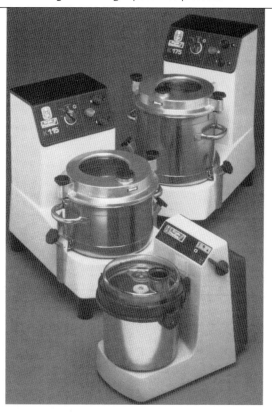

Figure 7.22 *High-speed food processor*

CHIPPER

The electric chipper should be thoroughly cleaned and dried after use, particular attention being paid to those parts which come into contact with food. Care should be taken that no obstruction prevents the motor from operating at its normal speed. Moving parts should be lubricated according to the maker's instructions.

MASHER (HAND OR ELECTRIC)

The hand type should be washed immediately after use, then rinsed and dried.

The electric masher should have the removable sections and the main machine washed and dried after use, extra care being taken over those parts which come into contact with food. The same care should be taken as with electric chippers regarding obstruction and lubrication.

ICE-CREAM MAKERS, JUICERS AND MIXERS

Ice-cream and sorbet machines are available from 1 litre capacity and enable establishments to produce home made ice-cream and sorbets using fresh fruit in season or frozen and canned fruits at all times of the year.

Juicers and mixers can provide freshly made fruit and vegetable juices, milk shakes and cocktails.

BOILERS
Water boiling appliances for tea- and coffee-making

There are two main groups of water boilers: bulk boilers from which boiling water can only be drawn when all the contents have boiled, and automatic boilers which provide a continuous flow of boiling water.

BULK BOILERS

These are generally used when large quantities of boiling water are required at a given time. They should be kept scrupulously clean, covered with the correct lid to prevent anything falling in, and when not used for some time they should be left filled with clean cold water.

AUTOMATIC BOILERS

These boilers have automatic waterfeeds and can give freshly boiled water at intervals. It is important that the water supply is efficiently maintained, otherwise there is a danger of the boiler burning dry and being damaged.

Pressure boilers

This is the type that operates many still sets, consisting of steam heating milk boilers and a pressure boiler providing boiling water. Care should be taken with the pilot light to see that it is working efficiently. As with all gas-fired equipment it is essential that regular inspection and maintenance is carried out by gas company fitters.

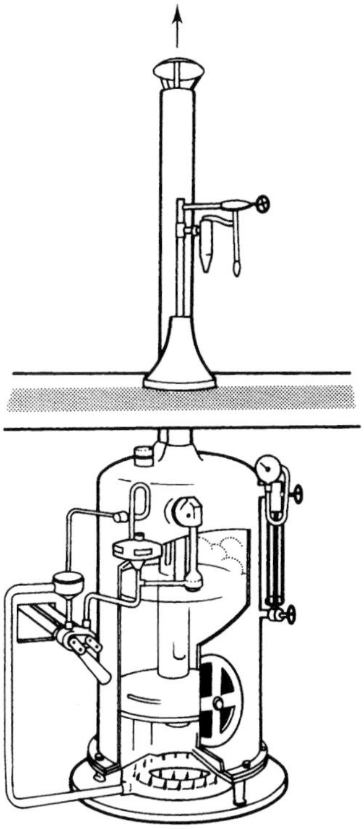

Coffee and milk heaters

Water-jacket boilers are made for the storage of hot coffee and hot milk with draw-off taps from the storage chamber. Inner linings may be of glazed earthenware, stainless steel or heat-resistant glass. It is very important that the storage chambers are thoroughly cleaned with hot water after each use and then left full of clean cold water. The draw-off taps should be cleaned regularly with a special brush.

Figure 7.23 *A pressure boiler*

Refrigerators, cold rooms, chill rooms, deep-freeze cabinets and compartments

Location

As adequate ventilation is vital, locate refrigeration equipment in a well-ventilated room away from:

○ sources of intense heat – cookers, ovens, radiators, boilers, etc.;

○ direct sunlight – from window or sky lights;

○ barriers to adequate air circulation.

In large establishments it is necessary to have refrigerated space at different temperatures. The cold rooms may be divided into separate rooms: one at a chill temperature for storing salads, fruits, certain cheeses; one for meats, poultry, game and tinned food which have to be refrigerated; one for deep-frozen foods. Frequently, the cold room storage is designed so that the chill room, the cold room and the deep-freeze compartment lead on from each other. Refrigerated cabinets, thermostatically controlled to various desired temperatures, are also used in large larders. Deep-freeze cabinets are used where a walk-in, deep-freeze section is not required and they maintain a temperature of $-18°C$ $(-0°F)$. Chest-type deep-freeze cabinets require defrosting twice a year. It is important to close all refrigerator doors as quickly as possible to contain the cold air.

Hygiene precautions

Refrigeration cannot improve the quality of foodstuffs and can only retard the natural process of deterioration.

For maximum storage of food and minimum health risk:

- Select the appropriate refrigerator equipment for the temperature requirement of the food.
- Always ensure refrigerators maintain correct temperature for food stored.
- Keep unwrapped foods, vulnerable to contamination and flavour and odour transfer, in separate refrigerators or in airtight containers and away from products such as cream, other dairy products, partly cooked pastry, cooked meat and delicatessen foods.
- Do not store foods for long periods in a good, general-purpose refrigerator because a single temperature is not suitable for keeping all types of food safely and at peak condition.
- Never keep uncooked meat, poultry or fish in the same refrigerator, or any other food which is not in its own sealed, airtight container.
- Never refreeze foods that have been thawed out from frozen.
- Always rotate stock in refrigerator space.
- Clean equipment regularly and thoroughly, inside and out.

Loading

- Ensure there is adequate capacity for maximum stock.
- Check that perishable goods are delivered in a refrigerated vehicle.
- Only fill frozen food storage cabinets with prefrozen food.
- Never put hot or warm food in a refrigerator unless it is specially designed for rapid chilling.
- Ensure no damage is caused to inner linings and insulation by staples or nails, in packaging.
- Air must be allowed to circulate within a refrigerator to maintain the cooling effect – do not obstruct any airways.

Cleaning

Clean thoroughly inside and out at least every two months as blocked drain lines, drip trays and air ducts will eventually lead to a breakdown.

- Switch off power.
- If possible transfer stock to available alternative storage.
- Clean interior surfaces with lukewarm water and a mild detergent. Do not use abrasives or strongly scented cleaning agents.
- Clean exterior and dry all surfaces inside and out.
- Clear away any external dirt, dust or rubbish which might restrict the circulation of air around the condenser.
- Switch on power, check when the correct working temperature is reached, refill with stock.

Defrosting

This is important as it helps equipment perform efficiently and prevents a potentially damaging build up of ice. Presence of ice on the evaporator or internal surfaces indicates the need for urgent defrosting; if the equipment is designed to defrost automatically this also indicates a fault.

Automatic defrosting may lead to a temporary rise in air temperature; this is normal and will not put food at risk.

For manual defrosting of chest freezers always follow suppliers' instructions to obtain optimum performance. Never use a hammer or any sharp instrument which could perforate cabinet linings – a plastic spatula can be used to remove stubborn ice.

Emergency measures

Signs of imminent breakdown include: unusual noises, fluctuating temperatures, frequent stopping and starting of the compressor, excessive frost build up, absence of normal frost.

Prepare to call a competent refrigeration service engineer, but first check that:

○ the power supply has not been accidentally switched off;

○ the electrical circuit has not been broken by a blown fuse or the triggering of an automatic circuit breaker;

○ there has been no unauthorised tampering with the user temperature control device;

○ any temperature higher than recommended is not due solely to routine automatic defrosting, to the refrigerator door being left open, or to overloading the equipment or to any blockage of internal passage of air;

○ there is no blockage of air to the condenser by rubbish, crates, cartons, etc. If you still suspect a fault, call the engineer and be prepared to give brief details of the equipment and the fault. Keep the door of the defective cold cabinet closed as much as possible to retain cold air. Destroy any spoilt food.

Monitoring refrigeration efficiency

The Energy Technology Support Unit (ETSU) estimates that businesses could save 20–25% of the energy currently consumed by refrigeration plants. The local energy efficiency advice centre may be able to provide consultancy services at subsidised or no cost.

All types of refrigerators, walk-in, cabinet with or without forced air circulation should be fitted with display thermometers or chart recorders that will enable daily monitoring to check that the equipment is working correctly. Sensors which can set off available alarms must be placed in the warmest part of the cabinet.

Chilled display units include:

○ multi-deck cabinets with closed doors used for dispensing sandwiches, drinks and other foods, used if food needs to be displayed for more than four hours;

○ open and semi-open display cabinets where food is presented on the base of the unit and cooled by circulating cooled air;

○ Gastronorm counters (see Figure 7.18, page 244).

Because of surrounding conditions it is unsafe to assume that refrigerated display cabinets will maintain the temperature of the food below 5°C (41°F) which is why these units should never be used to store food other than for display periods of not more than four hours.

Maintenance and servicing should be carried out regularly by qualified personnel.

Further information can be obtained from British Refrigeration Association, Henley Rd, Medmanham, Marlow, Buckinghamshire SL7 2ER www.fete.co.uk

DISHWASHING MACHINES

For hygienic washing up the generally recognised requirements are a good supply of hot water at a temperature of 60°C (140°F) for general cleansing followed by a sterilising rinse at a temperature of 82°C (180°F) for at least one minute. Alternatively low-temperature equipment is available which sterilises by means of a chemical, sodium hypochlorite (bleach). Further information can be obtained from Lever Industrial, Lever House, St James Road, Kingston-upon-Thames, Surrey KT1 2BA.

Dishwashing machines take over an arduous job and save a lot of time and labour, ensuring that a good supply of clean, sterilised crockery is available.

There are three main types:

○ Spray types pass-through dish washers – the dishes are placed in racks which slide into the machines where they are subjected to a spray of hot detergent water at 48–60°C (118–140°F) from above and below. The racks move on to the next section where they are rinsed by a fresh hot shower at 82°C (180°F). At this temperature they are sterilised, and on passing out into the air they dry off quickly.

○ Brush-type machines – use revolving brushes for the scrubbing of each article in hot detergent water; the articles are then rinsed and sterilised in another compartment.

○ Agitator water machines – baskets of dishes are immersed in deep tanks and the cleaning is performed by the mechanical agitation of the hot detergent water. The loaded baskets are then given a sterilising rinse in another compartment.

Dishwashing machines are costly and it is essential that the manufacturer's instructions with regard to use and maintenance are followed at all times.

MISCELLANEOUS EQUIPMENT

Food waste disposers

Food waste disposers are operated by electricity and take all manner of rubbish, including bones, fat, scraps and vegetable refuse. Almost every type of rubbish and swill, with the exception of rags and tins, are finely ground, then rinsed down the drain. It is the most modern and hygienic method of waste disposal. Care should be taken by handlers not to push waste into the machine with a metal object as this can cause damage.

Other equipment which may be found in a busy kitchen include an automatic pastry roller (see Figure 7.19, page 244) and toasters.

SMALL EQUIPMENT AND UTENSILS

Small equipment and utensils are made from a variety of materials such as non-stick coated metal, iron, steel, copper, aluminium, wood.

Iron

Items of equipment used for frying, such as movable fritures and frying-pans of all types, are usually made of heavy, black wrought iron.

Frying-pans are available in several shapes and many sizes, e.g.:

○ omelette pans;
○ oval fish frying-pans;
○ frying-pans;
○ pancake pans.

Baking sheets are made in various sizes of black wrought steel. The less they are washed the less likely they are to cause food to stick. New baking sheets should be well heated in a hot oven, thoroughly wiped with a clean cloth and then lightly oiled. Before being used baking trays should be lightly greased with a pure fat or oil. Immediately after use and while still warm they should be cleaned by scraping and dry-wiping. Hot soda or detergent water should be used for washing.

Tartlet and barquette moulds and cake tins should be cared for in the same way as for baking sheets.

Tinned steel

A number of items are made from this metal:

- conical strainer (*chinois*), used for passing sauces and gravies;
- fine conical strainer, used for passing sauces and gravies;
- colander, used for draining vegetables;
- vegetable reheating container;
- soup machine and mouli strainer, used for passing thick soups, sauces and potatoes for mash;
- sieves.

Copper

Tin lined copper pans are seldom used today because they are expensive, need periodic re-tinning which is also expensive, they also tarnish easily and look dirty.

Aluminium

Note: Minimum use of aluminium is recommended: stainless steel is to be preferred.

Saucepans, stockpots, sauteuses, sauté pans, braising pans, fish kettles and large, round deep pans and dishes of all sizes are made in cast aluminium. They are expensive, but one advantage is that the pans do not tarnish; also because of their strong, heavy construction they are suitable for many cooking processes.

A disadvantage is that in the manufacture of aluminium, which is a soft metal, other metals are added to make pans stronger. As a result certain foods can become discoloured (care should be taken when mixing white sauces and white soups). A wooden spoon should be used for mixing, then there should be no discoloration. The use of metal whisks or spoons must be avoided.

Water boiled in aluminium pans is unsuitable for tea-making as it gives the tea an unpleasant colour. Red cabbage and artichokes should not be cooked in aluminium pans as they will take on a dark colour, caused by chemical reaction.

Stainless steel

Heavy duty stainless steel pans, incorporating an extra thick aluminium base which gives excellent heat diffusion are available. They are suitable for all surfaces except induction hobs. Stainless steel is also used for many items of small equipment.

Non-stick metal

An ever-increasing variety of kitchen utensils (saucepans, frying pans, baking and roasting tins) are available and are suitable for certain types of kitchen operation, such as small scale or à la carte. Particular attention should be paid to the following points, otherwise the non-stick properties of the equipment will be affected:

Figure 7.24 *Non-stick pans*

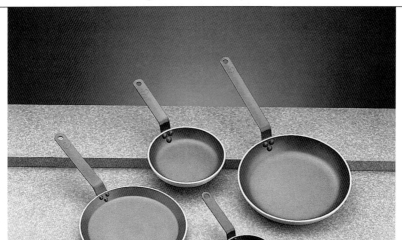

○ excessive heat should be avoided;
○ use plastic or wooden spatulas or spoons when using non-stick pans so that contact is not made to the surface with metal;
○ extra care is needed when cleaning non-stick surfaces; the use of cloth or paper is most suitable.

There are many small pieces of equipment made from metal of all types.

Figure 7.25 *Mouli; potato ricer; potato mashers; pestle; mortar*

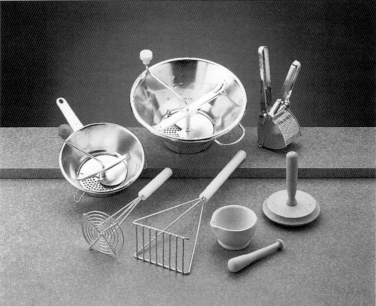

Figure 7.26 *Vegetable slicers (mandolines)*

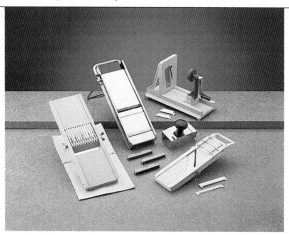

Wood and compound materials
Cutting boards *(See also page 214)*

These are an important item of kitchen equipment which should be kept in use on all table surfaces to protect the table and the edges of cutting knives.

Figure 7.27 *Modern chopping boards*

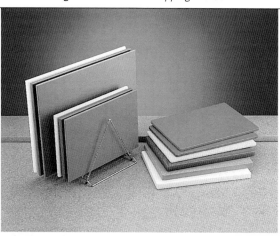

WOODEN CHOPPING BOARDS

To comply with current regulations, wooden boards should not splinter or leak preservatives. They should be of close-grained hard wood either in a thick, solid slab or separate pieces with close-fitting joints.

- Before using a new board, wash to remove wood dust.
- After use scrub with hot detergent water, rinse with clean water, dry as much as possible and stand on its longest end to prevent warping.
- Do not use for heavy chopping; use a chopping block instead.

CUTTING BOARDS OF COMPOUND MATERIALS

There are several types available. When selecting compound cutting boards it is essential to purchase those with a non-slip surface.

○ Polyethylene: six boards can be obtained marked in different colours along one edge. These can be kept in a special rack after washing and when not in use. This system is designed to cut down on cross-contamination by using one board exclusively for one type of food (see page 253).

○ Rubber: cutting boards are also made of hard rubber and rubber compounds (rubber, polystyrene and clay). These are hygienic because they are solid, in one piece and should not warp, crack or absorb flavours. They are cleaned by scrubbing with hot water and then drying or passing through a dishwasher.

ROLLING PINS, WOODEN SPOONS AND SPATULAS

These items should be scrubbed in hot detergent water, rinsed in clean water and dried. Rolling pins should not be scraped with a knife as this can cause the wood to splinter. Adhering paste can be removed with a cloth. Wooden spoons and spatulas are being replaced by a high-density plastic capable of withstanding very high temperatures. Wooden spoons/spatulas are considered unhygienic unless washed in a suitable sterilising solution such as sodium hypochloride solution (bleach) or a solution of Milton. Metal piping tubes are being replaced by plastic. These can be boiled and do not rust.

WOODEN SIEVES AND MANDOLINS

When these are being cleaned, care of the wooden frame should be considered taking into account the previous remarks. The blades of the mandolin should be kept lightly greased to prevent rust (stainless steel mandolins with protective guards are available).

CHINA AND EARTHENWARE

Bowls and dishes in china and earthenware are useful for serving and for microwaved dishes. They should be cleaned in a dishwasher with mild detergent and rinse aid, or by hand using the appropriate detergent for hand washing.

Figure 7.28 *Examples of flameproof china dishes*

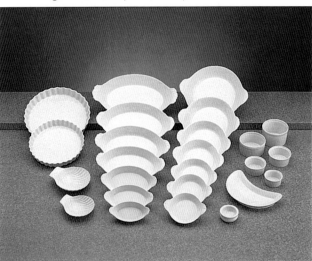

Materials

All materials should be washed immediately after use in hot detergent water, rinsed in hot, clean water and then dried. Tammy cloths, muslins and linen piping bags must be boiled periodically in detergent water. Kitchen cloths should be washed or changed frequently, otherwise accumulating dirt and food stains may cause cross-contamination of harmful bacteria/germs on to clean food.

○ Muslin may be used for straining soups and sauces.
○ Piping bags are made from linen, nylon or disposable plastic and are used for piping preparations of all kinds.
○ Kitchen cloths
  – General purpose – for washing up and cleaning surfaces.
  – Tea towel (teacloth) – for drying up and general-purpose hand cloths.
  – Bactericide wiping cloths – impregnated with bactericide to disinfect work surfaces. The cloths have a coloured pattern which fades and disappears when the bactericide is no longer effective; the cloth should then be discarded.
  – Oven cloths – thick cloths designed to protect the hands when removing hot items from the oven. Oven cloths must only be used dry, never damp or wet, otherwise the user is likely to be burned.

Papers

○ Greaseproof or silicone – for lining cake-tins, making piping bags and wrapping greasy items of food.
○ Kitchen – white absorbent paper for absorbing grease from deep-fried foods and for lining trays on which cold foods are kept.
○ General purpose – thick, absorbent paper for wiping and drying equipment, surfaces, food, etc.
○ Towels – disposable, for drying of hands.

Foils

○ Clingwrap – a thin, transparent material for wrapping sandwiches, snacks, hot and cold foods. Clingwrap has the advantage of being very flexible and easy to handle and seal. Due to risk of contamination, it is advisable to use a clingwrap that does not contain PVC, or is plasticiser-free.
○ Metal foil – a thin, pliable, silver-coloured material for wrapping and covering foods and for protecting oven roasted joints during cooking.

Topics for Discussion

1 List the essential requirements of kitchen equipment.
2 Discuss the respective advantages of a conventional oven, convection oven and a combination convection/steaming oven.
3 Compare induction cooking plates, halogen hobs or the conventional cooking tops.
4 Compare copper pans or stainless steel pans.
5 What are the benefits of the bratt pan?
6 What essential items of mechanical equipment are needed?
7 Discuss the importance of sufficient refrigeration.
8 What are the benefits of the food waste disposer or the advantages of a food compactor.

9   What is the argument for maintaining wooden chopping boards.

10   Discuss the design of equipment in relation to maintaining high standards of hygiene.

11   What factors should be considered by those designing kitchen equipment?

12   What faults, if any, do you wish to be remedied in any items of equipment?

13   What improvements could you suggest?

ENERGY EFFICIENCY
ENERGY AND THE ENVIRONMENT

The burning of fossil fuels to generate energy releases gases into the atmosphere. These include sulphur dioxide that gives rise to acid rain and carbon dioxide that is the main contributor to the threat of global warming.

Factors to convert consumption of fuels to emissions of carbon dioxide, in kg of carbon dioxide produced per kWh of fuel used are:

○ gas   0.21
○ oil   0.29
○ electricity   0.72

A typical hotel releases annually about 160 kg of CO_2 per square metre of floor area, equivalent to about 10 tonnes per bedroom.

WHO BENEFITS FROM ENERGY EFFICIENCY?

○ Hotel owners and management benefit because efficiency run buildings cost less to operate.

○ Guests benefit because an efficiently controlled hotel satisfies their needs and leads to repeat business.

○ Staff benefit through improved morale and better motivation, which in turn increase productivity.

○ The environment benefits because using energy efficiently reduces the adverse effects on the environment and preserves non-renewable resources for future generations.

Figure 7.29 *Analysis of delivered energy by cost*	**Figure 7.30** *Analysis of delivered energy by use*

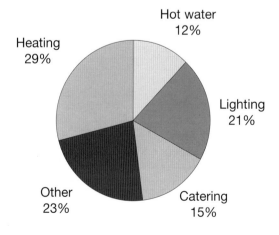

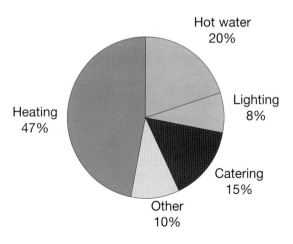

ENERGY EFFICIENCY MEASURES AND PERCENTAGE SAVINGS

Savings quoted are the *minimum* you can expect to achieve. Small percentage savings can mean appreciable cash benefits.

	BOILERS, CONTROLS AND HOT WATER	FOSSIL SAVING %	ELECTRICITY SAVING %	LIGHTING, CATERING AND OTHER SERVICES	FOSSIL SAVING %	ELECTRICITY SAVING %
No Cost	Ensure systems come on only when, where and to the extent they are needed.	1	2	Switch off lights and other equipment whenever possible. Label light switches.	0	0.5
	Establish a daily routine for checking control settings, especially where they may have been over-ridden in response to unexpected circumstances	1	1	Make maximum use of daylight. Place lights where they will be most effective. Clean light fittings and use translucent shades. Improve the reflection of light from walls and ceilings by using pale colours	0	0.5
	Use your existing equipment effectively. Check that timers, programmers, optimum start controls and weather compensation controls are set up and operating correctly.	3	1	Set illumination levels to the type of activity. Reduce lighting levels where possible and remove surplus lamps (but do not compromise safety).	0	0.5
	Isolate parts of systems which are not in use, for example, seasonally. Remove redundant pipework during refurbishment.	1	0	Provide training for catering staff about energy costs and correct use of equipment. Set energy targets for meals, monitor consumption and give feedback to staff.	0.2	0.2
	Ensure plant is regularly and correctly maintained	0.5	0.5	Ensure regular maintenance of cooking utensils, all appliances, burners, timers, controls and taps. Badly maintained equipment wastes energy.	0.2	0.2

continues

	BOILERS, CONTROLS AND HOT WATER	FOSSIL SAVING %	ELECTRICITY SAVING %	LIGHTING, CATERING AND OTHER SERVICES	FOSSIL SAVING %	ELECTRICITY SAVING %
	Review hot water thermostat accuracy and temperature settings periodically. Reducing temperatures will save energy – but take precautions to avoid the risk of Legionnaire's Disease.	1	0	Ensure optimum use of hot water, ventilation and lighting in the kitchen for various times of day and night. Do not use hobs or ovens for space heating. Run dishwashers only on full loads.	0.2	0.2
Low Cost	Fit draught stripping around windows and doors. Fit heavy curtains to guest and public rooms.	1	0	Where fittings allow, replace 38 mm fluorescent light tubes by 26 mm type, and install electronic starters and ballasts.	0	0.5
	Check boiler efficiency periodically and make improvements as required.	2	0	Consider replacement of tungsten lamps (including light fittings where necessary) by compact fluorescent types.	0	6
	Provide temperature and time controls for domestic hot water.	1	0	Consider installation of timers, dimmers, photocells and sensors so lighting operates only when, where and to the extent needed.	0	1
	Install showers and flow restrictors where possible. Reduce standing losses from hot water storage by lagging pipes and tanks	2	1	Consider installation of bedroom key fobs so lights and other electrical items operate only when rooms are occupied.	0	1

continues

BOILERS, CONTROLS AND HOT WATER	FOSSIL SAVING %	ELECTRICITY SAVING %	LIGHTING, CATERING AND OTHER SERVICES	FOSSIL SAVING %	ELECTRICITY SAVING %
Consider direct fired water heaters for hot water in place of boiler serving calorifier.	3	0	When replacing catering equipment, review current developments in appliance design to select the most energy efficient.	1	1
Establish a system for setting targets for energy consumption, monitoring actual consumption and assessing performance.	1	2	If you have a swimming pool, provide and use a cover to reduce heat losses at night.	0.5	0
Modernise heating and ventilation plant controls.	6	1	Ensure enough linen is available so that laundry equipment is run at full load.	0.5	0
Provide power factor correction, and consider load shedding to reduce maximum demand charges. This will not save fuel but will reduce electricity charges.	6	1	Use high efficiency lights for all external lights, including car parking areas, controlled by timers and/or photocells.	0	0.5

ELECTRICAL SAFETY

All electrical products must meet safety criteria laid out in European and National regulations.

FURTHER INFORMATION

HCIMA Techical brief no. 36. Energy Efficiency Office, Department of the Environment.

SERVICES AND ENERGY CONSERVATION

The supply of gas, electricity and water are of vital importance to the caterer. Any information required is best obtained up to date from the appropriate local board.

COMPARISON OF ELECTRICITY AND GAS

ADVANTAGES	DISADVANTAGES
Electricity	
○ Clean to use, low maintenance.	○ Time taken to heat up in a few instances.
○ Easily controlled, labour saving.	○ Particular utensils are required for some hobs, e.g. induction.
○ Good working atmosphere.	○ More expensive than gas.
○ Little heat loss, no storage space required.	
○ Low ventilation requirements.	
Gas	
○ Convenient, labour saving, no smoke or dirt	○ Some heat is lost in the kitchen.
○ Special utensils not required.	○ Regular cleaning required for efficient working.
○ No fuel storage required.	○ For gas to produce heat it must burn; this requires oxygen which is contained in the air and as a result carbon dioxide and water are produced.
○ Easily controllable with immediate full heat and the flames are visible.	○ As a result, adequate ventilation must be provided for combustion and to ensure a satisfactory working environment.
○ Cheaper than electricity.	

Gas

Gas is a safe fuel, but like all fuels it must be treated with respect.

What to do if you smell gas:

○ Open all doors and windows.

○ Check whether a gas tap has been left on, or if a pilot light has gone out. If so, turn off the appliance.

○ If in doubt, turn off the gas supply at the meter and phone for emergency service.

Electricity

Electricity cannot be heard, tasted or smelled. Installed and used correctly, it is a very safe source of energy, but misused can kill or cause serious injury. It is therefore essential that any electrical installation is undertaken by qualified engineers in accordance with British Standard 7671 and carried out by registered contractors of the National Inspection Council for Electrical Installation Contracting (NICIEC). A technical brief 'Guide to Electric Lighting, No 7/97' is available from the HCIMA.

Water

Water authorities are required, by law, to provide a supply of clean, wholesome water; water free from suspended matter, odour and taste; all bacteria which are likely to cause disease; and mineral matter injurious to health.

Comparison of fuels

Electricity and mains gas are most generally used in catering. Bottled gas, e.g. Calor is also used in some catering operations. Before deciding on the fuel to use (if there is a choice) the following factors should be considered:

○ safety;
○ cost;
○ efficiency;
○ storage requirements;
○ constancy of supply;
○ cleanliness and need for ventilation;
○ cost of equipment, installation and maintenance.

Energy conservation

At the Earth Summit in Rio de Janeiro in 1992 the UK signed an international agreement entitled the 'Climate Change convention', whereby it agreed that by the year 2000 the UK would reduce its fossil fuel emissions to the same levels as 1990. Energy conservation is not just an ethical or green issue but makes good business sense.

The costs of energy used in hotel and catering establishments varies widely according to the type of fuel used, the type and age of equipment, the way in which it is used and the tariff paid.

The basic principles of energy management are:

○ obtaining the best tariff available;
○ purchasing the most suitable energy efficient equipment;
○ reducing heat loss to a minimum;
○ matching heat and cooling loads on environmental systems whenever possible to the demands;
○ maintaining all equipment to optimum efficiency;
○ ensuring that the operating periods of systems and equipment are set correctly;
○ using heat recovery systems;
○ monitoring energy consumption;
○ training staff to be energy efficient.

Some factors to be considered in energy conservation

1 Always replace equipment with low energy rating equipment, by referring to wattage and running costs.

2 Ensure that all machinery is maintained at its optimum efficiency and that equipment needing regular cleaning is serviced in accordance with the maintenance manual requirements. This particularly applies to filters on ventilation and on conditioning systems, refrigeration plant condensers, cooking equipment and dishwashing machines.

3 When replacing equipment, its an opportune time to review the contents of the menu, the cooking and storage methods that menu requires. Can certain procedures be scaled down, omitted or can alternative procedures be used?

4 Check all preheating of equipment, over long pre-heating wastes fuel.

5 Constantly review all heating cooking procedures.

6 Is it possible to reduce operating hours?

7 Regularly check ventilation systems.

8 Regularly check that storage temperatures for hot water systems are not more than 65°C for central systems and 55°C for local units. Also ensure that this temperature is not less than 55°C to avoid the risk of legionnaires disease.

9 Regularly check all lighting systems, where possible use energy efficient compact fluorescent bulbs.

10 Train staff not to waste lighting or use lighting unnecessarily.

Some references to planning and equipment elsewhere in the book

Topics for Discussion

1 The advantages of gas or electricity for kitchen equipment.

2 How to effect economy in the consumption of energy by catering equipment.

3 Why maintenance of all services is essential.

4 How water conservation can be achieved.

5 Why hot water is more costly than cold water and how these costs can be reduced.

6 How could the use of the sun and wind be used to reduce costs in small establishments?

7 Discuss how training could reduce wastage of water, gas and electricity.

CHAPTER 8

Production Systems

QUALITY IN THE MANAGEMENT OF FOOD AND BEVERAGE PRODUCTION SYSTEMS

The British Standard Quality Award BS EN ISO 9002 : 1994, is a quality kitemark (standard or benchmark) in the fitness for purpose and safety in use sense, in the service provided and/or the products designed and constructed to satisfy the customer's needs.

It is concerned primarily with evidence of systematic processes, which are employed within an operation and which can demonstrate that there is a link between customer demand and the services and products on offer.

EUROPEAN FOUNDATION FOR QUALITY MANAGEMENT EXCELLENCE MODEL (1999)

The European Foundation for Quality Management Excellence Model is a non-prescriptive framework, which recognises that there are many approaches to achieving sustainable excellence in all aspects of performance. The model is based on nine criteria.

The model emphasises that results for customers, people (employees) and society are achieved through leadership driving policy and strategy, people management, partnership and resources and processes leading to business results.

Innovation and learning help to improve the enables, which in turn improve results.

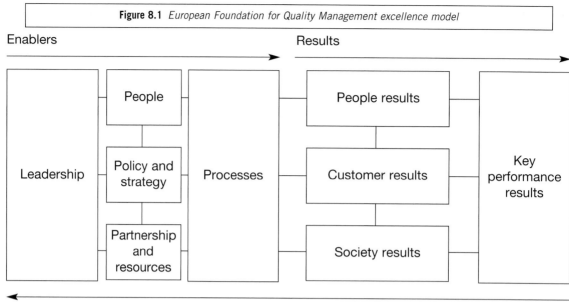

Figure 8.1 *European Foundation for Quality Management excellence model*

BRITISH STANDARD EN ISO 9002 : 1994

The British Standard scheme was introduced in 1979 with the aim of providing a method for organisations to assess the suitability of their supplier's products. The scheme aimed to rationalise the many schemes of supplier assessment used by various purchasing firms and organisations.

BS EN ISO 9002 identifies the systems, procedures and criteria that ensure that a product or service meets a customer's requirements. The key elements in quality management for most organisations in the hotel and catering (hospitality) industry include.

○ management responsibility – policy, objectives, identification of key personnel;

○ quality system procedures – all functions must be covered;

○ auditing the system – it must be audited internally;

○ quality in marketing – honest promotional activities;

○ material control and traceability – supplies must be traceable;

○ non-conformity – ensuring that faulty products/service do not reach the customer;

○ corrective action – identifying reasons for faults and subsequently implementing measures to correct them and records of the faults and measures, written and kept;

○ after-sales service – procedures for monitoring quality of after-sales service;

○ documentation and records – records of checks and inspections, action taken, audit reports;

○ personnel and training – identification of needs, provision and verification of training;

○ product safety and liability – procedures for handling, storing and processing materials, for example foods.

BS EN ISO 9002 can be important to food service operations for two reasons. First, when purchasing goods and services, BS EN ISO 9002 indicates that a supplier operates a quality system of a high standard. Secondly, food service operators, such as contract caterers, may find that they will not be considered as potential tenderers if they have not achieved BS EN ISO 9002. Additionally, BS EN ISO 9002 may even provide useful evidence that due diligence had been exercised, for example in the event of a food service operation being prosecuted under the Food Safety Act 1990.

In an increasingly competitive marketplace, and with increasing uniformity between operations, the level of service provided and its quality become ever more important. It is the front-line members of staff that offer this service: their training and development are crucial to the successful running of an operation. Total quality management offers a framework by which members of staff are given the scope to treat guests as individuals, and thereby offer superior service.

However, the costs involved in attaining the standard can be high, and therefore the introduction of BS EN ISO 9002 needs to be carefully assessed before implementation takes place. On the other hand, the reviews from many of the organisations moving towards BS EN ISO 9002 have suggested that it is cost-effective.

Further information on quality matters can be obtained from:

European Foundation for Quality Management
Brussels Representative Office
Avenue des Pleiades, 15
1200 Brussels
Belgium
http://www.efqm.org

The complete documents on BS EN ISO 9002: 1994 are available from:

British Standards Institution
Linford Wood
Milton Keynes
MK14 6LE

Also see *Managing Quality in the Catering Industry* (East 1993) and HCIMA Technical Brief no. 20/98, 'BSENISO 9002: 1994' (HCIMA, 1998).

PROBLEMS

Food production systems, such as cook-chill, cook-freeze and sous-vide, have been introduced into certain areas of catering in order to increase efficiency and productivity; changes have been made to maximise utilisation of equipment and to maintain high levels of output and viability.

The problems of the catering industry are as follows:

○ Staff
- unattractive work conditions;
- limited skilled staff;
- mobility of labour.

○ Food
- high cost;
- wastage.

○ Equipment
- high cost of replacement and maintenance;
- under-usage.

○ Energy
- wasteful high-cost traditional systems;
- availability.

○ Overheads
  – wage increases;
  – payments to National Insurance.
○ Space
  – most kitchens and services must be adequate for comfortable working while using space efficiently.
  – space is very costly.

The solution to these problems comes in the form of centralisation of production, using the skilled staff available to prepare and cook in bulk and then to distribute to finishing kitchens, which are smaller in size, employing semi-skilled and unskilled labour.

Cook-freeze and cook-chill systems have been developed to meet these requirements, each system having advantages over the other depending on the size and nature of the overall operation. For example, cook-freeze is not adaptable to very small units or to haute cuisine. Cook-chill can be adapted to any type of unit but cannot take advantage of seasonal, cheaper commodities.

Sous-vide, which is a method of working under vacuum-sealing, ice-water bath chilling and chilled storage, has also been developed as a production system.

Many catering operations face problems because of the growing shortage of skilled catering staff and the ever-increasing turnover of employees. Therefore:

○ It is essential that skilled staff are more fully utilised and given improved working conditions.
○ Certain catering tasks require deskilling so as to be carried out by a greater proportion of unskilled staff.
○ Better benefits and conditions of employment must be provided for fewer key staff in order to reduce levels of staff turnover and enhance job satisfaction.

Assured safe catering

This is a system developed for and with caterers to control food safety problems. It is based upon some of the principles of hazard analysis and critical control point (HACCP).

It involves looking at the catering operation step by step from the selection of ingredients right through to the service of food to the customer. With careful analysis or each step of the catering operation anything that may affect the safety of the food is identified. The caterer can then determine when and how to control that hazard. Assured Safe Catering helps prevent safety problems by careful planning in easy steps.

HYGIENE OF FOOD PRODUCTION SYSTEMS

Hygiene committees

It is generally recognised that one of the principal concerns of food production for caterers is to ensure that the food is safe when consumed. The need for special attention to be given to food hygiene is now well recognised. This involves everyone, whether directly or indirectly involved with food handling. In order for both to focus attention on the subject it is advisable for large caterers to set up hygiene committees. These should comprise those with an immediate responsibility for maintaining hygiene standards, quality control and training personnel, and also include representatives from all sections of the food production line, including the Food Service Personnel.

It is advisable that staff be seconded on to the committee for a set period of time, maximum two years, to encourage others in the organisation to show an interest. The objective is to set the pace in food hygiene standards. It can be useful from time to time to invite specialist speakers to talk on hygiene subjects relating to the industry on cleaning, equipment or transportation.

Figure 8.2 *The process of food hygiene management for production*

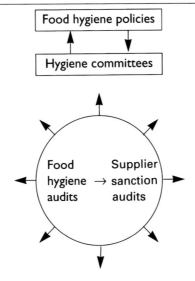

Food hygiene policies

Hygiene committees

Food hygiene audits → Supplier sanction audits

Hazard Analysis and Critical Control Point

Flow diagrams ——— hazards

Production details ——— hazards

Stages of the process

Management reports

Figure 8.3 *Elements of production*

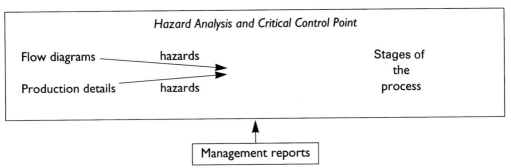

Food	Preparation	Cooking	Holding	Regeneration	Presentation
fresh	weigh/measure	blanche	chill	regithermic	bain marie
fresh cooked	clear/open	warm	sous vide	microwave	service flats
fresh prepared	chop/cut	simmer	freeze	convection	plates
canned	combine/mix	boil	tray	traditional	trays
frozen	blend	steam	hot cupboard		vending
chilled	shape/coat	grill	cold cupboard		buffet
vacuum	form	sauté			trolley
dehydrated		brown			dishes
smoked		bake			
salted		roast			
crystallized		broil			
acidified		fry			
pasteurized		microwave			
bottled					
UHT					

Foods in ←——————————— Process ——————————→ Ouput

Hazard analysis and critical control point (HACCP)

Developed in the USA in the mid 1970s HACCP is already used extensively in food manufacturing and processing. HACCP is a process which critically examines each stage of the process and where these may appear vulnerable in terms of producing a hazard into the food, then particular attention is given at that point. The process therefore critically examines the food production flow until the food is consumed. Once potential hazards in the food's journey are identified, whether it be in the kitchen or before, then particular attention can be given to eliminate or minimise the hazard. One of the advantages of HACCP is that a multi-disciplinary team is involved because it covers the entire range of activities associated with the product. The system does require the food preparation staff to be trained and committed to be effective.

For any caterer wishing to introduce HACCP the following need to be identified:

○ a flow diagram showing the path of the food throughout its manufacture;

○ product details so that any special characteristics that could cause a problem are noted;

○ where in each stage there is the likelihood of a hazard occurring; the risks should then be assessed as high, medium or low and then monitoring and control procedures can be implemented.

Food sampling and bacterial swabs are generally used to complement the HACCP programme.

Figure 8.4 *Work flow model*

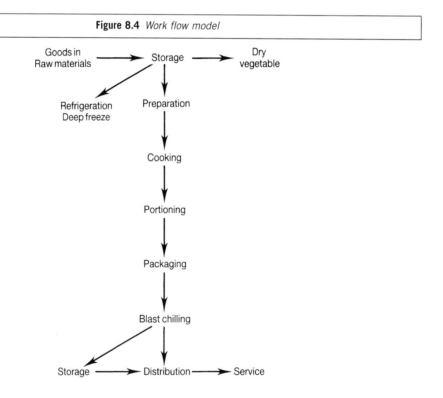

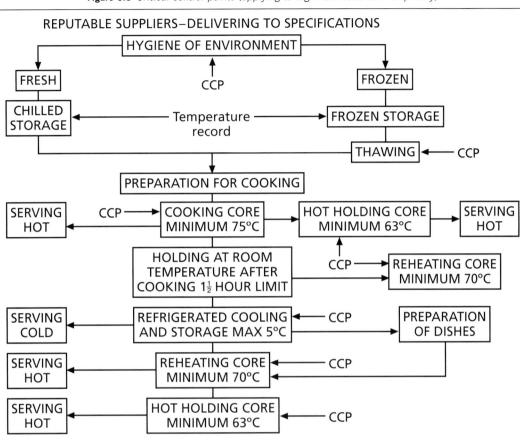

Figure 8.5 *Critical control points (applying to high-risk foods such as poultry)*

HACCP must not be seen as a sophisticated and thus complicated programme intended only for the larger operators. Every food has its critical point to some extent; this is why food production is so vulnerable. Those involved in food production must be aware of these stages where hazards occur and make every effort to eradicate or minimise them by paying extra attention to hygiene at the crucial stages in the production cycle. A programme of periodic monitoring will ensure that these parts of the food production chain will be properly monitored and safe.

EXAMPLES OF CRITICAL CONTROL POINTS

○ Inspection (including temperature checks) of goods on delivery and before use.
○ Separate storage and handling of ingredients and the finished product.
○ Correct temperature ranges of refrigerated and frozen goods.
○ Cleaning procedures for equipment and utensils.
○ Cross-contamination with other menu items in process.
○ Personal hygiene and health standards.
○ Proficiency in use and cleaning of equipment.

Further information: HCIMA Technical brief sheet No 5.

Food hygiene audits

Food hygiene audits are intended to scrutinise the food production operation with a view to recording deficiencies and areas for improvement, or simply to monitor performance at a certain point. These may be linked to any quality assurance criteria.

The approach to the audit may vary but it generally involves a suitably qualified person carrying out an in depth inspection of both premises, plant and the food production practices. There should be a report back procedure to management with both observations where necessary and any recommendations.

Caterers can change their techniques of operation for various reasons, without being aware of any hazards that are introduced and it is very easy for staff who are familiar with the production plant to fail to see problem areas that are emerging. It may be that staff are beginning to be lax in connection with a certain task. It could be that maintenance is required to parts of the building. Similarly, equipment may need attention. Day-to-day familiarity with the work and the operation often means that those closest to it simply do not notice problems and therefore a hygiene audit is one way of bringing in someone who can look critically, to the extent of picking up any problem areas or practices.

The frequency of these audits will vary. High intensity production will justify more frequent audits. It is important that whatever emerges from the in-depth inspections must be properly recorded and brought to the attention of the appropriate people, either the management or individual food handlers or both. Management must in turn ensure that the hygiene audit is acted upon, otherwise there is little value in the exercise.

Standards of hygiene

To ensure safe hygienic standards in any system the following points are crucial.

REFRIGERATION

Efficient refrigeration and temperature control are essential otherwise there is the danger of deterioration in structure, quality, appearance and nutritional value. Any rise in temperature will encourage the growth of micro-organisms and lead to poor quality food which may need to be destroyed.

It is vital that accurate temperature control and monitoring are carried out throughout the cook-freeze, blast-freeze, storage and regeneration process to ensure that food is always held at acceptable and safe temperatures.

Devices used to measure temperature (see Figure 8.7 on page 274) include:

○ hand-held probes, which provide a digital read-out for random checking at all stages;
○ audible alarms, fitted inside cold stores to warn of rises in temperature;
○ temperature gauges, which give a visible reading of the temperature.

PRODUCTION

In order to ensure that high quality, palatable food is produced at all times it is essential that working conditions are maintained to the highest possible standards, as laid down in the HMSO publication *Clean Catering*, such as:

○ stringent personal hygiene precautions against infection of the food;
○ all working surfaces and utensils thoroughly cleaned to minimise spread of bacteria;
○ clean equipment and utensils separated from used items awaiting cleaning;
○ separation of raw and cooked foods at all times;
○ strict control of cooking times and temperatures;
○ staff training in food hygiene;
○ consultation with medical and Public Health Officers when planning food production systems.

Further information: British Institute of Cleaning Science, 3 Moulton Court, Anglia Way, Moulton Park, Northampton NN3 6JA www.bics.org.uk

Figure 8.6 *Wheel-in refrigeration*

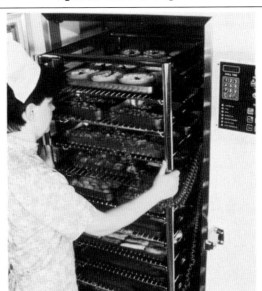

EQUIPMENT

The equipment used will vary according to the size of the operation but if food is batch-cooked then convection ovens, steaming ovens, bratt pans, jacketed boiling pans, tilting kettles, etc. may be used. Certain oven models are available in which a set of racks can be assembled with food and wheeled in for cooking.

The main difference between cook-freeze and cook-chill is the degree of refrigeration and the length of storage life. Other than these differences the information given in this chapter relates to both systems. (For details of cook-freeze, see page 283.)

COOK-CHILL

Cook-chill is a catering system based on normal preparation and cooking of food followed by rapid chilling storage in controlled low-temperature conditions above freezing point, 0–3°C (32–37°F) and subsequently reheating immediately before consumption. The chilled food is regenerated in finishing kitchens which require low capital investment and minimum staff. Almost any food can be cook-chilled provided that the correct methods are used during the preparation.

The cook-chill system is used in volume catering, in hospitals, schools and in social services. It is also used for banquets, in conference and exhibition catering, in vending machines where meals are dispensed to the customer, in factories, hospitals and services outside of main meal times.

Foods suitable for the cook-chill process
MEATS

All meat, poultry, game and offal can be cook-chilled. Meat dishes that need to be sliced, such as striploin of beef, is cooked, rapidly chilled, sliced and packaged for storage. The regeneration temperature must reach 70°C (158°F) in the centre of the produce for 2 minutes. Therefore, it is not possible to serve undercooked meats.

FISH

All precooked fish dishes are suitable for cook-chilling.

EGG DISHES

Omelets and scrambled eggs are now commonly used in this process especially on airlines. Omelets are now manufactured by companies who are able to supply the airline with the chilled product. The quality of the end product has greatly improved and continues to do so as more and more money is invested in product development.

SOUPS AND SAUCES

Most soups and sauces can now be successfully chilled. Those with a high-fat or egg-yolk content do need a certain amount of recipe modification to prevent separation on regeneration.

DESSERTS

There are a large number of desserts which chill well, especially the cold variety. Developments continue with hot sweets especially those which require a hot base and a separate topping.

Recipe modification

Successful production of chilled food does require a certain amount of recipe modification. These modifications may have to be introduced during the preparation or cooking or both.

BATTERED FISH

The batter should be made thicker, using a mixture with a higher fat content. This type of batter does not easily break away from the fish and will give a crisper end product.

STEWED/BRAISED ITEMS

Cut meat into smaller portions to avoid undue thickness. Flour-based sauces must be thoroughly cooked otherwise they will continue to thicken during regeneration.

SCRAMBLED EGGS

Cook until the egg begins to scramble, remove from heat and allow the product to continue to cook to a soft consistency. Chill immediately in shallow dishes, stir during chilling.

CREAMED AND MASHED POTATOES

More liquid is added than normal giving a loose and less dense product. This assists the chilling and regeneration stages as the potato absorbs more liquid when chilled.

The purpose of chilling food

The purpose of chilling food is to prolong its storage life. Under normal temperature conditions, food deteriorates rapidly through the action of micro-organisms and enzymic and chemical reactions. Reduction in the storage temperature inhibits the multiplication of bacteria and other micro-organisms and slows down the chemical and enzymic reactions. At normal refrigeration temperatures reactions are still taking place but at a much slower rate, and at frozen food storage temperatures, −20°C (−4°F) approximately, all reactions nearly cease. A temperature of 0–3°C

(32–37°F) does not give a storage life comparable to frozen food but it does produce a good product.

It is generally accepted that, even where high standards of fast chilling practice are used and consistent refrigerated storage is maintained, product quality may be acceptable for only a few days (including day of production and consumption). The storage temperature of 0–3°C (32–37°F) is of extreme importance to ensure both full protection of the food from microbiological growth and the maintenance of maximum nutritional values in the food. It is generally accepted that a temperature of 10°C (50°F) should be regarded as the critical safety limit for the storage of refrigerated food. Above that temperature, growth of micro-organisms may render the food dangerous to health.

In a properly designed and operated cook-chill system, cooked and prepared food will be rapidly cooled down to 0–3°C (32–37°F) as soon as possible after cooking and portioning and then stored between these temperatures throughout storage and distribution until required for reheating and service. Food prepared through the cook-chill system should be portioned and transferred to a blast chiller unit within 30 minutes. This will reduce the risk of the food remaining at warm incubation temperatures and prevent the risk of contamination and loss of food quality.

The cook-chill process

○ The food should be cooked sufficiently to ensure destruction of any pathogenic micro-organisms.

○ The chilling process must begin as soon as possible after completion of the cooking and portioning processes, within 30 minutes of leaving the cooker. The food should be chilled to 3°C (37°F) within a period of $1\frac{1}{2}$ hours (90 mins). Most pathogenic organisms will not grow below 7°C (45°F), while a temperature below 3°C (37°F) is required to reduce growth of spoilage organisms and to achieve the required storage life. However, slow growth of spoilage organisms does take place at these temperatures and for this reason storage life cannot be greater than five days.

○ The food should be stored at a temperature between 0–3°C (32–37°F).

○ The chilled food should be distributed under such controlled conditions that any rise in temperature of the food during distribution is kept to a minimum.

○ For both safety and palatability the reheating (regeneration) of the food should follow immediately upon the removal of the food from chilled conditions and should raise the temperature to a level of at least 70°C (158°F).

○ The food should be consumed as soon as possible and not more than 2 hours after reheating. Food not intended for reheating should be consumed as soon as convenient and within 2 hours of removal from storage. It is essential that unconsumed reheated food is discarded.

○ A temperature of 10°C (50°F) should be regarded as the critical safety limit for chilled food. Should the temperature of the chilled food rise above this level during storage or distribution the food concerned should be discarded.

Cook-chill is generally planned within a purpose-designed, comprehensive, new central production unit to give small, medium or large-scale production along predefined flow lines, incorporating traditional catering/chilling/post-chilling packaging and storage for delivery to finishing kitchens. Within an existing kitchen, where existing equipment is retained with possible minor additions and modifications, chilling/post-chilling packaging and additional storage for cooked chilled food are added.

Finishing kitchens

These can consist of purpose-built regeneration equipment plus refrigerated storage. Additional equipment, such as a chip fryer, boiling table and pressure steamer for chips, sauces, custard, vegetables, etc., can be added if required to give greater flexibility.

Where chilled food is produced to supply a service on the same premises, it is recommended that the meals should be supplied, stored and regenerated by exactly the same method as used for operations where the production unit and finishing kitchens are separated by some distance.

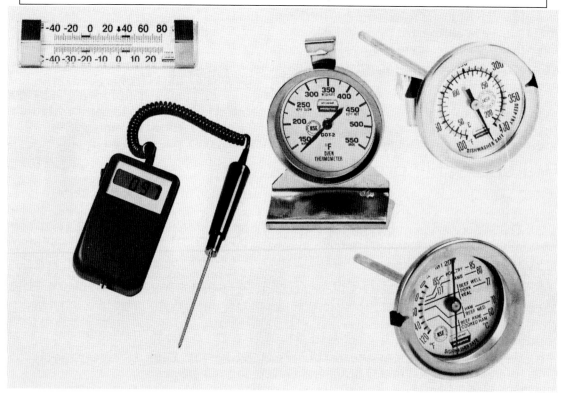

> **Figure 8.7** *A selection of temperature measuring devices (clockwise from top left): refrigerator/freezer thermometer; oven thermometer; confectionery/deep fat fry thermometer; meat thermometer; digital thermometer (general kitchen thermometer)*

Failure to adhere to just one procedure could result in disorganised production and reduced productivity. Once a decision is taken to sever production from service this method should be followed throughout the system.

Distribution of cook-chill

Distribution of the chilled food is an important part of the cook-chill operation. Fluctuations in storage temperature can affect the palatability and texture of food and lead to microbiological dangers requiring the food to be discarded. The distribution method chosen must ensure that the required temperature of below 3°C (37°F) is maintained throughout the period of transport. Should the temperature of the food exceed 5°C (41°F) during distribution the food ought to be consumed within 12 hours; if the temperature exceeds 10°C (50°F) it should be discarded (Department of Health guidelines). Because of this, refrigeration during distribution is to be encouraged in many circumstances.

In some cases the cook-chill production unit can also act as a centralised kitchen and distribution point. Food is regenerated in an area adjacent to the cook-chill production area and heat retention or insulated boxes are used for distribution. During transportation and service the food must not be allowed to fall below 62.8°C (145°F).

Know the legal requirements

Contravention of the Food Safety Act 1990 and the amendment regulations and lack of due diligence can be very costly if legal action is taken and proved against the caterer or food manufacturer. The labelling of food products, recording of temperatures, maintenance of hygiene standards and promotion of staff training is essential in defence of due diligence. For this defence to be successful, the caterer must convince the court that all the requirements under the law have been complied with and that the accepted customs and practices of the profession have been carried out. It is also of paramount importance that a caterer records that these systems have been adhered to by the submission of documentary evidence.

Avoiding the dangers of cook-chill

It is essential to:

○ maintain and record the correct temperatures;
○ maintain high standards of hygiene;
○ use fresh, high-quality ingredients avoiding raw materials which may contain excessive numbers of micro-organisms.

DELIVERIES

All food purchased must be of prime quality and stored correctly under the required temperatures.

PREPARATION

All food must be prepared quickly under the appropriate conditions avoiding any possible cross-contamination and at the correct temperature.

INITIAL COOKING AND PROCESSING

During the cooking process the centre of the food must reach a temperature of at least 70°C (158°F); preferably this temperature should reach 75°F or even 80°C (167–177°F) to achieve a greater safety margin.

PORTIONING

This should take place under appropriate conditions in a controlled environment, which is maintained to the highest hygiene standards. The depth of the food should be no more than approximately 5 cm (2 inch). The containers must be labelled with date of cooking, number of portions and reheating instructions.

CHILLING

All food must be chilled within 30 minutes of cooking and reduced to a temperature of 0–3°C (32–37°F) within 90 minutes.

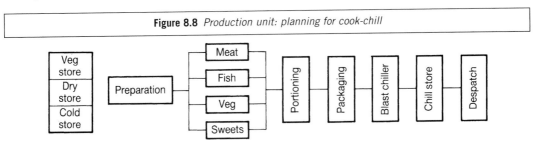

Figure 8.8 *Production unit: planning for cook-chill*

PORTIONING AFTER CHILLING

In some cook-chill systems the food is chilled in multiportion containers, then plated before reheating. The portioning process should be carried out in a controlled environment within 30 minutes of the food leaving the chilled store and before reheating commences at a temperature of 10°C (50°F). It is then transported under chilled conditions to the desired location, for example the hospital ward where it is reheated to at least 70°C (158°F) but preferably 80°C (177°F) on the plate on which it is to be served.

STORAGE

All chilled cooked food must be stored in its own special refrigeration area. Never store cooked chilled food under the same conditions as fresh products. Always monitor the temperature of the product regularly.

REHEATING

All cook-chill food must be reheated as quickly as possible to a minimum temperature of 70°C (158°F), ideally 75°C (167°F) but preferably 80°C (177°F).

Storage and quality of cook-chill foods

It has been found that during the storage period before reheating and consumption, certain products deteriorate in quality.

- The flavour of certain meat dishes, in particular white meats, veal and poultry, deteriorates after three days.
- Chilled meats without sauces can develop acidic tastes.
- Fatty foods tend to develop off flavours due to the fat oxidising.
- Fish dishes deteriorate more rapidly than meat dishes.
- Dishes containing meat tend to develop a flat taste and if spices have been used these can dominate the flavour of the meat by the end of the chilled storage period.
- Vegetables in general may discolour and develop a strong flavour.
- Dishes which contain large amounts of starch may taste stale after the chilled storage time.

CONTAINERS

The choice of containers must protect and in some cases enhance the quality of the product at all stages, it must assist in the rapid chilling, safe storage and effective reheating. Therefore the container must be:

- *sturdy:* to withstand chilling, handling and reheating;
- *safe:* not made of a substance that will cause harmful substances to develop in the food, nor react with the food to cause discolouring or spoilage;
- *have an easy-to-remove lid:* without damaging contents or causing spillage;
- *attractive:* to enhance the appearance of the product;
- *airtight and watertight:* so that moisture, flavours or odours do not penetrate the food or escape during storage and transportation.

There are various types of containers.

SINGLE-PORTION CONTAINERS

These can be of cardboard laminated with plastic; aluminium foil (unsuitable for microwave heating); plastic compounds; stainless steel and ceramic which are durable and reusable (stainless steel is, however, unsuitable for microwave ovens).

MULTIPORTION CONTAINERS

These can be of strong plastic compounds, stainless steel, ceramic or aluminium foil. Gastronorm containers are shown in Figure 8.14, page 281.

Figure 8.9 *Testing food with a hand-held thermometer*

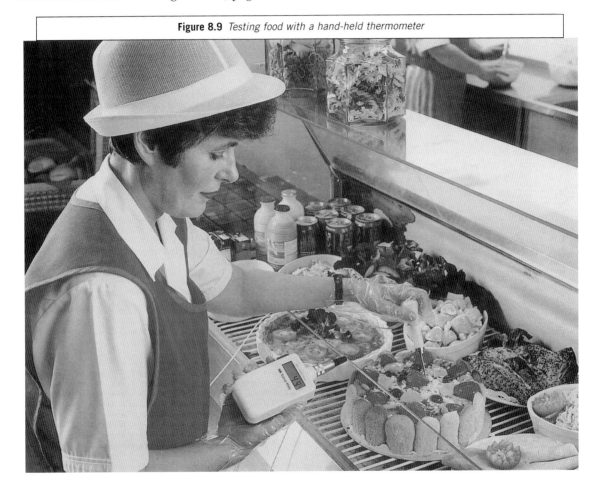

Figure 8.10 *A delivery temperature recorder which gives a print out of data*

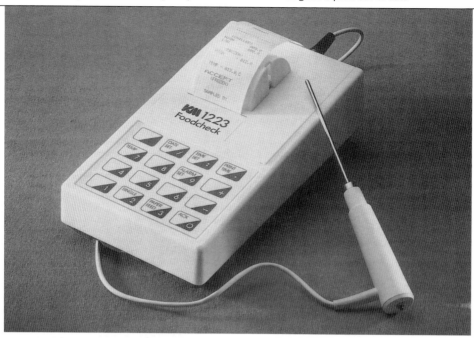

Figure 8.11 *A central monitoring alarm unit and an example of the areas it covers*

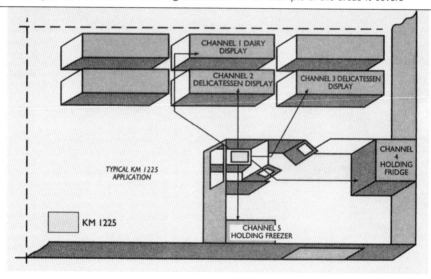

Labelling

Labels must stick securely to the containers and be easy to apply, clearly identifying the product. Colour coding is sometimes used to help identify the different days of product for example.

- *Sunday* – white
- *Monday* – red
- *Thursday* – orange
- *Saturday* – purple
- *Tuesday* – yellow
- *Wednesday* – blue
- *Friday* – green

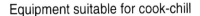

Figure 8.12 *Cook-chill equipment*

Equipment suitable for cook-chill

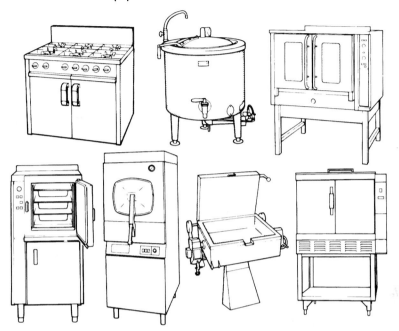

Chilling equipment

Only specially purpose built and designed equipment can take the temperature of cooked food down to safe levels fast enough.

BLAST CHILLERS OR AIR BLAST CHILLERS

These use rapidly moving cold air to chill the food evenly and rapidly. Some models have temperature probes so that the temperature of the food being chilled can be checked without opening the door.

CRYOGENIC BATCH CHILLERS

These use liquid nitrogen at a temperature of $-196°C$ ($-321°F$); this is sprayed into the chilling cabinet containing the warm food. In the warmer temperature of the cabinet, the liquid nitrogen turns to super cold gas absorbing the heat from the food as it does so. Fans move the cold gas over and around the food, once the gas has become warm it is removed from the cabinet. Some equipment uses carbon dioxide instead of nitrogen.

Reheating equipment

The caterer has the following choice of equipment for regenerating cook-chill products.

Figure 8.13 *A blast chiller*

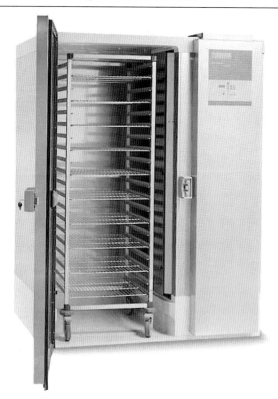

COMBINATION OVENS

These are ideally suited for bulk production, which can be used with steam which is very effective in producing quality products.

STEAMERS

These may be used for certain foods, especially vegetables.

MICROWAVE OVENS

These are used for small amounts of food.

INFRA-RED OVENS

These may be used for small or large quantities of food.

Points to remember to ensure a satisfactory product

○ Time and temperature are crucial.
○ The food should not wait longer than 30 minutes to be chilled.
○ The food should not be above 3°C (38°F) at the end of the chilling time. A higher temperature may be due to the food being packed too deep in the containers; the food may have been covered; there may be a malfunction in the equipment.

○ Food should not be stored beyond its 'use-by' date.
○ The temperature of the food rising above 3°C (38°F) during transportation this may be due to:
  – the journey taking too long using unrefrigerated transport;
  – the refrigerated van not operating correctly;

Figure 8.14 *Module sizes for gastronorm containers*

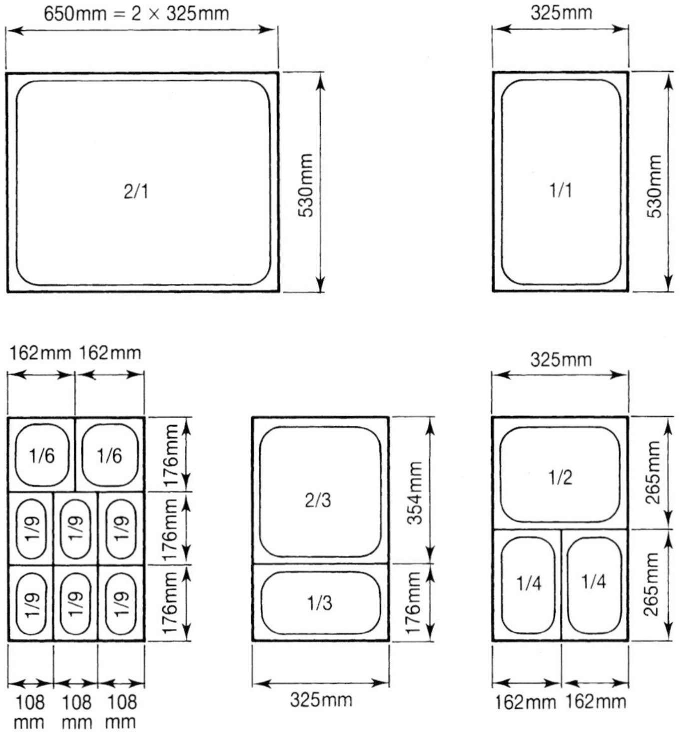

  – the insulated box (if used) not being precooled, or the lid not properly fitted. Whatever the cause, it must be recorded and the appropriate persons informed. If the temperature has not risen above 10°C (50°F) and the food is going to be served within 12 hours, the food may be allowed through. This will obviously depend on the type of food. Outside of these limits it should be discarded. If in doubt, throw it out.
○ Food should not be overcooked after reheating. This may be due to the food being heated too long or the temperature too high or faulty equipment being used.
○ Avoid food not reaching 70°C (158°F) within the 30 minutes allowed for reheating. This may be due to:
  – the label information not being followed correctly;
  – the label information not being correct;
  – the lid being taken off when it should have been left on;
  – faulty equipment.
  If the food temperature is unsafe, throw it away.
○ Avoid damaged containers. This may be due to:
  – mishandling during transportation;
  – badly stacked storage containers.

○ Observe high standards of personal hygiene and kitchen hygiene, to avoid product contamination or cross-contamination.
○ Portions must be controlled when filling packages in order to:
   – ensure efficient stock control;
   – control costs;
   – ensure that sufficient food is delivered to regenerating/finishing kitchens.
Check that the standard regeneration procedures are safe to use.
○ Food containers must be sealed correctly before storage in order to:
   – protect the food from airborne contamination;
   – enhance the presentation of dishes;
   – prevent the evaporation of moisture when heated;
   – reduce the dehydration effects chilling has on food;
   – avoid finishing products being tampered with.
○ All food products must be labelled correctly before storage to:
   – identify the product and the day of production by the colour coding and 'eat-by' date;
   – facilitate stock control;
   – maintain stock rotation;
   – enable visitors such as Environmental Health Officers to check that the food safety laws have and are being complied with;
   – ensure that quality tracking can be carried out.
○ Ensure that older stock is consumed before the new.
○ Ensure the security of storage areas against unauthorised access in order to:
   – prevent pilferage or damage by unauthorised persons;
   – prevent unnecessary opening of store doors which could destabilise storage temperature and thus may affect the temperature of the product rendering it unsafe.

Figure 8.15 *Refrigeration for cook-chill catering*

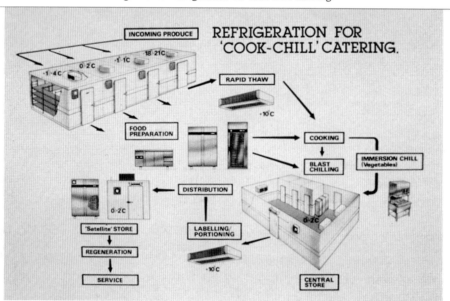

Further information, Chilled Food Association, PO Box 14811 London NW10 9ZR
www.chilledfood.org

Comparison of cook-chill and fast-food systems

The characteristics of each system are listed in the table on page 291.

COOK-FREEZE

Cook-freeze is a specialised food production and distribution system that allows caterers to take advantage of the longer life through blast freezing at -18 to $-20°C$ ($0°$ to $-32°F$) and stored at that temperature until required for resale or consumption for up to 3–6 months. Blast freezers have increasingly been introduced with success into catering operations. The ability to freeze cooked dishes and prepared foods, as distinct from the storage of chilled foods in a refrigerator or already frozen commodities in a deep-freeze, allows a caterer to make more productive use of kitchen staff. It also enables economies to be introduced into the staffing of dining rooms and restaurants.

The cook-freeze process

Cook-freeze uses a production system similar to that used in cook-chill. The recipes used have to be modified, enabling products to be freezer-stable, and modified starches are used in sauces so that on reheating and regeneration the sauce does not separate. Blast freezers are used in place of blast chillers. The freezing must be carried out very rapidly to retain freshness and to accelerate temperature loss through the latent heat barrier, thus preventing the formation of large ice crystals and rupturing of the cells.

Blast freezing takes place when low temperature air is passed over food at high speed, reducing food in batches to a temperature of at least $-20°C$ ($-4°F$) within 90 minutes. Blast freezers can hold from 20 to 400 kg (40–800 lb) per batch, the larger models being designed for trolley operation.

PREPARATION OF FOOD

The production menu for a month is drawn up and the total quantities of different foods required calculated. Supplies are then ordered, with special attention given to their being:

○ of high quality;

○ delivered so that they can immediately be prepared and cooked without any possibility of deteriorating during an enforced period of storage before being processed.

The dishes included in the menu must be cooked to the highest standards with rigid attention to quality control and to hygiene. Deep-freeze temperatures prevent the multiplication of micro-organisms but do not destroy them. If, therefore, a dish were contaminated before being frozen, consumers would be put at risk months later when the food was prepared for consumption. The exact adjustment of recipes to produce the best result when the food is subsequently thawed and reheated is still in process of being worked out by chefs, using numerous variations of the basic system. The single change needed in cookery recipes involving sauces is the selection of an appropriate type of starch capable of resisting the effect of freezing. Normal starches will produce a curdled effect when subsequently thawed and reheated.

In order to achieve rapid freezing with a quick reduction of temperature to $-18°C$ ($0°F$) or below, the cooked food must be carefully portioned (close attention being paid to the attainment of uniform portion size). Portions, each placed into a disposable aluminium foil container, may conveniently be placed into aluminium foil trays holding from 6 to 10 portions each, sealed and carefully labelled with their description and date of preparation.

FREEZING

The food thus divided into portions and arranged in trays is immediately frozen. An effective procedure is to place the trays on racks in a blast-freezing tunnel and expose them to a vigorous flow of cold air until the cooked items are frozen solid and the temperature reduced to at least −5°C (23°F). The quality of the final product is to a significant degree dependent on the rapidity with which the temperature of hot cooked food at say 80°C (176°F) is reduced to below freezing. The capacity of the blast freezer should be designed to achieve this reduction in temperature within a period of 1 to $1\frac{1}{2}$ hours.

STORAGE OF FROZEN ITEMS

Once the food items are frozen they must at once be put into a deep-freeze store maintained at −18°C (0°F). For a catering operation involving several dining rooms and cafeterias, some of which may be situated at some distance from the kitchen and frozen store, a 4 weeks' supply of cooked dishes held at low temperature allows full use to be made of the facilities.

TRANSPORT OF FROZEN ITEMS TO THE POINT OF SERVICE

If satisfactory quality is to be maintained, it is important to keep food, frozen in the cooked state, frozen until immediately prior to its being served. It should therefore be transported in insulated containers to *peripheral* or finishing kitchens, if such are to be used, where it will be reheated.

If frozen dishes are to be used in outside catering, provision should be available for transporting them in refrigerated transport and, if necessary, a subsidiary deep-freeze store should be provided for them on arrival.

THE REHEATING OF FROZEN COOKED PORTIONS

In any catering system in which a blast-freezing tunnel has been installed to freeze precooked food, previously portioned and packed in metal foil or other individual containers, it is obviously rational to install equipment that is particularly designed for the purpose of reheating the items ready to be served. The blast freezing system is effective because it is, in design, a specially powerful form of forced convection heat exchanger arranged to extract heat. It follows that an equally appropriate system for replacing heat is the use of a forced convection oven, specially for the reception of the trays of frozen portions. Where such an oven is equipped with an efficient thermostat and adequate control of the air circulation system, standardised setting times for the controls can be laid down for the regeneration of the various types of dishes that need to be reheated.

Quality control

Adequate control of bacterial contamination and growth, which are hazards in any kitchen, can be achieved by a survey of the initial installation by a qualified analyst, and regular checks taken on every batch of food cooked. Very large kitchens employ a full-time food technologist/microbiologist. In smaller operations the occasional services of a microbiologist from the public health authority should be used.

How freezing affects different foods
MEAT, POULTRY AND FISH

The tendency for the fat in meat to oxidise and go rancid even in frozen storage, means that lean meat is better than fatty meat for freezing. Chicken fat contains a natural antioxidant (vitamin E), therefore it will react to prevent rancidity occurring.

Fresh meat must always be used for cook-freeze dishes. Never use meat that has been previously frozen. This is because each time meat is thawed, even in cool conditions there is a chance for food poisoning bacteria to multiply.

Some loss of flavour in fish is unavoidable and any surfaces left exposed can suffer from oxidation thus producing a rancid taste. Deep-fried fish in batter has to be modified so that the batter does not peel off as a result of the freezing process. The batter should be made thicker or with a higher fat content.

Freezing does not stop the enzyme activity in the meat, poultry or fish that makes the fat present in the flesh go rancid. This particularly affects the unsaturated fats which are present in pork, poultry and fish. These items should therefore not be stored frozen for longer than 2 to 3 months. It is advisable therefore to trim all fat before processing these items.

FRUIT AND VEGETABLES

When fruit and vegetables turn brown, it is because of the action of enzymes present. These enzymes cause discoloration and gradually destroy the nutritive value of the fruit. Refrigeration slows this process down and freezing will further slow it down but not stop it completely. Therefore, fruit and vegetables should be blanched or completely cooked which will stop the enzymic processes.

The freezing process also has a softening effect on the texture of fruit and vegetables. This is accepted for hard fruits such as apples, unripened pears, etc. It is not suitable for soft fruits such as strawberries. Fruits like strawberries are only suitable for freezing if they are to be later used as a filling or in a sauce, but not for decorative purposes.

Only exceptionally fresh vegetables should be used for freezing. Avoid bruised vegetables which may produce the development of 'off' flavours. Blanch the vegetables to inactivate the enzymes, but avoid overblanching, otherwise vegetables will be overcooked. Blanch if possible in high pressure steamers as this will help reduce vitamin C loss.

Recipe modification

Generally, recipes have to be modified for the cook-freeze process.

Sauces, batters, thickened soups, stews and gravies will break down and separate unless the flour used in the recipes has an addition of waxy starch. Colflo and Purity 69 are two commercially manufactured starches which are used in cook-freeze recipes.

Jellies and other products containing gelatine are unsuitable because they develop a granular structure in the cook freeze process, unless the recipe is modified with stabilisers.

Packaging

Packaging is a very important consideration as this affects the storage and regeneration of the product. Containers must protect the food against oxidation during storage and allow for freezing and reheating. The containers must be:

○ watertight;
○ non-tainting;
○ disposable or reusable;
○ equipped with tight-fitting lids.

PACKAGING MATERIALS

There are a number of packaging materials available which include plastic compounds, aluminium foil and cardboard plastic laminates. These are available as single portion packs, complete meal packs and bulk packs.

CHOOSING THE CONTAINER

Various factors affect your choice of container:

○ Menu choice: single packs provide the greatest flexibility.
○ Food value: the overheating of complete meal packs or the edges of bulk packs, will damage the nutritional value.
○ Storage space: large bulk packs make the best use of space.
○ Handling time: after cooking, bulk packs are the quickest and easiest to fill whereas complete packs are the more difficult to fill. Bulk packs do, however, have to be portioned at the time of service and are therefore more time-consuming than if single packs are used.
○ Quality of the food.

Freezing time is obviously affected by the depth of the food; therefore, bulk packs, where the food is relatively deep, may not survive the freezing process as well as single portion packs. Bulk packs also rely on trained service staff to present the food attractively and portion it accurately.

Regeneration instructions can be complex if complete meal packs contain different food components which in theory may require different lengths of reheating time.

Freezing equipment

Specialist equipment is required in order to reduce the temperature of the food to the required storage temperature of $-18°C$ (0°F).

AIR BLAST FREEZERS OR BLAST FREEZERS

These take approximately 75–90 minutes to freeze food depending on how it is packaged. Extremely cold air between $-32°C$ and $-40°C$ ($-26°F$ and $-40°F$) is blown by fans over the cooked food. The warm air is constantly removed and recirculated through the heat exchange unit to lower its temperature. In the larger cook-freeze units the food is pushed in on a trolley at one end and then wheeled out at the other end frozen.

CRYOGENIC FREEZERS

These use liquid nitrogen with the freezing time taking on average 25 minutes, dependent on the food being frozen, provided the food is left uncovered. Liquid nitrogen at $-196°C$ ($-321°F$) is sprayed into the freezing chamber. Fans circulate the nitrogen so that the foods freeze evenly. The warm gas is pumped out of the cabinet as more cold nitrogen is pumped in. Some freezers used liquid carbon dioxide.

PLATE FREEZERS AND TUNNEL FREEZERS

These are used in food manufacturing and are less likely to be used in catering.

Transportation and distribution

Cook-freeze meals have to be delivered to finishing kitchens at the same temperature as they were held in storage. For short distances insulated containers are used. These are cooled down before being used. However, it is safer and more efficient to use refrigerated vans.

Finishing kitchen equipment

Thawing cabinets are similar to a forced air convection oven, but use a temperature of 10°C (50°F).

RAPID THAWING CABINET

This is used to defrost containers of frozen meals before they are placed in the oven; this has the effect of halving the reheating time. The temperature of the food is brought from $-20°C$ to $3°C$

(–4°F to 37°F) in approximately 4 hours, under safe conditions. Warming is kept at a steady controlled rate by a process of alternating low volume heat with refrigeration.

COMBINATION OVENS

These are suitable for large quantities of food.

MICROWAVE OVENS

These are only suitable for small amounts of food.

DUAL PURPOSE OVENS

These are microwave ovens which have a second heat source, for example an infrared grill, and a defrost control which switches the microwave power on and off.

FORCED AIR CONVECTION OVENS

These are suitable for large quantities of food.

Points to remember to ensure a satisfactory product

PREPARATION

○ Make sure that all preparation and cooking areas are clean and that the equipment is in working order.
○ Never use previously frozen food.
○ Avoid any delay between preparation and cooking.

COOKING

○ Check on the cooking process for the food that this process takes account of the overall effect on flavour, texture and nutritional value.
○ Always use temperature probes to check that the centre of the food has reached a safe temperature before the final cooking is complete.

PORTIONING AND PACKAGING

○ Make sure all areas are clean and hygienically safe.
○ Ensure that all packaging is ready and that it is of the correct size and material.
○ All reusable containers must be cleaned and thoroughly sterilised.
○ Make sure that all assistants who portion and package wear food-handling gloves.
○ Make sure that all general equipment used in this area is sterilised.
○ Accurately portion the food according to the recipe.
○ Do not pack the food to a depth greater than 5 cm (2 inches). For food which is to be microwaved the depth should be less.
○ Portions must be controlled when filling to:
  – standardise costs;
  – control costs;
  – facilitate stores control;
  – assist in food service;

○ – standardise the thawing and reheating process;
  – allow the sealing to be properly completed.
○ Food containers must be sealed correctly before storage in order to:
  – prevent spoilage due to contact with the cold air;
  – prevent spillage prior to freezing;
  – allow for safe stacking, helping to prevent damage to containers.
○ Cover the food before blast freezing.
○ Check and record the temperature of the food.

LABELLING

○ Label all food correctly.
○ Ensure labels have the right information which should include:
  – production date;
  – use-by date;
  – name of dish;
  – description of contents;
  – storage life;
  – number of portions;
  – instructions for reheating/regenerating with type of oven, temperature, time, and whether lid should be on or off.
○ Correct labelling will:
  – accurately identify the contents of the container;
  – enable quick and efficient stock-taking;
  – indicate important information regarding the packaging, date and the use-by date;
  – give information on the number of portions contained in the package.

FREEZING

○ Check all fast freezers are ready for use.
○ Freezing should be done immediately after cooking.
○ The foods must be frozen below −5°C (23°F) within 90 minutes.
○ There must be at least 2 cm ($\frac{3}{4}$ inch) air space between layers of containers in the freezer.
○ Immediately after freezing the food must be transported to the deep-freeze storage.

STORING

○ Store the food at the correct deep-freeze storage temperature of −20°C to −30°C (−4°F to −22°F) and at least below −18°C (0°F).
○ Monitor deep freezer temperatures at all times, keep accurate records.
○ Maintain the stock control rotation, keep all stock record systems up to date.
○ Store the food in the accepted manner on shelves and racks above the floor away from the door and with enough space around to allow the cold air to circulate.
○ Always wear protective clothing when entering the deep freeze store.
○ Destroy any foods that have passed their use-by date.
○ It is important to monitor and record food temperatures regularly in order to:

– prevent contamination from incorrect storage conditions;

– ensure flavour and texture is maintained.

○ Stock rotation procedures must be followed in order to:

– prevent damage or decay to stock;

– ensure that older stock is used before new stock.

○ Storage areas must be secured from unauthorised access in order to:

– prevent pilferage or damage by unauthorised persons;

– prevent injury to unauthorised persons;

– prevent unnecessary opening of store doors, which would destabilise the temperature.

DISTRIBUTION

○ Maintain freezer temperatures during distribution.

○ DHSS guidelines state that if the food is going to be regenerated within 24 hours, the permissible temperature range is between 0° and −18°C (32° and 0°F). Otherwise the temperature must be kept below −18°C (0°F).

○ All documentation and control systems for checking delivery should be carefully followed and implemented.

REGENERATION

○ Check that the work area is ready for operation.

○ Remove products from deep freeze for regeneration, check the labels.

○ Make sure equipment is at the correct temperature and in working order.

○ Follow the regeneration instructions on the label.

○ The foods must be reheated to at least 70°C (158°F) but to 75–80°C (167–177°F) immediately before service. Check temperature has been reached by using a sterilised calibrated temperature probe.

○ Serve the food as soon as possible after regeneration.

○ Food that has not been eaten within 2 hours should be thrown away. Food which has been allowed to cool must never be reheated.

GENERAL

○ To avoid separated sauces, the recipe must be modified correctly using the appropriate starches.

○ Meat and fish will taste rancid with badly prepared food or too long a storage period.

○ Soggy coated food will occur if the lid is not removed when regenerating.

○ A back log of food for freezing will occur with poor production planning.

○ Freezer burns are due to badly packaged food or when food is stored too long.

○ Standards of personnel hygiene and kitchen temperature are of paramount importance to maintain a clean and safe product.

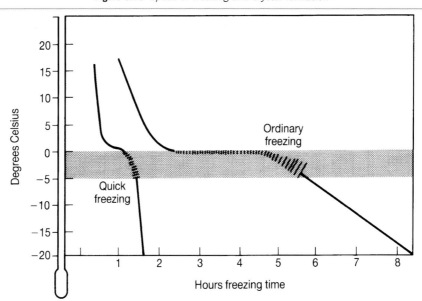

Figure 8.16 *Speed of freezing and crystal formation*

Overall benefits of cook-chill/cook-freeze

To the employer:

- ○ Portion control and reduced waste.
- ○ No over-production.
- ○ Central purchasing with bulk buying discounts.
- ○ Full utilisation of equipment.
- ○ Full utilisation of staff time.
- ○ Overall savings in staff.
- ○ Savings on equipment, space and fuel.
- ○ Fewer staff with better conditions – no unsociable hours, no weekend work, no overtime.
- ○ Simplified less frequent delivery to units.
- ○ Solves problem of moving hot foods. (EC regulations forbid the movement of hot foods unless the temperature is maintained over 65°C (149°F). Maintaining 65°C is regarded as very difficult to achieve and high temperatures inevitably will be harmful to foods.)

To the customer:

- ○ Increased variety and selection.
- ○ Improved quality, with standards maintained.
- ○ More nutritious foods.
- ○ Services can be maintained at all times, regardless of staff absences.

Advantages of cook-freeze over cook-chill

- ○ Seasonal purchasing provides considerable savings.
- ○ Delivery to units will be far less frequent.

Characteristics of cook-chill and fast-food systems

	COOK-CHILL	FAST-FOOD
Types of equipment	Flexible, general purpose	Single purpose
		Single function
Design of process	Functional	Product flow
Set-up time	Variable	Long
Workers	Variously skilled, partie system, limited flexibility	Low skill
		Flexible
Inventories for start of process	Vary, depending on 'foods in' required	High to meet potential demand.
	Limited in time by planning and forecasting	
	Limited by preplanning and forecasting	
Holding inventory	Five days max.	Ten mins max.
	Level forecasted	Level controlled
Lot sizes	Small to large (multiples of ten)	Individual
Production time	Variable depending on menu requirements	Short or constant
Product range	Fairly wide but within constraints of three or four course meals, lunch or dinner.	Very restricted
System structure	Stock/Customer/Operation	Stock/Queue/Operation
Capacity	Variable	Highly variable
Scheduling	Externally orientated	Externally orientated

○ Long-term planning of production and menus becomes possible.
○ Less dependence on price fluctuations.
○ More suitable for vending machines incorporating microwave.

Advantages of cook-chill over cook-freeze

○ Regeneration systems are simpler – infrared and steam convection ovens are mostly used and only 12 minutes is required to reheat all foods perfectly.
○ Thawing time is eliminated.
○ Smaller capacity storage is required: 3 to 4 days supply as opposed to up to 120 days.
○ Chiller storage is cheaper to install and run than freezer storage.
○ Blast chillers are cheaper to install and run that blast freezers.
○ Cooking techniques are unaltered (additives and revised recipes are needed for freezing).
○ All foods can be chilled so the range of dishes is wider (some foods cannot be frozen). Cooked eggs, steaks and sauces such as Hollandaise can be chilled (after some recipe modification where necessary).
○ No system is too small to adapt to cook-chill.

Further information can be obtained from the Electricity Association, 30 Millbank, London SW1P 4RD and the Department of Health.

VACUUM COOKING (SOUS-VIDE)

This is a form of cook-chill, using a combination of vacuum sealing in plastic pouches, cooking by steam and then rapidly chilling in an ice-water bath, as this most effective way of chilling. The objective is to rationalise kitchen procedures without having a detrimental effect on the quality of the individual dishes.

The process is as follows:

○ Individual portions of prepared food are first placed in special plastic pouches. The food can be fish, poultry, meats, vegetables, etc., to which seasoning, a garnish, sauce, stock, wine, flavouring, vegetables, herbs and/or spices can be added.

○ The pouches of food are then placed in a vacuum-packaging machine which evacuates all the air and tightly seals the pouch.

○ The pouches are next cooked by steam. This is usually in a special oven equipped with a steam control programme, which controls the injection of steam into the oven, to give steam cooking at an oven temperature below 100°C (212°F). Each food item has its own ideal cooking time and temperature.

○ When cooked, the pouches are rapidly cooled down to 3°C (37°F), usually in an iced water chiller or an air blast chiller for larger operations.

○ The pouches are then labelled and stored in a holding refrigerator at an optimum temperature of 3°C (37°F).

○ When required for service the pouches are regenerated in boiling water or a steam combination oven until the required temperature is reached, cut open and the food presented.

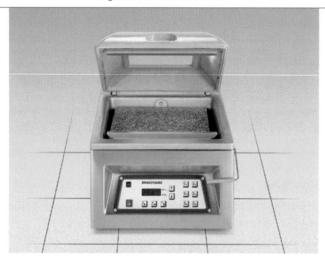

Figure 8.17 *Vacuum Packer*

Vacuum pressures are as important as the cooking temperatures with regard to weight loss and heat absorption. The highest temperature used in *sous-vide* cooking is 100°C (212°F) and 1000 millibars is the minimum amount of vacuum pressure used.

As there is no oxidation or discoloration it is ideal for conserving fruits, such as apples and pears (pears in red wine, fruits in syrup). When preparing meats in sauces the meat is preblanched then added to the completed sauce.

Sous-vide is a combination of vacuum sealing, tightly controlled *en papillotte* cooking and rapid chilling which can be used by almost any type of catering operation.

Advantages

- Long shelf-life, up to 21 days, refrigerated.
- Ability to produce meals in advance means better deployment of staff and skills.
- Vacuum-packed foods can be mixed in cold store without the risk of cross-contamination.
- Reduced labour costs at point of service.
- Beneficial cooking effects on certain foods, especially moulded items and pâtés. Reduces weight loss on meat joints.
- Full flavour and texture is retained as food cooks in its own juices.
- Economises on ingredients (less butter, marinades, etc.).
- Makes precooking a possibility for à la carte menus.
- Inexpensive regeneration.
- Allows a small operation to set up bulk production.
- Facilitates portion control and uniformity of standard.
- Has a tenderising effect on tougher cuts of meat and matures game without dehydration.

Disadvantages

- Extra cost of vacuum pouches and vacuum-packing machine.
- Unsuitable for meats (fillet steak) and vegetables which absorb colour.
- All portions in a batch must be identically sized to ensure even results.
- Most dishes require twice the conventional cooking time.
- Unsuitable for large joints as chilling time exceeds 90 minutes.
- Complete meals (meat and two vegetables) not feasible; meat component needs to be cooked and stored in separate bags.
- Extremely tight management and hygienic controls are imperative.
- Potentially adverse customer reaction ('boil-in-the-bag' syndrome).

Points to remember

- High standards of kitchen hygiene and personnel hygiene must be employed.
- Prime quality ingredients should be used.
- All aspects of the Food Safety Act must be adhered to.
- Where possible *sous-vide* should operate under a temperature controlled environment.
- All the basic principles of cook-chill apply to *sous-vide*.

Further information: Sous-vide Advisory Committee, New Hope Lodge, London Rd, Wendover, Aylesbury, Bucks HP22 6PN

CENTRALISED PRODUCTION

Why centralise?

Reasons for considering centralised production units are as follows:

- labour: reduction of kitchen preparation staff in end units;
- food cost: greater control over waste and portion sizes; competitive purchasing through bulk buying;

○ equipment: intensive central use of heavy equipment reduces commitment in individual units;
○ product: more control on product quality;
○ labour strategy: staff are employed at regular times (9am to 5pm) which can eliminate or lessen the difficulty of obtaining staff who will work shifts.

When considering a centralised production system it is essential that a detailed financial appraisal is produced and then looked at carefully, as each establishment has its own considerations. No general rule can be given as the profitability depends on the product, the size of each unit, the number of units and the method of preserving food.

Design

Centralised production systems can be designed in two ways:
○ using existing catering (operations) unit and modifying, etc.;
○ purpose-built.

Type of units

Centralised production units are grouped into four types:
○ units preparing fresh cooked foods which are then despatched;
○ cook-freeze: food is partly prepared or cooked, then frozen and regenerated when required;
○ cook-chill: food is cooked, then chilled and regenerated when required;
○ sous-vide: food is sealed in a special casing, vacuum-sealed, cooked and chilled.

Food production and preparation

The profitability of the production system depends largely upon contents of the end-unit menus.

MEAT

Careful purchasing is essential and the menu must be planned carefully:
○ The cut of meat required must be clearly specified in order to produce the exact dishes.
○ Strict portion control must be adhered to.
○ Trimmings/by-products must be fully utilised: meat trimming for cottage/shepherd's pie, bones for stock.

VEGETABLE PREPARATION

Because of increasing labour costs and difficulty in obtaining staff, a number of establishments now purchase: prepared potatoes, that are washed, peeled and in some cases shaped; prepared root vegetables; topped and tailed French beans; and ready prepared salads.

Reception and delivery

It is desirable to have two loading bays, one for receiving and one for delivery. They should be adjacent to the relevant store to facilitate loading. The receiving bay should be adjacent to the prime goods store for purchased meat, vegetables, etc., and the delivery bay near to the finished goods stores which contain items ready to go out to their end units.

Staff

Apart from a butcher some of the staff may not be highly skilled. The various processes involved in meat production can be divided as follows and staff trained for each procedure:

- machine operators: staff operating dicing machines, mincing machines, hamburger machines, to a strict procedure;
- trimmers: staff who are taught to trim carcasses and prime cuts;
- packers: who pack goods into foil cans, operate vacuum-packing machines, and label or pack finished goods into containers; caterers will have to consider if it is economically viable to have a butchery or whether to buy in prepared meats (this very much depends upon the range of menu).

Frequently, staff who are employed to carry out specific functions within a centralised kitchen may not have catering qualifications but will be trained by the organisation.

Method of operation

There are two types of operations:

- weekly production;
- daily total run.

Forecasts obtained from the end unit determine the quantity of the production run. This prepares items of a particular type on one occasion only. As soon as the run is completed the next run is then scheduled. The main advantage of this type of production is in the comparative ease with which a control system may be installed and operated.

A disadvantage is that, in the event of an error in production scheduling, it is wasteful and costly to organise a further production run of small volume. Another disadvantage is that the method leads to the building-up of stocks, both finished and unfinished, thereby affecting the profitability of the operation.

A daily total run is based upon the needs of items required by the end-unit. A disadvantage is that the forecast gap is shorter, so the end units are not able to provide accurate requisitions.

Purchasing

Any organisation depending for its existence on the economics of bulk purchasing must pay particular attention to the process of buying.

The following are the main objectives of the buyer:

- Quality and price of goods must be equalled with the size of purchase order.
- All purchase specifications must be met.
- Buying practice must supplement a policy of minimum stock holding.

Transport

The distribution of goods, routing and the maintenance of vehicles are very important to a centralised production operation. The usual practice is for transport to be under the control of a senior manager, who also has the complicated job of batching-up deliveries (normally weekly or bi-weekly). It is important that the senior manager has considerable administrative skill in order to prevent errors occurring.

Centralised production very often means that production is separated from the food service by distance, time or both. An example is in hospital wards; here there are satellite kitchens or regeneration kitchens. Other examples exist in aircraft catering and banqueting. Banqueting houses that use cook-chill either purchase from their own production unit or an independent company.

Fast food

Fast food is characterised by a smooth operation. The principal control adopted is 'door time': $3\frac{1}{2}$ minutes is the control average, $1\frac{1}{2}$ minutes queuing and 1 minute serving. Capital costs are high for production equipment. The menu range is narrow with the equipment often being specially developed to do one job. This is essentially one cell or family of related parts of one product.

Increases in volume required is met by increasing the speed of foods through the system. This is achieved by increasing labour and by duplicating the same cell. Workers are multi-functional but often of low skill. Staffing can be applied to a number of parts depending on volume of throughput. This type of staffing can give high job satisfaction (although short-term) similar to the rotation of chefs through the partie system.

This operation comes nearer to the continuous flow ideal and is often quoted as a classic just-in-time system.

The principles of manufacturing exist in both fast food and cook-chill systems. Other systems such as cook-freeze and *sous-vide* will take on a variety of cells relating to different parts of the meal. The fast-food system is primarily based upon one-cell systems. All systems use variations in the number of workers to control costs.

Small centralised operations

There are some very good examples of smaller centralised operations to be seen now in the catering industry. The purpose of installation is to provide ready-prepared goods which may be served to banquets or supplied to grills/coffee shops.

The preparation of the food takes place during the kitchen 'slack' period, principally after the luncheon service. The made-up items are put into polythene bags which contain from one to six portions. The packed items are marked with the date of packing, and the name of the item, and then blast frozen preparatory to storage. They are kept in store from 3 to 6 months and moved to a first-in, first-out basis. Some items have limited storage time so careful checking of dates is an important factor to consider. Refrigerators in the outlets are stocked up daily from the central code store.

When an item is ordered it is reheated by a simple boiling process which is operated by a timer. The cooked items are placed on the plate, with the garnish and vegetables being added separately. There are also, of course, many other refinements: carefully calculated production schedules and coloured photographs of the dishes to guide presentation, for example.

Ganymede dri-heat

This is a method of keeping foods either hot or cold. It is used in some hospitals as it ensures that the food which reaches the patients is in the same fresh condition as it was when it left the kitchens.

A metal disc or pellet is electrically heated or cooled and placed in a special container under the plate. The container is designed to allow air to circulate round the pellet so that the food is maintained at the correct service temperature.

This is used in conjunction with conveyor belts and special service counters and helps to provide a better and quicker food service.

IN-FLIGHT CATERING

In-flight catering is one of the most extensive food production operations within the catering industry (see Figure 8.18 on page 297). Some in-flight caterers may produce up to 36,000 meals a day during the peak season. This section describes a typical system that would be used by many in-flight caterers throughout the world. Caterers involved in large scale production are able to learn from the in-flight production system, in particular the production planning process, production scheduling and the production systems.

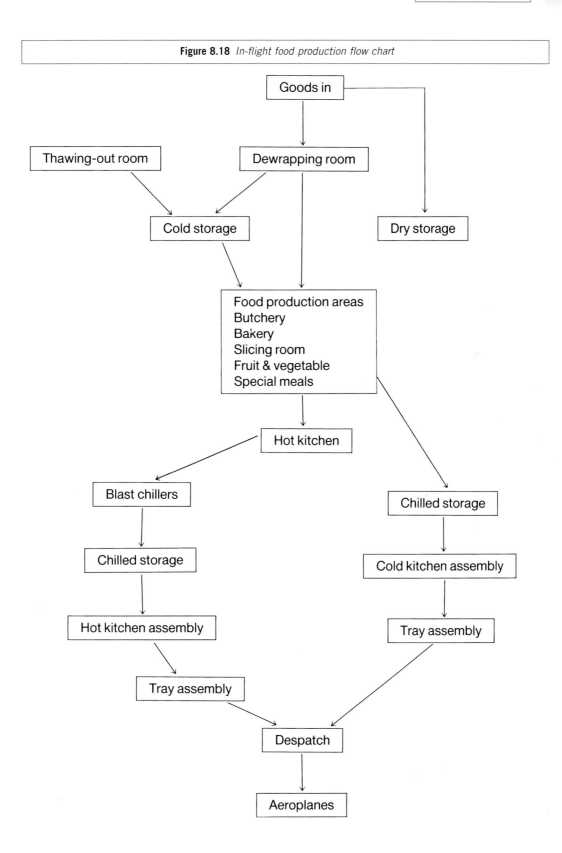

Figure 8.18 *In-flight food production flow chart*

Basic principles of the design of in-flight food production kitchens

Factors which will influence the design are similar to designing other food production systems:

○ the size and extent of the operations in terms of the maximum number of flight meals to be produced;

○ amounts of capital expenditure costs;

○ policy on the use of preprepared products;

○ the use of latest technology;

○ hygiene, food safety legislation;

○ the complexity of menus required by the airlines.

The flow process

Each kitchen should have a flow process chart detailing the materials (food) and labour, the chart will show the main parts of the process, demonstrating the flow of materials and labour, the transportation of products, storage and chilling. The chart will also clearly identify when the operator should temperature test and for how long.

Production planning

Good production planning for in-flight caterers involves a similar principle to JIT (just-in-time production techniques), meaning 'producing the necessary units, in the necessary quantities, at the necessary time'. This concept has in some way been used by large-scale caterers for some time, the difference being they have never referred to it as JIT, just good business practice. The principles of JIT are:

○ stock levels kept down to the level as and when required; order in as and when needed (stockless production);

○ elimination of waste;

○ enforced problem solving;

○ continuous flow manufacturing.

There is and has to be a strong emphasis on continual improvement rather than accepting the *status quo*.

BALANCING RESOURCES AND PASSENGER NEEDS IN A PRODUCTION PLAN

To achieve the tight balance between passenger needs and resources, the following need to be considered:

Orders

○ from the airline;

○ for stock;

○ broken down into details;

○ forecasting against budgeted figures and adapting to daily changing needs.

Continued on p304.

Figure 8.19 *The BA in-flight meal served to Club Europe passengers*

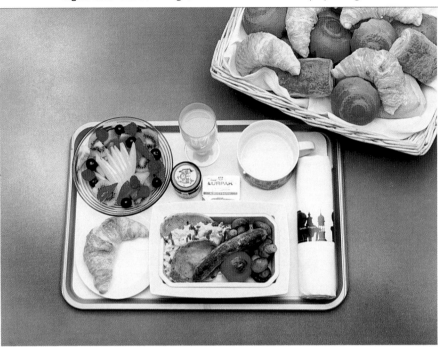

Figure 8.20 *WorldMarché*

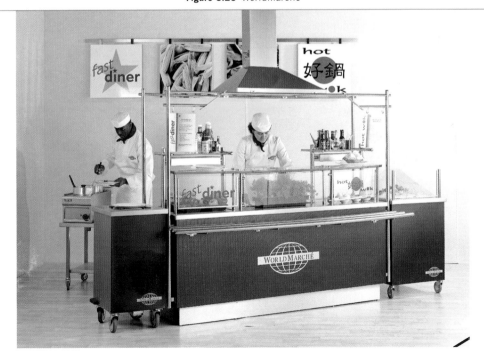

Figure 8.21 *WorldMarché*

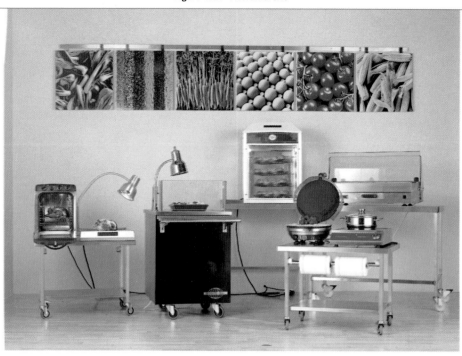

Figure 8.22 *Stir frying using the WorldMarché system*

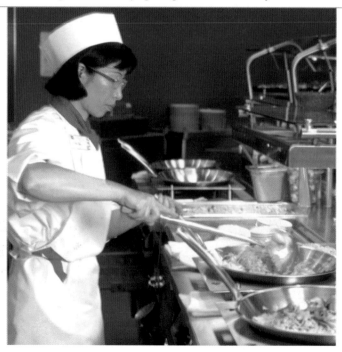

Figure 8.23 *Preparing food using the WorldMarché system*

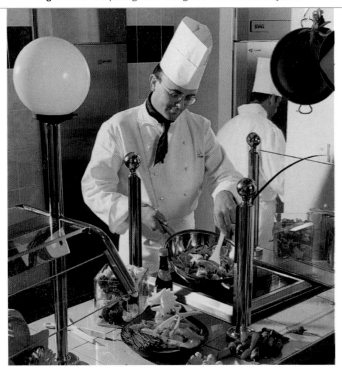

Figure 8.24 *Table set for tea*

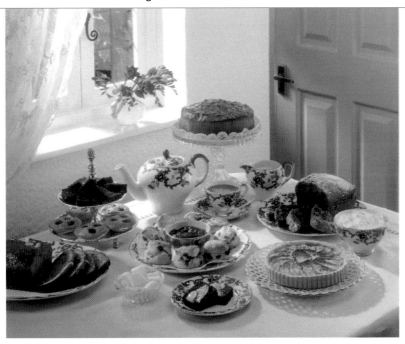

Figure 8.25 *Traditional English Breakfast*

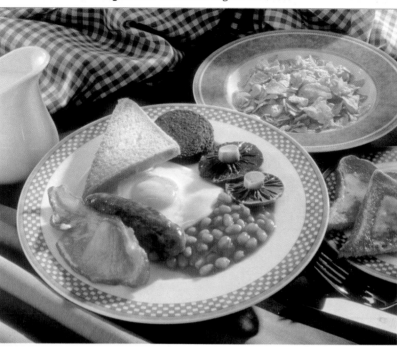

Figure 8.26 *A Children's Menu*

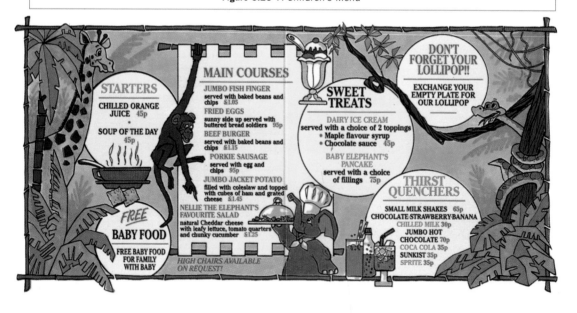

Figure 8.27 *A selection of gâteaux*

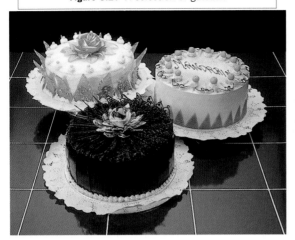

Figure 8.28 *A selection of pastries*

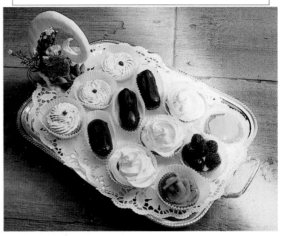

Figure 8.29 *Service of scones with clotted cream and jam*

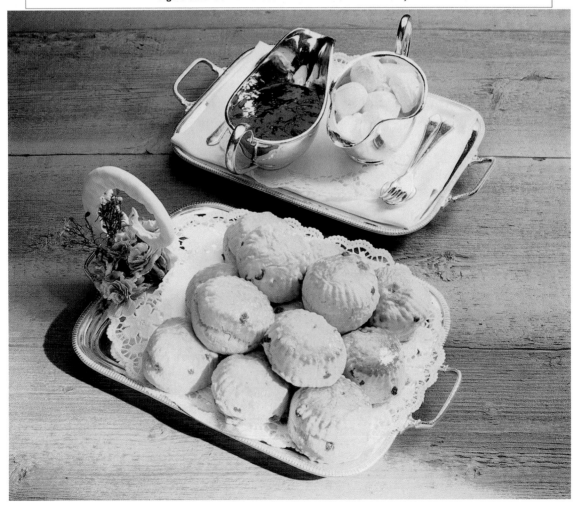

Figure 8.30 *A selection of petit fours*

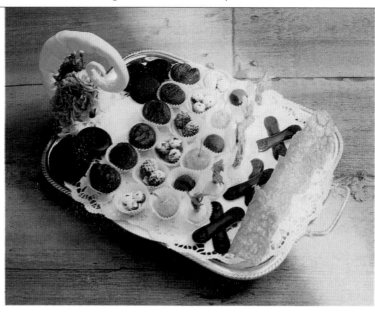

Priority
○ sequenced into date, time aircraft is due to take off;
○ special meal requirements identified;
○ evenly balanced work load where appropriate.

Availability
○ labour;
○ equipment;
○ outsourcing of quality and consistency can be guaranteed.

Cost
○ spend from airlines;
○ down-time costs from excessive change-overs;
○ cost of subcontracting.

Overall production control
A production plan is rarely, if ever, carried out in all its details. Equipment breaks down, staff can be off sick, suppliers fail to deliver, skilled people leave the company, etc.

The function of production control is to ensure that production is maintained in line with the production plan wherever possible and secondly, to respond to the things which do go wrong and rework the plan in to get back on schedule. However, the quality and consistency of the agreed specification must always be met.

Contd. on p307

Figure 8.31 *Control of hygiene in food preparation*

DEPARTMENT OF HEALTH
ASSURED SAFE CATERING · CRITICAL CONTROL POINTS

Step	Hazard	Action
1 **Purchase**	High-risk* (ready-to-eat) foods contaminated with food-poisoning bacteria or toxins (Poisons produced by bacteria).	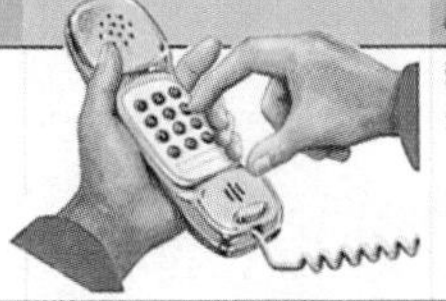 Buy from reputable supplier only. Specify maximum temperature at delivery.
2 **Receipt of food**	High-risk* (ready-to-eat) foods contaminated with food-poisoning bacteria or toxins.	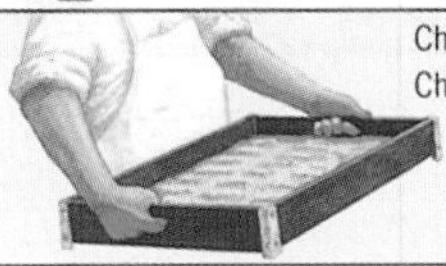 Check it looks, smells and feels right. Check the temperature is right.
3 **Storage**	Growth of food poisoning bacteria, toxins on high-risk* (ready-to-eat) foods. Further contamination.	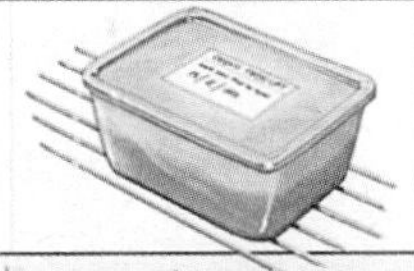 High-risk* foods stored at safe temperatures. Store them wrapped. Label high-risk foods with the correct 'sell by' date. Rotate stock and use by recommended date.
4 **Preparation**	Contamination of High-risk* (ready-to-eat) foods. Growth of food-poisoning bacteria.	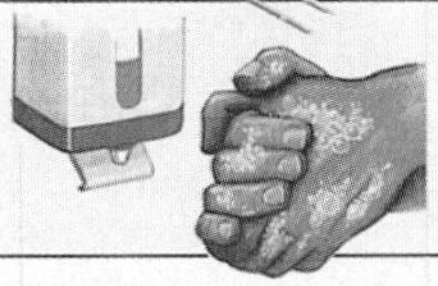 Wash your hands before handling food. Limit any exposure to room temperatures during preparation. Prepare with clean equipment, and use this for high-risk* (ready-to-eat) food only. Separate cooked foods from raw foods.
5 **Cooking**	Survival of food-poisoning bacteria.	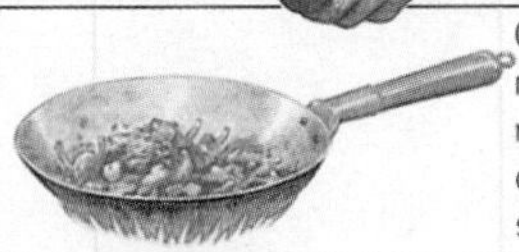 Cook rolled joints, chicken, and re-formed meats eg. burgers, so that the thickest part reaches at least 75°C. Sear the outside of other, solid meat cuts (eg. joints of beef, steaks) before cooking.
6 **Cooling**	Growth of any surviving spores or food poisoning bacteria. Production of poisons by bacteria. Contamination with food-poisoning bacteria.	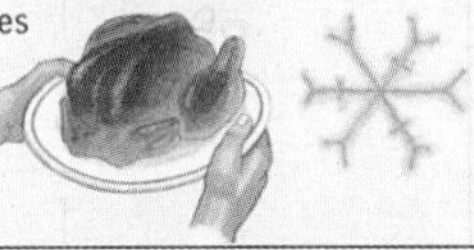 Cool foods as quickly as possible. Don't leave out at room temperatures to cool, unless the cooling period is short, eg place any stews or rice, etc, in shallow trays and cool to chill temperatures quickly.
7 **Hot-holding**	Growth of food-poisoning bacteria. Production of poisons by bacteria.	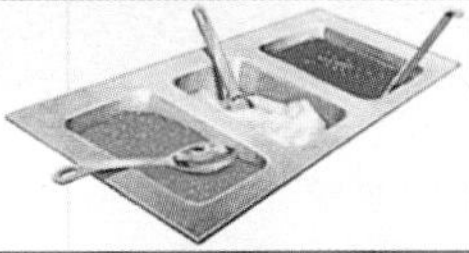 Keep food hot, above 63°C.
8 **Reheating**	Survival of food-poisoning bacteria.	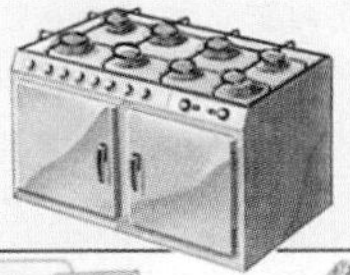 Reheat to above 75°C.
9 **Chilled storage**	Growth of food-poisoning bacteria.	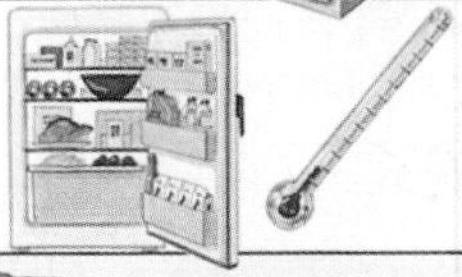 Keep temperature at right level. Label high-risk ready-to-eat foods with correct date code.
10 **Serving**	Growth of disease-causing bacteria. Production of poisons by bacteria. Contamination.	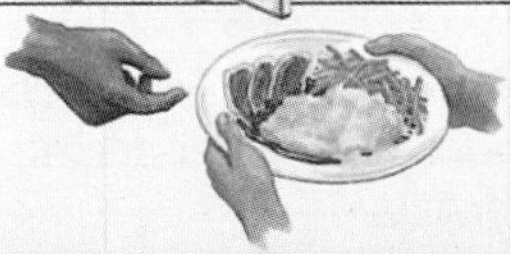 COLD SERVICE FOODS - serve high-risk foods as soon as possible after removing from refrigerated storage to avoid them getting warm. HOT FOODS - serve high-risk foods quickly to avoid them cooling down.

A. *High-risk foods are those which may easily support the growth of food poisoning organisms and won't be cooked any further before you serve them, for example: cooked fish, meat patés, cooked egg dishes, pre-prepared dairy products that may only be re-heated.
B. Some food-poisoning bacteria can form spores which may survive cooking.

If cooling is delayed or takes a long time, these spores may grow or produce toxins (poisons). After cooking, food should be cooled quickly to prevent or reduce this. The list above is not exhaustive but shows some of the hazards likely to be present in any operation. In your catering operation you may be able to identify other hazards not listed above. If you do so make sure you control these as well.

Figure 8.32 *Are you a healthy weight?*

ARE YOU A HEALTHY WEIGHT?

Take a straight line across from your height (without shoes) and a line up from your weight (without clothes). Put a mark where the two lines meet.

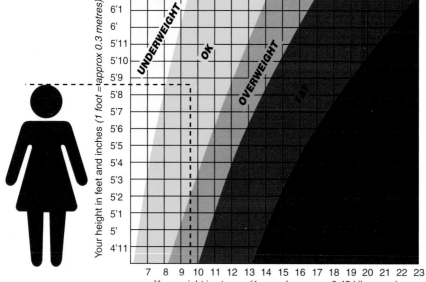

Your height in feet and inches (1 foot = approx 0.3 metres)

UNDERWEIGHT · OK · OVERWEIGHT · FAT

6'1 · 6' · 5'11 · 5'10 · 5'9 · 5'8 · 5'7 · 5'6 · 5'5 · 5'4 · 5'3 · 5'2 · 5'1 · 5' · 4'11

7 8 9 10 11 12 13 14 15 16 17 18 19 20 21 22 23
Your weight in stones *(1 pound = approx 0.45 kilograms)*

UNDERWEIGHT Maybe you need to eat a bit more. But go for well-balanced nutritious foods and don't just fill up on fatty and sugery foods. If you are very underweight, see your doctor about it.

OK You're eating the right quantity of food but you need to be sure that you're getting a healthy balance in your diet.

OVERWEIGHT You should try to lose weight.

FAT You need to lose weight.

■ You urgently need to lose weight. You would do well to see your doctor, who might refer you to a dietitian.

If you need to lose weight Aim to lose 1 or 2 pounds a week until you get down to the 'OK' range. Go for fibre-rich foods and cut down on fat, sugar and alcohol. You'll need to take regular exercise too.

Volumes of product used per year at a Gate Gourmet production centre for British Airways

Sausages (Assorted)	33.5 tonnes	Milk	602 250 pints
Fresh Salmon	67.25 tonnes	Double Cream	46 397 pints
Fillet Steaks 4.5oz	9.75 tonnes	Chocolate Boxes (Club)	557 507 boxes of 2 chocs
Bacon	15 tonnes	Bread Loaves	20 930 leaves
New Zealand Lamb	125 tonnes	Lettuce	182 736 lettuce
Chicken Breasts	40.5 tonnes	Melons	38 950 melons
Carrots	75 tonnes	Tomato Sauce	9 552 bottles
Cream Cheese	3.5 tonnes	Cornflakes	77 150 pkts small
Live Lobsters	39 tonnes	Tea	1 983 240 bags
Frozen Lobster Meat	30 tonnes	Fresh Eggs	2 700 000 eggs
Prawns	31 tonnes	Hard Boiled Eggs	1 421 550 eggs
Caviar	1.5 tonnes	Biscuits	50 154 tins
Flour	65.5 tonnes	Strawberry Jam	274 464 portions
Sugar	10.5 tonnes	Lemonade	1 204 752 cans
Smoked Salmon	22 tonnes	Coca Cola	2 868 728 cans
Fresh Strawberries	44.5 tonnes	Orange Juice	1 101 400 cups
Fresh Tomatoes	126.5 tonnes	Orange Juice	170 000 litres

The food production managers monitor the supply and production process to ensure that there is always up-to-date information on what has been achieved, or what further actions may be necessary to maintain the production flow and to achieve the airlines desired specification. Where deviations from the production plan are spotted, corrective action is then taken to overcome any shortfalls in the production.

Regular checks must be made on food availability and alternative suppliers must be identified in cases of emergency where a designated supplier fails to deliver on time or the exact quantity.

All food production managers and supervisors must be aware of what labour hours are available and how the operation is performing in terms of quality and productivity.

The production system

A large scale operation producing approximately 30 000 meals a day supplying 200 fully catered flights could well be dealing with over 300 food suppliers. In a typical system all stock would be on a 48-hour holding cycle, raw materials being held for no longer than 24 hours before being used in production.

The meal requirements are given to the food production manager and despatch control department. There is often a computer link which relays all flight details and eating requirements on each flight. The manager (usually the head chef of executive chef) gives the orders to the stores department. All orders to each supplier are on computer print-outs ready to be checked against a receipt of delivery.

The delivery should be systematically enrolled to avoid cross-contamination, segregating the delivery of each high risk food, for example poultry, meat and fish. The deliveries must be checked against the production requirements on the computer print-out, if there is any discrepancy the order should be refused.

The dry goods should be brought to the dry storage area. Any cold and frozen goods should be dealt with in a separate area where they can be unwrapped. This is to prevent any cardboard boxes or external wrappings entering into the food production or cold storage areas. These goods should be transferred to colour-coded plastic boxes. Computer-printed tags can be used to identify each plastic box. The tag attached to the box will normally have the day and date contents of each box. Frozen goods then pass into purpose-built thawing rooms. Chilled products are transferred to the cold storage areas. All storage rooms must be controlled and monitored 24 hours a day. When required these items are removed into the production areas where skilled operatives continue the production process.

Over the last few years there has been a move towards purchasing prepared and preprepared items; this is likely to accelerate in the future. A whole manufacturing industry has grown up around the supply of such products to other caterers. The advantage of using such products is that they provide greater cost control, reduce labour and processing costs, reduce hygiene costs and often give better standardisation, while giving the caterer greater flexibility in operations and purchasing power. Some manufacturers work directly with the airline to greater understand needs and this avoids a lot of re-working. It is also important to ensure that the airline recruits what it needs to deliver its own customer satisfaction rather than being led by its caterer who may want development for different reasons.

Some caterers still have their own bakery and pastry departments. Most buy in bread and bread rolls and therefore concentrate on sweets and pastries. Again the tendency is now towards purchasing preprepared sweets.

FUTURE DEVELOPMENTS

Industrial food service catering

Many different food delivery systems now operate with industrial catering. These concepts are developed by contract catering companies who have to work hard to retain old contracts and obtain new ones. Customers within these units have high expectations and demand high quality products, mirroring what is often available on the high street. One concept which has become increasingly used is the WorldMarché concept = The World Market!

WHAT IS WORLDMARCHÉ?

WorldMarché is a front of house, hot portable food delivery system that brings the full colour and flavour of the chef's theatre to customers. The system takes full advantage of new technological advances allowing the chef flexibility to use a number of different cooking methods to create innovative dishes freshly cooked to order **fast**.

WHY WAS WORLDMARCHÉ DESIGNED?

WorldMarché was designed to meet an ever-changing world. Customer's lifestyles have changed and we need to respond to this if we are going to retain and grow business. Customers now demand (Fig 8..20 page 299; 8.21, 8.22 page 300; Fig 8.23, page 301):

○ a greater variety of food offers including international cuisine;
○ use of fresh, quality ingredients;
○ food available quickly;
○ innovative approaches to food delivery;
○ value for money.

WHAT ARE THE BENEFITS OF WORLDMARCHÉ (WORLD MARKET)

For the Customer:
- Fresh quality food cooked to order fast
- Limitless choice of dishes
- Dishes cooked to customer requirements
- Food created in front of the customer in a fun way
- Value for money
- Food ready to go

For the contract caterer:
- Simple to operate
- Reduces wastage
- Builds customer and client loyalty
- Increases turnover and profit
- Increases spending per head
- Increases cooking skills
- Maximises the use of labour
- Reduces menu fatigue
- Reduces running costs
- Fits any servery
- Tried and tested
- Proven results

For the Client:
- WorldMarché will fit any space
- Innovative approach that will drive sales and profit
- Easy to implement
- Increases customer loyalty
- Delivering what the customer demands

HOW DOES WORLDMARCHÉ WORK?

WorldMarché comes in two sizes according to the space you have available. There is:
- GrandMarché – larger version
- MiniMarché – smaller version

To set you up there is a starter kit for each which is known as the WorldMarché platform which includes vario wok, ice box with eutectic plates, silesia contact grill, dry bain marie, extractor canopy etc. From here you can then mix and match to tailor the WorldMarché system to each unit's requirements. All the portable, interchangeable cookery equipment is designed to be powered from a 13 amp plug for ease and the extractor system has been designed to allow you to cook in the servery without setting off the fire alarm.

With the WorldMarché system you can cook *'Any food...Anytime...Anywhere'* and the options are limitless – you can create anything from traditional breakfasts through to crispy duck or Chinese noodles using the system. Every dish can be cooked freshly to order in minutes either using the wok or silesia grill, e.g. omelette 20 seconds, steak 2 minutes.

The system allows you to create a 'Call order' menu that will sell even more of your best sellers both during *and outside peak service times*. The fresh food offers will fulfil those parts of the day where more revenue should be realised.

What's more, because the "theatre" delivery adds real value, customers are prepared to pay a premium for a WorldMarché dish that's cooked 'exclusively' for them in front of their own eyes.

WHAT FOOD OFFERS ARE INCLUDED IN WORLDMARCHÉ?

Hot Wok
Oriental dishes – e.g. sizzling stir fry with crunchy vegetables and rice or noodles – choose from Chinese, Thai or Indonesian.

Go East
Aromatic dishes from India and Pakistan, using the colour and aromatic flavour of fresh spices.

Trad Favourites
Classics such as roast meat and two veg', bangers and mash, toasties and juicy grilled steaks.

Fast Diner
Fresh food FAST! Choose from North American, Tex Mex, Caribbean, Fusion.

Smart Start
Full English Breakfast – eggs: fresh fried or scrambled to order, fast bacon that is cooked to perfection, fresh fruit, fruit dishes, yoghurts and milk on ice.

Trattoria
Mediterranean foods from Italy to Greece – from home-cooked pasta to pizza with a wide range of mouthwatering toppings and sauces. Toasted panini of every kind.

To accompany this there are some simple 'slot in' food counter signage and Point of Sale materials which can be instantly changed according to the time of day and the food offer available.

WHAT IS THE BRAND PROPOSITION?

Any food...Anytime...Anywhere

○ Flexible, Exciting, Innovative 'Cooker Theatre'
○ Guarantees freshness and quality – FAST

The WorldMarché food delivery system has been developed and pioneered by the Compass Group of Companies.

The kitchen

The kitchen is a centre of creativity but it also creates much cost. The question is, how does the food and beverage manager get the cost of food preparation down to a level, or a percentage, which allows the profitable exploitation of the kitchen and the accompanying restaurant?

The answer is that the manager should know what it means to prepare traditional food in a modern, cost-saving way, making use of:

○ modern cooking and regeneration equipment;
○ new generations of high quality convenience-orientated, partly prepared food components;
○ new working methods in the kitchen.

In a traditional kitchen, whole products are prepared from scratch. This means that:

○ large storage rooms are needed for raw materials;
  storage rooms are needed for peeled/cooked preparations;
○ numerous preparation rooms are needed for: meat; fish; vegetables;
○ various preparation tools are needed: meat saw; chopper; vegetable peeler; cutter

○ traditional cooking equipment is needed:

  fry pan; grill; cooking pots; deep fryer; braising pan;

○ large stove top is needed for a large team.

The chef

The food and beverage manager's biggest challenge will certainly be to convince the tradition-orientated chef that the time has come to adopt new economical ways of preparing food.

The chef will no longer mainly excel in preparing food, but he will spend more time on:

○ selection of most suitable ingredients and meal components;

○ menu development, recipes;

○ controlling the correct cooking and regeneration procedures;

○ organising the kitchen staff.

The chef/pastry chef thus becomes the production manager who:

plans; organises; supervises; personalises.

Key questions

Will future employers be able to rely on their managers' know-how to organise or reorganise food and beverage systems which will contribute to the improved economical results needed and guarantee the quality level required?

For a regeneration-on-the-plate recipe, we have to answer the following questions:

○ *Who* makes the recipe? *Which* recipe? *Where* – work area?

○ *When* – 1, 2, 3 days ahead or the same day, in the morning, evening?

○ *How* – with what type of products?

      with what type of equipment?

      with what type of technique?

Important points to follow:

○ only regenerate what is needed; strictly follow recipes (measuring); produce at the right time; train the young chefs in this type of food preparation.

The assembly kitchen concept

Research – quality – production – tradition – innovation. This is a system based on accepting and incorporating latest technological development in manufacturing and conservation of food products. In the modern assembly kitchen, the chef does not automatically buy his ingredients. On the contrary, he will carefully choose from the 'five product types' (see page 313) what is best for him by asking himself:

○ Which fresh produce will I use?

○ Which semi-prepared food bases will I use?

○ Which finished products will I use?

The assembly kitchen still relies on skilled personnel. For it requires a thorough understanding of how to switch over from the traditional labour-intensive production method to a more industrial type of production, with some of the principles of the cook-chill, cook-freeze or *sous-vide* production systems taken on board. It realises the existence and availability of modern kitchen equipment and new generations of high quality convenience orientated food bases.

Thus, the concept includes:

○ preparing the food component in an appropriate kitchen, respecting the legislation;

○ arranging everything cold (even raw) onto the plate;
○ regenerating (even cooking) on the same plate as served;
○ if necessary, serving the sauce.

Success requires:
○ appropriate material and equipment;
○ very precise preliminary preparations (mise en place);
○ support by well trained team (kitchen+service staff).

Advantages include:
○ less staff needed for arranging;
○ the regeneration can be done near the consumer;
○ different types of plates can be regenerated at the same time;
○ hygiene and consequently safety is guaranteed;
○ storage rooms only needed for 5 types of products (see page 313);
○ large preparation areas disappear;
○ smaller equipment is needed.

Inconveniences include:
○ very hot plates;
○ some additional investments (trolleys, etc.);
○ some products cannot be prepared (French fries, etc.).

A planning schedule would envisage:
○   2 days   – cooking and chilling;
                – storing at +3°C (37°F) in labelled, dated gastronorm containers.
○   12 hours – arrange food onto plates;
                – storage at +3°C (37°F) on trolley.
○   30 mins – taking the trolley out of storage;
                – setting of regeneration equipment;
                – regeneration.
○   2 min   – taking out and finishing of plates;
                – sauce, garnish;
                – serving;
                – cleaning of equipment.

The principal investments will be for:
○ multi-purpose equipment which are covering most of the cooking methods;
○ storage for dry, chilled, frozen products;
○ equipment to chill or freeze;
○ equipment to regenerate:
   – on plates;
   – gastronorm pans.

The new generation equipment must be:
○ easy to handle;   ○ gastronorm;
○ easy to clean;   ○ good service (maintenance).

The five types of products are:

1 FRESH (RAW PRODUCT):

- meat with bones;
- whole fish;
- vegetables, potatoes, fruits, unpeeled;
- milk.

2 SHELF-STABLE:

- sterilised, pasteurised:
  - vegetables, potatoes, fruits;
  - dairy products, meat products.
- dehydrated products, partly elaborated:
  - stocks, sauces;
  - bouillons, soups, purées;
  - mousses, creams, custards;
  - culinary aids.

3 FROZEN:

- meat, fish, vegetables, potatoes, fruits;
- pastry products, ice cream.

4 CHILLED ('FRESH' PRODUCTS, PARTLY ELABORATED):

- meat or fish, boned, cut into pieces or portioned;
- washed, peeled and cut vegetables, potatoes, fruits, etc.

5 CHILLED (PRODUCTS, NORMALLY COOKED AND PACKED OR SOUS-VIDE):

- meat, fish, vegetables, desserts (with or without sauce).

METHODS OF FOOD PRODUCTION

NO.	METHOD	DESCRIPTION
1	Conventional	Term used to describe production utilising mainly fresh foods and traditional cooking methods
2	Convenience	Method of production utilising mainly convenience foods
3	Call order	Method where food is cooked to order either from customer (as in cafeterias) or from waiter. Production area often open to customer area
4	Continuous flow	Method involving production line approach where different parts of the production process may be separated (e.g. fast food)
5	Centralised	Production not directly linked to service. Foods are 'held' and distributed to separate service areas
6	Cook-chill	Food production storage and regeneration method utilising principle of low temperature control to preserve qualities of processed foods
7	Cook-freeze	Production, storage and regeneration method utilising principle of freezing to control and preserve qualities of processed foods. Requires special processes to assist freezing
8	Sous-vide	Method of production, storage and regeneration utilising principle of sealed vacuum to control and preserve the quality of processed foods
9	Assembly kitchen	A system based on accepting and incorporating the latest technological development in manufacturing and conservation of food products

Some references to production systems elsewhere in the book

Topics for Discussion

1 The advantages and disadvantages of cook-chill and cook-freeze system.

2 Essential hygiene and food safety requirements for cook-chill and cook-freeze systems.

3 The reason for quality control, temperature control, microbiological control when producing cook-chill and cook-freeze foods.

4 Types of operation suitable for using cook-chill and cook-freeze foods.

5 For and against a centralised production system with examples.

6 The food production system and its main advantages.

7 The principles of in-flight catering.

8 Catering on board the trains travelling through the Channel Tunnel.

9 What do you consider to be the future of food production systems?

CHAPTER 9

MENU PLANNING, DEVELOPMENT AND STRUCTURE

EVOLUTION

Initially menus were lists of food, in seemingly random fashion with the food being raw, prepared or cooked. Individual menus came into use early in the 19th century and courses began to be formulated. For special occasions seven or so courses might be served e.g. hors-d'œuvre, soup, fish, entree, sorbet, roast, sweet, savoury.

With the formulation of menus, artistry and flair began to influence the various ways of cooking and dishes were created after 'the style of' e.g. à la francaise or/and given names of important people for whom they had been created e.g. Peach Melba, a simple dish of poached fresh peach, vanilla ice-cream and fresh raspberry pureé created by Escoffier at the Savoy for Dame Nellie Melba, a famous opera singer.

As the 20th century advanced and more people of the world moved and settled from country to country so began the introduction of styles of food and service from a wide variety of nations resulting in the number of ethnic dishes and ethnic restaurants which abound today.

Eating at work, at school in hospitals and institutions led to a need for healthy, budget conscious food.

Rapid air transport made it possible for foods from all corners of the globe to be available which together with domestic and European produce gives those who compose menus a tremendous range of choice.

ESSENTIAL CONSIDERATIONS PRIOR TO PLANNING THE MENU

○ **Competition** – be aware of any competition in the locality, including prices and quality. As a result it may be wiser to produce a menu quite different.

○ **Location** – study the area in which your establishment is situated and the potential target market of customers.

○ **Analyse** – the type of people you are planning to cater for, e.g. office workers in the city requiring quick service.

○ **Outdoor Catering** – are there opportunities for outdoor catering or take-away food.

○ **Estimated customer spend per head** – important when catering, for example for hospital staff and patients, children in schools, workers in industry. Whatever level of catering a golden rule should be 'offer value for money'.

○ **Modern trends in food fashions** – should be considered alongside popular traditional dishes.

○ Decide the range of dishes to be offered and the pricing structure. Price each dish separately? Or offer to set 2 to 3 course menus? Or a combination of both?

○ **Space and equipment in the kitchens** will influence the composition of the menu e.g. overloading use of deep frying pan, salamanders and steamers.

○ **Number and capability of staff** – over-stretched staff can easily reduce the standard of production envisaged.

○ **Availability of supplies and reliability of suppliers** – seasonal foods and storage space.

○ **Food Allergies** (see page 342).

○ **Cost factor** – is crucial if an establishment is to be profitable. Costing is essential for the success of compiling any menu. Modern computer techniques can analyse costs swiftly and daily.

TYPES OF MENU

○ **Table d'hôte or set-price menu** – a menu forming a meal usually of two or three courses at a set price. A choice of dishes may be offered at all courses.

○ **A la carte** – a menu with all the dishes individually priced. The customers can therefore compile their own menu, which may be one, two or more courses. A true á la carte dish should be cooked to order and the customer should be prepared to wait.

○ **Special party or function menus** – menus for banquets or functions of all kinds.

○ **Ethnic or speciality menus** – these can be set price or dishes individually priced specialising in the food (or religion) of the country or in a specialised food itself: ethnic – Chinese, Indian, kosher, African Caribbean, Greek; speciality – steak, fish, pasta, vegetarian, pancakes.

○ **Hospital menus** – these usually take the form of a menu card given to the patient the day before service so that his or her preferences can be ticked. Both National Health Service and private hospitals cater for vegetarians and also for religious requirements.

○ **Menus for people at work** – menus which are served to people at their place of work. Such menus vary in standard and extent from one employer to another due to company policy on the welfare of their staff and work-force.

○ There may also be a call-order à la carte selection charged at a higher price. The food will usually be mainly British with some ethnic dishes and vegetarian dishes.

Menus may consist of soup, main course with vegetables, followed by sweets, cheese and yogurts. According to the policy of the management and employee requirements, there will very often be a salad bar and healthy eating dishes included on the menu. When there is a captive clientele who face the same surroundings daily and meet the same people, then no matter how long the menu cycle or how pleasant the people, or how nice the decor, boredom is bound to set in and staff then long for a change of scene. So, a chef or manager needs to vary the menu constantly to encourage customers to patronise the establishment rather than going off the premises to eat. The decor and layout of the staff restaurant plays a very important part in satisfying the customer's needs. The facilities should be relaxing and comfortable so that he or she feels that the restaurant is not a continuation of the work-place. Employees who are happy, well-nourished and know that the company has their interests and welfare at heart will tend to be well-motivated and work better.

○ Menus for children – in schools there is an emphasis on healthy eating and a balanced diet particularly in boarding schools. Those areas with children of various cultural and religious backgrounds have appropriate items available on the menu. Many establishments provide special children's menus which concentrate on favourite foods and offer suitably sized portions.

Cyclical menus

These are menus which are compiled to cover a given period of time: one month, three months, etc. They consist of a number of set menus for a particular establishment, such as an industrial catering restaurant, cafeteria, canteen, director's dining-room, hospital or college refectory. At the end of each period the menus can be used again thus overcoming the need to keep compiling new ones. The length of the cycle is determined by management policy, by the time of the year and by different foods available. These menus must be monitored carefully to take account of changes in customer requirements and any variations in weather conditions which are likely to affect demand for certain dishes. If cyclical menus are designed to remain in operation for long periods of time, then they must be carefully compiled so that they do not have to be changed too drastically during operation.

ADVANTAGES OF CYCLICAL MENUS

○ They save time by removing the daily or weekly task of compiling menus, although they may require slight alterations for the next period.

○ When used in association with cook/freeze operations, it is possible to produce the entire number of portions of each item to last the whole cycle, having determined that the standardised recipes are correct.

○ They give greater efficiency in time and labour.

○ They can cut down on the number of commodities held in stock, and can assist in planning storage requirements.

DISADVANTAGES

○ When used in establishments with a captive clientele, then the cycle has to be long enough so that customers do not get bored with the repetition of dishes.

○ The caterer cannot easily take advantage of 'good buys' offered by suppliers on a daily or weekly basis unless such items are required for the cyclical menu.

Preplanned and predesigned menus
ADVANTAGES

- Preplanned or predesigned menus enable the caterer to ensure that good menu planning is practiced.
- Before selecting dishes that he or she prefers, the caterer should consider what the customer likes, and the effect of these dishes upon the meal as a whole.
- Menus which are planned and costed in advance allow banqueting managers to quote prices instantly to a customer.
- Menus can be planned taking into account the availability of kitchen and service equipment, without placing unnecessary strain upon such equipment.
- The quality of food is likely to be higher if kitchen staff are preparing dishes that they are familiar with and have prepared a number of times before.

DISADVANTAGES

- Preplanned and predesigned menus may be too limited to appeal to a wide range of customers.
- They may reduce job satisfaction for staff who have to prepare the same menus repetitively.
- They may limit the chef's creativity and originality.

STRUCTURE OF MENUS
Menu structure
LENGTH

The number of dishes on a menu should:

- Offer the customer an interesting and varied choice.
- In general, it is better to offer fewer dishes of good standard than a long list of mediocre quality.

DESIGN

Should complement the image of the dining room and be designed to allow for changes (total or partial) which may be daily, weekly, monthly etc. An inset for dishes of the day or of the week gives the customer added interest.

LANGUAGE

- Accuracy in dish description helps the customer to identify the food they wish to choose.
- Avoid over-elaboration and flowery choice of words.
- Wherever possible use English language. If a foreign dish name is used then follow it with a simple, clear English version.

PRESENTATION

Ensure the menu is presented in a sensible and welcoming way so that the customer is put at ease and relaxed.

An off-hand brusque presentation (written or oral) can be off-putting and lower expectations of the meal.

PLANNING

Consider the following:

1 Type and size of establishment: pub, school, hospital, restaurant etc.
2 Customer profile: different kinds of people have differing likes and dislikes.
3 Special requirements: Kosher, Muslim, Vegetarian.
4 Time of the year: certain dishes acceptable in summer may not be so in winter.
5 Foods in season: are usually in good supply and reasonable in price.
6 Special days: Christmas, Hogmanay, Shrove Tuesday etc.
7 Time of day: breakfast, brunch, lunch, tea, high tea, dinner, supper, snack, special function.
8 Price range: charge a fair price and ensure good value for money, customer satisfaction can lead to recommendation and repeat business.
9 Number of course.
10 Sequence of course.
11 Use menu language that customers understand.
12 Sensible nutritional balance.
13 No unnecessary repetition of ingredients from dish to dish.
14 No unnecessary repetition of flavours and colours.
15 Be aware of the Trades Description Act 1988 'Any person who in the course of a trade or business: applies a false trade description to any goods or supplies or offers to supply any goods to which a false trade description is applied shall be guilty of an offence.'

PRICE MARKING (FOOD AND DRINK ON PREMISES) ORDER 1979

The wording and pricing of food and drink on menus and wine lists must comply with the law and be accurate. However by offering dishes on the menu there is no legal obligation to serve the customer if he or she may cause a nuisance to other customers or due to demand the dish had sold out and was 'off' the menu. But for establishments providing accommodation there is an obligation to provide refreshment providing the customer is able to pay and is in an acceptable state e.g. sober.

CONSUMER PROTECTION ACT 1987

This Act contains recommendations in the form of a Code of Practice regarding a service charge. This should be incorporated in the inclusive price where practicable and indicated e.g. price includes service.

Non-optional charges e.g. cover charges or minimum charges should be prominently displayed.

SALE OF GOODS AND SERVICES ACT 1982

This Act is to ensure that goods sold are of satisfactory quality and fit for the purpose intended. This would especially apply to equipment as well as commodities.

Menu policy – summary

○ Provide a means of communication.
○ Establish the essential and social needs of the customer.
○ Accurately predict what the customer is likely to buy and how much he or she is going to spend.

- ○ Purchase and prepare raw materials to preset standards in accordance with predictions and purchasing specifications.
- ○ Skilfully portion and cost the product in order to keep within company profitability policy.
- ○ Effectively control the complete operation from purchase to service on the plate.
- ○ Customer satisfaction is all-important: remember who pays the bill.

Consumer protection

There is a comprehensive set of legislation concerned with protecting the consumer. This can be divided into that which is concerned with health and safety, economic protection such as weights and measures, and others which deal with unfair contract terms.

Fundamentally, however, all consumer protection starts with the basic contract. If a supplier fails to supply what a consumer has contracted to purchase, the supplier may be in breach of contract. However, because breach of contract cases can be difficult to prove and expensive, the government over the years has introduced legislation to improve protection for the consumer.

There is a whole range of law concerned with consumer protection. Some is concerned with health and safety and others such as weights and measures law is concerned with economic protection.

Fundamentally however, all consumer protection starts with the basic contractor. If a supplier does not supply what a consumer has contracted to purchase, the supplier may be in breach of contract. However, because breach of contract, cases can be difficult to prove.

The main consumer protection acts
TRADE DESCRIPTIONS ACT 1968

This Act makes it a criminal offence to falsely describe goods or services, or to supply or offer for sale any goods or services to which a false description applies. It is also an offence to make reckless statements, e.g. statements without the knowledge to support the claims made about the goods or services. Examples of offences include describing pork as veal or frozen foods as fresh.

There are also offences under the Food and Safety Act 1990.

SUPPLY GOODS AND SERVICES 1982

This Act is concerned with 'implied' terms in a contract.

SALE AND SUPPLY OF GOODS ACT 1994

This is an amending Act that mainly amends the Sale of Goods Act 1979.

SALE OF GOODS ACT 1979

This Act supplies to the Sale of Goods only. From the caterer's viewpoint this Act works mainly to his or her advantage whereas the *Supply of Goods and Services Act 1982* works mainly to the customer's advantage. In essence the Act is concerned with ensuring that customers receive goods which are of satisfactory quality and are fit for the purpose.

Goods may be defined as of satisfactory quality 'if they are as fit for the purpose or purposes for which goods of that kind are commonly bought as it is reasonable to expect having regard to any description applied to them, the price (if relevant) and all the other circumstances'.

In addition to goods being of satisfactory quality they must also be fit for the purpose. This means that if a purchaser makes known a specific purpose for their goods, then the goods should be able to satisfy that purpose.

CONSUMER PROTECTION ACT 1987

This act deals with three main subjects, liability for defective products, consumer safety and misleading price indications.

Code of practice on price indications
THE CONSUMER PROTECTION ACT 1987

Authorised the issue of a code of practice on prices. This covers the Code of Practice for Traders on Price Indications, contains recommendations on service, cover and minimum charges in hotels, restaurants and similar establishments.

It states: "if your customers in hotels, restaurants or similar places must pay a non-optional charge e.g. a 'service charge'.

1   Incorporate the charge within the fully inclusive prices wherever practicable.

2   Display the fact clearly on any price list or priced menu whether displayed inside or outside (e.g. by using statements like all prices include service."

Do not include suggested optional sums, whether for service or any other item, in the bill presented to the customer.

The code concedes that it is not practical to include some non-optional extra charges, for example cover charges or minimum charges in a quoted price. In these cases the charge should be shown as prominently as other prices on any list or menu whether displayed inside or outside.

DATA PROTECTION ACT 1984

The Data Protection Act 1984 regulates the use of personal data.

Data being information recorded in a form in which it can be processed by equipment operating automatically in response to instructions given to it.; 'personal data' being data consisting of information which relates to a living individual who can be identified from that information (or from that and other information held by the data user.

The Act imposes specific duties on data users and those carrying en computer bureaux and gives certain rights to individuals including employees on whom personal data is held.

DATA PROTECTION PRINCIPLES

1   Personal data information must be fairly and lawfully obtained and processed.

2   Personal data can be held only if there are one or more specified and lawful purposes.

3   Personal data held for any purpose or purposes shall not be used or disclosed in any manner incompatible with that purpose or purposes.

4   Personal data held should be adequate, relevant and not excessive in relation to that purpose or purposes.

5   Personal data should be accurate and kept up to date.

6   Personal data should not be kept longer than for the purpose or purposes for which it is required.

7   An individual shall be entitled

    a)   at reasonable intervals and without undue delay or expense

        i)   to be informed by any data user whether he/she holds personal data of which that individual is subject;

ii) to access any such data held by a data user and

b) where appropriate to have such data corrected or erased.

8 Appropriate security measures should be taken against unauthorised access to, or alteration, disclosure or destruction of, personal data and against accidental loss or destruction of personal data.

MENU COPY

Items or groups of items should bear names people recognise and understand. If a name does not give the right description, additional copy may be necessary. Descriptions can be produced carefully, helping to promote the dish and the menu. However, the description should describe the item realistically and not mislead the customer. Interesting descriptive copy is a skill; a good menu designer is able to illuminate menu terms, specific culinary terms and in doing so is able to draw attention to them. Simplicity creates better understanding and endorses the communication process.

Some menus can be built around a general descriptive copy featuring the history of the establishment or around the local area in which the establishment is located. Descriptive copy can alternatively be based on a speciality dish which has significant cultural importance to the area or the establishment. In doing so the description may wish to feature the person responsible for creating and preparing the dish, especially if the chef is reasonably well known and has appeared on national or local television or radio. The chef may have also had his/her recipes featured in the local press. This too may be included in the menu to further create interest.

Menu copy should be set in a style of print which is easily legible and well spaced. Mixing type face is often done to achieve emphasis; if overdone the overall concept is likely to look a mess and therefore unattractive to the eye.

Emphasis may be easily achieved by using boxes on the menu. Also menu paper and colour of the print can be carefully chosen to make certain dishes stand out.

Some mistakes in menu copy are as follows:

○ Descriptive copy is left out when it is required (confusing to the customer).
○ The wrong emphasis is given.
○ Emphasis is lost because print size and style are not correctly used.
○ The menu lacks creativity (boring).
○ The menu is designed for the wrong market.
○ Much needed information is omitted.
○ Pricing is unclear.
○ Menu sequence is wrong.
○ Customers do not see valuable copy because added sheets such as 'dish of the day' or 'today's specials' cover up other parts of the menu or cover up essential information.

Menu cover

The cover of the menu should reflect the identity or the decor of the operation and should ideally pick up the theme of the restaurant. A theme can be effective in creating the right image of the restaurant. The cover design must therefore reflect this overall image. The paper chosen must be of good quality, heavy, durable and grease-resistant.

MENU FLEXIBILITY

In times of inflation and recession when prices rise or the amount of disposable income decreases, customer demands change and therefore menus become outdated and obsolete.

Some operations use the menu of the day on a wall board or chalk board to provide flexibility in items offered and pricing. This custom started in Paris. A neatly written wall board told customers as they entered the restaurant what was on offer that day. Some establishments change part of their menus, daily or weekly while the main core of the menu remains the same. Changes can be made on paper insert and this added to the hard printed menu. Hors-d'œuvre, side dishes, salads, desserts and beverages do not change frequently. These dishes are printed on the main copy while the speciality dishes, which do change more frequently are placed on the paper insert.

Nothing becomes obsolete faster to the regular customer than the same menu. Menu fatigue sets in and you begin to lose customers. Even fast-food establishments which have a basic menu on offer year in year out, still have to create interest by advertising certain new products or new recipes to existing products in order to keep interest alive. Menus should change at least every three months.

Menu engineering

Chefs and Food and Beverage Managers operating in a competitive environment require a knowledge of menu engineering in order to maximise business potential.

One approach to sales analysis which has gained some popularity is the technique known as 'menu engineering'. This is a technique of menu analysis that uses two key factors of performance in the sales of individual menu items: the popularity and the gross profit contribution of each item. The analysis results in each menu item being assigned to one of four categories:

○ Items of high popularity and high cash gross profit contributions. These are known as the *Stars*.

Figure 9.1 *Menu engineering matrix (based on Kasavana and Smith 1982)*

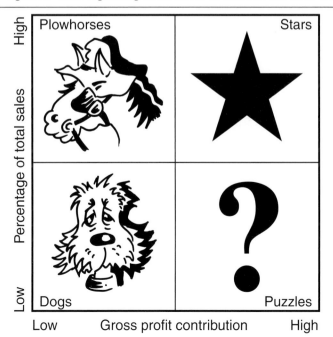

○ Items of high popularity but with low cash gross profit contribution. These are known as the *Plowhorses*.

○ Items of low popularity but with high cash gross profit contributions. These are known as the *Puzzles*.

○ Items of low popularity and low cash gross profit contribution. These are the worst items on the menu, and are known as the *Dogs*.

The advantage of this approach is that it provides a simple way of graphically indicating the relative cash contribution position of individual items on a matrix as in the figure.

There are a variety of computer-based packages which will automatically generate the categorisation, usually directly using data from electronic point-of-sale (EPOS) control systems. The basis for the calculations is as follows.

In order to determine the position of an item on the matrix, two things need to be calculated. These are:

○ the cash gross profit;

○ the sales percentage category.

The cash gross profit category for any menu item is calculated by reference to the weighted average cash gross profit. Menu items with a cash gross profit which is the same as or higher than the average are classified as high. Those with lower than the average are classified as low cash gross profit items. The average also provides the axis separating Plowhorses and Dogs from Stars and Puzzles.

The sales percentage category for an item is determined in relation to the menu average; taking into account an additional factor. With a menu consisting of ten items one might expect, all other things being equal, that each item would account for 10 per cent of the menu mix. Any item which reached at least 10 per cent of the total menu items sold would therefore be classified as enjoying high popularity. Similarly, any item which did not achieve the rightful share of 10 per cent would be categorised as having a low popularity. With this approach, half of the menu items would tend to be shown as being below average in terms of their popularity. This would potentially result in the frequent revision of the composition of the menu. It is for this reason that Kasavana and Smith (1982) have recommended the use of a 70 per cent formula. Under this approach, all items which reach at least 70 per cent of their rightful share of the menu mix are categorised as enjoying high popularity. For example, where a menu consists of, say, 20 items, any item which reached 3.5 per cent or more of the menu mix (70 per cent of 5 per cent) would be regarded as enjoying high popularity. Whilst there is no convincing theoretical support for choosing the 70 per cent figure rather than some other percentage, common sense and experience tend to suggest that there is some merit in this approach.

INTERPRETING THE CATEGORIES

There is a different basic strategy which can be considered for items that fall into each of the four categories of the matrix.

○ *Stars* These are the most popular items which may be able to yield even higher gross profit contributions by careful price increases or through cost reduction. High visibility is maintained on the menu, and standards for these dishes should be strictly controlled.

○ *Plowhorses* These again are solid sellers which may also be able to yield greater cash profit contributions through marginal cost reduction. Lower menu visibility than Stars is usually recommended.

○ *Puzzles* These are exactly that – puzzles. Items such as flambé dishes or a particular speciality can add an attraction in terms of drawing customers, even though the sales of these items may be low. Depending on the particular item, different strategies might be considered, ranging from accepting the current position because of the added attraction that they provide to increasing the price further.

○ *Dogs* These are the worst items on a menu and the first reaction is to remove them. An alternative, however, is to consider adding them to another item as part of a special deal. For instance, adding them in a meal package to a Star may have the effect of lifting the sales of the Dog item and may provide a relatively low-cost way of adding special promotions to the menu.

The menu engineering methodology is designed to categorise dishes into good and poor performers.

Dishes with High Popularity and High Contribution – 'Stars'

○ do nothing;
○ modify price slightly – up or down;
○ promote through personal selling or menu positioning.

Dishes with High Popularity and Low Contribution – 'Plowhorses'

○ do nothing;
○ increase price;
○ reduce dish cost – modify recipe by using cheaper commodities or reducing the portion size.

Dishes with Low Popularity and High Contributions – 'Puzzles'

○ do nothing;
○ reduce price;
○ rename dish;
○ reposition dish on menu;
○ promote through personal selling;
○ remove from menu.

Dishes with Low Popularity and Low Contribution – 'Dogs'

○ do nothing;
○ replace dish;
○ redesign dish;
○ remove dish from menu.

Some Potential Limitations

○ *Elasticity of demand* One of the practical difficulties with price-level adjustment is not knowing enough about the elasticity of demand. The effect of demand (number of covers) of any one change in the general level of menu prices is usually uncertain. Also, what applies to one menu item applies equally to the menu as a whole. There is an additional problem of cross-elasticity of demand, where the change in demand for one commodity is directly affected by a change in the price of another. Even less is known about the cross-elasticity of demand for individual menu items than is known about the elasticity of demand for the menu as a whole. Any benefit arising from an adjustment in the price of one item may therefore be offset by resultant changes in the demand for another item. Price-level adjustments must therefore be underpinned by a good deal of common sense, experience and knowledge of the particular circumstances of the operation.

○ *Labour intensity* In menu engineering the most critical element is cash gross profit. Whilst this may be important, the aspect of labour intensity cannot be ignored. The cash gross profit on a flambé dish, for example, may be higher than on a more simple sweet; however, when the costs of labour are taken into account – especially at peak periods – it may well be that the more simple sweet is the more profitable overall.

○ *Shelf-life* The food cost of an item used to determine the cash gross profit may not take account of cost increases which are the result of food wastage through spoilage, especially at slack times.

○ *Fluctuations in demand* Another factor is the consistency of the buying of the consumer. The approach assumes that changes can be made to promote various items and that this will be reflected in the buying behaviour of the customer. The approach will work well where the potential buying pattern of the consumer is fairly similar over long periods. However, where the customers are continually changing, as for instance in the restaurant of an hotel, popularity and profitability can be affected more by changes in the nature of the customer and the resultant change in demand than as a result of the operation's attempting to manipulate the sales mix.

* See page 343 for note on price elasticity of demand.

GLOSSARY OF FRENCH MENU AND KITCHEN TERMS

Universal respect for French traditions of classical cookery has left a repertoire of French words and terms which are understood and accepted by most professionals. As Italian has been the traditional language for music so French has been the traditional international language for food, drink and writing menus. Current trends however indicate that the vast majority of menus are written in English. Because certain French words and terms remain and are in everyday use in many establishments, the following glossary is included. Some examples are given in brackets.

l'aile (f)	wing of poultry or game birds e.g. phesant or chicken
à la	in the style of (*à la mode*)
à la française	dishes prepared in the French way (boiled beef); see *Practical Cookery*
à l'anglaise	in the English style (roast duck)
à la broche	cooked on a spit (chicken)
à la diable	devilled, a highly seasoned dish (kidneys)
à la carte	dishes on a menu prepared to order and individually priced
l'aloyau (m)	sirloin of beef (on the bone)
en aspic (m)	in savoury jelly (breast of chicken)
assorti	an assortment (*fromages assortis*)
au bleu	when applied to meat it means very underdone (fillet steak)
au four	cooked in the oven (*pomme au four*)
au gratin	sprinkled with breadcrumbs and/or cheese and browned (cauliflower)
au vin blanc	with white wine sauce (fillets of sole)
la blanquette	a white stew cooked in stock from which the sauce is made (*blanquette de veau*)
la bordure	a ring, sometimes of rice or potatoes as a border to a plate or dish.
les bouchées	small puff-pastry cases
bouilli	boiled

le bouquet garni	a faggot or bundle of herbs, usually parsley stalks, thyme and bay leaf, tied inside pieces of celery and leek
braisé	braised (beef)
la braisière	braising pan
en branche	a term denoting vegetables, such as spinach, cooked and served as whole leaves
la brioche	a light yeast cake
la broche	a roasting spit
la brochette	a skewer
brouillé	scrambled (*œufs brouillés*)
le buffet	a sideboard of food, or a self-service table
le canapé	a cushion of toasted or fried bread on which are served various hot or cold foods (as a base for savouries); when served cold the base may be toast, biscuit or short or puff-paste with the food on top
la carte du jour	menu, or bill of fare for the day
en casserole	in a fireproof dish (chicken)
la charlotte	name given to various hot and cold sweet dishes which have a case of biscuits, bread, sponge, etc. (apple charlotte)
le chateaubriand	the head of the fillet of beef
chaud	hot
le chaud-froid	a creamed velouté or demi-glace with gelatine or aspic added, used for masking cold dishes
le civet	a brown stew of game, usually hare (jugged hare)
la cloche	a bell-shaped cover, used for special *à la carte* dishes (*suprême de volaille sous cloche*)
la cocotte	porcelain fireproof dish
la compote	stewed fruit (*compote des poires*)
concassé	coarsely chopped (parsley, tomatoes)
le consommé	basic clear soup
le contrefilet	boned sirloin of beef
le cordon	a thread or thin line of sauce
la côte	rib (*côte de bœuf*)
la côtelette	cutlet (*les côtelettes d'agneau*)
coupe	cut; also dish in which ice-cream is served
le court-bouillon	a cooking liquor for certain foods (oily fish, etc.); it is water containing vinegar, sliced onions, carrots, herbs and seasoning
la crème fouetée	whipped cream
la crème Chantilly	sweetened, whipped vanilla-flavoured cream (*meringue Chantilly*)
la crêpe	pancake (*crêpes à l'orange*) (orange pancakes)
le croquette	cooked foods moulded cylinder shape, egg and crumbed and deep fried (*croquette de volaille* or chicken croquettes)
la croûte	a cushion of fried or toasted bread on which are served various hot foods, (savouries, game stuffing, etc.)
le croûton	cubes of fried bread served with soup, also triangular pieces which may

	be served with spinach and heart-shaped ones which may be served with certain braised vegetables and entrées
les crustacés (m)	shellfish
la cuisse de poulet	leg of chicken (grilled, devilled)
la darne	a slice of round fish cut through with the bone (*darne de saumon*)
le déjeuner	lunch
le petit-déjeuner	breakfast
le dîner	dinner
du jour (plat du jour)	special dish of the day
duxelles	a basic preparation of finely chopped mushrooms cooked with chopped shallots
émincé	sliced (*chicken à la king*)
l'entrecôte (f)	a steak from a boned sirloin
l'escalope (f)	thin slice of meat (*escalope de veau Holstein*)
étuvée	cooked in its own juice (*braised endives*)
la farce	stuffing
farci	stuffed
fécule	a thickening agent made from potato or rice
le feuilletage	puff paste
les fines herbes	chopped parsley, tarragon and chervil
flambé	flamed or lit (*poire flambée*)
le flan	open fruit tart (apple, banana)
le fleuron	small crescent pieces of puff paste used for garnishing certain dishes (fish and vegetable)
le foie	liver (*foie de veau lyonnaise* or calves' liver and onions)
le foie gras	fat goose liver
le fondant	a soft icing for cakes
fondu	melted (butter served with asparagus)
le four	oven
frappé	chilled (*melon frappé*)
les friandises	petits fours, sweetmeats, etc.
la fricassée	a white stew in which the poultry or meat is cooked in the sauce
frisé	curled (*endive frisée*)
fumé	smoked (*saumon fumé*)
le fumet	a concentrated stock or essence
la garniture	the trimmings on the dish
le gâteau	cake (of a number of portions)
la gelée	jelly (*gelée des fruits*)
le gibier	game (*salmis de gibier*)
la glace	ice or ice-cream
glacé	iced or with ice-cream (*meringue glacé*)
glacer	to glaze under the salamander

gratiner	to colour or gratinate under the salamander or in a hot oven using grated cheese or breadcrumbs
grillé	grilled (sole)
hacher	to chop finely or very finely dice; to mince
les herbes (f)	herbs
hors-d'œuvre	preliminary dishes of an appetising nature, served hot or cold
le jambon froid	cold ham
jardinière	cut into batons
julienne	cut into fine strips
le jus-lié	gravy thickened with arrowroot or cornflour or *fécule*
liaison	yolks of eggs and cream when used as a binding or a thickening (soup or sauce)
lier	to thicken (*jus-lié*)
la longe	loin (*longe de veau*)
macédoine	either a mixture of fruit or vegetables (*macédoine de fruits*); or cut into 6mm ($\frac{1}{2}$ inch) dice
macérer	to steep, to soak, to macerate (peaches in brandy)
la marinade	a richly spiced pickling liquid for enriching the flavour and tenderness of meats before braising
mariné	pickled (as in roll mops)
la madère	Madeira wine
masquer	to mask or coat (with a sauce)
médaillon	foodstuffs prepared in a round, flat shape (*médaillon de veau*)
le menu	bill of fare
mignonette	coarse ground or crushed pepper
les mille-feuilles (f)	'thousand leaves', a puff-pastry cream slice
à la minute	cooked to order
mirepoix	roughly cut onions, carrots, celery and a sprig of thyme and bay leaf
mollet	soft (*œuf mollet* or soft boiled egg)
le moule	mould; also *les moules*, mussels
la mousse	a hot or cold dish of light consistency, sweet or savoury
la moutarde	mustard
moutarder	to smear with mustard, or to add mustard to a sauce
mûr	ripe, mature
natives (f)	a menu term denoting English oysters
navarin	a brown lamb or mutton stew
le nid	nest; imitation nest made from potatoes or sugar, etc.
la noisette or *noisette*	a hazelnut used in confectionery; or small round potatoes cut with a special scoop; or as for noisette butter (nut-brown butter); or a cut of loin of lamb
la noix	nut, also the name given to the cushion piece of the leg of veal (*noix de veau*)
les nouilles (f)	noodles

œuf brouillé	a scrambled egg
œuf en cocotte	egg cooked in an egg cocotte
œuf à la coque	egg boiled and served in its shell
œuf dur	a hard-boiled egg
œuf mollet	a soft-boiled shelled egg
œuf poché	a poached egg
œuf sur le plat	egg cooked in an egg dish
œuf à la poêle	a fried egg
l'oignon (m)	onion
l'orge (f)	barley
oseille (f)	sorrel
les pailles (f)	straws (*pommes pailles*) or straw potatoes
les paillettes de fromage (f)	cheese straws
le pain	bread
panaché	mixed (*salade panaché*)
pané	flour, egg and crumbed
panier	basket
papain	a proteolytic enzyme sometimes called vegetable pepsin, used as a meat tenderiser
papillote	foods cooked *en papillote* are cooked in greased greaseproof paper or foil in their own steam in the oven
la pâte	a dough, paste, batter, pie or pastie
la pâtisserie	a pastry
la paupiette	a strip of fish, meat or poultry stuffed and rolled
paysanne	cut into even thin triangles, round or square pieces
le pilon	the drumstick of a leg of chicken
le piment	pimento
piquant	sharp flavour
piqué	studded (*onion piqué*)
poivre	pepper
poêlé	pot roasted (beef fillet)
les pointes d'asperges	asparagus tips
la praline	chopped grilled almonds or hazelnuts or crushed almond toffee
primeurs	early vegetables (*navarin aux primeurs*)
printanière	garnish of spring vegetables (as for *consommé*)
profiteroles	small balls of *choux* paste for garnishing soups or as a sweet course
la purée	a smooth mixture obtained by passing food through a sieve
la quennelle	forcemeat of poultry or fish, pounded, sieved, creamed and shaped, then poached
la râble	the back (*râble de lièvre* or the saddle of a hare)
le ragoût	stew (*ragoût de bœuf*)

le ravioli	an Italian paste, stuffed with various ingredients (meat, spinach, cheese, etc.)
le risotto	Italian rice stewed in stock
le ris	sweetbread (*ris de veau*)
rissolé	fry to a golden brown
rôti	roast
le sabayon	yolks of eggs and a little liquid cooked till creamy
sauté	tossed in fat or turned in fat; also a specific meat dish e.g. *Sauté de veau*
soubise	an onion purée
le soufflé	a light dish, sweet or savoury, hot or cold; whites of eggs are added to the hot basic preparation and whipped cream to the cold
le suprême	when applied to poultry it means whole wing and half the breast of the bird (there are two *suprêmes* to a bird); for other foods it is applied to a choice cut
table d'hôte	a fixed price meal of several courses, which may have a limited choice
la terrine	an earthenware utensil with a lid; a terrine also indicates a pâté cooked and served in a terrine
tomaté	preparations to which tomato purée has been added to enhance the flavour and colour
tourné	turned, shaped (barrel or olive shape)
la tranche	a slice
le tronçon	a slice of flat fish cut with the bone (*tronçon de turbot*)
le velouté	basic sauce; or soup of velvet or cream consistency
vert	green (*sauce verte*) sometimes served with cold salmon
voiler	to veil or cover with spun sugar
la volaille	poultry
le vol-au-vent	puff-pastry case

EXAMPLES OF DIFFERENT MENUS

Breakfast menu

Breakfast menus can be compiled from the following foods and can be offered as a continental, Table d'Hôte, A la Carte or Buffet. For buffet service customers can self serve the main items they require with assistance from counter hands. Ideally eggs should be freshly cooked to order.

○ Fruits, Fruit juices, Stewed fruit, Yogurts, Cereals: porridge, etc, Eggs: fried, boiled, poached, scrambled; omelettes with bacon or tomatoes, mushrooms or sauté potatoes.

○ Fish: kippers, smoked haddock, kedgeree.

○ Meats (hot): fried or grilled bacon, sausages, kidneys, with tomatoes, mushrooms or sauté potatoes, potato cakes.

○ Meats (cold): ham, bacon, pressed beef with sauté potatoes.

○ Preserves: marmalade (orange, lemon, grapefruit, ginger), jams, honey.

○ Beverages: tea, coffee, chocolate.

○ Bread: rolls, croissants, brioche, toast, pancakes, waffles.

Figure 9.2 *Example of a Continental breakfast*

Fruit Juice – Orange, Grapefruit or Tomato
Fresh Grapefruit or Orange Segments

Stewed Fruits – Prunes, Figs or Apricots

Fresh Fruit Selection, Fresh Fruit Salad

Yogurts

Choice of Cereals, Porridge or Mix your own Muesli

Baker's Selection

Croissant, White and Wholemeal Rolls, Continental Pastry

Your choice of White or Brown Toast

Marmalade, Preserve, Honey, Country Butter or Flora
Margarine

Assorted Cold Meats and Cheese

English Breakfast Tea with Milk or Lemon

Coffee – Freshly Brewed or Decaffeinated
with Milk or Cream

Hot Chocolate, Cold Milk

Chilled Ashbourne Water

Figure 9.3 *Example of an English à la carte breakfast menu*

A LA CARTE

FRUITS & JUICES

Fresh Orange or Grapefruit Juice £.... Large £....

Pineapple, Tomato or Prune Juice £.... Large £....

Chilled Melon £.... Stewed Prunes 3.... Half Grapefruit £....

Stewed Figs £.... Fresh fruit in Season £....

BREAKFAST FAVOURITES

Porridge or Cereal £....

Eggs, any style: one £..... Two £....

Ham, Bacon, Chipolata Sausages or Grilled Tomato £....

Omelette, Plain £.... with Ham or Cheese £....

Grilled Gammon Ham £.... Breakfast Sirloin Steak £....

A Pair of Kippers £.... Smoked Haddock with a Poached Egg £....

Pancakes with Maple Syrup £....

FROM OUR BAKERY

Croissants or Breakfast Rolls £.... Brioche £....

Assorted Danish Pastries £.... Toast £....

BEVERAGES

Tea, Coffee, Sanka, Chocolate or Milk £....

Service Charge 15%

Points to consider when compiling a breakfast menu:

○ It is usual to offer three of the courses previously mentioned:

fruit, yogurt, or cereals; fish, eggs or meat; preserves, bread, coffee or tea.

○ As large a choice as possible, should be offered, depending on the size of the establishment, bearing in mind that it is better to offer a smaller number of well-prepared dishes than a large number of hurriedly prepared ones.

○ A choice of plain foods such as boiled eggs or poached haddock should be available for the person who may not require a fried breakfast.

Buffet breakfast – offers a choice of as many breakfast foods as is both practical and economic. Can be planned on a self-service basis or part self-service and assisted service e.g. hot drinks and freshly cooked eggs.

Luncheon and dinner menus
TYPES OF MENU

○ A set price one, two, or three-course menu with ideally a choice at each course.

○ A list of well varied dishes each priced individually so that the customer can make up his/her own menu of whatever number of dishes they require.

○ Buffet which may be all cold or hot dishes, or a combination of both, either to be served or organised on a self-service basis. Depending on the time of year and location, barbecue dishes can be considered.

○ Special party, which may be either:

a) set menu with no choice;

b) set menu with a limited choice such as soup or melon, main course, choice of two sweets;

c) served or self-service buffet.

Figure 9.4 *Luncheon menu*

Luncheon Menu

Ginger Crab Cakes

Rack of Lamb with a Herb and Shallot crust
Boulangère Potatoes
French Beans

Chocolate and Rum Pie

Figure 9.5 *Luncheon (top) and dinner menu*

Dinner Menu

Smoked Fish Ravioli with Dill and Mustard Cream

Rump of Lamb with Fried Celeriac, Reform Sauce

Calvados and Apple Brulée with Palmiers

Only offer the number of courses and number of dishes within each course that can be satisfactorily prepared, cooked and served.

A vegetarian menu may be offered as an alternative to or as part of the à la carte or table d'hôte menus.

Figure 9.6 *Vegetarian menu*

VEGETARIAN MENU
Iced Cucumber Soup
(Flavoured with mint)
Avocado Waldorf
(Filled with celery & apple bound in mayonnaise, garnished with walnuts)
* * *
Vegetable Lasagne
(Layers of pasta & vegetables with melted cheese, served with salad)
Mushroom Stroganoff
(Flamed in brandy, simmered in cream with paprika & mustard, served with rice)
Chilli con Elote
(Seasonal fresh vegetables in a chilli & tomato fondue, served with rice)
Poached Eggs Elizabeth
(Set on buttered spinach, coated in a rich cream sauce)

Figure 9.7 *Vegetarian menu*

Friday 24th June

Crostini with Roasted Tomato & Pesto

★★★

Courgette & Coriander Soup

★★★

Red Pepper Plait
Potatoes Dauphinoise & Green Beans

★★★

Strawberry & Rhubarb Compote
or
Vegan "Ice Cream"

★★★

Coffee, Tea or Herbal Tea

Tea menus

These vary considerably, depending on the type of establishment. For example:

○ Assorted sandwiches.
○ Bread and butter (white, brown, fruit loaf). Assorted jams.
○ Scones with clotted cream, pastries, gâteaux.
○ Tea (Indian, China, iced, fruit, herb).

The commercial hotels, tea rooms, public restaurants and staff dining rooms will offer simple snacks, cooked meals and high teas. For example:

○ Assorted sandwiches.
○ Buttered buns, scones, tea cakes, Scotch pancakes, waffles, sausage rolls, assorted bread and butter, various jams, toasted tea-cakes, scones, crumpets, buns.
○ Eggs (boiled, poached, fried, omelettes).
○ Fried fish; grilled meats; roast poultry. Cold meats and salads.
○ Assorted pastries; gâteaux.
○ Various ices, coupes, sundaes.
○ Tea; orange and lemon squash.

Light buffets (including cocktail parties)

Light buffets can include:

○ Hot savoury pastry patties of e.g. lobster, chicken, crab, salmon, mushrooms, ham.
○ Hot chipolatas; chicken livers, wrapped in bacon and skewered.
○ Bite-sized items: quiche and pizza, hamburgers, meat balls with savoury sauce or dip, scampi, fried fish en goujons, tartare sauce.
○ Savoury finger toast to include any of the cold canapés; these may also be prepared on biscuits of shaped pieces of pastry.
○ Game chips, gaufrette potatoes, fried fish balls, celery stalks spread with cheese.
○ Sandwiches; bridge rolls, open or closed but always small.
○ Fresh dates stuffed with cream cheese; crudités with mayonnaise and cardamon dip; tuna and chive Catherine wheels; crab claws with garlic dip; smoked salmon pin wheels; choux puffs with camembert.
○ Sweets e.g. trifles, charlottes, bavarois, fruit salad, gâteaux.

FORK BUFFETS

All food must be prepared enabling it to be eaten with a fork or spoon.

Fast-food menus

Although some people are scornful of the items on this type of menu, calling them 'junk food', nevertheless their popularity and success is proven by the fact that from the original McDonald's, opened in Chicago in 1955, there are many thousands of outlets world-wide. McDonald's offer customers a nutrition guide to their products, and also information for diabetes sufferers.

Banquet menus

When compiling banquet menus, consider:

○ The food, which will possibly be for a large number of people, must be dressed in such a way that it can be served fairly quickly. Heavily garnished dishes should be avoided.

○ If a large number of dishes have to be dressed at the same time, certain foods deteriorate quickly and do not stand storage, even for a short time in a hot plate.

A normal menu is used, bearing in mind the number of people involved. It is not usual to serve farinaceous dishes, eggs, stews or savouries. A luncheon menu could be drawn from the following and would usually consist of three courses. Dinner menus, depending on the occasion, generally consist of three to five courses.

○ *First course:* soup, cocktail (fruit or shellfish), hors-d'œuvre, assorted or single item, a small salad.

○ *Second course:* fish, usually poached, steamed, roasted or grilled fillets with a sauce.

○ *Third course:* meat, poultry or game, hot or cold, but not a stew or made-up dish; vegetables and potatoes or a salad would be served.

○ *Fourth course:* if the function is being held during the asparagus season, then either hot or cold asparagus with a suitable sauce may be served as a course on its own.

○ *Fifth course:* sweet, hot or cold, and/or cheese and biscuits.

Figure 9.8 *Example of a banquet dinner menu*

Avocado filled with cream cheese and two fruit sauces

* * *

Seafood filled fish mousse with crayfish sauce

* * *

Butter cooked fillet of beef with sliced mushrooms and
tongue in Madeira sauce
A selection of market vegetables
Potatoes garnished with cream cheese

* * *

Light soft meringue topped with fruit

* * *

Coffee
Sweetmeats

The meal experience

If people have decided to eat out then it follows that there has been a conscious choice to do this in preference to some other course of action. In other words, the foodservice operator has attracted the customer to buy their produce instead of another product, for example the theatre, cinema or simply staying at home. The reasons for eating out may be summarised under seven headings:

○ *Convenience*, for example being unable to return home as in the case of shoppers, people at work or those involved in some leisure activity

○ *Variety*, for example trying new experiences or as a break from home cooking.

○ *Labour*, for example getting someone else to prepare, serve food and wash up or simply the impracticality of housing special events at home.

○ *Status*, for example business lunches or people eating out because others of their socio-economic group do so.

○ *Culture/tradition*, for example special events or because it is a way of getting to know people.

○ *Impulse*, a spur-of-the-moment decision.

○ *No choice*, for example those in welfare, hospitals or other forms of semi- or captive markets.

People are, however, a collection of different types, as any demographic breakdown will show. Whilst it is true that some types of foodservice operation might attract certain types of customer, this is by no means true all the time; for example, McDonald's is marketed to the whole population, and customers are attracted depending on their needs at the time.

The decision to eat out may also be split into two parts: first, the decision to do so for the reasons given above, and then the decision as to what type of experience is sought after. It is generally agreed that there are a number of factors influencing this latter decision. The factors that affect the meal experience may be summarised as follows:

○ *Food and drink on offer* This covers the range of foods, choice, availability, flexibility for special orders and the quality of the food and drink.

○ *Level of service* Depending on the needs people have at the time, the level of service sought should be appropriate to these needs. For example, a romantic night out may call for a quiet table in a top-end restaurant, whereas a group of young friends might be seeking more informal service. This factor also takes into account services such as booking and account facilities, acceptance of credit cards and the reliability of the operation's product.

○ *Level of cleanliness and hygiene* This relates to the premises, equipment and staff. Over the past decade this factor has increased in importance in the customers' minds. The recent media focus on food production and the risks involved in buying food have heightened public awareness of health and hygiene aspects.

○ *Perceived value for money and price* Customers have perceptions of the amount they are prepared to spend and relate these to differing types of establishment and operation. However, many people will spend more if the value gained is perceived to be greater than that obtained by spending slightly less.

○ *Atmosphere of the establishment* Composed of a number of factors such as: design, décor, lighting, heating, furnishings, acoustics and noise levels, the other customers, the staff and the attitude of the staff.

Identifying these factors is important because it considers the product from the point of view of the customer. All too often, foodservice operators can get caught up in the provision of food and drink, spend several thousands on design, décor and equipment, but ignore the actual experience the customer might have. Untrained service staff are a good example of this problem. Operations can tend to concentrate on the core product and forget the total package. A better understanding of the customer's viewpoint or the nature of customer demand leads to a better product being developed to meet it.

MANAGING A FUNCTION

A function can be described as the service of food and drink at a specific time and place, for a given number of people at a known price.

Examples of hospitality functions:

○ **Social functions** – Weddings, Anniversaries, Dinner dances.

○ **Business functions** – Conferences, Meetings, Working lunches, Working dinners.

○ **Social and business functions** – Corporate entertaining.

Sometimes functions are called banquets, however the word banquet is normally used to describe a large formal occasion.

The variety of function events ranges from simply providing bar facilities in a conference reception area before the meeting, to the more formal occasion catering for 1500 to 2000 people. Many establishments concentrate and market themselves as specialist function caterers. The function business may be the company's sole business; on the other hand it may be part of the product range, for example in a hotel, you may well find rooms, restaurants, conferences facilities and banqueting.

The type of function facilities found in an establishment will also depend on the level of market for which it is catering.

Function catering is found in the commercial and public sector of the Hospitality Industry. The types of function suites and variety of functions on offer in all establishments will often differ considerably.

Policy decisions relating to function catering are determined by a number of characteristics inherent to this type of catering. Firstly, depending where the establishment is located there will be a banqueting season, this is where the main business is concentrated, for example from May to September depending on the location this is known as the 'Wedding Season'.

A considerable amount of information is available to the caterer in advance of the function. This includes:

- number of guests;
- menu requirement;
- type of menu.
- price per couvert (head or cover);
- drink required;

This information allows the manager to assess the resource requirement, for example:

- staffing;
- food and drink;
- linen;
- equipment.

The manager is then also able to assess the profit margins to be achieved. This will then aid the control procedures and help to establish yardsticks against which the performance of a function may be measured.

Financial considerations

Function catering is most commonly associated with the commercially orientated sector of the Hospitality Industry. Gross profit margins in function catering tend to be higher than those achieved in hotel restaurants and coffee shops.

An average gross profit percentage of 65% and 75% is usually required in function catering depending on the type of establishment, types of customers, level of service etc.

The types of customers and their spending power can in most cases be determined in advance. The average spending power will comprise the cost of the meal and will generally include the beverages served during the function. Items that may not be included in the list of the meal are pre-dinner drinks, liqueurs etc.

The financial policy will also determine the pricing structures of the different types of functions and different menus on offer. Some establishments will also make a separate charge for room hire.

The pricing structure for an establishment's function catering will be determined by its cost structure, with reference to its semi-fixed and variable costs. There are a variety of pricing structures that may be used for costing functions, the adoption of any one being determined by such factors as the type of establishment, the food and beverage product on offer and the cost structure of the establishment.

Marketing considerations

The marketing policy of a function establishment will focus on the market which the business aims to capture, and how best to promote the special characteristics of the establishment. Different selling techniques will be used to sell the establishment.

An establishment's marketing policy should contain a review relating to the competition in the area in order to keep abreast of fashions and trends in the function market. To assist in this review it is important that information and quotations are obtained from other establishments. A manager must be constantly aware of the types of products and services on offer in the market place. Every consideration must be given to customers' needs and matching these needs to the establishment's facilities.

In the marketing of an operation's function facilities the function manager should be aware of who is buying the 'product' in a particular organisation being contracted. Arrangements should be made to show the client the facilities and every effort should be made to create a good impression.

The function manager should devise a marketing plan based on the marketing policy for a given period. This plan should take into account:

- **Finance:** Targets of turnover, profit for a given period.
- **Productivity:** Targets of productivity and performance of the banqueting function department.
- Promotions:

   General – How to increase the business and how it is to be achieved.

   Special – Specially devised promotions to be launched in a given period. Often aimed at different groups, clubs etc.
- **Facilities:** Focused on selling certain facilities, for example recently refurbished.
- **Development:** The promotion of a new development or concept. The launch of new conference/seminar rooms.
- **New Product Lines:** Launch of weekend breaks for clubs, groups etc. with special rates.
- **Research:** Ongoing market research, project research etc.

Every organisation needs to advertise and promote its functions. There are a number of ways in which an organisation can promote the business:

- special brochures;
- photographs;
- press releases about function to local newspapers' magazines etc.

Brochures have to be designed carefully using professional designers, printers etc. The menus should be clear and easily understood with the prices stated. All photographs must be clear and accurate, they should be in no way misleading.

Brochures or folders should ideally contain the company logo. The pack should also contain the following:

- a letter from the Banqueting Manager to the client;
- details of all function rooms, with size and facilities on offer;
- sample menus;
- rates and prices;
- wine lists;
- maps.

The menus which have been compiled would have been carefully constructed by the chef with pre-determined gross profits, recipe specifications and purchasing specifications.

Pricing

Function menus are usually pre-listed with the desired profit margins added to them. These menus will generally have a standard set of purchasing and operational specifications added to them. However there is normally a flexible element added to it. It is not unusual for a banqueting manager to offer additions to the menu at no additional cost to the client in order to capture the business in a competitive environment.

The relationship between price and value for money is an important aspect of pricing. Value for money extends far beyond the food to be served. It takes into account the whole environment in which the food is consumed – the atmosphere, decor and surroundings of the establishment and the level of service.

In order to be successful and to obtain a satisfactory volume of sales, pricing has to consider three basic factors:

○ The nature of demand for the product.

   Firstly we have to think of the elasticity of demand, this means how sensitive is price to affect demand. The menus are said to have an elastic demand when a small decrease in the price brings about a significant increase in sales, and alternatively if an increase in price would bring about a decrease in sales. Menus with an inelastic demand a small increase in decrease in price does not bring about any significant increase or decrease in sales.

○ The level of demand for the product.

   Most catering operations experience fluctuations in demand for their products. The change in demand affects the volume of sales which results in the under utilisation of the premises and staff. Fluctuation in demand makes it necessary to take a flexible approach to pricing, to increase sales. For example, during certain times of the year it may be possible to obtain certain deals on functions.

○ The level of the competition for the product.

   Competition is an important function in pricing. Establishments commonly monitor the prices in competitors' establishments recognising that customers have a choice. Monitoring competition is not just examining the price, but the facilities, decor, services etc.

The exact method of pricing used by an establishment will depend on the exact market the establishment is operating in. The price in itself can be a valuable selling tool and a great aid in achieving the desired volume of sales.

Every business whatever its size can choose to set its prices above its proper costs or at or below the prices of its competitors. More often establishments are forced to fix their price by the competition. This is the discipline of the market place. The challenge then is to get the costs below the price which has to be set. The danger here is that managers tend to subconsciously alter the costs. This happens when the fixed costs such as wages, heating etc. are split over all the sales to arrive at the unit cost. It is always tempting then to over estimate the sales, thereby reducing the unit cost.

No one should attempt to sell anything until they have calculated the break-even point. This is the point which the amount of sales (menus, portions) at a certain price have to reach to cover their variable costs and all the fixed costs. Profit only starts when the break even point is reached.

Pricing is as much psychology as it is accounts. Establishments also need to market research price. Too low a price, although enabling to produce profit on paper, may fail as the customers may perceive the product to be cheap and of poor quality. Some people expect to pay high prices for some goods and services.

PLANNING A FUNCTION

Collecting the function details

Customers are usually invited for a detailed view of the venue, in some establishments this will include a menu tasting. During the menu tasting the customer is encouraged to discuss their requirements, the food and beverage manager will gather this information. The customer will also be advised of the different options available, for example:

○ different room layouts;

○ choice of menu, vegetarian or allergy requirements;

○ order of service;

○ flowers;

○ cloakroom requirements;

○ technical requirements, overhead projectors, public address system etc.

The customer requirements are then summarised in a function sheet and divided into departmental responsibilities.

The function sheet may be issued to the customer one week before the function.

Ideally the function sheets should be colour coded for each department one week before the function. The date for the confirmation of the final catering numbers is noted in the function sheet.

Internal communication procedures

Internal communication is especially important within any organisation. Frequent meetings are essential to inform the staff of the forthcoming events and the expected working hours for the following week.

Often more detailed and user-friendly, internal function sheets are compiled so that the key people are aware of the customer requirements.

Internal function sheets should be given to the relevant staff at least one week in advance of the function. It is then up to each department to assess their own responsibility and needs relating to the event so that the work can be planned in advance. These sheets will determine the amount of staff that is required for the function, how much linen, crockery, glassware etc. is required.

Such decisions will have to be made taking account of the price the customer is paying and the overall budget. Final numbers should be confirmed from the client at least 48 hours before the event.

An example of costs and resources

Different services provided may be priced separately, e.g. menu price may comprise of the internal costs:

    30%   food cost

    30%   labour

    30%   operational costs

             e.g. linen, cleaning etc.

    10%   profit

Usually each department has its own budget to reach. Resources for each department must be deployed and used effectively in order to maximise profitability.

All revenue earned and costs are summarised on a weekly basis in the form of a weekly cost breakdown report. This is then passed on to the Control Office, Manager or Director.

Expenditure for each function is usually controlled on a daily basis. The Head chef must be aware of the total food expenditure target for each function. All costs must be controlled through the careful management of resources. Staffing needs to be kept to a minimum without compromising the quality.

The importance of timing

The accurate timing of functions is vital for the following reasons:

- Each department needs time to prepare for the function. Some departments will require more time than others, for example the kitchen needs the most time to prepare the menu, whilst the technician only requires a few minutes to prepare the video playback machine.
- The timing of deliveries is most important as late deliveries can cause severe problems to the kitchen. It is also important that the deliveries meet the required specification.
- In high quality banqueting houses much of the service and presentation is finished at the last minute.
- Any delays in the function will result in hourly paid staff being paid extra time thus pushing up costs.
- Timing can affect the smooth running of the function, also whether it is possible to turn the room around in enough time for a second function, e.g. lunch, then dinner.

The importance of communication and information

Communication and flow of information in any organisation is paramount to a successful organisation.

Information needs to be broken down and allocated to the appropriate departments and it is vital that there is a two way communication between departments. Any changes to the function must be immediately communicated to all those concerned.

Information firstly is obtained by the first point of customer contact, i.e. the Event Organiser, the Food and Beverage manager, Conference and Function Organisation. At a later stage more specialist information is gathered by the individual department heads by using various means of communication:

- telephone;
- fax;
- e-mail;
- meetings.

This information is recorded in different stages:

- telephone enquiry;
- bookings diary;
- hire contract;
- function sheet;
- internal function sheet;
- invoice;
- feedback form;
- weekly report;
- thank you letter.

Information may be presented in different ways, either formally or informally.

FORMAL CORRESPONDENCE

Information relating to client's function must be professionally presented, accurate and reflect the company's image.

INTERNAL INFORMATION

Must also be accurate and well presented so that staff are able to understand clearly what is expected of them. All instructions should be in detail leaving nothing to chance or guesswork.

CUSTOMER INFORMATION

All information relating to the needs of the customers must be recorded throughout the booking process using appropriate documentation:

○ hire contract;

○ function sheets, etc.

SPECIAL REQUIREMENTS

In small establishments the services on offer can be tailored-made to the needs of the customer.

○ Dietary needs must be catered for.

○ Access, it is important that if wheelchair access is required it is made available.

○ Where it is difficult to accommodate certain special requirements, the customer should be given, where possible alternatives.

FOOD ALLERGIES

When planning menus for a large function the chef must think of the danger of any food allergies. All waiting staff must be informed of the contents of the dishes, e.g. shellfish, gluten, peanuts.

LEGAL REQUIREMENTS

All functions must be planned within the legal framework. Consideration must be given to the welfare of the staff. Provide training in Health, Safety and Hygiene. The employees must understand the fire regulations and evacuation procedures. Training is important in risk assessment, handling dangerous equipment, handling chemical products.

Companies have a legal responsibility to the customer, e.g. the customer needs to be aware of the maximum number of guests permitted in the building due to the Fire Regulations and similarly whether or not a licence extension or the evacuation procedures in the event of a fire or a bomb threat are in place.

The issuing of Contract Forms, forms a legal bond between the customer and the venue.

The event

The staff are required to familiarise themselves with the function sheets identifying any special requirements that are needed by the organiser. Staff also require a full briefing so that they understand exactly what is required of them and to reconfirm the function details. It is important that the client feels that they are being looked after and that they can feel at ease. The function must be executed as planned in line with the client's needs.

At the end of the function it is essential to gain feedback from the client to ensure that if the client was not satisfied a follow up letter apologising or offering some compensation be sent. This client evaluation should then be passed on to the staff.

A final calculation on the incurred costs for each department needs to be done to check the efficiency of the budget management. Invoices are then raised.

Some companies will contact the client one to three days after the function to obtain constructive feedback, using a standard evaluation form for them to fill in.

Well organised functions that give customer satisfaction can not only be profitable but may also lead to repeat business.

* [see page 326] Price elasticity of demand – if a price change results in a more than proportionate change in demand, demand is said to be elastic. Similarly, if the change in demand is less than proportionate, demand is inelastic.

Cross-elasticity of demand describes the complementary or substitute relationship between two commodities.

Some references to menus elsewhere in the book

Speciality restaurants	13	Computers	565
Transport catering	25	Diets	185

Topics for Discussion

1 A sensible menu policy.

2 The advantages and disadvantages of a cyclical menu.

3 The advantages of using English menus. When would you consider using another language?

4 The essentials of menu design and construction.

5 The various styles of buffet menus.

6 The implications of menu fatigue.

7 How would you promote your menu for a 50 seater high street bistro in the centre of town?

8 Each member of the group to obtain a number of differing menus e.g. breakfast, lunch, dinner, special party, from different types of catering e.g. school meals, industrial catering, small, medium and large hotels and restaurants for discussion and critique.

9 How have menus changed over the last 20 years, discuss why they have changed.

10 What menu changes do you envisage, explain why you think they will occur.

11 Specify the essential menu requirements and state your reasons for children, teenagers and senior citizens.

CHAPTER 10

FOOD PURCHASING, STORAGE AND CONTROL

LIAISON WITH FOOD SUPPLIERS

There are certain important factors involved in a successful working relationship with food suppliers. Both parties have responsibilities that must be carried out to ensure proper food safety and quality. Food-borne illness incidents, regardless of the cause, have an impact on the reputation of caterers and suppliers' business will be lost. A good working relationship and knowledge of each other's responsibilities is a major help in avoiding such incidents.

Suppliers must be aware of what is expected of the product. They must also make sure that the caterer is aware of any food safety limitations associated with the product. These are usually stated on all labelling. Such statements may just simply say 'keep refrigerated' or 'keep frozen', others might well include a graph or chart of the projected shelf-life at different storage temperatures. The responsibility for meeting these specifications is an important factor in a successful catering operation.

The Purchasing Cycle

The purchasing cycle is pivotal to overall business performance and a firm purchasing policy is the initial control point of the catering business.

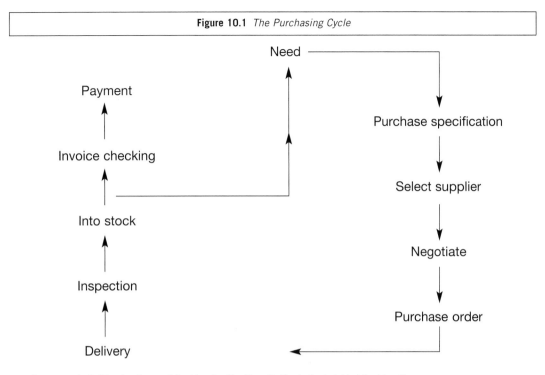

Figure 10.1 *The Purchasing Cycle*

Source: Drummond, D *'Purchasing and Costing for the Hospitality Industry'*, Hodder Headline.

FOOD PURCHASING

Once a menu is planned, a number of activities must occur to bring it into reality. One of the first and most important stages is to purchase and receive the materials needed to produce the menu items. Skilful purchasing with good receiving can do much to maximise the results of a good menu. There are six important steps to remember:

- know the market;
- determine purchasing needs;
- establish and use specifications;
- design the purchase procedures;
- receive and check the goods;
- evaluate the purchasing task.

Knowing the market

Since markets vary considerably, to do a good job of purchasing a buyer must know the characteristics of each market.

A market is a place in which ownership of commodity changes from one person to another. This could occur using the telephone, on a street corner, in a retail or wholesale establishment or at an auction.

It is important that a food and beverage purchaser has knowledge of the items to be purchased, such as:

- where they are grown;
- seasons of production;
- approximate costs;
- conditions of supply and demand;

○ laws and regulations governing the market and the products;
○ marketing agents and their services;
○ processing;
○ storage requirements;
○ commodity and product, class and grade.

The buyer

This is the key person who makes decisions regarding quality, amounts, price, what will satisfy the customers but also make a profit. The wisdom of the buyer's decisions will be reflected in the success or failure of the operation. The buyer must not only be knowledgeable about the products, but must have the necessary skills required in dealing with sales people, suppliers and other market agents. The buyer must be prepared for hard and often aggressive negotiations.

The responsibility for buying varies from company to company according to the size and management policy. Buying may be the responsibility of the chef, manager, storekeeper, buyer or buying department.

A buyer must have knowledge of the internal organisation of the company, especially the operational needs and to be able to obtain the product needs at a competitive price. Buyers must also acquaint themselves with the procedures of production and how these items are going to be used in the production operations, in order that the right item is purchased. For example, the item required may not always have to be of prime quality, for example tomatoes for soups and sauces.

A buyer must also be able to make good use of market conditions. For example, if there is a glut of fresh salmon at low cost, has the organisation the facility to make use of the extra salmon purchases? Is there sufficient freezer space? Can the chef make use of salmon, by creating a demand on the menu?

Buying methods

These depend on the type of market and the kind of operation. Purchasing procedures are usually formal or informal. Both have advantages and disadvantages. Informal methods are suitable for casual buying, where the amount involved is not large and speed and simplicity are desirable. Formal contracts are best for large contracts for commodities purchased over a long period of time. Prices do not vary much during a year, once the basic price has been established. Prices and supply tend to fluctuate with informal methods.

INFORMAL BUYING

This usually involves oral negotiations, talking directly to sales people, face to face or using the telephone. Informal methods vary according to market conditions.

FORMAL BUYING

Known as competitive buying, formal buying involves giving suppliers written specifications and quantity needs. Negotiations are normally written.

Selecting suppliers

Selecting suppliers is important in the purchasing process. Firstly consider how a supplier will be able to meet the needs of your operation. Consider:

○ price; ○ delivery; ○ quality/standards.

Information on suppliers can be obtained from other purchasers. Visits to suppliers' establishments are to be encouraged. When interviewing prospective suppliers, you need to question how reliable a supplier will be under competition and how stable under varying market conditions.

Principles of purchasing

A menu dictates an operation's needs. Based on this the buyer searches for a market that can supply the company. After the right market is located, the various products available that may meet the needs are then investigated. The right product must be obtained to meet the need and give the right quality desired by the establishment. Other factors that might affect production needs include:

- type and image of the establishment;
- style of operation and system of service;
- occasion for which the item is needed;
- amount of storage available (dry, refrigerated or frozen);
- finance available and supply policies of the organisation;
- availability, seasonability, price trends and supply.

The skill of the employees, catering assistants, chefs, must also be taken into account as well as condition and the processing method; the ability of the product to produce the item or dish required; the storage life of the product.

THREE TYPES OF NEEDS

- **Perishable:** fresh fruit and vegetables, dairy products, meat and fish; prices and suppliers may vary; informal needs of buying are frequently used; perishables should be purchased to meet menu needs for a short period only.
- **Staple:** supplies canned, bottled, dehydrated, frozen products; formal or informal purchasing may be used; because items are staple and can be easily stored, bid buying is frequently used to take advantage of quantity price purchasing.
- **Daily use needs:** daily use or contract items are delivered frequently on par stock basis; stocks are kept up to the desired level and supply is automatic; suppliers may be daily, several times a week, weekly or less often; most items are perishable, therefore supplies must not be excessive but only sufficient to get through to the next delivery.

WHAT QUANTITY AND QUALITY

Determining quantity and quality of items to be purchased is important. This is based on the operational needs. The buyer must be informed by the chef or other members of the production team of the products needed. The chef and his or her team must establish the quality and they should be required to inspect the goods on arrival. The buyer with this information then checks out the market and looks for the best quality and best price. Delivery arrangements and other factors will be handled by the buyer. In smaller establishments the chef may also be the buyer.

When considering the quantity needed, certain factors should be known:

- the number of people to be served in a given period;
- the sales history;
- portion sizes (this is determined from yield testing a standard portion control list drawn up by the chef and management teams).

Buyers need to know production, often to be able to decide how many portions a given size may yield. He or she must also understand the various yields. Cooking shrinkage may vary causing problems in portion control and yield.

The chef must inform the buyer of quantities. The buyer must be aware also of different packaging sizes, such as jars, bottles, cans and the yield from each package. Grades, styles, appearance, composition, varieties, quality factors must be indicated, such as:

- colour;
- texture;
- size;
- absence of defects;
- bruising;
- irregular shape;
- maturity.

Quality standards should be established by the chef and management team when the menu is planned. Menus and recipes may be developed using standardised recipes which directly relate to the buying procedure and standard purchasing specifications.

Buying tips

The following is a list of suggestions to assist the buyer:

- Acquire, and keep up-to-date, a sound knowledge of all commodities, both fresh and convenience, to be purchased.
- Be aware of the different types and qualities of each commodity that is available.
- When buying fresh commodities, be aware of part-prepared and ready-prepared items available on the market.
- Keep a sharp eye on price variations. Buy at the best price to ensure the required quality and also an economic yield. The cheapest item may prove to be the most expensive if waste is excessive. When possible order by number and weight:

$$20\,kg\ plaice\ could\ be \quad 80 \times 250\,g\ (8\,oz)\ plaice$$
$$40 \times 500\,g\ (1\,lb)\ plaice$$
$$20 \times 1\,kg\ (2.2\,lb)\ plaice$$

It could also be 20kg total weight of various sizes and this makes efficient portion control difficult. Some suppliers (butchers, fishmongers) may offer portion control service by selling the required number of a given weight of certain cuts:

$$100 \times 150\,g\ (6\,oz)\ sirloin\ steaks$$
$$25\,kg\ (50\,lb)\ prepared\ stewing\ beef$$
$$200 \times 100\,g\ (4\,oz)\ pieces\ of\ turbot\ fillet$$
$$500 \times 100\,g\ (4\,oz)\ plaice\ fillets.$$

- Organise an efficient system of ordering with copies of all orders kept for cross checking, whether orders are given in writing, verbally or by telephone.
- Compare purchasing by retail, wholesale and contract procedures to ensure the best method is selected for your own particular organisation.
- Explore all possible suppliers: local or markets, town or country, small or large.
- Keep the number of suppliers to a minimum. At the same time have at least two suppliers for every group of commodities, when possible. The principle of having competition for the caterer's business is sound.
- Issue all orders to suppliers fairly, allowing sufficient time for the order to be implemented efficiently.
- Request price lists as frequently as possible and compare prices continually to make sure that you buy at a good market price.
- Buy perishable goods when they are in full season as this gives the best value at the cheapest price. To help with the purchasing of the correct quantities, it is useful to compile a purchasing chart for 100 covers from which items can be divided or multiplied according to requirement. Indication of quality standards can also be inserted in a chart of this kind.

○ Deliveries must all be checked against the orders given for quantity, quality and price. If any goods delivered are below an acceptable standard they must be returned either for replacement or credit.

○ Containers can account for large sums of money. Ensure that all the containers are correctly stored, returned to the suppliers and the proper credit given.

○ All invoices must be checked for quantities and prices.

○ All statements must be checked against invoices and passed swiftly to the office so that payment may be made in time to ensure maximum discount on the purchases.

○ Foster good relations with trade representatives because much useful up-to-date information can be gained from them.

○ Keep up-to-date trade catalogues, visit trade exhibitions, survey new equipment and continually review the space, services and systems in use in order to explore possible avenues of increased efficiency.

○ Organise a testing panel occasionally in order to keep up to date with new commodities and new products coming on to the market.

○ Consider how computer application can assist the operation (see Chapter 17, page 565).

○ Study weekly Fresh Food price lists.

PORTION CONTROL

Portion control means controlling the size or quantity of food to be served to each customer. The amount of food allowed depends on the three following considerations:

○ **The type of customer or establishment:** there will obviously be a difference in the size of portions served, such as to those working in heavy industry or to female clerical workers. In a restaurant offering a three-course table d'hôte menu for £x including salmon, the size of the portion would naturally be smaller than in a luxury restaurant charging £x for the salmon on an à la carte menu.

○ **The quality of the food:** better quality food usually yields a greater number of portions than poor quality food: low quality stewing beef often needs so much trimming that it is difficult to get six portions to the kilo, and the time and labour involved also loses money. On the other hand, good quality stewing beef will often give eight portions to the kilogramme with much less time and labour required for preparation and more customer satisfaction.

○ **The buying price of the food:** this should correspond to the quality of the food if the person responsible for buying has bought wisely. A good buyer will ensure that the price paid for any item of food is equivalent to the quality – in other words a good price should mean good quality, which should mean a good yield, and so help to establish a sound portion control. If, on the other hand, an inefficient buyer has paid a high price for indifferent quality food then it will be difficult to get a fair number of portions, the selling price necessary to make the required profit will be too high and customer satisfaction can be affected.

Portion control should be closely linked with the buying of the food; without a good knowledge of the food bought it is difficult to state fairly how many portions should be obtained from it. To evolve a sound system of portion control each establishment (or type of establishment) needs individual consideration. A golden rule should be 'a fair portion for a fair price'.

Convenient portioned items are available, such as individual sachets of sugar, jams, sauce, salt, pepper; individual cartons of milk, cream and individual butter and margarine portions.

Portion control equipment

There are certain items of equipment which can assist in maintaining control of the size of the portions:

○ Scoops, for ice-cream or mashed potatoes.
○ Ladles, for soups and sauces.
○ Butter pat machines, regulating pats from 7 g upwards.
○ Fruit juice glasses, 75–150 g.
○ Soup plates or bowls, 14, 16, 17, 18 cm.
○ Milk dispensers and tea-measuring machines.
○ Individual pie dishes, pudding basins, moulds and coupes.

As examples of how portion control can save a great deal of money the following instances are true:

○ It was found that 0.007 litre of milk was being lost per cup by spilling it from a jug; 32000 cups = 224 litres of milk lost daily; this resulted in a loss of hundreds of pounds per year.
○ When an extra pennyworth of meat is served on each plate it means a loss of £1000 over the year when 1000 meals are served daily.

Portion amounts

The following list is of the approximate number of portions that are obtainable from various foods:

○ Soup: 2–3 portions to the $\frac{1}{2}$ litre.
○ Hors-d'œuvre: 120–180 g per portion.
○ Smoked salmon: 16–20 portions to the kg when bought by the side; 20–24 portions to the kg when bought sliced.
○ Shellfish cocktail: 16–20 portions per kg.
○ Melon: 2–8 portions per melon, depending on the type of melon.
○ Foie gras: 15–30 g per portion.
○ Caviar: 15–30 g per portion.

FISH

○ Plaice, cod, haddock fillet	8 portions to the kg
○ Cod and haddock on the bone	6 portions to the kg
○ Plaice, turbot, brill, halibut, on the bone	4 portions to the kg
○ Herring and trout	1 per portion (180–250 g fish)
○ Mackerel and whiting	250–360 g fish
○ Sole for main dish	300–360 g fish
○ Sole for filleting	500–750 g best size
○ Whitebait	8–10 portions to the kg
○ Salmon (gutted, but including head and bone)	4–6 portions to the kg
○ Crab or lobster	250–360 g per portion

(A 500 g lobster yields about 150 g meat; a 1 kg lobster yields about 360 g meat).

SAUCES

8–12 portions to $\frac{1}{2}$ litre:

○ Hollandaise
○ Béarnaise
○ Tomato
○ Any demi-glace, reduced stock or jus-lié

○ Custard
○ Apricot
○ Jam
○ Chocolate

10–14 portions to $\frac{1}{2}$ litre:

Apple, Cranberry, Bread

15–20 portions to $\frac{1}{2}$ litre:

Tartare, Vinaigrette, Mayonnaise

MEATS

Beef

○ Roast boneless	6–8 portions per kg
○ Boiled or braised	6–8 portions per kg
○ Stews, puddings and pies	8–10 portions per kg
○ Steaks	
– Rump	120–250 g per one portion
– Sirloin	120–250 g per one portion
– Tournedos	90–120 g per one portion
– Fillet	120–180 g per one portion

Offal

○ Ox-liver	8 portions to the kg
○ Sweetbreads	6–8 portions to the kg
○ Sheep's kidneys	2 per portion
○ Ox-tongue	4–6 portions per kg

Lamb

○ Leg	6–8 portions to the kg
○ Shoulder boned and stuffed	6–8 portions to the kg
○ Loin and best-end	6 portions to the kg
○ Stewing lamb	4–6 portions to the kg
○ Cutlet	90–120 g
○ Chop	120–180 g

Pork

○ Leg	8 portions to the kg
○ Shoulder	6–8 portions to the kg
○ Loin on the bone	6–8 portions to the kg
○ Pork chop	180–250 g

Ham

○ Hot	8–10 portions to the kg

- Cold   10–12 portions to the kg
- Sausages are obtainable 12, 16 or 20 to the kg
- Chipolatas yield approximately 32 or 48 to the kg
- Cold meat   16 portions to the kg
- Streaky bacon   32–40 rashers to the kg
- Back bacon   24–32 rashers to the kg

Poultry

- Poussin   1 portion 360 g (1 bird)
  2 portions 750 g (1 bird)
- Ducks and chickens   360 g per portion
- Geese and boiling fowl   360 g per portion
- Turkey   250 g per portion

VEGETABLES

- New potatoes   8 portions to the kg
- Old potatoes   4–6 portions to the kg
- Cabbage   6–8 portions to the kg
- Turnips   6–8 portions to the kg
- Parsnips   6–8 portions to the kg
- Swedes   6–8 portions to the kg
- Brussels sprouts   6–8 portions to the kg
- Tomatoes   6–8 portions to the kg
- French beans   6–8 portions to the kg
- Cauliflower   6–8 portions to the kg
- Spinach   4 portions to the kg
- Peas   4–6 portions to the kg
- Runner beans   6 portions to the kg

METHODS OF PURCHASING

There are three main methods for buying, each depending on the size and volume of the business.

- **The primary market:** raw materials may be purchased at the source of supply, the grower, producer or manufacturer, or from central markets such as Smithfield (meat), Nine Elms (fruit and vegetables) or Billingsgate (fish) in London. Some establishments or large organisations will have a buyer who will buy directly from the primary markets. Also, a number of smaller establishments may adopt this method for some of their needs (the chef patron may buy his fish, meat and vegetables directly from the market).
- **The secondary market:** goods are bought wholesale from a distributor or middle man; the catering establishment will pay wholesale prices and obtain possible discounts.
- **The tertiary market:** the retail or cash and carry warehouse is a method suitable for smaller companies. A current pass obtained from the warehouse is required in order to gain access. This method also requires the user to have his or her own transport. Some cash and

carry organisations require a VAT number before they will issue an authorised card. It is important to remember that there are added costs:

– running the vehicle and petrol used;

– the person's time for going to the warehouse.

Cash and carry is often an impersonal way of buying as there are no staff to discuss quality and prices.

Standard purchasing specifications

Standard purchasing specifications are documents which are drawn up for every commodity describing exactly what is required for the establishment. These standard purchasing specifications will assist with the formulation of standardised recipes. A watertight specification is drawn up which, once approved, will be referred to every time the item is delivered. It is a statement of various criteria related to quality, grade, weight, size and method of preparation, if required, such as washed and selected potatoes for baking. Other information given may be variety, maturity, age, colour, shape, etc. A copy of standard specification is often given to the supplier and the storekeeper who are left in no doubt as to what is needed. These specifications assist in the costing and control procedures.

Commodities which can be specified include:

○ Grown (primary): butchers meat; fresh fish; fresh fruit and vegetables; milk and eggs.

○ Manufactured (secondary): bakery goods; dairy products.

○ Processed (tertiary): frozen foods including meat, fish and fruit and vegetables; dried goods; canned goods.

It can be seen that any food product can have a specification attached to it. However, the primary specifications focus on raw materials, ensuring the quality of these commodities. Without quality at this level, a secondary or tertiary specification is useless. For example, to specify a frozen apple pie, this product would use:

○ a primary specification for the apple;

○ a secondary specification for the pastry;

○ a tertiary specification for the process (freezing).

But no matter how good the secondary or tertiary specifications are, if the apples used in the beginning are not of a very high quality, the whole product is not of a good quality.

EXAMPLES OF STANDARD PURCHASING SPECIFICATION

Tomatoes

○ Commodity: round tomatoes.

○ Size: 50 g (2 oz) 47–57 mm diameter.

○ Quality: firm, well formed, good red colour, with stalk attached.

○ Origin: Dutch, available March–November.

○ Class/grade: super class A.

○ Weight: 6 kg (13 lb) net per box.

○ Count: 90–100 per box.

○ Quote: per box/tray.

○ Packaging: loose in wooden tray, covered in plastic.

○ Delivery: day following order.

○ Storage: temperature 10–13°C (50–55°F) at a relatively humidity of 75–80%.

○ Note: avoid storage with cucumbers and aubergines.

EXTRACT FROM A PURCHASE SPECIFICATION
SCHEDULE B: SUPPLIER'S QUALITY AND PREPARATION SPECIFICATION

PRODUCT: BEEF AND VEAL

GENERAL:

1   All products supplied to SODEXHO must comply with the provisions of the Weights and Measures Act 1976 and 1985, Trade Descriptions Act 1968, Food Safety Act 1990 and any amendments that are enforced from time to time.

2   No meat from cow (including that designated as 'commercial') or bull carcasses will be supplied.

3   Cuts, joints and steaks of fresh beef are to be prepared from the chilled unfrozen carcasses or primal cuts of 'clean' steers and heifers of English, Irish or Scottish origin.* Beef of intervention storage and from imported chilled and frozen meat can also be supplied if they originated from animals which conformed to the standards of home killed graded beef.

4   No cuts from excessively lean or fat carcasses to be supplied.

5   Unfrozen beef carcasses and primal cuts from the hindquarter must be stored at chilled temperatures for 7–10 days prior to preparation, to allow for maturation.

6   Cuts, joints and steaks of veal are to be prepared from the chilled unfrozen carcass of English or Dutch milk fed beasts.

7   Beef and veal other than that supplied frozen must be kept chilled (below 5°C) throughout preparation, storage and distribution.

8   Prepared cuts of chilled beef and veal that are supplied frozen must be fully frozen to a temperate of not higher than $-18°C$ by mechanical blast freezers. Meat that has not been frozen by such means cannot be supplied to SODEXHO. The exception to this is stewing steak that has been frozen to much higher temperatures to allow mechanical dicing.

9   Fresh beef and veal that has been designated as frozen must be delivered by transport that has frozen storage capacity. The temperature of the meat must not reach a value of more than $-10°C$ during distribution.

10   Meat purchased as frozen and then thawed for the preparation of joints, steaks, mince or stewing steak, must not be refrozen.

11   Prepared cuts must be wrapped and sealed in polythene bags and delivered in a rigid impervious receptacle or tray of good hygienic standard.

12   Suppliers of fresh beef and veal to SODEXHO must adhere to the purchasing and Supply specification of Schedule D.

Home-killed beef to conform to the Meat and Livestock Commission (MLC) grading system.

- outline of the quantities and quality of goods required
- whether supplier has 'sole' status
- incorporation of the purchase specification
- the way in which unsatisfactory goods will be treated
- the collection arrangements for returnable containers
- a disputes procedure and an indemnity clause
- delivery arrangements and invoicing procedures a termination and review clause.

For most perishable items, rather than entering into a long term contract, a daily or monthly quotation system is more common. This is essentially a short term contract regularly reviewed to ensure that a competitive situation is maintained.

The standard recipe

Standard recipes are a written formula for producing a food item of a specified quality and quantity for use in a particular establishment. It should show the precise quantities and qualities of the ingredients together with the sequence of preparation and service. It enables the establishment to have a greater control over cost and quantity.

Objective

To predetermine the following:

○ the quantities and qualities of ingredients to be used stating the purchase specification;
○ the yield obtainable from a recipe;
○ the food cost per portion;
○ the nutritional value of a particular dish.

To facilitate:

○ menu planning; purchasing and internal requisitioning; food preparation and production; portion control.

Also the standard recipe will assist new staff in preparation and production of standard products, which can be facilitated by photographs or drawings illustrating the finished product.

Cost control

It is important to know the exact cost of each process and every item produced, so a system of cost analysis and cost information is essential.

The advantages of an efficient costing system are:

○ It discloses the net profit made by each section of the organisation and shows the cost of each meal produced.
○ It will reveal possible sources of economy and can result in a more effective use of stores, labour, materials, etc.
○ Costing provides information necessary for the formation of a sound price policy.
○ Cost records provide and facilitate the speedy quotations for all special functions, such as special parties, wedding receptions, etc.
○ It enables the caterer to keep to a budget.

No *one* costing system will automatically suit every catering business, but the following guidelines may be helpful:

○ The co-operation of all departments is essential.
○ The costing system should be adapted to the business and not vice versa. If the accepted procedure in an establishment is altered to fit a costing system then there is danger of causing resentment among the staff and as a result losing their co-operation.
○ Clear instructions in writing must be given to staff who are required to keep records. The system must be made as simple as possible so that the amount of clerical labour required is kept to a minimum. An efficient mechanical calculator or computer should be provided to save time and labour.

To calculate the total cost of any one item or meal provided it is necessary to analyse the total expenditure under several headings. Basically the total cost of each item consists of three main elements:

○ **Food or materials costs:** known as variable costs because the level will vary according to the volume of business; in an operation that uses part-time or extra staff for special occasions, the money paid to these staff also comes under variable costs; by comparison, salaries and wages paid regularly to permanent staff are fixed costs.

○ All cost of **labour and overheads:** regular charges which come under the heading of fixed costs; labour costs in the majority of operations fall into two categories: **direct labour** cost, which is salaries and wages paid to staff such as chefs, waiters, barstaff, housekeepers, chambermaids and where the cost can be allocated to income from food, drink and accommodation sales; **indirect labour** cost, which would include salaries and wages paid, for example, to managers, office staff and maintenance men who work for all departments (so their labour cost should be charged to all departments). **Overheads** consist of rent, rates, heating, lighting and equipment.

Cleaning materials

An important group of essential items that is often overlooked when costing are cleaning materials. There are over 60 different items that come under this heading, and approximately 24 of these may be required for an average catering establishment. These may include: brooms, brushes, buckets, cloths, drain rods, dusters, mops, sponges, squeegees, scrubbing/polishing machines, suction/vacuum cleaners, wet and wet/dry suction cleaners, scouring pads, detergents, disinfectants, dustbin powder, washing-up liquids, fly sprays, sacks, scourers, steel wool, soap, soda, etc.

It is important to understand the cost of these materials and to ensure that an allowance is made for them under the heading of overheads.

Profit

It is usual to express each element of cost as a percentage of the selling price. This enables the caterer to control his profits.

Gross profit or kitchen profit is the difference between the cost of the food and the net selling price of the food. Net profit is the difference between the selling price of the food (sales) and total cost (cost of food, labour and overheads).

Sales – Food cost = gross profit (kitchen profit)

Sales – total cost = net profit

Food cost + gross profit = sales

Example	Food sales for 1 week	=	£25,000
	Food cost for 1 week	=	£12,000
	Labour and overheads for 1 week	=	£9,000
	Total costs for 1 week	=	£21,000
	Gross profit (kitchen profit)	=	£13,000
	Net profit	=	£4,000

Food sales – food cost	£25,000 – £12,000 = £13,000 (gross profit)
Food sales – net profit	£25,000 – £4,000 = £21,000 (total costs)
Food cost + gross profit	£12,000 + £15,000 = £25,000 (food sales)

Profit is always expressed as a percentage of the selling price.

∴ the percentage profit for the week is:

$$\frac{\text{Net profit}}{\text{Sales}} \times 100 = \frac{£4000 \times 100}{25,000} = 16\%$$

A breakdown shows:

		Percentage of sales (%)
Food cost	£12,000	44
Labour	£6,000	25
Overheads	£3,000	18
	£21,000	
Net profit	£4,000	13
Sales	£25,000	

If the restaurant served 1000 meals then the average spent by each customer would be:

$$\frac{\text{Total sales £25,000}}{\text{No. of customers 1000}} = £25.00$$

As the percentage composition of sales for a month is now known, the average price of a meal for that period can be further analysed:

Average price of a meal = £25.00 = 100%

25p = 1%

which means that the customer's contribution towards:

Food cost	= 25 × 48	= £12.00
Labour	= 25 × 24	= £6.00
Overheads	= 25 × 12	= £3.00
Net profit	= 25 × 16	= £4.00
Average price of meal		= £25.00

A rule that can be applied to calculate the food cost price of a dish is: let the cost price of the dish equal 40% and *fix the selling price* at 100%.

$$\text{Cost of dish} = 400\text{p} = 40\%$$

$$\therefore \text{Selling price} = \frac{400 \times 100}{40} = £10.00$$

Selling the dish at £10, making 60% gross profit above the cost price, would be known as 40% food cost. For example:

Sirloin steak (250 g (8 oz))

250 g (8 oz) entrecote steak at £10.00 a kg = £2.50

$$\text{To fix the selling price at 40% food cost} = \frac{2.50 \times 100}{40} = £6.25$$

The table below will help you with various food costings:

If food costing is controlled accurately the food cost of particular items on the menu and the total expenditure on food over a given period are worked out. Finding the food costs helps to control costs, prices and profits.

An efficient food cost system will disclose bad buying and inefficient storing and should tend to prevent waste and pilfering. This can help the caterer to run an efficient business and enable him to give the customer adequate value for money.

The caterer who gives the customer value for money together with the desired type of food is well on the way to being successful.

FOOD COST AND OPERATIONAL CONTROL

As food is expensive, efficient stock control levels are essential to help the profitability of the business. The main difficulties of controlling food are as follows:

○ Food prices fluctuate frequently because of inflation and falls in the demand and supply, through poor harvests, bad weather conditions, etc.

○ Transport costs rise due to wage demands and cost of petrol.

FOOD COSTINGS

FOOD COST (%)	TO FIND THE SELLING PRICE MULTIPLY THE COST PRICE OF THE FOOD BY:	IF THE COST PRICE OF FOOD IS £4 THE SELLING PRICE IS:	IF THE COST PRICE IS £1.20 THE SELLING PRICE IS:	GROSS PROFIT (%)
60	1.66	£6.64	£1.92	40
55	1.75	£7.00	£2.04	45
50	2	£8.00	£2.40	50
45	2.22	£8.88	£2.64	55
40	2.5	£10.00	£2.88	60
$33\frac{1}{3}$	3	£12.00	£3.60	$66\frac{2}{3}$

○ Fuel costs rise, which affects food companies' and producers' costs.

○ Any food subsidies imposed by governments are removed.

○ Changes occur in the amount demanded by the customer; increased advertising increases demand; changes in taste and fashion influence demand from one product to another.

○ Media focus on certain products which are labelled healthy or unhealthy will affect demand; for example butter being high in saturated fats, sunflower margarine being high in polyunsaturates.

Each establishment should devise its own control system to suit the needs of that establishment.

Factors which affect a control system are:

○ regular changes in the menu;

○ menus with a large number of dishes;

○ dishes with a large number of ingredients;

○ problems in assessing customer demand;

○ difficulties in not adhering to or operating standardised recipes;

○ raw materials purchased incorrectly.

Factors assisting a control system include:

○ menu remains constant, (McDonald's, Harvester, Pizza Hut, Burger King);

○ standardised recipes and purchasing specifications used;

○ menu has a limited number of dishes.

Stocktaking is therefore easier and costing more accurate.

In order to carry out a control system, food stocks must be secure, refrigerators and deep freezers should be kept locked, portion control must be accurate. A book-keeping system must be developed to monitor the daily operation.

VAT

Value Added Tax is the tax which is charged as a percentage of the value added to a product by each and every supplier who handles it.

In the hospitality and catering industry it is collected by the operator from the customer to be forwarded to the VAT department of Her Majesty's Customs and Excise office.

This applies to all food and drink sales for consumption on the premises of businesses which have a taxable turnover of £55,000 in 12 months.

If food is sold to be taken away and consumed off the premises, it is standard-rated or zero-rated depending on whether the food is hot.

The control cycle of daily operation

PURCHASING

It is important to determine yields from the range of commodities in use which will determine the unit costs. Yield testing indicates the number of items or portions obtained and helps to provide the information required for producing, purchasing and specification. Yield testing should not be confused with product testing which is concerned with the physical properties of the food – texture, flavour, quality. In reality tests are frequently carried out which combine these objectives.

RECEIVING

Goods must be checked on delivery to make sure they meet the purchase specifications.

Before items are delivered, it is necessary to know what has been ordered, both the amount and quality, and when it will be delivered. This is essential so that persons requiring items will know when foods will be available, particularly perishable items and that on arrival they can be checked against the required standard. It is also helpful for the storekeeper to know when to expect the goods so that he or she can plan the working day and also inform staff awaiting arrival of items.

The procedure for accepting deliveries is to ensure that:

1 adequate storage space is available;
2 access to the space is clear;
3 temperature of goods where appropriate is checked;
4 perishable goods are checked immediately;
5 there is no delay in transporting items to cold storage;
6 all other goods are checked for quantity and quality and stored;
7 any damaged items are returned;
8 items past their 'use by' or 'best before' dates are not accepted;
9 receipts or amended delivery notes record returns;
10 one part of the delivery note is retained;
11 the other part is kept by the supplier;
12 a credit note is provided for any goods not delivered;
13 should there be any discrepancies, the person making the delivery and the supplier are informed.

ORGANISATION OF CONTROL

Introduction

Control in every catering organisation is crucial: in small restaurants and tea shops, in hospital kitchens, large hotels; on contract and airline catering, in school meals, in fact in every establishment.

The role of potential managers and managers, whether they are called Food and Beverage Managers or Assistant F&B Managers, Executive Chefs, Chef de Cuisine, Sous Chef, Head Chef, Chef de Parti or whatever, is to organise:

- themselves;
- their time;
- other people;
- physical resources.

An essential factor of good organisation is effective control of oneself, of those responsible to you, and of physical resources which often includes financial control. The amount and how it is administered will vary from establishment to establishment. However, successful control applies to all aspects of catering, namely:

- purchasing of food etc.;
- storage of food etc.;
- preparation of food;
- production of food;
- presentation of food;
- hygiene;
- safety;
- security;
- waste;
- energy;
- first Aid;
- equipment;
- maintenance;
- legal Aspects.

Control of resources

The effective and efficient management of resources requires knowledge and, if possible, experience. In addition, it is necessary to keep up-to-date. This may require attending courses on management, computing, hygiene, legislation and so on. Membership of appropriate organisations such as HCIMA, or former student associations, can also be valuable, as is attending exhibitions and trade fairs.

How the controlling of resources is administered will depend partly on the system of the organisation but also on the way the person in control operates. Apart from knowledge and experience, respect from those for whom one is responsible is earned, not given, by the way staff are handled in the situation of the job. Having earned the respect and co-operation of staff a system of controls and checks needs to be operated which is smooth running and not disruptive. Training and delegation may be required to ensure effective control and periodically it is essential to evaluate the system to see that the recording and monitoring are being effective.

The purpose of control is to make certain:

1 that supplies of what is required are available;
2 that the supplies are of the right quality and quantity;
3 that they are available on time;
4 there is the minimum of wastage;
5 there is no overstocking;
6 there is no pilfering;
7 that legal requirements are complied with.

Means of control

Checks need to occur spontaneously, without previous warning of the check being made, at regular intervals which may be daily or weekly. These checks may involve one item, several items or all items. Records need to correspond with the physical items, for example if records indicate 40 packets of sugar at 1 kilo, then those 40×1 kilo packets need to be seen. It is necessary to know to whom any discrepancies should be reported and what action should be taken. Therefore the policy of the establishment should be clear to all members of staff.

A system of authorisation regarding who may purchase and who may issue goods to whom, with the necessary suitable documents and records, needs to be established and inspected to see that it works satisfactorily.

Checklist for control

Goods inwards

○ Are deliveries correct re:

quality; quantity, hygiene, temperature.

Storage

○ Items issued in rotation, Accurate recording.

○ Correct standards of hygiene: temperature, security, minimum wastage.

Food Preparation ⎫ proper standard of
Production ⎭ hygiene and safety

Presentation Accurate portion control

Back door Measures to prevent pilfering

Recording ⎫
Monitoring ⎬ Is it effective, adequate
Checking ⎭

The following topics in *The Theory of Catering* are essential reading:

○ Food purchase and control; Energy conservation; Health.

○ Legal aspects; Supervision; Computers; Hygiene.

INTRODUCTION TO THE ORGANISATION OF RESOURCES

Organisation chart

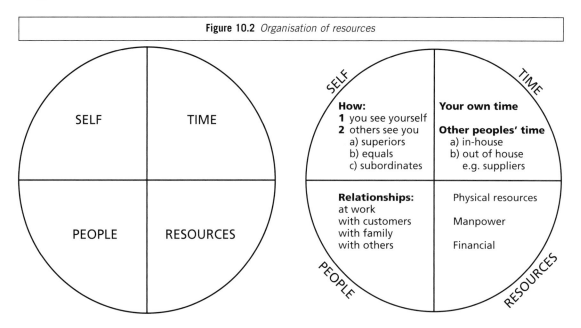

Figure 10.2 *Organisation of resources*

Control of resources

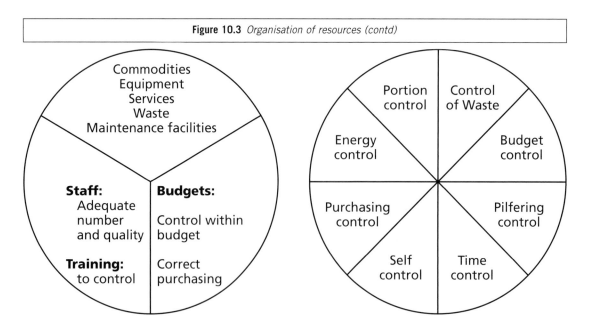

Figure 10.3 *Organisation of resources (contd)*

HEALTH AND SAFETY REQUIREMENTS

To comply with the regulations it is essential to observe these practices not only because of the legal requirement but for the benefit of all who use the storage areas of the premises.

○ Receiving areas must be clean and free from litter.

○ Waste bins, empty return boxes, etc. should be kept tidy and safe.

○ Waste bins (rubbish and swill) must be kept with lids on and emptied frequently and kept clean.

○ All storage areas must be kept clean and tidy.

○ Trolleys and stacking shelves should be suitable for heavy items.

○ The trolley should not be overloaded; accidents can occur due to careless loading such as heavy items on top light items.

○ Lifting of heavy items should be done in a manner to prevent injury.

○ Cleaning equipment and materials must be available and kept separate from food items.

○ All items should be stored safely, shelves not overloaded, heavier items lower than lighter items, with suitable steps to reach higher items.

○ Stores should have a wash hand basin, towel, soap and nail brush.

○ Unauthorised persons should not have access to the stores or areas where goods are delivered.

○ Be prepared for the unexpected, accidents can occur due to:

    – delivery vehicles and trolley movement;

    – breakages of containers, glass jars, etc.;

    – undue waste by delivery or storekeeping staff.

○ Know where the first aid box is.

○ Know the procedures to follow in the event of an accident.

TEMPERATURE OF FOOD ON DELIVERY

Procedures must be laid down for checking the temperature of foods on arrival at the establishment. Delivery vehicles are subject to legislation and food should be at these temperatures when delivered.

DOCUMENTATION OF DELIVERIES

Goods are ordered from the supplier for the amounts required and when it is to be delivered. The quality and details of the foods will have been specified by the establishment so that when delivered the goods should comply with what is ordered.

STORING AND ISSUING

Raw materials should be stored correctly under the right conditions, temperature, etc. A method of pricing the materials must be decided, and one of the following should be adopted for charging the food to the various departments. The cost of items does not remain fixed over a period of time; over a period of one year a stores item may well have several prices. The establishment must decide which price to use:

○ actual purchase price;

○ simple average price;

○ weighted average price;

○ inflated price (price goes up after purchase);
○ standard price (fixed price).

Weighted average price example (of dried beans)

$$= 10\,\text{lb} \;(5\,\text{kg}) \times 80\text{p} \quad = \quad £4.00$$
$$20\,\text{lb} \;(10\,\text{kg}) \times 100\text{p} \quad = \quad \underline{£10.00}$$

Total £14.00

$\therefore 14.00 \div 30\,\text{lb}\;(15\,\text{kg}) = 93\text{p}$ per kg = weighted average price.

PREPARING

This is an important stage of the control cycle. The cost of the food consumed depends on two factors:

○ the number of meals produced;
○ the cost per meal.

In order to control food costs we must be able to:

○ control the number to be catered for;
○ control the food cost per meal in advance of production and service by using a system of precosting, using standardised recipes, indicating portion control.

SALES AND VOLUME FORECASTING

This is a method of predicting the volume of sales for a future period. In order to be of practical value the forecast must:

○ predict the total number of covers (customers);
○ predict the choice of menu items.

Therefore it is important to:

○ keep a record of the numbers of each dish sold from a menu;
○ work out the average spent per customer;
○ calculate the proportion, expressed as a percentage, of each dish sold in relation to total sales.

Forecasting is in two stages:

○ **Initial forecasting** – this is done once a week in respect of each day of the following week. It is based on sales histories, information related to advance bookings and current trends, and when this has been completed, the predicted sales are converted into the food/ingredients requirements. Purchase orders are then prepared and sent to suppliers.

○ **The final forecast** – this normally takes place the day before the actual preparation and service of the food. This forecast must take into account the latest developments, such as the weather and any food that needs to be used up; if necessary suppliers' orders may need to be adjusted.

Sales forecasting is not a perfect method of prediction, but does help with production planning. Sales forecasting, however, is important when used in conjunction with cyclical menu planning.

PRECOSTING OF DISHES

This method of costing is associated with standardised recipes which give the total cost of the dish per portion and often with a selling price.

Summary of factors which will affect the profitability of the establishment

These include:

- overcooking food resulting in portion loss;
- inefficient preparation of raw materials;
- poor portion control;
- too much wastage, insufficient use of raw materials; left-over food not being utilised; see HCIMA Technical brief No 9.
- theft;
- inaccurate ordering procedures;
- inadequate checking procedures;
- no reference mark to standardised recipes and yield factors;
- insufficient research into suppliers;
- inaccurate forecasting;
- bad menu planning.

STOREKEEPING

A clean, orderly food store, run efficiently, is essential in any catering establishment for the following reasons:

- Stocks of food can be kept at a suitable level, so eliminating the risk of running out of any commodity.
- All food entering and leaving the stores can be properly checked; this helps to prevent wastage.
- A check can be kept on the percentage profit of each department of the establishment.

This control may be assisted by computer application, see Chapter 17, page 565. A well-planned store should include the following features:

- It should be cool and face the north so that it does not have the sun shining into it.
- It must be well ventilated, vermin proof and free from dampness (dampness in a dry store makes it musty, and encourages bacteria to grow and tins to rust).
- It should be in a convenient position to receive goods being delivered by suppliers and also in a suitable position to issue goods to the various departments.
- A wash hand basin, soaps, nail brush and hand drier must be provided for staff; also a first-aid box.
- A good standard of hygiene is essential, therefore the walls and ceilings should be free from cracks, and either painted or tiled so as to be easily cleaned. The floor should be free from cracks and easy to wash. The junction between the wall and floor should be rounded to prevent the accumulation of dirt. A cleaning rota should clearly show daily, monthly and weekly cleaning tasks.
- Shelves should be easy to clean.
- Good lighting, both natural and artificial, is very necessary.
- A counter should be provided to keep out unauthorised persons, thus reducing the risk of pilfering.

- The storekeeper should be provided with a suitable desk.
- There should be ample, well-arranged storage space, with shelves of varying depths and separate sections for each type of food). These sections may include deep-freeze cabinets, cold rooms, refrigerators, chill rooms, vegetable bins and container stores. Space should also be provided for empty containers.
- Efficient, easy-to-clean weighing machines for large and small-scale work should be supplied.
- Stores staff must wear clean overalls at all times, and suitable shoes to help prevent injury if a heavy item is dropped on the feet.
- Steps to help staff reach goods on high shelves and an appropriate trolley should be provided.

Store containers

Foods delivered in flimsy bags or containers should be transferred to suitable store containers. These should be easy to wash and have tight-fitting lids. Glass or plastic containers are suitable for many foods, such as spices and herbs, as they have the advantage of being transparent; therefore it is easy to see at a glance how much of the commodity is in stock.

Bulk dry goods (pulses, sugar, salt, etc.) should be stored in suitable bins with tight-fitting lids. These bins should have wheels so that they can be easily moved for cleaning. All bins should be clearly labelled or numbered.

Sacks or cases of commodities should not be stored on the floor; they should be raised on duck boards so as to permit a free circulation of air.

Some goods are delivered in containers suitable for storage and these need not be transferred. Heavy cases and jars should be stored at a convenient height to prevent any strain in lifting.

Special storage points

- Always comply with 'best by' or 'use by' dates.
- All old stock should be brought forward with each new delivery.
- Commodities with strong smells or flavours should be stored as far away as possible from those foods which readily absorb flavour; strong-smelling cheese should not be stored near eggs.
- Bread should be kept in a well-ventilated container with a lid. Lack of ventilation causes condensation and encourages moulds. Cakes and biscuits should be stored in airtight tins.
- Stock must be inspected regularly, particularly cereals and cereal products, to check for signs of mice or weevils.
- Tinned goods should be unpacked, inspected and stacked on shelves. When inspecting tins, these points should be looked for:
  - blown tins – this is where the ends of the tins bulge owing to the formation of gases either by bacteria growing on the food or by the food attacking the tin-plate; all blown tins should be thrown away as the contents are dangerous and the use of the contents may cause food-poisoning;
  - dented tins – these should be used as soon as possible, not because the dent is an indication of inferior quality but because dented tins, if left, will rust and a rusty tin will eventually puncture;
  - storage life of tins varies considerably and depends mainly on how the contents attack the internal coating of the tin which may corrode and lay bare the steel.
- Due to fewer preserving additives, many bottled foods now need to be refrigerated once they are opened.

○ Cleaning materials often have a strong smell; therefore they should be kept in a separate store. Cleaning powders should never be stored near food.

Storage accommodation

Foods are divided into three groups for the purpose of storage: perishable foods, dry foods and frozen foods.

○ Perishable foods include: meat, poultry, game, fish; dairy produce and fats; vegetables and fruit.

○ Dry foods include: cereals, pulses, sugar, flour, etc.; bread, cakes; jams, pickles and other bottled foods; canned foods; cleaning materials.

○ Frozen foods must be placed immediately into a deep freeze at a temperature of $-20°C$.

TEMPERATURES AND STORAGE TIMES FOR FREEZERS

SYMBOL	TEMPERATURE MAXIMUM	SAFETY STORAGE TIME
*	$-6°C$ (21°F)	7 days
**	$-12°C$ (10°F)	1 month
***	$-18°C$ (0°F)	3 months
****	$-18°C$ (0°F)	more than 3 months

STORAGE TEMPERATURES FOR FROZEN ITEMS OF FOODS

meat	$-20°C$ to $-16°C$
fish	$-20°C$ to $-16°C$
frozen foods	$-20°C$ to $-16°C$
ice-cream	$-22°C$ to $-18°C$

STORAGE TEMPERATURES OF REFRIGERATED FOOD ITEMS

cooked pies, pasties, sausage rolls	7°C
pies containing gelatine	5°C
other cooked foods	8°C
milk and cream	5°C
eggs	4°C

These are temperatures which must not be exceeded; lower temperatures down to 1°C (34°F) are preferable

REFRIGERATED PRODUCTS IN THE RIGHT CABINET

TYPE	TEMPERATURE	PRODUCTS
refrigerator	1°–4°C (34°–39°F)	cooked meats (ham, pork, beef, lamb, etc.); cooked poultry and game (chicken, turkey, duck. etc.); dairy products (milk, butter, fats, eggs, cheese); prepared salads, sandwiches
meat cabinet	−2°–0°C (28°–32°F)	fresh lamb, beef, pork, chicken, turkey, duck, etc.
fish cabinet	−2°–0°C (28°–32°F)	fresh fish (cod, plaice, haddock, skate, etc.)
freezer	−18°– −20°C (0°– −4°F)	frozen meat; poultry; vegetables; prepared meals; ice-cream, etc.

Storage of perishable foods
MEAT AND POULTRY

○ Meat joints should be hung on hooks with drip tray to collect any blood.
○ Temperature of refrigerator should be between −1°C (30°F) and 1°C (34°F).
○ Humidity level should be approximately 90%.
○ Meat and poultry should ideally be stored in separate places.
○ Cuts of meat may be brushed with oil or wrapped in oiled greaseproof paper, wrapped in cling film or vacuum packed.
○ Drip trays and other trays used for meat or poultry should be cleaned daily.
○ Frozen meat and poultry must be stored at −18°C – 20°C.

FISH

○ Store in ice in fish refrigerator or fish drainer at between −1°C (30°F) to 1°C (34°F).
○ Keep types of fish separated.
○ Smoked fish should be separate from fresh fish.
○ Frozen fish should be stored at −18°C.

VEGETABLES

○ Ideally have a cool dry vegetable store with racks.
○ As a safety precaution do not stack sacks too high.
○ Leave potatoes in sacks.
○ Place root vegetables on racks.
○ Store green vegetables on racks.
○ Store lettuces leave as delivered in a cool environment.
○ Remove any vegetables that show decay.
○ Leave onions and shallots in nets or racked.
○ Place cauliflower and broccoli on racks.

○ Leave courgettes, peppers, avocado pears and cucumbers in delivery containers.

○ Leave mushrooms in containers.

FRUIT

○ Soft fruits should be left in punnets and placed in refrigeration.

○ Hard fruits and stone fruits are stored in cold store.

○ Do not refrigerate bananas as they will turn black. If possible hang by the stems to slow down ripening.

EGGS

○ Store refrigerated at 1–4°C.

○ Keep away from other foods; their shells are porous and they can absorb strong smells.

○ Keep in their delivery boxes; handle as little as possible.

○ Use in rotation.

MILK AND CREAM

○ Store in the refrigerator below 5°C.

○ Partially used containers should be covered.

○ Use in rotation.

CHEESE AND BUTTER

○ Refrigerate at a temperature below 5°C.

○ Cut cheeses should be wrapped.

○ Use in rotation.

BREAD, ETC.

○ Use in rotation, first in first out.

○ Store in well-ventilated cool store.

○ Avoid overstocking.

○ Take care that biscuits are stacked carefully to avoid breaking.

○ Frozen gâteaux should be kept frozen.

○ Cakes containing cream must be refrigerated.

SANDWICHES

○ All sandwiches must be sold within 4–24 hours of preparation.

○ They must be stored at a maximum temperature of 8°C (46°F).

○ Sandwiches to be sold within 4 hours are not covered by this legislation.

Storage of dry goods

○ Storage must be cool, well lit, ventilated.

○ Storage should be off the floor or in bins.

○ Issue goods in rotation, last in last out.

○ Stack items so that stock rotation is simple to operate.

○ Arrange items in such a way that they can easily be checked.

Storage of ice-cream and frozen goods

○ Store immediately on receipt.
○ Storage temperature must be at −20°C.
○ Use in rotation.
○ Keep chest lid closed as much as possible.

Cleanliness and safety of storage areas

High standards of hygiene are essential in the store.

○ Personnel must:
  – wear clean clothing;
  – be clean in themselves;
  – be particular with regard to hand washing;
  – have clean hygienic habits.
○ Floors must:
  – be kept clear;
  – be cleaned of any spillage at once;
  – be in good repair.
○ Shelving must:
  – be kept clean;
  – not be overloaded.
○ Cleaning material must be:
  – kept away from foods;
  – stored with care and marked dangerous if they are dangerous chemicals.
○ Windows and, where appropriate, doors must be fly- and bird-proof.
○ Walls should be clean and where any access by rodents is possible, sealed.
○ Equipment such as knives, scales, etc., must be:
  – thoroughly cleaned;
  – stored so that cross-contamination is prevented.
○ Cloths for cleaning should be of the disposable type.
○ Surfaces should be cleaned with an antibacterial cleaner.
○ All bins should have lids and be kept covered.
○ All empties should be stacked in a safe area with care.
○ Waste and rubbish should not be allowed to accumulate.
○ Empty bottles, waste paper, cardboard, etc. should be recycled.

The cold room

A large catering establishment may have a cold room for meat, with possibly a deep-freeze compartment where supplies can be kept frozen for long periods. The best temperature for storing fresh meat and poultry (short term) is between 4° and 6°C (39–43°F) with a controlled humidity (poultry is stored in a cold room). Fish should have a cold room of its own so that it does not affect other foods. Game, when plucked, is also kept in a cold room.

Chill room

A chill room keeps food cold without freezing, and is particularly suitable for those foods requiring a consistent, not too cold, temperature, such as dessert fruits, salads, cheese. Fresh fruit, salads and vegetables are best stored at a temperature of 4–6°C (39–43°F) with a humidity that will not result in loss of water from the leaves causing them to go limp. Green vegetables should be stored in a dark area to prevent leaves turning yellow. Certain fruits such as peaches and avocados are best stored at 10°C (50°F), while bananas must not be stored below 13°C (55°F) otherwise they will turn black. Dairy products (milk, cream, yogurt and butter) are best stored at 2°C (35°F). Cheese requires differing storage temperatures according to the type of cheese and degree of ripeness. Fats and oils are best stored at 4–7°C (39–45°F) otherwise they are liable to go rancid.

Refrigeration

Because spoilage and food poisoning organisms multiply most rapidly in warm conditions, there is a need for refrigeration through every stage of food delivery, storage, preparation, service and in certain situations onward distribution. Refrigeration does not kill micro-organisms but prevents them multiplying. Many cases of food poisoning can be tracked back to failure to control food temperatures or failure to cool food properly.

Temperature control is so important that statutory measures have been extended by the Food Hygiene Regulations whereby all food must be stored at or below 8°C (46°F) and some foods at lower temperatures. Chilling at 0°–3°C (32–37°F) and freezing at −18° to −22°C (0° to −7.6°F) is the easiest and most natural way of preserving food and maintaining product quality because it:

○ cuts down on wastage (reducing operating costs);
○ allows a wider variety of food to be stacked;
○ gives flexibility in delivering, preparation and use of foods.

To maintain the quality and freshness of food, refrigeration at correct temperatures must be provided:

○ at delivery;
○ for storage;
○ for preparation;
○ for onward distribution;
○ for holding, display and service.

TYPES OF REFRIGERATION

○ Mise en place – these are smaller refrigerators placed near to or under specific working areas. Some types have bain-marie style containers which allow for the storage of the many small prepared food items required in a busy à la carte kitchen.
○ Separate cabinets are essential for such foods as pastry; meat and fish; and cold buffets where food is displayed for more than 4 hours.
○ Quick chillers – as the slow cooling of cooked food can allow rapid bacterial growth, rapid chillers are available.
○ Display cabinets incorporating forced circulation of chilled air.

TEMPERATURE CHECKS

In addition to the legal requirements for food to be stored at the correct temperature, the maintenance of correct temperature display should be specified on each cabinet and should be monitored regularly, with the use of probes, thermometers, etc.

Further information can be obtained from Electricity Association, 30 Millbank, London SW1P 4RD.

Temperatures and storage times are listed on page 367.

POINTS TO NOTE ON REFRIGERATION

○ All refrigerators, cold rooms, chill rooms and deep-freeze units should be regularly inspected and maintained by qualified refrigeration engineers.

○ Defrosting should take place regularly, according to the instructions issued from the manufacturers. Refrigerators usually need to be defrosted weekly; if this is not done, then the efficiency of the refrigerator is lessened.

○ While a cold unit is being defrosted it should be thoroughly cleaned, including all the shelves.

○ Hot foods should never be placed in a refrigerator or cold room because the steam given off can affect nearby foods.

○ Peeled onions should never be kept in a cold room because the smell can taint other foods.

Vegetable store

This should be designed to store all vegetables in a cool, dry, well-ventilated room with bins for root vegetables and racking for others. Care should be taken to see that old stocks of vegetables are used before the new ones; this is important as fresh vegetables and fruits deteriorate quickly. If it is not convenient to empty root vegetables into bins they should be kept in the sack on racks off the ground.

Ordering of goods within the establishment

In a large catering establishment the stores carry a stock which for variety and quantity often equals a large grocery store. Its operation is similar in many respects, the main difference being that requisitions take the place of cash. The system of internal and external accountancy must be simple but precise.

The storekeeper

The essentials which go to making a good storekeeper are:

○ experience;

○ knowledge of how to handle, care for and organise the stock in his or her charge;

○ a tidy mind and sense of detail;

○ a quick grasp of figures;

○ possibly computer literate;

○ clear handwriting;

○ a liking for his or her job;

○ honesty.

There are many departments which draw supplies from these stores – kitchen, still room, restaurant, grill room, banqueting, floor service. A list of these departments should be given to the storekeeper, together with the signatures of the heads of departments or those who have the right to sign the requisition forms.

All requisitions must be handed to the storekeeper in time to allow the ordering and delivery of the goods on the appropriate day. Different coloured requisitions may be used for the various departments if desired.

DUTIES OF A STOREKEEPER

○ To keep a good standard of tidiness and cleanliness.

○ To arrange proper storage space for all incoming foodstuffs.

○ To keep up-to-date price lists of all commodities.

- To ensure that an ample supply of all important foodstuffs is always available.
- To check that all orders are correctly made out, and dispatched in good time.
- To check all incoming stores – quantity, quality and price.
- To keep all delivery notes, invoices, credit notes, receipts and statements efficiently filed.
- To keep a daily stores issue sheet.
- To keep a set of bin cards.
- To issue nothing without receiving a signed chit in exchange.
- To check all stock at frequent intervals.
- To see that all chargeable containers are properly kept, returned and credited, that is all money charged for sacks, boxes, etc. is deducted from the account.
- To obtain the best value at the lowest buying price.
- To know when foods are in or out of season.

Types of records used in stores control

BIN CARD

Figure 10.4 *Example of a bin card*

BIN CARD

PRICE

UNIT (lbs, Tins, etc) ________________ MAX STOCK _____

COMMODITY ________________________ MIN STOCK _____

DATE	RECEIVED	ISSUED	STOCK IN HAND	

There should be an individual bin card for each item held in stock. The following details are found on the bin card:

- name of the commodity;
- issuing unit;
- date goods are received or issued;
- from whom they are received and to whom issued;
- maximum stock;
- minimum stock;
- quantity received;
- quantity issued;
- balance held in stock.

STORES LEDGER

This is usually found in the form of a loose-leaf file giving one ledger sheet to each item held in stock. The following details are found on a stores ledger sheet:

○ name of commodity;
○ classification;
○ unit;
○ maximum stock;
○ minimum stock;
○ date of goods received or issued;
○ from whom they are received and to whom issued;
○ invoice or requisition number;
○ quantity received or issued and the remaining balance held in stock;
○ unit price;
○ cash value of goods received and issued and the balancing cash total of goods held in stock.

Figure 10.5 *Example of a daily stores issue sheet*

Commodity	Unit	Stock in hand	Monday In	Monday Out	Tuesday In	Tuesday Out	Wednesday In	Wednesday Out	Thursday In	Thursday Out	Friday In	Friday Out	Total pur-chases	Total issues	Total stock
Butter	kg	27		2						3				5	22
Flour	Sacks	2		1		1							1	1	2
Olive oil	Litres	8		1						½				1½	6½
Spices	30g packs	8		4			8						8	4	12
Peas, tin	A10	30		6						3				9	21

.... CANTEEN Week ending .... No. meals served .... Cost per meal ....

Commodity	hand B/F	Stock received during week M.	Tu.	W.	Th	F.	Total	Stock used during week M.	Tu.	W.	Th.	F.	S.	Total	@*	Cost*	in hand C/F
Apples, canned																	
Apples, dried Apricots, etc – dried																	
Baking powder																	
Baked beans																	

* The cost of stock used can also be checked by using two extra columns

Figure 10.6 *Example of a stores ledger sheet*

BIN No   DESCRIPTION   CLASSIFICATION   CODE UNIT MAXIMUM MINIMUM

Date	DETAIL	Invoice or Req No	QUANTITY Received	Balance	Issued	UNIT PRICE	VALUE Received	Balance	Issued

Every time goods are received or issued the appropriate entries should be made on the necessary stores ledger sheets and bin cards. In this way the balance on the bin card should always be the same as the balance shown on the stores ledger sheet.

DEPARTMENTAL REQUISITION BOOK

Figure 10.7 *Example of a stores requisition sheet*

DEPARTMENTAL REQUISITION BOOK   267

Date _____   Class _____

Description	Quan	Unit	Price per Unit	Issued if Different	Quan	Unit	Price per Unit	Code	£	

One of these books should be issued to each department in the catering establishment which needs to draw goods from the store. These books can either be of different colours or have departmental serial numbers. Every time goods are drawn from the store a requisition must be filled out and signed by the necessary head of department – this applies whether one or 20 items are needed from the store. When the storekeeper issues the goods he or she will check them against the requisition and tick them off; at the same time the cost of each item is filled in. In this way the total expenditure over a period for a certain department can be quickly found. The following details are found on the requisition sheet:

○ serial number;
○ name of department;
○ date;
○ description of goods required;
○ quantity of goods required;
○ unit;
○ price per unit.
○ issue, if different;
○ quantity of goods issued;
○ unit;
○ price per unit;
○ cash column;
○ signature;

ORDER BOOK

This is in duplicate and has to be filled in by the storekeeper every time he or she wishes to have goods delivered. Whenever goods are ordered, an order sheet must be filled in and sent to the supplier, and on receipt of the goods they should be checked against both delivery note and duplicate order sheet. All order sheets must be signed by the storekeeper. Details found on an order sheet are as follows:

○ name and address of catering establishment;
○ name and address of supplier;
○ serial number of order sheet;
○ quantity of goods;
○ description of goods to be ordered;
○ date;
○ signature;
○ date of delivery, if specific day required.

STOCK SHEETS

Stock should be taken at regular intervals of either one week or one month. Spot checks are advisable about every three months. The stock check should be taken where possible by an independent person, thus preventing the chance of 'pilfering' and 'fiddling' taking place. The details found on the stock sheets are as follows:

○ description of goods;
○ quantity received and issued, and balance;
○ price per unit;
○ cash columns.

The stock sheets will normally be printed in alphabetical order.

All fresh foodstuffs such as meat, fish and vegetables, will be entered in the stock sheet in the normal manner, but as they are purchased and used up daily a NIL stock will always be shown on their respective ledger sheets.

Commercial documents

Essential parts of a control system of any catering establishment are delivery notes, invoices, credit notes and statements.

Delivery notes

These are sent with goods supplied as a means of checking that everything ordered has been delivered. The delivery note should also be checked against the duplicate order sheet.

INVOICES

These are bills sent to clients, setting out the cost of goods supplied or services rendered. An invoice should be sent on the day the goods are despatched or the services are rendered or as soon as possible afterwards. At least one copy of each invoice is made and used for posting up the books of accounts, stock records and so on. (See Figure 10.8, page 377.)

Invoices contain the following information:

○ name, address, telephone numbers (as a printed heading), fax numbers, of the firm supplying the goods or services;
○ name and address of the firm to whom the goods or services have been supplied;
○ the word *invoice*;
○ date on which the goods or services were supplied;
○ particulars of the goods or services supplied together with the prices;
○ a note concerning the terms of settlement, such as 'Terms 5% per month', which means that if the person receiving the invoice settles his or her account within one month he or she may deduce 5% as discount.

CREDIT NOTES

These are advices to clients, setting out allowances made for goods returned or adjustments made through errors of overcharging on invoices. They should also be issued when chargeable containers such as crates, boxes or sacks are returned. Credit notes are exactly the same in form as invoices except that the word *credit note* appears in place of the word *invoice*. To make them more easily distinguishable they are usually printed in red, whereas invoices are always printed in black. A credit note should be sent as soon as it is known that a client is entitled to the credit of a sum with which he or she has been previously charged by invoice.

Figure 10.8 *Example of an invoice and statement*

INVOICE

Phone: 0208 574 1133	No. 03957
Fax: 0208 574 1123	Vegetable Suppliers Ltd.,
Email: greend@veg.sup.ac.uk	D. Green
Website: http//www.greend.com	5 Warwick Road,
Messrs. L. Moriarty & Co.,	Southall,
597 High Street,	Middlesex
Ealing,	
London, W5	Terms: 5% One month

Your order No. 67 Dated 3rd September, 19...	£

Sept 26th	10 kg Potatoes beg 6.00	6.00
	5 kg Sprouts, net 8.00	2.10
		14..00

STATEMENT

Phone: 0208 574 1133	Vegetable Suppliers Ltd.,
Fax: 0208 574 1123	D. Green
Email: greend@veg.sup.ac.uk	5 Warwick Road,
Website: http//www.greend.com	Southall,
Messrs. L. Moriarty & Co.,	Middlesex
597 High Street,	
Ealing,	
London, W5	Terms: 5% One month

19...		£
Sept 10th	Goods	45.90
17th	Goods	32.41
20th	Goods	41.30
26th	Goods	16.15
		135.76
28th	Returns credited	4.80
		130.96

STATEMENTS

These are summaries of all invoices and credit notes sent to clients during the previous accounting period, usually one month. They also show any sums owing or paid from previous accounting periods and the total amount due. A statement is usually a copy of a client's ledger account and does not contain more information than is necessary to check invoices and credit notes.

When a client makes payment he or she usually sends a cheque, together with the statement he or she has received. The cheque is paid into the bank and the statement may be returned to the client duly receipted.

CASH DISCOUNT

This is a discount allowed in consideration of prompt payment. At the end of any length of time chosen as an accounting period, such as one month, there will be some outstanding debts. In order to encourage customers to pay within a stipulated time, sellers of goods frequently offer a discount. This is called cash discount. By offering cash discount, the seller may induce his or her customer to pay more quickly, so turning debts into ready money. Cash discount varies from $1\frac{1}{4}$ to 10%, depending on the seller and the time: $2\frac{1}{2}$% if paid in 10 days; $1\frac{1}{4}$% if paid in 28 days, for example.

TRADE DISCOUNT

This is discount allowed by one trader to another, a deduction from the catalogue price of goods made before arriving at the invoice price. The amount of trade discount does not therefore appear in the accounts. For example, in a catalogue of kitchen equipment, a machine listed at £250 less 20% trade discount shows:

Catalogue price	£250
Less 20% trade discount	£50
Invoice price	£200

The £200 is the amount entered in the appropriate accounts.

In the case of purchase tax on articles, discount is taken off *after* the tax has been deducted from list price.

Gross price is the price of an article before discount has been deducted.

Net price is the price after discount has been deducted; in some cases a price on which no discount will be allowed.

CASH ACCOUNT

The following are the essentials for the keeping of a simple cash account:

- all entries must be dated;
- all monies received must be clearly named and entered on the left-hand or debit side of the book;
- all monies paid out must also be clearly shown and entered on the right-hand or credit side of the book;
- at the end of a given period – either a day, week or month or at the end of each page – the book must be balanced; that is, both sides are totalled and the difference between the two is known as the balance; if, for example, the debit side (money received) is greater than the credit side (money paid out), then a credit or right-hand side balance is shown, so that the two totals are then equal; a credit balance then means cash in hand;
- a debit balance cannot occur because it is impossible to pay out more than is received.

An example is given in the following table.

GENERAL RULE

Debit – monies coming in.

Credit – monies going out.

CASH ACCOUNT

DR. Date	Receipts	£	FIRST WEEK Date	Payment	CR. £
Oct 3	to lunches	400	Oct 1	by repairs	80
4	,, teas	100	2	,, grocer	100
5	,, tax rebate	60	6	,, butcher	120
				,, balance c/fwd	260
		560			560

DR. Date	Receipts	£	SECOND WEEK Date	Payment	CR. £
Oct	to balance b/fwd	260	Oct 8	by fishmonger	50
9	,, sale of pastries	100	10	,, fuel	50
11	,, goods	200	11	,, tax	40
			12	,, greengrocer	60
				,, balance c/fwd	360
		560			560

DR. Date	Receipts	£	THIRD WEEK Date	Payment	CR. £
Oct	to balance b/fwd	360	Oct 19	by butcher	80
15	,, teas	120	21	,, grocer	60
17	,, pastries	110		,, balance c/fwd	650
24	,, goods	60			
26	,, goods	80			
29	,, goods	60			
		790			790

EXAMPLE

Make out a cash account and enter the following transactions:

Oct.	1	Paid for repair to stove	£109.00
	2	Paid to grocer	200.00
	3	Received for lunches	750.00
	4	Received for teas	200.00
	5	Received tax rebate	97.84
	6	Paid to butcher	120.00
Oct.	8	paid to fishmonger	72.60
	9	Received for sale of pastries	112.90
	10	Paid for fuel	80.00
	11	Paid tax	60.00
	11	Received for goods	500.00
	12	Paid to greengrocer	112.36
Oct.	15	Received for teas	150.20

Continues

17	Received for pastries	150.00
19	Paid to butcher	100.80
21	Paid to grocer	95.00
24	Received for goods	130.00
26	Received for goods	150.00
29	Received for goods	140.00

Some references to storage and control elsewhere in the book

Safety	479, 486	Computers	565
Each commodity	61	Pricing	338
Costing	340, 355	Management control	431
Waste	527	People control	440
Hygiene	510		

Topics for Discussion
FOOD PURCHASING

1 A food-buying policy.
2 Is there a need for portion control?
3 The relationship between food quality and price.
4 The reasons for using standard purchasing specifications.
5 The use of standardised recipes.
6 How you would implement a cost control system.
7 The advantages of a computerised stockkeeping system.
8 How the role of the storekeeper may change in the future.

STORAGE AND CONTROL

1 Why control of goods from receipt (delivery) to final destination (the customer) is essential.
2 What controls are needed regarding goods, staff and the preparation and service of food?
3 The need to be knowledgeable regarding the cost and quality of foods in relation to selling price.
4 The implication of setting the selling price too low and also of setting it too high.
5 How do you consider a fair % profit is arrived at, specify the establishment you have in mind.
6 What do you understand to be a "suitable portion". Give examples and explain your reasoning.

CHAPTER 11

AN OVERVIEW OF FOOD AND BEVERAGE SERVICE

WHAT IS FOOD AND BEVERAGE SERVICE?

Detailed information can be found in *Food and beverage service*, 6th edition, Lillicrap, D., Cousins, J. and Smith, R., 2002, Hodder and Stoughton, London

Food and beverage service is the essential link between the menu, beverages and the other services on offer in an establishment, and the customers. For a particular food and beverage (or foodservice) operation the choices on how the food and beverage service is designed, planned, undertaken and controlled are made taking into account a number of organisational variables. These include taking account of:

○ customer needs;
○ level of customer demand;
○ the type and style of the food and beverage operation;
○ the nature of the customers (non-captive, captive or semi-captive);
○ prices to be charged;
○ production process;
○ volume of demand;
○ volume of throughput;
○ space available;
○ availability of staff;
○ opening hours;
○ booking requirements;
○ payment requirements;
○ legal requirements.

Figure 11.1 *Stock taking*

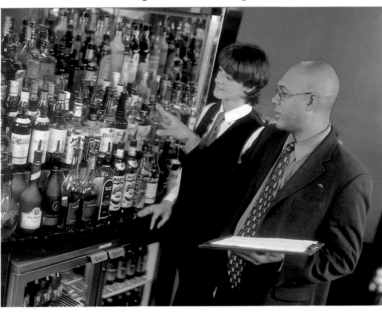

For food and beverage service staff the four key requirements are:

1 sound product knowledge;
2 competence in technical skills;
3 well developed social skills;
4 the ability to work as part of a team.

Whilst there have been changes in food and beverage service in some sectors, with less emphasis on the high level technical skills, these four key requirements remain for all staff. However the emphasis on these key requirements varies according to the type of establishment and the particular service methods being used.

Food and beverage service was traditionally seen primarily as a delivery system. However, food and beverage service actually consists of two separate systems, which are operating at the same time. These are:

1 **The service sequence** – which is primarily concerned with the delivery of food and beverages to the customer
2 **The customer process** – which is concerned with the experience the customer undertakes

The service sequence

The service sequence is essentially the bridge between the production system, beverage provision and the customer process (or experience). The service sequence consists of seven stages. These are:

1 preparation for service;
2 taking food and beverage orders;
3 the service of food and beverages;
4 billing;
5 clearing;

6 dishwashing;

7 clearing following service.

Within these seven elements, there are a variety of alternative ways of achieving the service sequence.

1. PREPARATION FOR SERVICE

Within the service areas, there are a variety of tasks and duties which need to be carried out in order to ensure that adequate preparation has been made for the expected volume of business and the type of service which is to be provided. These activities include:

○ taking and checking bookings;

○ checking and ensuring the cleanliness of glassware, crockery, flatware and cutlery;

○ dealing with linen and paper items;

○ undertaking housekeeping duties;

○ arranging and laying up the service areas;

○ stocking hotplates, workstations, display buffets;

○ setting up bars and bar areas;

○ arranging and laying up lounge areas;

○ briefing of staff to ensure that they have adequate knowledge of the product and the service requirements.

2. TAKING FOOD AND BEVERAGE ORDERS

Taking orders from customers for the food and drink they wish to have, takes time. The order-taking process is part of a longer process, which feeds information to the food production or bar areas and provides information for the billing method. Whatever type of system is used whether manual or electronic it will be based on one of the three basic order-taking methods. These are:

1 Duplicate: Order taken and copied to supply point and second copy retained by server for service and subsequent billing.

2 Triplicate: Order taken and copied to supply point and cashier for billing, third copy retained by server for service.

3 Service with order: Taking order and serving to order, as used in e.g. bar service or take-away methods.

Within the order-taking procedure there are many opportunities for exploiting the potential for personal selling that can be carried out by service staff. Personal selling refers specifically to the ability of the staff to contribute to the promotion of sales. This is especially important where there are specific promotions being undertaken. Service staff must therefore be trained in selling and also be well briefed on the special offers (see The Customer Process page 389).

3. THE SERVICE OF FOOD AND BEVERAGES

The various service methods available are given on page 390 of this Chapter. The choice of service method will depend as much on the customer service specification (see page 390) as on the capability of the staff, the capacity of he operation and the equipment available. Differing service methods will also determine the speed of service and the time the customer takes to consume the meal, which in turn will have an impact on the throughput of customers.

Good food and beverage service is achieved where management continually reinforces and supports service staff in the maintenance of good standards of achievement. Additionally the provision and maintenance of good service is primarily dependent on teamwork, not only among service staff but also amongst and between staff in other departments.

Figure 11.2 *Informal dining (Brasserie)*

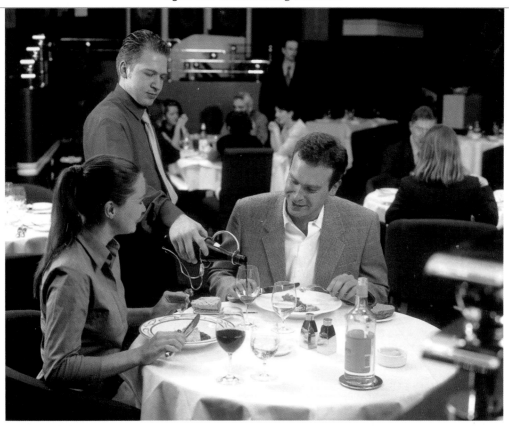

Figure 11.3 *Gastro-pub dining*

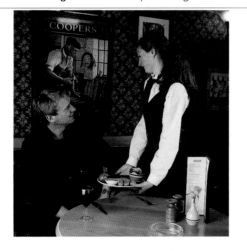

Figure 11.4 *Fine dining*

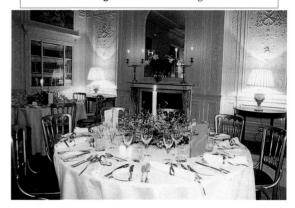

Figure 11.6 *Feeding at work*

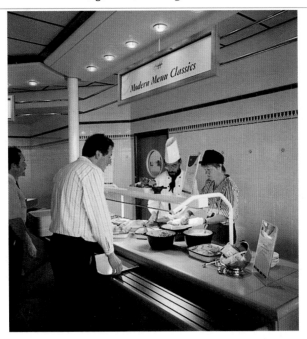

Figure 11.5 *Carvery*

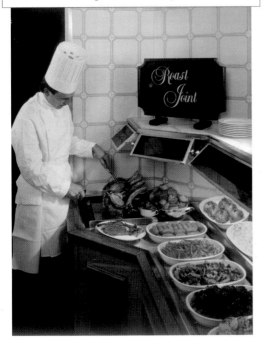

Figure 11.7 *Hospital catering*

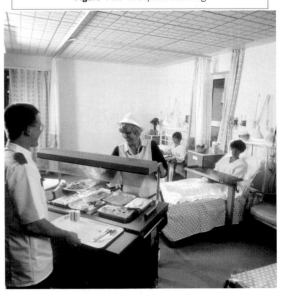

Figure 11.8 *Restaurant receptionist*

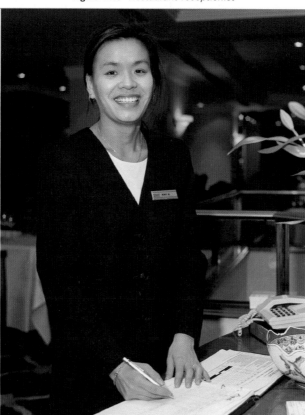

Figure 11.9 *Large scale production*

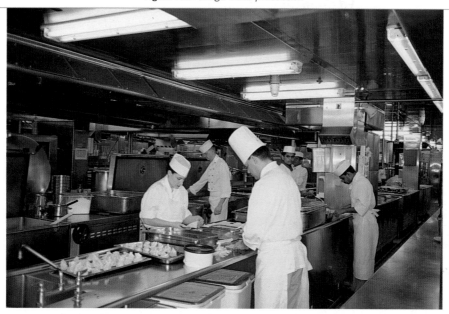

Figure 11.10 *School meals service*

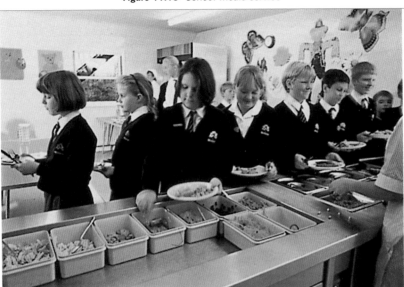

Figure 11.11 *Outdoor catering service*

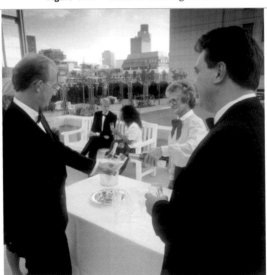

Figure 11.12 *Fast food service*

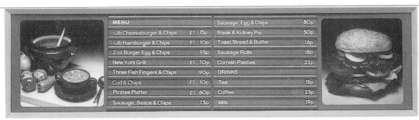

4. BILLING

The various billing methods found in food service operations are as follows:
- Bill as check: Second copy of order used as bill.
- Separate bill: Bill made up from duplicate check and presented to customer.
- Bill with order: Service to order and billing at same time, e.g. bar or take-away methods.
- Prepaid: Customer purchases ticket or card in advance either for specific meal or specific value.
- Voucher: Customer has credit issued by third party, e.g. luncheon voucher or tourist agency voucher for either specific meal or specific value.
- No charge: Customer not paying.
- Deferred: e.g. function-type catering where bill paid by organiser.

The actual choice of billing method will be dependent on the type and style of the operation. However, the billing system is also part of a longer process linked first to the order-taking method and second to the revenue control procedures.

5. CLEARING

The various clearing methods found in food service operations may be summarised as follows:
- Manual 1: The collection of soiled ware by waiting staff to dishwash area.
- Manual 2: The collection and sorting to trolleys by operators for transportation to dishwash area.
- Semi-self-clear: The placing of soiled ware by customers on strategically placed trolleys within dining area for removal by operators.
- Self-clear: The placing of soiled ware by customers on conveyor or conveyorised tray collecting system for mechanical transportation to dish wash area.
- Self-clear and strip: The placing of soiled ware into conveyorised dishwasher baskets by customer for the direct entry of baskets through dishwash.

The choice of clearing method, whether manual by staff or involving customers, will be dependent not only on the type of operation but also on the nature of the demand being met.

6. DISHWASHING

The capacity of the dishwashing system should always be greater than the operational maximum required. This is because slow dishwashing increases the amount of equipment required to be in use at a particular time and increases the storage space required in service areas.

The various dishwashing systems are as follows:
- Manual: The manual washing of soiled ware by hand or brush.
- Semi-automatic: The manual loading by operators of a dishwash machine.
- Automatic conveyor: The manual loading by operators of soiled ware within baskets mounted on conveyor for automatic transportation through the dishwash machine.
- Flight Conveyor: The manual loading by operators of soiled ware on pegs mounted on a conveyor for automatic transportation through the dishwasher.
- Deferred wash: The collection, stripping, sorting and stacking of ware by operators for transportation through dishwash at a later stage.

Essentially, the potential volume that can be accommodated increases, as well as potential efficiency, from the manual method to the flight conveyor method. The choice of method will be largely dependent on the scale of the operation. It is also often necessary to employ more than one method.

For hygienic washing up the generally recognised requirements are a good supply of hot water at a temperature of 60°C (140°F) for general cleansing followed by a sterilising rinse at a temperature of 82°C (180°F) for at least one minute. Alternatively low-temperature equipment is available which sterilises with the chemical sodium hypochlorite (bleach). Further information can be obtained from Lever Industrial, Lever House, St James Road, Kingston-upon-Thames, Surrey KT1 2BA.

Dishwashing machines take over an arduous job and save a lot of time and labour, ensuring that a good supply of clean sterilised crockery is available.

There are three main types:

○ Spray types – the dishes are placed in racks which slide into the machines where they are subjected to a spray of hot detergent water at 48–60°C (118–140°F) from above and below. The racks move on to the next section where they are rinsed by a fresh hot shower at 82°C (180°F). At this temperature they are sterilised, and on passing out into the air they dry off quickly.

○ Brush-type machines – revolving brushes are used for the scrubbing of each article in hot detergent water; the articles are then rinsed and sterilised in another compartment.

○ Agitator water machines – baskets of dishes are immersed in deep tanks and the cleaning is performed by the mechanical agitation of the hot detergent water. The loaded baskets are then given a sterilising rinse in another compartment.

Dishwashing machines are costly and it is essential that the manufacturer's instructions with regard to use and maintenance are followed at all times.

8. CLEARING FOLLOWING SERVICE

After the service periods, there are a variety of tasks and duties to be carried out; partly to clear from the previous service and partly to prepare for the next. The efficient management of the clearing stage can have a dramatic impact on the potential reuse of an area.

Included in this stage of the service sequence is the requirement for the management of cleaning programmes. Detailed cleaning schedules need to be developed to ensure that all cleaning activities are coordinated. These can be daily, weekly, monthly and for other periods. Alongside these cleaning schedules, it is desirable to incorporate maintenance checks. These, together with the operation of cleaning schedules, can help to ensure that equipment and facilities are always available and in working order.

THE CUSTOMER PROCESS

The customer receiving the food and beverage product is required to undertake or observe certain requirements: this is the customer process. If food and beverage service is viewed as primarily a delivery process, then the customer can often be seen as a passive recipient of the service. As a result, systems and procedures tend only to be designed from the delivery perspective. However, a customer service specification cannot be achieved if it does not take account of both the infrastructure supporting the specification as well as the ability to implement standards within the interactive phase.

In food and beverage operations there are five basic processes which customers undertake. these are:

1 **Table service** (service at a laid cover).
2 **Assisted service** (part service at a laid cover and part self-service).
3 **Self-service**.
4 **Service at a single point** (ordering, receipt of order and payment).
5 **Specialised service or service *in situ***.

In the first four of these customer processes, the customer comes to where the food and beverage service is offered and the service is provided in areas primarily designed for the purpose. However in the fifth customer process the service is provided in another location and where the area is not primarily designed for the purpose.

A summary of the five customer processes is shown in the chart below and a listing of all food and beverage service methods is given below.

A SUMMARY OF THE FIVE FOOD AND BEVERAGE SERVICE CUSTOMER PROCESSES

SERVICE METHOD	FOOD AND BEVERAGE SERVICE AREAS	ORDERING AND SELECTION	SERVICE	DINING CONSUMPTION	CLEARING
Table service	Customer enters food service area and is seated	Orders from the menu	By staff to customer	Seats at a laid table (cover)	By staff
Assisted service	Customer enters food service area and is usually seated	Orders from the menu, the buffet or passed trays	By staff and the customer helping him/herself	Usually at laid table (cover)	By staff
Self service	Customer enters food service area and is not seated by staff	Customer selects own tray and food	Customer carries own tray	Dining area or take-away	By staff / By customer or both
Single point service	Customer enters food service area	Orders meal at single point	Customer carries own meal	Dining area of take-away	By staff / By customer or both
Specialised or in situ	In situ	Orders from menu or food is pre-determined	Brought to customer	Where food is served	By staff or by customer

CUSTOMER SERVICE SPECIFICATIONS

Like the food/product specifications there must also be customer service specifications. For food and beverage operations the customer service specification is focused as much on identifying the procedures that need to be followed (as summarised in the notes on the *service sequence* and the *customer process* above) as they are on the way they are carried out. This is because food and beverage is more than a delivery system; it also requires customers to be assisted in following various procedures such as being seated at a table, and also to enable a positive interaction between staff and customers.

Customer service specifications can be defined by five characteristics. These are:

1 **Service level:** the method of service and the extent of the individual personal attention give to customers.
2 **Availability of service:** e.g. the opening times, variations in the menu and wine and drinks lists on offer.
3 **Level of standards:** e.g. food quality, decor, equipment cost, staff professionalism.
4 **Reliability of the service:** the extent to which the product is intended to be consistent in practice.
5 **Flexibility of the service:** the provision of alternatives, or variations in the standard product on offer.

In designing a foodservice operation to meet a customer service specification, care is taken to ensure profitability by considering the efficiency of the use of resources. The resources used in foodservice operations are:

○ **Materials:** commodities and equipment.
○ **Labour:** staffing and costs.
○ **Facilities:** basically the premises and the volume of business that the premises are able to support.

The management of the operation must therefore take account of the effect that the level of business has on the ability of the operation to maintain the service while at the same time ensuring a high productivity of all the resources being used.

The operation must be physically capable of supporting the customer service specifications otherwise it will always be the cause of difficulties.

In addition the staff must be capable of supporting the intended customer service specification into account their technical and interpersonal skills, product knowledge and team working capability of the staff.

As well as the interaction with customers service staff also interact with customers outside the service areas, e.g. kitchen staff, bill office staff dispense bar staff, stillroom staff. It is important that the provision of the food and beverage product within an establishment is seen as a joint effort between all departments, with each department understanding the needs of the others in order to meet the customers' demands.

In order to minimise problems with customer relations there has to be equal concern over the physical aspects of the service, the way in which the service is operated, and with the interpersonal interaction between customers and staff. Knowing what the potential for customer satisfaction is from the food and beverage products can help to ensure that there are procedures in place for dealing with any difficulties that might arise. The potential for satisfaction should already have been built into the design of the product so that it meets the needs the customers have at the time. Obviously there is also the potential for dissatisfaction. Potential dissatisfactions fall into two categories: those which are controllable by the establishment, such as scruffy, unhelpful staff, or customers, the weather, and those which are uncontrollable, such as behaviour of other customers, the weather, or transport problems. Being able to identify all of these possibilities enables an operation to have procedures in place to deal with them when they occur.

FOOD AND BEVERAGE SERVICE METHODS

TABLE SERVICE

This is service of food and beverages to a customer at a laid cover.

1 **Waiter service**
   a) Silver/English Service: Presentations and service of food to a customer by waiting staff from a food flat or dish.
   b) Family Service: Main courses plated with vegetables placed in multi-portion dishes on tables for customers to help themselves. Any sauces are usually offered.
   c) Plated/American service: Service of pre-plated foods to customers, now widely used in many establishments and in banqueting.
   d) Butler/French Service: Presentation of food individually to customers by food service staff for customers to serve themselves.
   e) Russian Service: Table laid with food for customers to help themselves. (Also sometimes confusingly used to indicate Guéridon or Butler service).
   f) Guéridon Service: Food served onto customer's plate at a side table or from a trolley. Also may include carving, cooking and flambé dishes, preparation of salads and dressings.

2 **Bar counter service**
Service to customers seated at a bar counter (usually U shaped) on stools.

ASSISTED SERVICE

This is a combination of table service and self-service.

3 **Assisted**
   a) Commonly applied to 'carvery' type operations, some parts of the meal are served to seated customers; the customers collect other parts. Also used for breakfast service.
   b) Buffets where customers select food and drink from displays or passed trays, consumption is either at tables, standing or in lounge area.

SELF-SERVICE

Self-service of customers

4 **Cafeteria service**
   a) Counter: Customers line up in a queue at a service counter and choose the menu items they require. The customer places their items on a tray. Some establishments use a 'carousel', a revolving stacked counter saving space.
   b) Free Flow: Selection as in a counter service. Customers move at will to random service points exiting via a payment point.
   c) Echelon: This is a series of counters at angles to customer flow within a free flow area, thus saving space.
   d) Supermarket: Island service points within a free-flow area. Call order may also feature in some cafeterias.

SINGLE POINT SERVICE

This is the service of customers at a single point where they consume on the premises or they take away.

5 **Take away**

Customer orders are served from a single point usually at a counter, hatch or snack-stand and the customer normally consumes the food off the premises although some take-away establishments provide limited seating. This service method is commonly used for *fast-food* operations and also includes *drive thrus* where the customer drives a vehicle past order, payment and collection points.

6 **Vending**

Automatic retailing of food and beverage products.

7 **Kiosks**

Service provided by outstations during peak demand in specific locations.

8 **Food Court**

This is a group of autonomous counters where customers may either order and eat or buy from a number of counters and cut in separate eating area or take away.

9 **Bar**

A selling point for the consumption of intoxicating liquor in licensed premises.

SPECIALISED (OR IN SITU) SERVICE

Service to customers in areas not primarily designed for service.

10 **Tray Service**

Service of a meal or part of a meal in a tray to the customer in situ, e.g. in hospitals or in an aircraft.

11 **Trolley**

Service of food and beverage from a trolley away from dining areas to customers at their seats or desks. Used, for example on an aircraft, on trains and in offices.

12 **Home Delivery**

Food and beverage delivered to a customer's home or place of work e.g. Pizza delivery, meals-on-wheels, or sandwiches to offices.

13 **Lounge service**

Service of food and beverages in a lounge area e.g. an hotel lounge.

14 **Room service**

Service of food and beverages in guest apartments or meeting rooms.

15 **Drive in**

Customers are served food and beverages to their vehicles.

(**Note:** Banquet/function catering is a term used to describe food and beverage operations that are providing service for a specific number of people at specific times in a variety of dining layouts. Service methods also vary. The term banquet/function catering therefore refers to the organisation of service rather than a specific service method.)

RESTAURANT PLANNING

Planning a restaurant needs to focus on the market it is aiming to attract, its customers, the theme the restaurant will take, type of food and service it is going to offer, and customer turnover each sitting.

Reception

The best place for taking bookings, receiving customers and processing the bills, is near the restaurant entrance.

Bar/Coffee Lounge

Space permitting there should be a separate bar and/or coffee lounge. This will help increase restaurant sales by giving customers somewhere to order their meals while the restaurant is full.

Circulation

The style of the restaurant will determine how customers will go to their table or are served.

The number of covers each session, each day and peak demands at certain times, needs to be considered to ensure space, facilities and employees are used effectively and that all delay and any congestion is avoided.

Physical barriers such as floral decorations and cutlery stands direct circulation in a self-service restaurant.

Space

The amount of space required per customer depends on the type of standard expected from the style and theme of the operation. Consideration has to be given to comfort versus the maximum number of customers you are trying to fit into the restaurant. The more 'up market' the restaurant, the more comfortable and spacious it should be.

A diner, when seated, will occupy up to 2 ft [61 cm] of floor space from the table therefore to give customers plenty of room and to allow for comfortable service, a 6 ft [183 cm] square space is normally required for a four seat table.

To create a bustling and busy bistro atmosphere you may require the tables to be closer together, which may mean a little discomfort for the customer. In this type of restaurant, often lower spend, you do not want to encourage the customer to stay too long. In many fast food restaurants the chairs are usually uncomfortable; this is to ensure that once the customers finish their meal, they leave.

A large restaurant with a huge expanse of tables and chairs can look boring and uninteresting. In such cases a better atmosphere and environment can be created by dividing the room into sections using panels or using raised sections.

Kitchen/Restaurant relationship

In most restaurants the storage and preparation of the food will be done in the kitchens, away from the dining area. All seating in the restaurant should be arranged away from the doors into the kitchen. The customers should not be able to see into the kitchen from the restaurant where the kitchen is not a feature of the meal experience. Often a screen is placed in front of the kitchen doors, with subdued lighting at this point, and the use of double doors will considerably help to keep hidden all the kitchen activity.

Bistros and brasseries often feature the cooking area; this is on full view of the customer and contributes to the customer's meal experience. In this case the kitchen is a central feature with some of the cooking smells and noise going in to the restaurant.

Types of internal fittings

The choice of tables, chairs, decor and furnishings will depend on the theme and style of the restaurant, also the market and type of customer it is going to attract. It is important to remember that the decor must be pleasing to the eye. The lighting is also extremely important; if done well it will enhance the overall appearance of the restaurant and the food being served.

LICENSING

Intoxicating liquor (alcohol) is licensed because excessive consumption of alcoholic drinks can seriously affect people's health and their wellbeing, and the same can result in anti-social behaviour. For this reason the sale of alcohol is controlled by law and holding a license to sell alcohol is a responsibility for the acts of the public and employees.

Therefore intoxicating drinks may only be sold and consumed on **licensed premises** during certain times of the day known as permitted hours of opening. At the end of the permitted hours, a time is allowed for drinking up time.

Liquor licensing

The Licensing Act of 1964 is the basis of liquor licensing law at the present time. The Licensing (Restaurant Meals) Act 1987 permitted licensed establishments serving bona fide meals to serve alcoholic beverages throughout the afternoon. This Act was followed by the Licensing Act 1988 which, among other provisions, permitted holders of licences to serve alcoholic drinks for up to 12 hours a day.

The retail of intoxicating drinks cannot be undertaken without a Justices' Licence.

Justices' Licences are granted by Licensing Committees. Justices of the Peace acting within a designated area appoint, from themselves, Licensing Justices, and they together form a Licensing Committee.

TYPES OF JUSTICES' LICENCES

There are two types of Justices' Licences.

On Licence

This licence authorises the person to whom it is granted to sell intoxicating drinks for consumption either on or off the premises of a named public house.

Off Licence

This licence authorises the person to whom it is granted to sell intoxicating drinks from named premises but for consumption away from those premises.

There are also limited On Licences, known as Part IV licences, which are needed to serve intoxicating drinks in a restaurant or boarding house. The licensing justices can only refuse an application for such a licence on specified grounds. In order to qualify for these types of licences the following conditions have to be fulfilled.

A RESTAURANT LICENCE

The premises must be used as intended to be used for the serving of meals at lunch or dinner or both. Intoxicating drinks (alcohol) can only be supplied for consumption with a table meal.

A RESIDENTIAL LICENCE

The premises must be suitable and used for boarding purposes, including breakfast and at least one other main meal.

Intoxicating drinks (alcohol) can only be supplied to residents or their private friends entertained by them at their expense.

A RESIDENTIAL AND RESTAURANT LICENCE

Such a licence is subject to the conditions applying to both Residential and Restaurant Licences.

A NEW LICENCE

Licensing Justices will only grant a new licence to a person considered fit to operate the licence they have applied for. The duration of the licence is normally three years.

RENEWAL OF AN EXISTING LICENCE

Applications for the renewal of existing licences must be made to every third General Annual Licensing Meeting. Application may be made in writing and attendance is not required unless the licensee of the licence has received notice of objection to the renewal. Any new licence granted during the three year period between renewal meetings falls due for renewal at the next triennial General Annual Licensing Meeting. If a license is not renewed, it lapses on 4 April in that year.

OCCASIONAL LICENCES

Sometimes it is necessary to apply for a special licence to run a bar at a function. This is called an occasional licence, which is granted by the Magistrates' Court.

PENALTY

The penalty for selling intoxicating drinks by retail without a licence is imprisonment for up to six months and/or a fine. On a second or subsequent conviction, disqualification from holding a licence for a specified period is possible.

HOURS OF OPENING IN ENGLAND FOR ON-LICENSED PREMISES

Weekdays

11.00 a.m.–11.00 p.m.

Sundays

12 noon–11.00 p.m.

Christmas Day

12 noon–3.00 p.m. 7.00 p.m.–10.30 p.m.

DRINKING UP TIME

Licensing Justices or the Magistrates' Court can adjust permitted hours. At the end of the permitted hours, 20 minutes is allowed for customers to finish their drinks, 30 minutes is allowed for drinks purchased with a meal.

SPECIFIC EXCEPTIONS TO PERMITTED HOURS

Permitted hours do not apply to residents (including resident staff) who may be supplied with, and consume, intoxicating drinks at any time. Residents may also entertain their private friends with alcoholic drink.

LICENSEES

A person holding a licence may entertain their friends at their own expense at any time. paying customers may not become 'guests' at the end of the permitted hours.

EMPLOYEES

May be given intoxicating drinks for consumption on the premises outside the permitted hours provided that the employer pays.

PENALTY

The penalty for selling intoxicating liquor outside the permitted hours is a fine.

LICENSING AND YOUNG PEOPLE

Because of the possible effects of the excessive consumption of alcohol in social behaviour, personal health or individuals, restrictions are placed on the sale of intoxicating drinks to young people. It is assumed that young people under a certain age do not have the sense of responsibility to act with moderation.

Children under the age of 14 are not allowed in a bar during permitted hours unless they are:

○ the children of the licensee;

○ resident in the public house but not employed on the premises;

○ passing through the bar from one part of the establishment to another, when there is no other convenient way; or

○ the establishment has a children's licence.

Although young persons aged 14 and under 18 are allowed in a bar during permitted hours at the licensee's discretion, it is an offence:

○ for licensees and their employees to sell intoxicating drinks to a person under 18 or allow such a person to consume drinks in the bar;

○ for a person under 18 to buy or attempt to buy any intoxicating drinks or to consume them in the bar;

○ for any person to buy or attempt to buy intoxicating drinks for consumption in the bar by a person under 18.

PENALTIES

Penalties for breach of the law relating to the sale and consumption of intoxicating drinks by young persons and presence in bars are listed below.

○ Allowing a child under 14 to be in a bar during permitted hours is an offence subject to a fine.

○ Selling intoxicating drinks to a person under age or allowing consumption by a person under 18 in a bar is also subject to a fine. A second or subsequent conviction could result in the license being forfeited.

○ Where the selling of intoxicating drinks to young people has been alleged, only evidence of the actual sale and the age of the purchaser is required to prove the offence.

If the holder of the licence is also charged because of the action of an employee, it is also a defence for the licensee to show that 'all due diligence' was exercised by seeking to ensure that staff knew the law and were careful to apply it whenever necessary.

Public entertainment

In order to provide the following public entertainment legally, an Entertainment Licence is needed:

○ live music by more than two performers;

○ dancing;

○ karaoke (may also require a Cinema Licence);

○ the operation of a Special Hours Certificate requires an Entertainment Licence.

Entertainment licences are granted by the local council or district council. A Performing Rights Society (PRS) licence is needed for the live performance or public playing of copyright music by any means.

PENALTIES

Penalty for infringement is a fine or imprisonment.

Weights and measures

In addition to laws regulating when, where and to whom intoxicating drinks may be sold, there are also laws which specify the measures governing the dispensing of drinks and the type of glasses which certain drinks must be sold in.

BEER AND CIDER

The Weights and Measures Act (Intoxicating Liquor) Order 1988 requires:

○ Draught beer and cider be sold in measures of $\frac{1}{3}$ pint, $\frac{1}{2}$ pint or multiples of $\frac{1}{2}$ pint. A measure of these drinks served in brim measure glasses may consist of liquid and a reasonable head. The Brewers and Licensed Retailers Association recommends that the liquid content of beer and cider served in brim measure glasses, once the head has collapsed, should not be less than 98% of any of the permissible measures.

○ When draught beer and cider are to be served in a glass which corresponds to any of these measures and which is government stamped to confirm this.

This does not apply when such drinks are dispensed by a stamped measuring instrument designed to dispense predetermined quantities. In this case, however, the drink must be dispensed in front of the customer who has ordered the drink. This does not apply to beer and cider when they are sold in a mix of drinks, for example a shandy. It is permissible to use pint and half pint glasses to serve such drinks and they may be described in the price list using imperial measures without reference to the metric equivalent.

WHISKY, GIN, RUM AND VODKA

The Weights and Measures Act (Intoxicating Liquor) Order 1988 further requires that whisky, gin, rum and vodka be sold for consumption in measures of 25 ml or multiples thereof, or 35 ml or multiples thereof. A licensee must display a notice showing the quantity in which these drinks are served on his/her premises.

WINE

When wine is sold by the glass the wine must be in measures of 125 ml and/or 175 ml or multiples thereof. The licensee must display a statement setting out the measures that are in use. This statement must be included on the menu or wine list. There is no requirement to serve the wine in a lined glass.

Wine sold in carafes or other open vessels not intended to be used for drinking, the permissible measures are 25 cl, 50 cl, and 1 litre.

The licensee is required to display a statement setting out the quantities contained in such carafes or vessels. This statement may be included on the menu or wine list.

PRICE LISTS

Customers must be able to know the prices of food and drink being served for sale and so the Price Marking (Food and Drink on Premises) Order 1979 requires price lists to be displayed in a way in which they can be clearly seen.

PENALTIES

For contravention of the law a fine is imposed on summary conviction.

NOTICES TO BE DISPLAYED IN ON-LICENSED PREMISES

It is mandatory to display the following information as a notice on lists on-licensed premises.

- The name of the licensee along with the details of the licence held. This is usually displayed above the main entrance.
- Details of hours subject to a Restriction Order.
- A Supper Hour Certificate and Extended Hours Order.
- A Special Hours Certificate.
- Details of hours under a General Order of Exemption.
- The measure used for the sale of whisky, gin, rum and vodka and the measures used for the sale of wine by the glass and in carafes.
- Price lists.
- A tobacco sales notice under the provision of the Children and Young Persons (Protection from Tobacco) Act 1991.
- A Children's Certificate notice where applicable.

Intoxicating drinks

Drink containing alcohol is classified as intoxicating for the purposes of licensing law if it contains more than 0.5% of alcohol by volume (0.5%) and requires a Justices' Licence for its retail sale.

THE STRENGTH OF INTOXICATING DRINKS

The strength of an intoxicating drink depends on how much alcohol it contains. The amount of alcohol contained is expressed as a percentage of volume – percentage alcohol by volume, abv for short. The formula for expressing abv on labels is alcohol % volume on % volume. For so a fortified wine, such as sherry or vermouth labelled as alcohol 18% volume means 18% of any given quantity is pure alcohol.

FOOD AND BEVERAGE STAFF

In food and beverage establishments today, there are many different ways of using and deploying staff. Also differing terminology is used to describe what people do.

Food and beverage staff are at the delivery end of the production cycle, it is these staff who are responsible for the customers' well being in the restaurant.

Food and beverage staff must be given appropriate training in social skills and social interaction. They must have the ability to respond to customer needs and to observe the overall dynamics of a restaurant. Good food and beverage staff should through experience be able to anticipate the individual needs of customers and able to read their body language. Customers want individual attention, good food and beverage professionals will be able to anticipate the individual need of the customer before the customer themselves has.

Food and beverage staff play an important role in the customer overall meal experience and this aspect of the delivery system must not be underestimated.

Examples of some positions
FOOD AND BEVERAGE MANAGER

Depending on the size of the establishment, the food and beverage manager is responsible for the implementation of agreed policies or for contributing to the setting of catering policies. The larger the organisation, the less likely the manager is to be involved in policy setting. In general food and beverage managers are responsible for:

○ ensuring that the profit margins are achieved for each food and beverage outlet;
○ updating and compiling new wine lists according to availability of stocks, current trends and customer needs;
○ liaising with the head chef on the instruction of menus for special occasions;
○ supervising the purchasing of all food and drink;
○ maintaining quality standards in food and beverage;
○ employing staff;
○ holding regular meetings with section heads to ensure all areas are working effectively, efficiently and are well co-ordinated.

RESTAURANT MANAGER/SUPERVISOR

A person who has overall responsibility for the organisation and administration of a food and beverage area. Responsible also for staff training duty rotas, the maintaining of an efficient and smooth service.

RECEPTION HEAD WAITER

Responsible for booking and keeping the booking diary up to date; allocation of tables and will greet the guests as they arrive.

HEAD WAITER/SUPERVISOR (MAÎTRE D'HÔTEL)

Overall responsibility for the staff team, allocating duties in the service area. The head waiter will liaise with the person responsible for table allocation (Reception Head Waiter). Responsible also for duty rotas.

STATION HEAD WAITER/SECTION SUPERVISOR

Responsible for a team serving on set number of tables, known as a station.

STATION WAITER

Known also as a chef de rang. Works under the direction of the station head waiter. There may also be an Assistant Station Waiter.

WAITER/WAITRESS (COMMIS AND APPRENTICES)

Works under the direction of the station waiter.

Bar staff are also employed in the floor service of a hotel and in other public areas of the lounge.

WINE BUTLER/WINE WAITER/SOMMELIER

Responsible for the service of all alcoholic drinks during the service of meals. This person must have a detailed knowledge of wine and be able to 'sell' wine to customers.

COCKTAIL BAR STAFF

Should be trained in cocktail making with a detailed knowledge of alcoholic beverages. In addition to other staff, cashiers are employed.

FUNCTION AND BANQUETING STAFF

There is normally a small number of banqueting staff in establishments which have facilities for banqueting who are employed on a permanent basis. These include Banqueting Managers, Banqueting Head Waiters, a Banqueting Secretary. Banqueting service staff are normally employed on a casual basis.

Food and wine harmony

The enjoyment of food and wine together is very much a matter of personal taste. Today there is a relaxed attitude. People have broken away from the very rigid approach to the marriage of food and wine. People tend to drink what they like, when they like and tend to be much more open and honest about their wine preferences. Customers should not feel intimidated by wine waiters when they order unconventional food and wine accompaniment.

When selecting a wine to accompany a meal, it is important to understand the compatibility of flavours and textures. This can be gleaned through trial and error. However, there are some general guidelines for the selection of wine to accompany food.

○ Dry wines should be served before sweeter wines.

○ White wines come before red wines.

○ Lighter wines should be served before heavier wines.

○ Good wines should appear before great wines.

Wine can be difficult with certain foods like chocolate, eggs, salads with vinegar dressings, mint sauce and very hot and spicy foods such as curries. If an accompaniment is desired with these foods, then something inexpensive such as light beer, could be chosen.

However, when contemplating possible food and wine partnerships, remember that no guidelines exist to which there are no exceptions. For example, although fish is usually served with white wine, some dishes, such as salmon served with a red wine sauce can be served with a slightly chilled red, e.g. Saint Emilion or Pomerol. The combinations that prove most successful are those that please the customer!

Clearly, the matching of food and wine is very subjective. The overall intention is to provide food and wine which harmonise well together.

Apéritifs

The word apéritif comes from the Latin aperitifs, meaning to open out. In the case of food and wine, this means to stimulate and open out the gastric juices which are opened out to give an appetite for the meal to come. e.g.

○ Champagne, Sherry, Dry white wine, Italian Vermouth, French Vermouth.

EXAMPLES OF WINE ACCOMPANIMENTS

Hors-d'œuvre	Manzanilla sherry, Gewurtztraminer
	Sancerre
Clear soups	Madeira
Pasta	Italian wines
	Valpolicella, Chianti, Barolo
Fish – shellfish	Champagne, Chablis, Muscadet, Soave, Frascati
Smoked fish	White Rioja, Hock, White Graves, Verdicchio
Fish dishes with sauces	Vouvray, Montrachet, Riesling
Shallow fried	Vinho Verde
Poached	Moselle
Grilled fish	Californian Chardonnay
	Australian Sémillon or Chardonnay

White meats

The type of wine to serve is dependent on whether the white meat (chicken, turkey, rabbit, veal or pork) is served hot or cold.

Hot with sauce or savoury stuffing	Rosé Anjou, Beaujolais, New Zealand Pinot Noir
	Californian Zinfandel, Saint Julien, Bourg and Burgundy
Served cold	Fuller wines such as Hocks, Gran Viña Sol, Sancerre
	Rosés from Provence and Tavel

OTHER MEATS

Duck and goose	Châteauneuf-du-Pape, Hermitage, Barolo,
	Australian Cabernet, Shiraz
Roast lamb	Medoc, Saint Emilion, Pomerol
Roast beef – grilled steaks	Burgundies, Rioja, Barolo
Meat stews	Lighter reds, Zinfandel
	Côtes du Rhone, Clos du Bois, Vino Nobile di Montepulciano
Game	Côte Rotie, Rioja, Chianti, Australian Shiraz
	Californian Cabernet Sauvignon, Chilean Cabernet Sauvignon
Oriental foods – Peking duck	Gewürztraminer
Mild curry	Lutomer Riesling
Tandoori	Vinho Verde
Shish kebab	Mateus Rosé, Anjou Rosé

CHEESE

Light cream cheeses – full bodied whites, rosés, and light reds, strong

Pungent and blue vein cheeses – Bordeaux and Burgundy reds, Ports or luscious sweet wines

Sweets	Champagne, Muscats – de Beaumes-de-Venise, de Setúbal de Frontignan, Samos

	Sainte – Croix du Mont, Sauternes, Banyuls, Monbazillac
Dessert (fresh fruit and nuts)	Sherry, Port Madeira, Málaga, Marsala
Coffee	Cognac, Armagnac, Grappa
	Calvados, Liqueurs and ports

Some references to food and beverage service elsewhere in the book

Marketing	337, 450	Customer care	468
Menus	315	Economics	1
Managing people	440	Establishments	10
Beverages	136		

Topics for Discussion

1 Discuss the relationship between the kitchen staff and waiting staff. Explain how good relations may be developed.

2 Discuss the merits of six methods of service and the kind of establishment for which they would be suitable.

3 Why should food service staff be knowledgeable about the food dishes they will serve and why should the kitchen staff appreciate the role of the waiting staff?

4 Explain your reasons for what you consider to be a suitable selection for a wine list. State the kind of establishment you have in mind.

5 Discuss the statement *Every chef should serve as a waiter and every waiter work as chef for a period of time*.

6 What is your opinion of the kitchen being on view to the customers? What do you think is the opinion of customers?

CHAPTER 12

CHEMISTRY IN THE KITCHEN AND PRODUCT DEVELOPMENT

UNDERSTANDING BASIC CHEMISTRY

Modern day chefs are encouraged to be creative, to use their flair and imagination to create interesting and appetising dishes. An understanding of the basic chemistry of food products will help chefs in their work to produce dishes that are practically feasible. A knowledge of how ingredients perform under different conditions is also valuable in development work.

PH AND WATER *(see also page 189)*

Pure water has a pH of 7.0. Water is seldom pure. Rain water and distilled water sometimes contain dissolved materials. All water contains dissolved gases from the air. Distilled water has enough dissolved carbon dioxide to make it distinctly acidic. The pH of distilled water is approximately 5.5 and rainwater can be even lower when it washes certain industrial pollutants out of the atmosphere. This is known as acid rain.

Dissolved gases contribute to the flavour of water. The nature of water often affects the food we cook in it. For example, hard water causes difficulties when cooking pulses since magnesium and calcium interfere with tenderising these foods. Likewise an acidic cooking medium will stop dried beans from absorbing water and soften properly.

Not only is water a component of all foods, but it contributes significantly to the physical differences among foods and to the changes that foods undergo.

PROTEINS

Proteins are an important part of many foods and ingredients that a chef uses. Amino acids are the structural units of proteins. There are some twenty different amino acids found in proteins. The nature of the protein is determined both by the proportions of each amino acid and by the order in which they are arranged. A typical protein may contain 500 amino acids; this means that there can be much variation between different types of protein.

Proteins are the most complex substances known. For example, glucose has a simple molecular weight of 180 daltons (dalton is the measurement of the relative molecular mass devised by John Dalton in 1808) whereas a simple amino acid such as lactoglobulin has a molecular weight of 4200. Some proteins have a molecular weight of several million.

The structure of an amino acid can affect its chemical properties. The general structure is shown below:

R represents residual
part of molecule

AMINO GROUP
(NH$_2$)
reacts with acid

H   R   O
\ | //
N— C — C
/ | \
H   H   OH

CARBONYL GROUP
(COOH)
reactions with alkali

The majority of amino acids have only one carbonyl and amino group. They are termed **neutral**. If more than one amino group is present the amino acid is called **basic**. If more than one carbonyl group is present it is called **acidic**. Development chefs do not need to know about the proportion or order of the amino acids in a protein. What they should be concerned with is the shape of the protein, and how this shape can be changed.

The amino acids are held together in their long chains by what are called 'strong bonds' which are very hard to break. To split up the proteins into amino acids requires conditions such as heating in the presence of a strong acid or by certain enzymes. The procedures in the kitchen are unlikely to break these strong bonds. Cooking has a much greater effect on what is known as secondary structure. Since proteins are long chains, they can double back on themselves to form loops. These loops are held in place by 'weak bonds' to give a secondary structure.

Protein shapes

When developing new products it is advisable to understand the shape of the protein molecule. Many of the cooking processes used by chefs will break the weak bonds and thus change the shape of the molecule. The effect of changing the shape of the protein molecule may be useful but in some cases it may be undesirable. There are two main protein shapes: fibrous and globular.

FIBROUS PROTEINS

Fibrous proteins are insoluble, resistant to acids and alkali and are uneffected by moderate heating. They maintain their strand-like shape. They are often coiled like springs and can be elastic or stretchy. Sometimes two or more strands are twisted together and are held together by weak bonding. Fibrous proteins are generally very tough and are found in animal tissue.

GLOBULAR PROTEINS

These are usually water soluble and affected by acid and alkali. They are shaped like tiny balls with weak bonding. These proteins are not usually part of the structure of the plant or animal, but tend to be functional proteins such as enzymes or storage proteins.

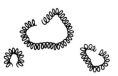

Figure 12.1 *Fibrous protein*

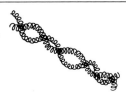

Figure 12.2 *Globular protein*

Denaturing protein

It is important to understand what happens to protein when it is cooked, mixed with other ingredients, or treated by different methods such as whipping. The protein is denatured during cooking. Proteins are denatured when their properties are completely altered; the bonds which hold the protein are broken, these bonds are replaced by other weak bonds not normally present and a new shape is formed. Solubility is decreased, visibility increased and it is an irreversible change.

Proteins can be denatured in many different ways:

○ Heat: normal cooking methods;
○ Salting: by adding salt;
○ Mechanical action: whipping egg whites;
○ Enzymes: meat tenderisers;
○ Acid: by adding acid, yogurt, sour cream.

EFFECT OF HEAT ON GLOBULAR PROTEINS

Making an egg custard is an example. The main ingredients are milk, sugar and eggs. They are beaten together before the cooking process. As it cooks the mixture thickens. The thickening is due to the heat denaturation of the egg proteins. First the egg albumen molecules, in this case

Figure 12.3 *Food analysis*

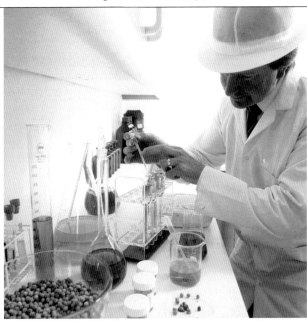

the globular proteins, are moved about by the input of heat energy. As this movement becomes more vigorous, the weak bonds that hold the globules in place start to break up. Secondly, the protein chains start to unfold and may come into contact with other chains and form new weak bonds. Thirdly, a stable three-dimensional mesh of large molecules is formed. This mesh traps many small pockets of water and limits the movement of the water. The effect is a thick smooth texture. If the egg custard is allowed to continue cooking the protein mesh will contract or coagulate and squeeze out the pockets of water. The custard will then curdle and resemble lumps of scrambled egg suspended in milk. This loss of water is known as syneresis. The presence of salt or acid will speed up the process of coagulation. This is evident if vinegar is added to water for poaching eggs.

EFFECT OF HEAT ON FIBROUS PROTEINS

Although fibrous proteins do not dissolve in water they do have capacity to attract and bind water. This is often important in meat cooking particularly when producing chopped meat or minced products that require moisture to be added to them.

When fibrous proteins are heated they contract and squeeze out the associated water. For example when fillet steak is cooked the protein called myosin coagulates at 71°C (160°F). If the temperature continues to increase, the protein contracts, squeezes out much of the water associated with it and thus becomes drier and the eating quality is impaired. For a tender, juicy fillet steak the chef would heat the steak just sufficiently to sear the outside. This will also melt any fat, acting as a lubricant and improving the overall tenderness and eating quality.

Cuts of meat can consist of large amounts of connective tissue, for example collagen and elastin. Collagen is tough and chewy. Elastin is stretchy and heating has little effect on it except helping to produce a tougher product. Meat that contains high proportions is naturally tougher and therefore not usually suitable for prime cooking. Collagen will denature becoming water soluble when heated in water. This then becomes gelatine.

TYPES OF PROTEIN FOUND IN FOOD

TYPE	PROTEIN	WHERE FOUND
fibrous	collagen	connective tissue
fibrous	elastin	connective tissue
fibrous	gluten	wheat flour
fibrous	albumen	egg white, milk
fibrous	casein	milk
fibrous	enzymes	many tissues
fibrous	myosin	muscle

EFFECTS OF ACIDS ON PROTEINS *(See page 189 for information on pH)*

Acids play an important part in cooking procedures:
○ as a component in raising agents in baking powder;
○ as a preservative in yogurt;
○ as a tenderising agent in meats.

The citric acid in lemon juice will slow down any browning reaction on cut fruit.

Proteins can also be denatured by acids. The albumen in milk is a globular protein. In its natural

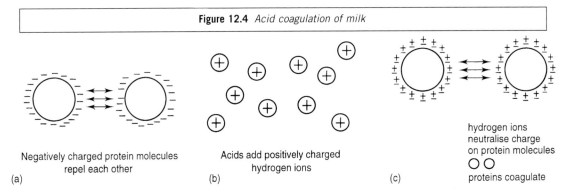

Figure 12.4 *Acid coagulation of milk*

Negatively charged protein molecules repel each other
(a)

Acids add positively charged hydrogen ions
(b)

hydrogen ions neutralise charge on protein molecules

proteins coagulate
(c)

state, each albumen molecule carries a negative electrical charge. Charged particles are similar to north and south poles on magnets, that is like repels like: whenever a negative particle gets near another negative particle they repel each other and remain separate.

If acid is added to milk (see Figure 12.4), then we are adding hydrogen ions which are very small positively charged particles. The hydrogen ions (positively charged) are attracted to the albumen globules (negatively charged) and the two neutralise each other. The albumen is then electrically neutral, and any globules that come in contact stick together or coagulate and form a mass with a gel-like, semisolid consistency. This process is useful in food preparation, for example in cheese making, yogurt and sour cream.

EFFECT OF MECHANICAL ACTION ON PROTEIN

The bonds that maintain the shape of protein molecules are so weak that we are able to break them by agitating the molecules, for example meringues, which are foams (relatively stable masses of air bubbles which are pockets of gas surrounded by a thin film of water). Foams in beer are less stable because there is no stabiliser present.

By whipping egg whites we are adding air and physically agitating the egg white globular proteins. The mechanical stresses resulting from the physical agitation and contact with air act to unfold the globular proteins. The unfolded proteins associate to form a sort of mesh reinforcement of the bubble walls. (This can be considered as the culinary equivalent of quick-setting cement). The egg white foam is relatively stable because it is held together by proteins, while the foam in a head of beer quickly deflates.

Gluten gives bread dough both its elasticity and plasticity. Gluten is formed by two proteins, gliadin and glutenin, coming together in the presence of water; they form a tangled mass of protein molecules. During kneading, the gluten molecules are physically rearranged from a tangled mass to a series of parallel sheets. The molecules in the sheets of gluten are shaped like tiny springs and account for the stretchy nature of bread dough. The sheets of gluten act to trap the gas formed by the yeast growing in the dough and allow the bread to rise.

Enzymes

Enzymes are proteins which are catalysts, meaning that they speed up chemical reactions. Enzymes catalyse a wide range of chemical reactions that take place in all living things. Some enzymes are useful while others lower the quality of foods. An example of one enzyme is rennet added to milk to produce junket.

Each enzyme requires an optimum temperature in which to work. At lower temperatures they will act more slowly and at higher temperatures they will gradually be destroyed. The optimum temperature for an enzyme that comes from a mammal is often close to 37°C (98.6°F) (body temperature). Enzymes are also affected by acidity and can sometimes be controlled by changing the pH. An example of this is using lemon juice to stop the enzyme-catalysed browning of apples.

EFFECT OF HEAT ON MATERIALS FOUND IN MEAT

MEAT MATERIAL	WHAT HAPPENS	EFFECT
muscle protein (myosin)	fibres shrink and lose water	meat becomes tougher and
connective tissue (collagen)	heat plus water causes collagen to denature	drier gelatine is formed
fat	fat melts and acts as a lubricant	meat seems more tender

AGEING OF MEAT – THE ROLE OF ENZYMES

Like cheese and wine, meat benefits from a period of 'ageing' or slow chemical change, before it is consumed. The flavour improves and it becomes more tender. As lactic acid accumulates in the tissue after slaughter, it begins to break down the walls of lysosomes, the cell bodies that store protein-attacking enzymes. As a result, these enzymes will digest proteins indiscriminately. Flavour changes result from the degradation of proteins into individual amino acids, which generally have a strong flavour. It is not clear whether these same enzymes also tenderise the meat by breaking up the actin–myosin complex.

Glycogen, a carbohydrate energy reserve, is stored by the animals. It is glycogen which is converted to the lactic acid required in the ageing process. Glycogen cannot be converted to carbon dioxide and water as it would be in the living animal due to the lack of oxygen, instead it is converted to lactic acid. The lactic acid lowers the pH of the muscle from about 7.0 in the living animal to 5.6 in the dead animal. The lactic acid breaks down the structures in the cells that contain enzymes capable of digesting protein. Protein muscle fibres are partly digested. As a result of these changes the meat is softer and more tender. It has been partially degraded by its own enzymes.

For these changes to occur during ageing it is necessary to have an adequate supply of glycogen in the muscle when the animal is slaughtered. If the animal is not fed or subjected to

stress before slaughter the glycogen will have been used up, and the desirable post-mortem changes will not take place. This meat will be darker in colour and tougher in texture.

ENZYME EFFECTS ON FOODS

FOOD	CHANGE	ENZYME SOURCE
Desirable changes		
black tea	oxidation similar to browning of apples	naturally present
beef	tenderising during ageing	naturally present
bananas and apples	conversion of starch to sugar during ripening	naturally present
meat	tenderisers	paw paw, pineapple
Cheddar cheese	conversion of milk to 'curds and whey'	calves' stomach
starch	conversion of starch to glucose syrups	moulds
Undesirable Changes		
fatty meats	development of rancidity	naturally present
fruit jellies	failure to set when using fresh pineapple or paw paw	present in fruit
fruits and vegetables	development of brown colour where exposed to air	naturally present

CARBOHYDRATES

These can be sugars and non-sugars:

Carbohydrates are an extremely diverse group of substances. Simple sugars are the first products of the photosynthetic process in plants. Plants trap energy from sunlight using the green pigment called chlorophyll and use it to produce sugars from carbon dioxide and water. In this way plants are the ultimate source of all our food. Sugars may be more or less sweet. Generally the more complex carbohydrates lack a sweet flavour. The number in the chart below under 'sweetness' for simple sugars compares the relative sweetening power of a sugar to sucrose. Values greater than 100 are sweeter and values less than 100 are less sweet than an equal weight of sugar. Some substances are considerably sweeter than sugar. For example saccharin would have a value of 3000. This means that 1 g of saccharin has the sweetening power of 300 g of sucrose.

Fructose and glucose are monosaccharides. Sucrose, maltose and lactose are disaccharides.

Complex carbohydrates are composed of long chains of sugars up to 1000 units in length.

Sugars in cooking

The first concentrated sweetener was honey. Bees produce honey from nectar (a weak solution of sucrose produced by flowers). The bees use an enzyme in their saliva to break down the sucrose into fructose and glucose, and concentrate the nectar by evaporating some of the water. Honeys can contain small amounts of other substances found in the nectar from some plants which can be poisonous. Honey is used as a flavouring agent, sweetener and as a humectant (water-holding property). Products which contain honey stay moist longer than those made with sugar.

Sugar is also used for volume as it gives bulk to baked goods, ice-creams, jams and confectionery. It assists in the leavening of some cakes by assisting the incorporation of air. Air is incorporated into cake-making during the creaming process by the physical action of the sugar crystals dragging pockets of air into the fat. The size of crystals affects the properties of the sugar. If the crystals are too large, few pockets of air will be incorporated. If too fine the sugar will dissolve rather than remain in discrete crystals. Sugar is also necessary for the action of pectin for the setting of jams and preserves.

Sugar can contribute to the colour of cooked food products by caramelisation or through the Maillard reaction. Both processes require high temperatures. The Maillard reaction requires the presence of sugar and protein. Both react together at relatively low temperatures, but this is only significant at above 149°C (300°F). The high temperatures required for both these reactions to occur explain why steamed foods are often blander than roasted foods. The Maillard reaction is responsible for colour and flavour in foods such as roasted meats, nuts, coffee beans, bread crusts, etc. Lactose is more likely to participate in the Maillard reaction than some other sugars. Lactose and protein are found in milk. Thus bread brushed with milk before baking will have an attractive brown crust on removal from the oven.

The viscosity of many liquids is affected by sugar.

TYPES OF CARBOHYDRATES

SUGARS	NON-SUGARS
monosaccharides	polysaccharides (starch)
disaccharides	complex polysaccharides
trisaccharides	(pectin, alginates)
tetrasaccharides	

SIMPLE CARBOHYDRATES FOUND IN FOOD

NAME	SIMPLE SUGARS SWEETNESS	OCCURRENCE IN FOODS
fructose (fruit sugar)	170	fruits, jams, honey
sucrose (table sugar)	100	many foods
glucose (blood sugar)	70	grapes, honeys, jams
lactose (milk sugar)	40	milk, milk products
maltose (malt sugar)	30	malt, glucose syrup

COMPLEX CARBOHYDRATES FOUND IN FOOD

NAME	OCCURRENCE IN FOODS
starch	flours, potatoes, corn
inulin	Jerusalem artichokes
cellulose	vegetables, whole grain cereals
pectin	fruits, jams

Complex carbohydrates

These are important in product development because they have a major influence on the texture of foods.

STARCH

Starch is found in foods that come from plants. It consists of long straight or branched chains of glucose molecules. The plant makes starch as a means of storing glucose. Starch is found in seeds, roots and tubers and stored in the form of granules or grains. The starch granules from different sources show characteristic sizes and shapes. Starch molecules in the granules are of two types. One is a long chain of glucose units called *amylose*, accounting for 20–30% of the starch. The rest is a branched molecule shaped rather like a bush called *amylopectin*.

Figure 12.5 *Types of starches*

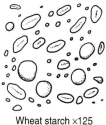

Wheat starch ×125

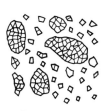

Oat starch ×125

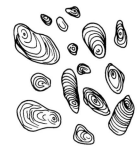

Potato starch ×125

When starch granules are mixed with cold water, they will only absorb water and swell to a limited extent. The water cannot penetrate between the strongly attached starch chains. As the water is heated, the molecules of water move more rapidly, and thus begin to penetrate the starch grains; the water causes the grain to swell. As swelling occurs the mixture thickens. Some of the starch molecules burst out from the granule and form a tangled mass that contributes to the thickening process known as gelatinisation.

The temperature at which gelatinisation occurs depends upon the type of starch used and generally varies from 60°C (140°F) for potato starch, 83°C (181.4°F) for corn starch. As a rule large starch granules gelatinise at lower temperatures than small starch granules.

Starch grains must be separated before any heat is applied. The chef is able to do this in three ways.

○ disperse the starch in cold liquid;
○ mix the starch grains with sugar;
○ coat the grains with solid or melted fat as in the making of a roux.

The thickening capacity of starches depends on the following facts.

○ The type of starch used is important. Arrowroot has a greater thickening capacity than corn or potato starch. High amylose starches have better thickening properties because of the long chain-like molecules which are more likely to become tangled than the compact amylopectin molecules.
○ Thickening properties are changed by heat treatment. For example, the browning of flour in the oven has less thickening power because of the chemical changes caused by using this method of heating.
○ Sugar decreases the thickness of starch-thickened fillings. The effect of sugar is related to its water-attracting ability; available water is reduced and this allows the starch granules to swell.
○ Acid reduces the thickening power of starch. The acid breaks down the starch chains. This breakdown occurs faster if the reaction takes place at high temperature. Therefore any acid required for flavour should be added at the end of gelatinisation to minimise the acid hydrolysis of the starch.

COMPLEX CARBOHYDRATES IN PLANT CELL WALLS

Pectin, cellulose, hemicellulose are found in plants. Cellulose and hemicellulose form the rigid walls around each cell. Pectin is found between the cell walls and acts as a glue-like substance which holds the cells together. All three substances contribute to the fibre in our diets. Rigid cellulose in the cell walls provides much of the crunchiness in vegetables. Cellulose is not water-soluble and is not affected much by cooking. Pectins, however, can be particularly dissolved by hot water. This is exactly what happens when vegetables are cooked and accounts for the softer texture of cooked vegetables and fruit.

Hemicellulose will dissolve in the presence of alkali. Vegetables cooked in the presence of carbonate of soda lose their structure and will become mushy if cooking is continued.

Pectins are used to set jams and jellies and are in flan gel and commercial dessert mixes. Fruits can be divided into high pectin and low pectin types. The low pectin types require the addition of pectin or may be mixed with a high pectin fruit to allow gelling. Pectins are long chains of sugars, which form a network trapping water to form the gel.

A firm gel depends on:

○ percentage of pectin;
○ molecular weight of the pectin;
○ percentage of methyl ester groups;
○ amount of sugar;
○ pH of the mix.

Most gels are made with about 65% sugar; in excess of this crystallisation will occur on the surface.

Most pectin products will not form gels until the pH is lowered to about 3.5. The firmness of the gelling increases as the pH is lowered. A pH lower than the optimum will cause a weak gel and water separating (syneresis).

TYPES OF PECTIN USED TO DEVELOP FOOD PRODUCTS

○ *Rapid-set pectins:* degree of methyl group 70%, forming gels with acid and sugar; optimum pH is 3.5; starts to gel on cooling to 88°C (190.4°F).

○ *Slow-set pectins:* degree of methyl groups 50–70%, gels with sugar and acid; pH 2.8–3.2; starts to gel at 54°C (129°F).

○ *Low methoxyl pectins:* degree of methyl ester groups <30%; these do not form gels with acid and sugar but will gel in the presence of calcium ions or other polyvalent ions (milk).

Pectin is added to natural juice products to give a permanent cloudiness. Pectin is used as a stabiliser in ice-cream products to prevent large crystals forming. It may also be used in mayonnaise as an emulsifying agent.

LIPIDS

Lipids include fats, oils, cholesterol and certain emulsifying agents known as phospholipids. An example is lecithin found in egg yolk. An important feature of these materials is that they are 'hydrophobic' or repel water.

Lipids are important in food production. They contribute to the eating quality of cakes, pastries, biscuits; they affect the texture of yeast products by separating the gluten layers and, in pastry making, by shortening the gluten strands.

Lipids in culinary work

○ Cooking medium – provides heat transfer; used as a lubricant.

○ Texture – gives goods a 'shorter texture'; provides smooth mouth feel; aids aeration; aids moistness; provides volume in bread.

○ Emulsification – emulsifies sauces, ice-creams, etc.

○ Flavour – provides a flavouring agent (butter, olive oil, peanut oil); acts as a solvent for some flavour components of foods.

SOURCES OF FATTY ACID TYPES

TYPE OF FATTY ACID	NUMBER OF DOUBLE BONDS	WHERE FOUND
saturated	0	palm oil coconut oil butter beef fat mutton fat lard
monosaturated	1	olive oil peanut oil lard
polyunsaturated	2 or more	corn oil soya bean oil sunflower oil walnut oil

Lipid structure

In order to use lipids effectively in food production we must know something about their behaviour, or their molecular structure. Fats and oils are triglycerides, meaning they are comprised of three molecules of fatty acids, bonded to one molecule of glycerol.

$$
\text{glycerol}
\left\{
\begin{array}{l}
\text{fatty acid} - 1 \\
\text{fatty acid} - 2 \\
\text{fatty acid} - 3
\end{array}
\right.
$$

The way fats and oils behave is affected by the nature of the fatty acid. The fatty acids consist of chains of carbon atoms that vary in length from 4 to about 20 carbon atoms. Molecules with short-chain fatty acids will have a lower melting point than those with long-chain fatty acids. These fatty acids may also be divided up into saturated and unsaturated groups. All fats contain a mixture of saturated and unsaturated fatty acids. The difference between a saturated fat and an unsaturated fat is based on their individual chemistry. The chains of carbon atoms that make up fatty acids may be joined together with what is known as a 'single bond' or with a double bond.

```
      H   H   H   H
      |   |   |   |
...— C — C — C — C —...
      |   |   |   |
      H   H   H   H
         Single bond
```

```
   H   H           H
   |   |           |
   C — C — C = C — C
   |   |   |   |
   H   H   H   H
        Double bond
```

If the fatty acid contains no double bonds it is called a saturated fatty acid. If it contains one double bond it is monounsaturated and if there is more than one double bond it is called polyunsaturated.

The saturated fatty acids are found in animal fats and in a few oils from tropical plants such as palm oil and coconut oil. Olive oil is mostly monounsaturated, while sunflower, corn and peanut oils and margarine made from these oils are highly unsaturated.

Types of fatty acids

○ Never in fats
- Formic methanoic   – Acetic ethanoic   – Propionic

○ Only found in butter
- Butyric   – Caproic   – Caprillic

○ Most common
- Capric   – Myristic   – Stearic
- Lauric   – Palmitic

FACTORS AFFECTING THE DEVELOPMENT OF RANCIDITY IN FATS

FACTOR	EFFECT
water	necessary for development of rancidity by hydrolysis
heat	speeds up most chemical reactions including development of rancidity
lipases (enzymes which split fats)	present in certain foods and can cause rancidity
metal ions (iron)	speeds up development of rancidity in fats, e.g. cast iron pans
light	speeds up oxidation
salt food particles	speeds up development of rancidity

Important facts in the chemistry of fats

○ Most fats contain at least five different sorts of fatty acids in their make-up.

○ The number of triglycerides is large.

○ Oleic acid is the most important of all the fatty acids occurring in fats. Often it is more than 50% of the total fatty acids in a fat and it is always present in a fat.

○ If a particular saturated acid is present, then it very often happens that the acids immediately above and below it in the fatty acid series also occur.

Spoilage of fats and oils

Fats require care to maintain quality. They may deteriorate because of:

○ odours: many compounds that have a strong aroma can dissolve in fats; if fats are stored in an open container they are able to absorb these odours.

○ rancidity: this is caused by the presence of free fatty acids which have an unpleasant smell; for example, butyric acid accounts for the smell of rancid butter; caproic acid has a very strong smell; rancid fats are able to impart their smell to any foods they are used in or are cooked in.

One way that rancidity develops is when some of the fat molecules are split by a reaction with water that releases fatty acids and glycerol. The action involves an enzyme and is called hydrolysis.

Oxidation will also cause rancidity. This involves the reaction of unsaturated fatty acids with oxygen to release small fatty acids and other molecules that affect the flavour and aroma. The development of rancidity by hydrolysis or oxidation occurs faster under certain conditions.

Other factors can slow down the development of fat oxidation. These are known as antioxidants. They can be naturally occurring or artificial. Examples include vitamin E, ascorbic acid, and certain herbs such as sage and rosemary. Artificial antioxidants include butylated hydroxyanisole (BHA) and butylated hydroxytoluene (BHT). These are added to many commercial fats. Antioxidants only slow the development of rancidity in fats. They cannot prevent it totally.

EMULSIONS

The hydrophobic nature of fats and oils presents problems when developing recipes in attempting to make a stable dispersion of an oil and water. Emulsifiers stabilise dispersion of the immiscible liquids. The stable dispersion is called an emulsion. Emulsifiers can be proteins, plant gums or resins, starch, or very small particles such as ground mustard. Thus mustard added to a vinaigrette acts as an emulsifying agent as well as a flavouring agent.

The type of emulsion formed by an oil-water system depends upon a number of factors:

○ the composition of the oil and water phases;
○ the chemical nature of the emulsifying agent;
○ the proportions of the oil and water present.

If the polar group of an emulsifier is more effectively adsorbed than the non-polar group, adsorption by the water is greater than by the oil. The extent of adsorption at a liquid surface depends upon the surface area of liquid available, and increased adsorption of emulsifier by water is favoured by the oil–water interface becoming convex towards the water, thus giving an oil–water emulsion.

The relative proportions of oil and water also help to determine which type of emulsion forms. If more oil than water is present, the water tends to form droplets and a water–oil emulsion is formed. If more water than oil is present an oil–water emulsion is favoured.

Artificial emulsifiers are added during the preparation of many emulsions. An example is GMS (glyceryl monostearate). GMS is a monoglyceride which is formed when one hydroxyl group of glycerol is esterified with stearic acid.

For example:

$$CH_2OH$$
$$|$$
$$CHOH + CH_3(CH_2)_{16}COOH \quad \rightarrow$$
$$|$$
$$CH_2OH$$

$$CH_2OH$$
$$|$$
$$CHOH + H_2O$$
$$|$$
$$CH_2O—CO(CH_2)_{16}CH_3$$

hydrophobic portion

of glyceril monostearate

One part of the GMS molecule is hydrophilic because it contains hydroxyl groups and the rest of the molecule, as indicated, is hydrophobic. When GMS is added to a water–oil emulsion the hydrophilic parts of the molecules are absorbed into the surface of the water droplets and the lipophilic parts are absorbed into the surface of the oil round drops as shown in Figure 12.6, page 417.

Lecithin is the phospholipid emulsifier found in egg yolk and is also extracted from vegetable oils. The structure of lecithin is a triglyceride of two fatty acids and phosphoric acid.

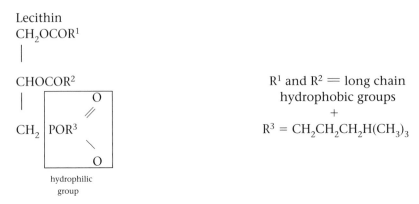

Lecithin
$$CH_2OCOR^1$$
$$|$$

$$CHOCOR^2$$

$$CH_2 \; | \; POR^3$$

hydrophilic
group

R^1 and $R^2 =$ long chain hydrophobic groups

$+$

$R^3 = CH_2CH_2CH_2H(CH_3)_3$

In many recipes, stabilisers are added to products in addition to emulsifiers. Stabilisers are proteins, carbohydrates, starches, gums. Their function is to hold the emulsion together once it has been formed. Such substances improve the stability of emulsions mainly by increasing their viscosity. Viscosity increases, the freedom of movement of the dispersed droplets of the emulsion is reduced, and this lessens the chance of their coming into contact and coalescing.

If you add oil or butter when making hollandaise or mayonnaise, the sauce may curdle because the lecithin has had insufficient time to coat the droplets. This can be rectified by adding the broken sauce to more egg yolks.

The most important characteristic of emulsions is that they require energy for their formation.

Figure 12.6 *Molecules of emulsifier absorbed at a water – oil interface forming a complete protective film around a water droplet*

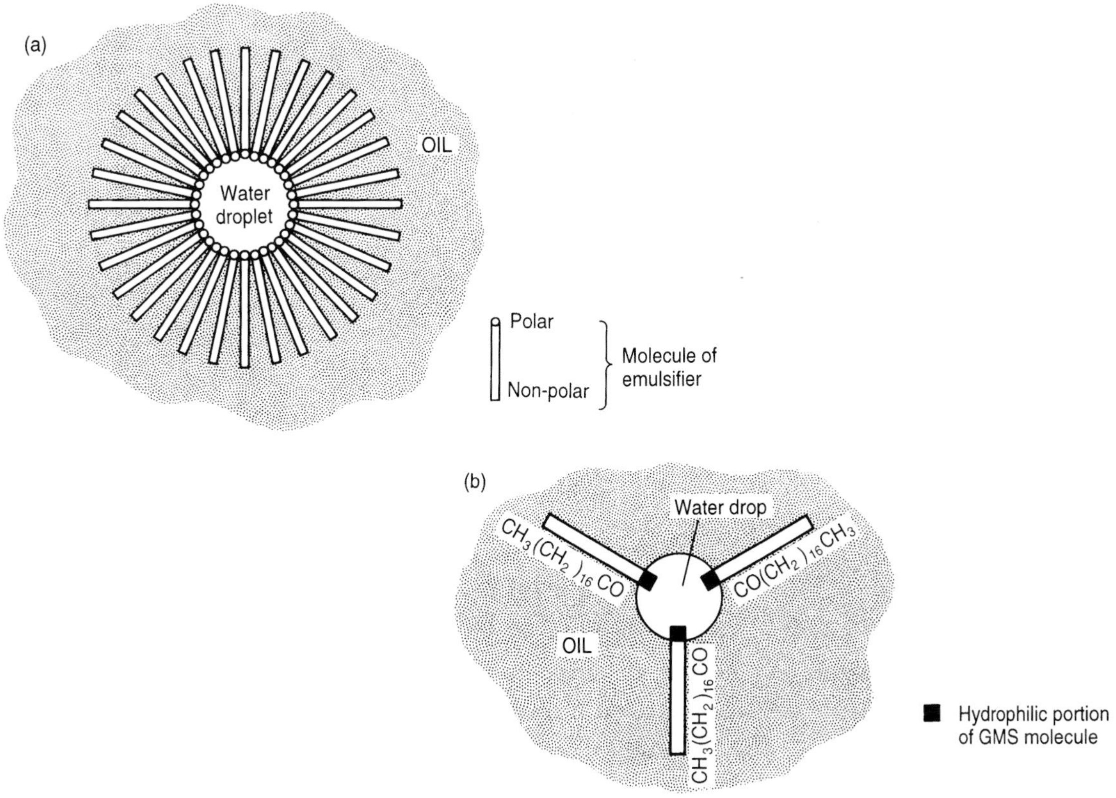

SENSORY EVALUATION OF FOOD

The most important thing to remember when applying chemistry to food products is that the food must ultimately give pleasure to the consumer. This is dependent on appearance, flavour, smell and texture. These are assessed by our senses. Scientists use complex and expensive equipment to measure the factors in food that determine the taste, aroma or tenderness. The process is based on objective assessment and is vital in product development.

When referring to our senses we are concerned with vision, hearing, smell, touch and taste. Some scientists add three more: temperature, pain and balance. Except for balance, all these senses are used to relay messages about the food.

Taste and smell are the most important chemical receptors and are often used with the most expensive equipment found in food laboratories. Vision and smell operate at a distance, meaning that the individual does not have to come into contact with the food to use these senses.

Examples of the messages that a sense tells us about food.

- Vision
  - colour
  - size
  - shape
  - freshness
  - maturity
  - quality
- Smell
  - freshness
  - ripeness
  - character
  - identification
- Hearing
  - sizzling related to temperature
  - texture, crispness, crunchiness
- Touch
  - texture
  - consistency
  - ripeness
  - mouth-feel
- Taste
  - salt
  - sweet
  - sour
  - bitter
- Temperature
  - hot/cold
  - chilled
- Pain
  - chilli pepper

EXAMPLES OF TYPES OF TASTE

TASTE	EXAMPLE
sweet	sugar, saccharin, aspartame, cyclamates
salt	sodium chloride
bitter	alkaloids (in caffeine)
sour	acids, vinegar, lemon juice
metallic	potassium chloride found in some salt substitutes
soapy	after-taste in baking powder goods

When we eat and enjoy food the messages we receive by our senses are harmonious and from a much more complicated picture than that gained by one sense on its own. Flavour is a combination of smell, taste and mouth-feel. If any one of these components is missing, for example smell when we have a cold, the overall impact is changed.

Cooking and processing food is the use of chemical technology to create a harmonious product using colour, smell, taste, texture and mouth-feel. A knowledge of basic food ingredients and their chemistry will help the chef both develop new recipes, dishes and give him/her a knowledge of how to correct dishes when things go wrong.

Vision

Colour has an effect on the eye appeal, having an overall effect on the presentation of the food.

The colour of food is extremely important to our enjoyment of it. People are sensitive to the colour of the food they eat and will reject food that is not considered to have the accepted colour. For example, strawberries that have been preserved in sulphite lose all their natural colour and appear white. If strawberries are to be canned or used in jam, artificial colour must be added before they are considered acceptable to eat. Colour is added to a wide range of food products to enhance attractiveness.

There is a strong link between the colour and the flavour of food. An ability to detect flavour of food is very much connected with its colour and if the colour is unusual our sense of taste is confused. For example, if a fruit jelly is red, it is likely that the flavour detected will be that of a red coloured fruit such as a strawberry even if the true flavour is lemon or banana.

The depth of colour in food also affects our sense of taste. We associate strong colours with strong flavour. For example, if a series of jellies all contain the same amount of given flavour, but are of different shades of the same colour, then those having a stronger colour will appear also to have a stronger flavour.

Smell

Smell is a chemical sense that acts over a distance. Chemicals are detected by their volatile compounds, this means that they must evaporate and become airborne easily. Smell receptors are located in the back of the nasal cavity known as the olfactory area.

The air is able to reach the olfactory area through both the nose and the mouth. Many of the characteristics are associated as flavours actually are related to smell rather than taste. When we eat food, the volatile components evaporate and reach the olfactory area through the back of the throat that connects the mouth and nasal cavity. When we have a cold, the membranes of the nasal cavity swell and prevent access to the area containing the smell receptors. We say we cannot taste when we mean we actually cannot smell the food.

The sense of smell is very sensitive, it may be divided into the following basic types:

- pungent;
- putrid;
- camphoric;
- musky;
- floral;
- peppermint;
- ethereal.

Figure 12.7 *The olfactory area*

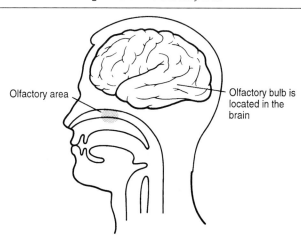

Olfactory area

Olfactory bulb is located in the brain

EXAMPLES OF TEXTURES ENCOUNTERED IN FOOD

FOOD	TEXTURE	FOOD	TEXTURE

cheese	solid
	   elastic
	   crumbly
	   creamy
	melted
	   liquid
	   viscous
		sauces
		
		vegetables
		
		soups
			thick
			thin
			lumpy
			crisp
			crunchy
			soft
			thick
			thin
			lumpy

Taste

Taste is another chemical sense, but unlike smell it does not work at a distance. The messages we receive from taste are simpler than those of smell. There are four basic tastes: salt, sweet, sour and bitter; metallic and soapy tastes may also be included.

Taste buds are located on the tongue. Babies and children have more taste buds than adults, the number decreases with age.

For a substance to give a sensation of taste it must be soluble in water. When we eat food, some of it dissolves in saliva which contributes to the taste sensation we experience.

Our reactions to taste differ considerably. Many taste preferences are learnt in childhood. We generally are much more sensitive to bitter than to any other tastes, meaning we are able to taste smaller amounts of bitter substances than of sweet, salty or sour substances.

Taste is affected by several factors. Flavour enhancers, for example MSG (monosodium glutamate), increase the intensity of both salt and bitter tastes and of 'meatiness'.

The temperature of food also affects the way we perceive taste. We are most sensitive to taste when the food is between 22° and 41°C (71.6–105.8°F). Temperatures above and below this range decrease the sensitivity of the taste buds.

Touch

Touch referring to sensory evaluation is mouth-feel, the way food feels in the mouth. Mouth-feel is very important when we assess or develop food products, recipes and dishes. Mouth-feel adds to the food acceptability. Texture is a message we receive from mouth-feel. This includes consistency, chewiness, brittleness, crunchiness, astringency, etc. These sensations add greatly to our enjoyment of food.

THE COOKING PROCESSES AND THE EFFECTS ON FOODS

There are twelve ways of cooking foods.

METHOD	EFFECT ON FOODS
1 Boiling	Gentle boiling helps to break down the tough fibrous structure of certain foods which would be less tender if cooked by other methods. When boiling meats for long periods the soluble meat extracts are dissolved in the cooking liquid. Cooking must be slow to give time for the connective tissue in tough meat to be changed into soluble gelatine, so releasing the fibres and making the meat tender. If the connective tissue gelatinises too quickly the meat fibres fall apart and the meat will be tough and stringy. Gentle heat will ensure coagulation of the protein without hardening. Vegetables should be boiled for the shortest time possible otherwise the nutrient content will be reduced or lost.
2 Poaching	Helps to tenderise the fibrous structure of the food and the raw texture of the food becomes edible by chemical action.
3 Stewing	In the slow process of cooking in gentle heat, the connective tissue in meat and poultry is converted into a gelatinous substance so that the fibres fall apart easily and become digestible. The protein is coagulated without being toughened.
4 Braising	Causes the breakdown of tissue fibre in the structure of certain foods which softens the texture, thus making it tender and edible.
5 Steaming	The structure and texture of food is changed by chemical action and becomes edible.
6 Baking	Chemical action caused by the effect of heat on certain ingredients, e.g. yeast, baking powder, changes to raw structure of many foods to an edible texture (pastry, bread).
7 Roasting and spit-roasting	The surface protein of the food is scaled by the initial heat of the oven, thus preventing the escape of too many natural juices. When the food is highly browned, the oven temperature is reduced to cook the inside of the food without hardening the surface.
8 Grilling	Because of the speed of cooking there is maximum retention of nutrients and flavour because the effect of fierce heat on the surface of meat rapidly coagulates and seals the surface protein thus helping to retain the meat juices.
9 Shallow frying	The high temperature produces almost instant coagulation of the surface protein of the food and prevents the escape of natural juices. Some of the frying medium will be absorbed by the food being fried which will change the nutritional content.

continued

METHOD	EFFECT ON FOODS
10 Deep frying	Foods coated with flour, eggs, milk, breadcrumbs or a batter absorb the minimum amount of fat because the surface is sealed by the coagulation of the protein. Uncoated foods such as chips absorb a huge amount of fat thus affecting the texture and nutritional content.
11 Paper bag cookery	Because the food is tightly sealed in oiled greaseproof paper or foil, no steam escapes during cooking and maximum natural flavour and nutritive value is retained.
12 Microwave cookery	A method of cooking and heating food by using high frequency power. The microwave disturbs the molecules or particles of food and agitate them, thus causing friction which has the effect of cooking the whole of the food. This method of cooking causes the food to become edible by the heat generated. Proteins become denatured, starches are gelatinised, with most of the moisture and flavour being retained.

GENETICALLY MODIFIED FOOD

Scientists can create plants that nature itself has never created – plants that are resistant to chemicals that kill weeds (herbicides), plants that produce chemicals to kill insects (pesticides) and plants that last longer after harvesting. The methods used to produce these new crops involves the crops genes changing or modifying. Genes are contained in the cells of all living things. They guide how living things are made and how they function.

What are genes?

Genes are the recipe for all living things. They act as codes for different traits such as the size or colour of fruit. These traits are passed from one generation to the next. Genes are carried in a chemical called DNA.

DNA stands for deoxyribonucleic acid. Its secret lies in its structure – a long, ladder-like molecule that winds like a spiral staircase.

The rungs of the ladder are made up of chemicals.

Figure 12.8 the DNA ladder

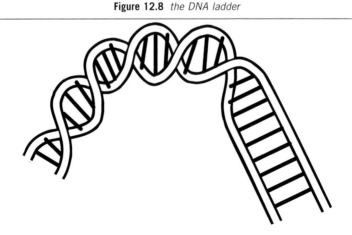

The order of the chemicals along the DNA spiral forms a code that spells out the cell's job, just like letters of the alphabet spell out the words in this book.

Chromosomes

In the nucleus (middle) of a cell there are a certain number of chromosomes. Chromosomes are packages of tightly coiled DNA. In a human the DNA in a single cell, stretched out, would be two metres long; in a whole body, this would make a hundred billion kilometres of DNA. All living things have chromosomes, though not all have the same number; humans have 46 per cell and tomatoes have 24. Half the chromosomes come from the father and half from the mother, so there are two copies of each chromosome, one from each parent.

Genes

There are many, many genes in a chromosome. Each gene is a section of the DNA spiral that is responsible for making a particular protein. Proteins determine what plants and animals look like and how they work. Seen close up DNA looks like a double spiral.

Swapping genes

The secret of swapping genes lies in rings of DNA called plasmids which are found in bacteria. Plasmids seem to be nature's way of moving genes between different organisms. By cutting open the ring and putting in an extra piece of DNA – a gene – the plasmid's genetic message can be changed.

The first experiments were done in bacteria called Esherichia Coli (E.Coli). By modifying the plasmids in these E.Coli cells and growing them in a petri dish, they could be turned into bacterial factories able to make any protein. Different proteins are needed to build the different tissues of living things.

Figure 12.9 *Proteins*

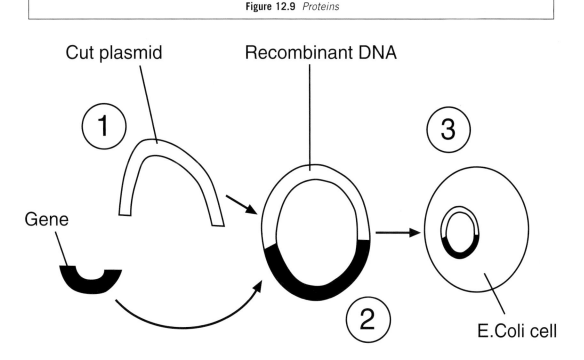

Plasmids can be cut open using enzymes. The cutting process leaves the plasmid with sticky ends. If another stretch of DNA – a gene – is added, it sticks and completes the ring. The result is called recombinant DNA. The new plasmid is then put back into the E.Coli cell.

How is genetic modification done?

Now scientists are going beyond using recombinant DNA in bacteria. By adding genes or stopping existing genes working, they can create crops that resist weed-killers, plants that produce their own insecticides, or tomatoes that go soft more slowly because the gene that makes them rot has been deactivated.

The desired gene is chosen and isolated. This might be a gene that makes strawberries sweeter by producing more sugar. The gene is cut into the plasmid of a bacterium called Agrobacterium Tumefaciens. Cells are taken from the strawberry plants. The bacterium containing the plasmid is mixed with the strawberry cells in a dish which contains a nutrient jelly (Agar) to keep the cells alive. The cells are tested to see which of them have been infected by the bacterium and have accepted the plasmid. The modified cells are encouraged to grow into plants which are then planted in large nurseries to create more plants or seed for sale to farmers.

Some plants, including cereals, cannot be modified by the Agrobacterium method. To modify these plants, genes are coated onto tiny gold pellets which are then fired like a shot from a gun, into plant cells. Some of the genes work inside the cells to produce a modified plant.

Type of modification

The most common GM crops grown at the moment are those that resist herbicides. The second most common are the crops which can kill pests. Some crops have been given both these genes.

A bacterium called Bacillus Thuringiensis (Bt) which is found in the soil, produces a toxin that kills insects but is harmless to people. Putting the Bt toxin gene into maize plants allows them to make their own poison which kills a crop pest called the corn borer.

In future, GM crops that grow in poor, dry or salty soils may be developed. This would make huge areas of worthless land productive.

Potatoes modified to contain less starch could make healthier chips because they do not absorb so much fat in the cooking. GM vegetables produced with added nutrients may help to fight off heart disease and cancer.

Effects on nature

GM plants could have unexpected effects on nature. The poisons intended to kill pests could damage other insects while genes put into the plants could escape in their pollen.

Laboratory experiments in the United States have shown that the Bt toxin intended to kill pests can also kill Monarch butterflies which are harmless to crops. Recent research has shown that GM crops are leaking toxins from their roots into the soil. This affects the soil and may even produce new strains of pests.

Pollen from GM crops may be carried a long distance by wind and cross-pollinate with wild plants or other crops. This may create odd breeds and affect organic crop farmers.

PRODUCT DEVELOPMENT

Introduction

Why produce new recipes and new menus? In order to create or develop customer or consumer satisfaction it is essential to prevent menu apathy and to produce interest, enabling the discovery of new flavours and combinations.

The exercise is two-fold, to satisfy the customer *and* management. Therefore the prime consideration is cost of the development and the selling price. It is essential to consider the style or type of establishment and the kind of clientele for whom the changes are intended, as well as regional variations and food fashions.

The reasons for change could include:

- menu fatigue;
- changes in clientele;
- food fashion changes;
- availability of supplies;
- need to stimulate business;
- new chef and staff;
- opening of similar local establishment etc.

Whatever the cause, it is necessary to introduce new recipes and menus in relation to the organisation's objectives. It follows that in every sphere of catering, whether it is school meals, in hospitals, speciality outlets, exclusive restaurants, recipe and menu changes may need to occur. If new developments are intended it is essential to evaluate:

- the cost of development;
- the effect the change or changes will have on the existing situation;
- the ability of the staff to cope;
- that there is adequate equipment and suitable suppliers;
- the presentation of the dishes;
- the format of the menu.

Recipe development: preparation

Preparation prior to the practical aspects of producing new recipes includes the need to construct a method of recording accurate details of ingredients, their cost, quality and availability. Time needed for preparation, production and yield must also be recorded. Space should be made on the chart to specify several attempts, so that comparison can be made and to ensure that there is adequate space for making notes.

An evaluation sheet is required so that a record is made of the opinions of the tasting panel or persons consulted. This sheet will, as appropriate, be constructed to include space for flavours, colour, texture, presentation, etc.

Developing new ideas

The developing of new recipes is challenging, stimulating and creates new interest, but where do original ideas come from? Many are triggered by creations of others. It is therefore particularly worthwhile to keep abreast of what is happening around us.

PUBLISHING

- Chef magazine in the Caterer and Hotel Keeper;
- books produced by leading chefs;
- magazines, including women's magazines;
- newspaper articles;
- libraries, etc.

TV AND RADIO

- 'Master Chef' competition;
- 'Junior Master Chef' competition;
- 'Ready Steady Cook', for example;
- food programmes.

CONTACTS

- visiting other establishments;
- visiting catering exhibitions;
- lectures, demonstrations;
- competitors;
- catering organisations etc.

Extra care needs to be taken when introducing new recipes to patients in hospitals and nursing homes and in the provision of meals in schools and residential establishments, to ensure the nutritional content is suitable. Dieticians can provide advice on the dietary requirements of these persons.

COMMUNICATION

Information sources for recipes are available everywhere. Every kind of establishment from the local Chinese restaurant to the 5-star hotel can present innovative ideas. Overseas travel can be influential in bringing new dishes to the UK. Department stores, exhibition centres, outdoor events and so on may well also stimulate ideas. The range of ingredients available from catering suppliers is immense, but local markets and supermarkets should not be ignored as other sources of supply.

With new developments in mind, it is necessary to pass on these proposals to both senior management (who will be responsible for their implementation) and to fellow members of the kitchen brigade (for their constructive comments). If possible, put your ideas to the test with respected members of the catering profession with whom you are acquainted. The proposals should include estimated food costing, times to produce, labour costs, equipment and facilities needed and details of staff training if required. Knowledge of the establishment's organisation is important so that the right person or persons are involved.

QUALITY OF MATERIALS

The highest possible standards of ingredients should be used so that a true and valid result is available for assessment of the recipe.

STAFF ABILITIES

The staff's craft skills should be appraised in order to assess their capability in coping with innovations. Failure to do so could jeopardise the whole project. Also their cooperation to put new ideas into practice should be sought; and encouragement given when the outcome is successful.

EQUIPMENT FACILITIES

New recipes can affect the utilisation of existing equipment by overloading at peak times. The capacity of items such as pastry ovens, deep fat fryers or salamanders can already be fully used. New items can affect the production of the present menu; this fact should be borne in mind so that service is not impaired.

COOKING

It goes without saying that accurate cooking is essential with any development and *Practical Cookery* gives guidance on this aspect of the project.

IMPLEMENTATION

Having tested and arrived at the finished recipe staff may need to practise production and presentation of the dish. This may include both small and large quantities depending on the establishment. In all cases careful recording of all aspects of the operation can help in the smooth running of the exercise, in particular basic work study should be observed. Constructive comments by the staff should be asked for, in particular any problems should be discussed.

The results of such trial runs should be conveyed to senior personnel and any problems that have been identified should be resolved.

Having validated the recipe, checked on a reliable supplier, and ensured the capability of the staff, it is important that all concerned know when the dishes will be included on the menu.

Storekeepers, kitchen staff and serving staff need to be briefed and any other departments involved, as to the time and date of implementation.

PRESENTATION

Of particular importance is how the customer sees the dish; when it is received it needs to appeal to the senses of sight and smell – even before taste. Consideration needs to be given early in the development of the idea; what dish or plate will be used, what will accompany it and the skill needed to serve it. Foods in some establishments are prepared and cooked in front of the customer, while some require the dish to be cooked fresh while the customer waits. Therefore, details of presentation must be recorded and where possible a test made in the actual situation.

Should the new recipe be for a food service operation which involves preparation, cooking and presentation before the customer so that the all or part is seen by the potential consumer, then attention needs to be paid to the skills of the chef and extra training, not only culinary skills but customer handling skills may be needed as well as particular attention to hygiene. These factors need to be observed at the development stage so that customer satisfaction occurs immediately.

ORGANISATION

To implement new dishes, adequate time needs to be allowed to test and develop the recipe, to train the staff, to appraise comments and modify recipes if necessary. Staff must be briefed on the composition of the dish, particularly serving staff, as well as being told when it will be included on the menu. They need to be asked if there are any problems and if required this could be in a written form. Senior personnel need to be informed verbally or in writing of the implementation of the new items.

Should the new dish or dishes require skills which are unfamiliar to some staff, then the workload of individuals may need to be changed so as to accommodate staff with the appropriate skill. In estimating how long it will take to implement the new dish factors to take account of are: the skills of the staff, that suitable equipment is available, that suppliers can produce the required ingredients in the right quantity at the desired quality at a suitable price.

Clear written instructions may need to be provided – which means the sequence in which the ingredients are to be used with the appropriate amount (for example 10 portions or 50 portions).

The introduction of a salad bar or sweet trolley including new dishes can affect the service of the usual dishes. If the clientele require, say, vegetarian dishes or those with cultural or religious needs have special requests, then adaptations may be necessary to accommodate this in the existing set-up.

In addition to obtaining feedback from staff, it is just as important, if not more so, to obtain comments from the customer or consumer.

MANAGING RESOURCES WHEN DEVELOPING RECIPES

The following points should be considered:
○ the elimination of waste;
○ the control of materials and ingredients;

○ the careful use of energy;
○ the most effective use of time.

Ensure that a record is kept so that no resources are misused. Failure to control and monitor resources can be expensive in time, materials and effort.

SPECIFIC CONSIDERATIONS

When considering any development, it is necessary to take into account current problems and issues which may affect the outcome. It is essential to keep up-to-date on issues such as the BSE scare and the effect on consumers' choice or rejection of beef. The increasing use of 'organic foods' may encourage customer demand for such foods to be used; all foods are organic but the term has become restricted to mean those grown without the use of pesticides or processed without the use of additives. There is little difference nutritionally between organic and non-organic produce. *The Manual of Nutrition*, published by HMSO, is a most useful reference book for information on nutrition.

Certain groups of people have restrictions on their eating habits which must be observed when producing new recipes for them:

○ **Vegetarians** – no meat, most eat no fish, most eat cheese, eggs and milk.
○ **Vegans** – no food of animal origin.
○ **Hindus** – no beef, mainly vegetables, no alcohol.
○ **Muslims** – no pork, no alcohol, no shellfish, meat: halal (meat killed according to Muslim custom).
○ **Sikhs** – no beef, no alcohol, only meat killed with one blow of head.
○ **Jews** – no pork, meat must be kosher, only fish with fins and scales, meat and dairy produce not to be eaten together.
○ **Rastafarians** – no animal products except milk, no canned or processed foods, no salt added, foods should be organic.

MENU DESIGN

The function of a menu is to inform potential customers what dishes are available and, as appropriate, the number of courses, the choice on the courses and the price. The wording should make clear to the kind of customer using the establishment what to expect. The menu may also be used to promote specific items, such as when an ingredient is in season, childrens' menus, reductions for senior citizens or served at particular times.

If printed, the type should be clear and of readable size; if hand-written, the script should be of good quality so as to create a good impression. Menus are expensive to produce but when attractive and fulfil the function of informing, they may enhance the reputation of the establishment and increase custom.

Some references to chemistry elsewhere in the book

Nutrition	162, 181	pH	189
Preservation	191	Hygiene	510
Bacteria	530		

Further information
Vegan Society, www.vegansociety.com
Vegetarian Society UK Ltd
www.vegsoc.org

Topics for Discussion

1 What advantages does a chef have in understanding basic food science?
2 Why product development is important to food production outlets.
3 How emulsions are formed and stabilised.
4 The effect of heat on proteins and carbohydrates.
5 Current product development in the food and catering industry.
6 How working in a product development kitchen differs from a production kitchen.

PART 5

Organisation and business development

CHAPTER 13

MANAGING RESOURCES

INTRODUCTION

To effectively manage people and resources it is essential to manage oneself; to manage oneself it is essential to analyse oneself truthfully, assess one's weaknesses and take positive action to improve. This is necessary so that self-development improves.

'Know Yourself and to yourself be true' is a maxim which assists the potential manager to develop and earn the respect of those he or she will manage. It is not easy to assess one's own personality, nor is it easy to improve or change it. The following self-analysis guide may be helpful:

Having assessed your strengths and weaknesses, what need or needs do you require to be self-fulfilled or self-satisfied to develop into a successful manager? In catering, because of the variety of roles, most people's needs can be met. These needs include the need:

○ to achieve; to be friendly, to show off; to be tenacious; to be free of controls; to have power; to need sympathy; to seek knowledge; to be orderly; to show care.

Having concluded the kind of person you think you are (which may not be the same as others see you) list your qualities and your failings and endeavour to change those you think should be changed. To be successful in achieving this it is essential to be positive and really want to improve. Be clear about the benefits of what you hope to gain. Know what you want and when things do not go as expected have other options and seek advice and help of others.

Key skills for management

These include:

○ self management;
○ time management;
○ decision making;
○ communication;
○ resource management.

Self management

Effective management starts with how one sees oneself, how superiors see you and how those you are responsible for see you. First impressions and following impressions are vital to successful development as a manager. Firstly what constitutes a good manager, what qualities, attitudes and values are desirable to form the basis from which to improve?

○ Honesty and integrity.
○ Loyalty and conscientiousness.
○ Willingness and cooperativeness.
○ Courteous and caring.
○ Orderly and of neat appearance.
○ Able to lead and set an example.
○ Enthusiastic and punctual etc.

Direction

To progress it is essential to be able to clarify roles, to focus on key issues and to specify targets and standards; that is, to know what direction you are going and how you intend to get there.

Teamwork

When working in a team it is essential to plan, to use the ideas of the team members so that you can be effective.

Actions

Actions need to be taken. Prevarication, hesitancy and lethargy do not help decision-making.

CATEGORY OR TYPE OF PERSON		MANAGEMENT SKILLS WHICH MAY NEED IMPROVING
Confident Bold Arrogant	Self-centred Authoritative Independent	May be too bossy and aggressive, need to develop patience
Optimistic Cheerful Enthusiastic	Sociable Articulate Persuasive	May be too friendly and require greater self discipline in difficult management situations
Relaxed Patient Laid back	Stable Passive Calm	You may be unwilling to change and lack sense of urgency to change

CATEGORY OR TYPE OF PERSON		MANAGEMENT SKILLS WHICH MAY NEED IMPROVING
Careful Neat Perfectionist	Self-disciplined Accurate Aggressive	You may find difficulty in delegating, worry too much and be defensive
Agreeable	Peaceful	May find leadership hard and become
Self-effacing	Unassuming	discouraged in difficult situations
Frustrated	Easily discouraged	
Reserved Quiet Pessimistic	Distant Imaginative Remote	May be shy and unsociable and not good at dealing with people
Restless Erratic Tense	Impetuous Quick Highly strung	May be seen as impatient and intolerantand aggressive, may need to learn to calm down
Independent Stubborn Argumentative	Informal Uninhibited	May be an effective delegator but unreliable and not good at making decisions

However, act by having priorities right and using resources, manpower, financial and equipment and commodities efficiently.

Results

Analyse problems, give and receive feedback and use the information to persuade others, thus improving your own performance.

Positive balanced management

To improve performance clear positive thinking and the ability to generate enthusiasm may be helpful. A flexible approach, sensitive to others' feelings and expectations and capable of inspiring them may well develop confidence in one's own ability.

Decision making

1 Define the aim.
2 Collect the information.
3 List possible courses of action.
4 Evaluate the pros and cons and examine the consequences and make the decisions.
5 Act on the decision, monitor and review it.

Firstly know why a decision has been made and consider the situation and possible solutions. Evaluate how the aim will be achieved, how long it will take and what is its cost? Moreover, is it acceptable? If it is not acceptable, reconsider.

Thinking requires three aspects to make it effective:

○ **Analysing:** breaking the whole into small parts and the complex into simple elements.

○ **Holistic thinking:** thinking of the entirety, the opposite to analysing.
○ **Valuing:** the judgmental and critical aspect.

To make decisions fully effective it is necessary to use all three thought processes. Decisions based on intuition, instinct, or emotion will not produce logical decision-making.

Before making a decision, ensure you have the facts and then decide what to do. Value judgements are effective only if you are aware of your prejudices that may affect your decision and acknowledge them and learn not to be prejudiced.

Also you need to know of any codes of values which are needed by the establishment such as legal requirements and any social behaviour codes and company procedures.

Decision-making styles

AUTOCRATIC

The manager solves the problem based on the information he has.

INFORMATION FINDING

When a manager does not have enough information or skill, he or she asks other people, then makes a decision.

CONSULTATION

The situation is explained to the group who generate and evaluate solutions and make recommendations. The leader makes the decision.

NEGOTIATION

The group are provided with information. They then negotiate a solution which is acceptable.

DELEGATION

Responsibility for the decision rests with a group or an individual. The manager may guide the discussion that leads to the decision, which is then implemented.

Implementation of decision

Having made a decision, determine clear objectives and consider what can be delegated, to whom, the time needed and if further training is necessary.

To action the decision define it in writing, set details of progress report backs.

Time management

To organise oneself efficiently so as to be an effective manager requires attention controlling one's time. Determining priorities is an essential step to this end and can be aided by producing lists and categorising jobs to be done, as well as using a diary effectively.

Time needs to be allocated for tasks such as thinking and planning, as well as using a diary effectively. A good organiser plans both for the expected and the unexpected. Be prepared for problems but allow time to prevent them if possible and allot time for solving them.

It is important to realise that good managers need adequate quality sleep, and exercise, so as to be healthy and alert at work. Time is also needed for leisure, and self development. Control of good eating and drinking habits may not be easy in the catering industry but they require time to be allocated sensibly, not too long, too short or erratic.

Time is the substance life is made of; time is money, time past has gone forever, today's newspaper tomorrow is history. You cannot buy time but an efficient manager can organise his own time and that of those for whom he is responsible advantageously.

Unfortunately a lot of time is wasted by being punctual because others are not on time. Always be punctual and expect others to be so. Be well organised before a meeting, know what you expect from it and what others expect from you. Set objectives which are:

- clear;
- specific;
- measurable;
- worthwhile;
- attainable;
- challenging;
- timed.

If no time limit is stated then time could be wasted. Ideally agreement for whom the objectives are set and the person setting them should agree on the time factor.

1 Plan each day, and decide on priorities.
2 Identify immediate, short-term and long-term goals, and organise office and paperwork.
3 Avoid distractions; prevent interruptions.
4 Delegate, and make list and delete when done.
5 Be organised; develop routines.
6 Do important jobs when you are at your best. Set time limits and keep to them.
7 Do not put off unpleasant or difficult tasks, let others know you have a quiet time.
8 Do one thing at a time and finish it if possible; plan phone calls.
9 Arrange breaks; keep a notebook for ideas.
10 Learn to say no; think before acting.

Communication and information

To develop managerial skills it is important to communicate effectively with senior management and other departmental managers and with those for whom you are responsible. It is essential to realise that what is communicated is understood in the way it is intended. Likewise it is very important that information, suggestions, commands, decisions, requests etc. are clear, cannot be misconstructed or are ambiguous. Listening is an art which needs particular attention for this is a vital aspect of effective communication.

Information may be communicated by oral or visual means, depending on the establishment's policy, personal preference and the matter to be conveyed. The advantage of speech is that questions and discussions can clarify the issues immediately and intonation and emphasis convey more accurately what is intended. Whilst the telephone is invaluable there is no eye contact which makes face to face communication more effective. Body language conveys much to both communicators which naturally can only occur in direct contact situations.

Written instructions, reports etc. have an advantage that there is tangible evidence of what is communicated. However care must still be taken that what is written is understood by the recipient, that which is written may be clear to the person writing the instructions, it is essential that it is specific, unambiguous and not wordy, so that there are no misunderstandings.

Self-assessment

In order to improve performance it is desirable to review one's current situation and how to develop into the future. Appropriate others such as colleagues in the establishment, comparison with people in similar situations in other organisations, members of professional associations, tutors at colleges and persons who have experience or experienced management in catering may all provide constructive advice. Keep abreast of developments by reading journals and visiting trade fairs.

Balanced organisation

Evaluate responsibilities objectively so that you understand, appreciate and can act effectively in an efficient but balanced lifestyle.

○ **Assess your responsibilities for:**   people; finance; development; administration and communication.

○ **People to consider are:**   yourself; your subordinates; your family and your department.

○ **Finance:**   your own; the department's; budgeting; authorisation of expenditure and control of expenditure.

○ **Development in:**   the organisation; the department; your own and new ideas.

○ **Administration may include:**   an office; secretary; your department; other departments and customers.

○ **Communication: ensure it is effective:**   to others and from others.

DEVELOPING TRUST AND SUPPORT WITH MANAGERS

Trust and support with one's immediate manager will simply not appear in an ad hoc fashion. For a chef this may be the food and beverage manager or the general manager. Serious attention has to be paid to developing a communication channel with one's immediate manager in order to encourage an effective relationship which will help to achieve the departmental or organisation goals. The better the communication then it is likely that the relationship will become better and more efficient.

It is important that the departmental head consults with his or her line manager on a regular basis to genuinely seek his or her views, ideas and feelings which may improve the quality of decisions. This will stimulate better co-operation between managers.

Conflict with your immediate line manager can be very damaging. However, it is one of the main areas in which conflict can and does take place at work. Section heads may often feel dissatisfied with their line manager perhaps over pay, working conditions etc. Another issue may be one of the communication between the section head and the line manager.

The section head should take time to find out about his/her line manager by discussing, observing and talking to him/her and other managers in the organisation.

It also helps if a close relationship is developed with the manager and an understanding of all the issues the organisation is faced with. Provide the manager with ideas, give definitions of problems and your views on solutions.

A manager will generally have:

○ another view or alternative view on things;

○ more information on the overall picture;

○ advice on difficult issues;

○ guidance on appropriate policies;

○ support, protection (through consultation with him or her).

The departmental head must in turn provide:

○ clear documentation;

○ clear definition of issues;

○ identified courses of action and views on the various strategies available;

○ reasoned arguments on how/why he or she has arrived at the recommendations;

○ predictions about likely outcomes and contingencies if a recommendation he or she actions is unsuccessful;

○ information on his or her team's progress.

Your line manager is expecting you to produce results and to organise your team. This will strengthen your relationship with the line manager. Your manager will often, in turn, take a certain amount of credit for what you do well!

Consider also your own relationship with your subordinates. If the relationship works well, then what are the reasons? Are these relevant to establishing a working relationship with your line manager?

Assess your line manager

○ Understand what he or she wants for themselves.

○ What are his or her values?

○ Is he or she able to accept criticism?

○ Is he or she ambitious?

○ How does he or she measure himself/herself?

○ Who are the people that he or she admires?

○ Does the manager like open, frank discussion?

○ Does the manager take risks? or is he or she a protector?

○ Is the manager an autocratic leader, expecting you to do as he or she says, or intuitive, expecting you to follow, broad informal indications or signs?

Try to analyse why situations produce conflict or stalemate. Is it because your views differ or because you both manage the situations badly? Does this help you to decide if you have the qualities he or she values? What does your manager expect from you? Do his or her goals match yours? If not, can you live with the resulting difficulties?

Learn to understand your manager's strengths and weaknesses

○ Does the manager need time and lengthy explanations?

○ Is the manager good at one-to-one communication?

○ Is the manager able to see essentials, and keen to resolve issues?

○ Does the manager contribute to good ideas?

○ Is he or she able to see practical solutions?

○ Is the manager able to handle conflict, or does he or she seek to avoid it.

Once these strengths and weaknesses have been identified you should seek to complement them. You may need to modify your behaviour to ensure your relationship with him/her is legitimate, not a sell out and can be productive, taking care not to go too far in compromising.

Analyse his or her style

○ Does your manager prefer written detailed reports? If so, you should provide them and check them thoroughly.

○ He or she may prefer verbal briefings. If so, provide them but follow up with a memo.

- He or she may prefer formal meetings with itemised agendas.
- Assess the circumstances within the environment you are both working in.
- What are the pressures on you both?
- What are his or her own dealings with his or her peers and more senior managers?
- What is expected of your manager? Where does he or she look for success?
- What are the rewards for succeeding? Could this reflect on your relationship?
- Salary increase?
  - Promotion?
  - Bonus?
- How are you contributing to what he or she is trying to achieve?
- How do people view the manager in the organisation?

Making decisions

Decision making is a very important part of the management process. No matter how good you are as a section manager, how well you motivate your staff or how good your ideas are, you will be judged by your manager and on your staff on the quality of the decisions you make.

Quantity can be no substitute for quality. An excess of bad or short-term decisions will lead to a serious backlog of niggling problems.

Decisions are your judgement choices between alternative courses of action. To be effective, often this means keeping our decision making to a minimum but ensuring the decisions that have to be made are timed correctly, after taking into account all the facts and information at our disposal.

Managing the team and its performance in a regular series of tasks and a number of various projects involves decisions relating to routine, individuals and the team.

- Different strategies and styles of working/interaction which encourage effective working relationships with senior staff.
- Range of methods to keep the immediate manager informed and how to select an appropriate method according to a range of issues and contexts.
- The types of emerging threats and opportunities about which the manager needs to be informed and the degree of urgency attached to this.
- How to develop and present proposals in a way which is realistic, clear and likely to influence the immediate manager's decision making positively.
- Handling disagreements positively.

Assess the likely reaction from both the team and individuals.

- Avoid making decisions on impulse.
- Collect all information, not just the material that supports your view.
- Discuss decisions with more experienced senior staff, but retain responsibility for the final decision.
- Do not take premature or unnecessary decisions.

Routine decision making is often delegated by a departmental head to a junior. This encourages and develops them in the decision making process and allows the head to concentrate on more strategic issues.

Certain decisions remain with the departmental manager.

- These which focus an overall direction.
- Staff resourcing.

○ Organisation structure in the section to achieve objectives and cope with the workload.

○ Skills, forecasting.

○ Planning to achieve operational objectives.

Avoid using one style of dealing with everything. Use 'unswerving flexibility'.

Managing projects means making hard decisions about money, materials, time and staff.

○ All team members must know their roles.

○ Progress must be frequently reviewed to spot potential problems and to note what time and resources are available.

○ Continually feedback to your line manager to avoid misunderstandings or conflict if things go wrong.

○ Consult experts when necessary before any emergency.

○ Refer any decisions to your line manager that fall outside your sphere of authority, responsibility or flexibility. Referrals should be accompanied with a clear statement of possible choices, together with your recommendations.

Steps to effective decision making

CLASSIFY THE PROBLEM

If it is generic, it is probably one of those everyday problems that has to be solved by adapting the appropriate generic rule, policy or principle. If it is extraordinary, the problem must be dealt with on its individual merits.

DEFINE THE PROBLEM

State precisely the nature of the problem and check your definition against all the observable facts. Beware the plausible but incomplete definition that does not embrace all the known facts.

SPECIFY THE CONDITIONS

Clarify exactly what the decision must accomplish. These are the so-called boundary conditions, or specifications, that must be satisfied by the solution to the problem.

DECIDE ON THE RIGHT ACTION

Decide first of all what is right to do rather than what is acceptable in the circumstances. Make the decision that satisfies all the specifications.

COMPROMISE THE DECISION

In reality there usually has to be some form of compromise, so make the best decision possible by adapting it to the circumstances.

IMPLEMENT THE DECISION

Assign the responsibility of carrying out the decision to those staff who are capable of doing so. Inform everyone who needs to know about the decision and the effects of the decision.

REVIEW THE EFFECTIVENESS OF THE DECISION

The implementation process should involve feedback and monitoring. Receive reports on the results of the decision, how does the decision measure up to its expectations? All positive facts should be incorporated into the classifying, defining and specifying process of making decisions.

MANAGING PEOPLE

Developing the trust and support of colleagues and team members

As individuals working within an organisation, we can achieve very little but working within a group we are able to achieve a great deal more. Good effective teamwork is an important feature of human behaviour and organisational performance.

Each member in a group must:

1 regard themselves as being part of that group;

2 interact with one another;

3 perceive themselves as part of the group and;

4 share the purpose of the group.

This will help build trust and support and will result in an effective performance. Co-operation is therefore important.

People in groups will influence one another, within the group there may be a leader and/or a hierarchical system. The pressures within the group may have a major influence over the behaviour of individual members and their performance. The style of leadership within the group has an influence on the behaviour of members within the group.

Groups help share the work pattern of organisations, and the attitudes and behaviour of members to their jobs.

Two types of team can be identified within an organisation.

The **formal** team is the department or section created within a reorganised structure to pursue specified goals.

The **informal** teams deal with a particular situation, members have fewer fixed organisational relationships and are disbanded after performing their function.

Both groups have to be developed and lead. Thought has to be given to relationships and the tasks and duties the team has to carry out.

Selecting and shaping teams to work within a department is very important. This is the job of the departmental head. It requires management skills. Matching each individual's talent to the task or job has to be considered.

A good developed team will mean that the group will be able to carry out the following:

○ analyse problems effectively and create useful ideas;

○ communicate with each other and get things done;

○ good leadership will result in skilled operations with technical precision and ability;

○ evaluate logically and equate control systems.

The group will never become a team unless personalities are able to relate to and communicate with one another, and value contribution each employee or team member makes.

The team leader has a strong influence on his or her team or brigade, and is expected to set examples that have to be followed particularly when under pressure, dealing with conflict, personality clash, change and stress.

People's behaviour is affected by many factors, e.g.:

○ individual characteristics, cultural attributes and social skills.

The head must lead rather than drive and encourage the team to practise reasonable and supportive behaviour so that any problems are dealt with in an objective way and the team's personal skills are harnessed to achieve their full potential.

Every team has to deal with:

○ the egos and the weaknesses and strengths of the individuals;

○ the self-appointed experts within the group;

○ relationships/circumstances constantly changing.

The head is able to manage the team successfully by pulling back from the task in hand. He or she must examine the processes that create efficient teamwork, finding out what it is that makes them greater than the sum of its parts. To assist this process the following is necessary:

○ have a consistent approach to solving problems;

○ take into account people's characters as well as their technical skills;

○ encourage supportive behaviour in the team;

○ create an open, healthy climate;

○ make time for the team to appraise its progress.

Supportive team practices
LISTENING SKILLS

○ Pay attention, responding positively.

○ Looking interested, avoid interrupting.

○ Build on proposals, asking for clarity on questions.

○ Summarise to check your understanding.

CO-OPERATING

○ Encouraging others to give their views.

○ Complimenting on good ideas.

○ Avoiding coercion and acrimony.

○ Careful consideration giving to different proposals.

○ Offering new ideas openly.

CHALLENGING

○ Any assumptions are questioned in a reasonable manner.

○ Continually refer back to the problem-solving process and aims.

○ Review progress of the objectives and aims, in relationship to the team and time taken.

Motivation and the team

An understanding of what motivates staff is crucial to the creation of productivity and the realisation of profits. People's needs and wants are complex and often difficult to define.

Money and status are important but they cannot be relied upon exclusively. Behavioural scientists have provided useful ways of thinking about people's needs and wants.

F. W. Taylor established a scientific management approach. This involved breaking down jobs into simple but repetitive tasks, providing training, isolating individuals from distractions and each other and paying good wages, which included bonuses for productivity over target levels.

In the short term, productive gains were significant, in the long run, these gains were less than significant as people reacted against the area of being treated as a machine.

The scientific approach may have been discredited because some managers give too much attention to pay and insufficient to personnel needs and the needs of groups and teams.

Maslow concentrated on human needs, which are defined as five-fold:

1 **PHYSIOLOGICAL NEEDS**

   The need for food and shelter.

2 **SAFETY NEEDS**

   The security of home and work.

3 **SOCIAL NEEDS**

   The need for a supportive environment.

4 **ESTEEM NEEDS**

   Gaining the respect of others.

5 **SELF-FULFILMENT**

   The need to realise one's potential.

As each goal is achieved, the next is sought. Thus, at different stages of career development, each individual has different values depending on their progress through the 'hierarchy of needs'.

In 1959 Frederick Herzberg added to Taylor's and Maslow's work by introducing the idea of 'hygiene' factors. If these hygiene factors are absent they will lead to dissatisfaction and will prevent effective motivation. The hygiene factors can be identified as follows.

1 The organisational policy and rules.

2 The management styles and controls.

3 Retirement and sickness policies.

4 Pay and recognition of status.

○ Hygiene factors, although considered important, do not have lasting effects on motivation, as other positive motivating factors must be present.

○ Money obviously plays an important role in motivation. There are a number of non-financial motivators, and these are considered to be highly important, to achieve the organisational goals.

○ Most people want to achieve – those in charge of teams must recognise this and provide opportunities for others to attain levels of achievement that celebrate ability.

○ People also want recognition. Praise and feedback spur people on to achieve even more.

○ People generally want to move on to more challenging situations. The team should aim to challenge its members.

○ Certain workers, e.g. chefs, want to practice their skill and use their intelligence to maintain interest.

○ Most workers want to accept responsibility and authority.

MOTIVATING A TEAM

A leader must motivate his or her team, by making their work interesting, challenging and demanding. People must also know what is expected of them and what the standards are. Rewards are linked to effort and results.

Unless these factors go towards fulfilling the organisational needs and the expectations of team members, if pay and prospects within the establishment are bad, the system should be improved and performance should be recognised. Therefore, the leader should attempt to intercede on behalf of his or her staff. This, in turn, will help to increase their motivation and their commitment to the team.

For the leader to manage his or her staff effectively, it is important to get to know them well, understand their needs and aspirations, and help them achieve their personal aims.

Communication

Successful communication is vital when working to build working relationships. Training and developing the team is about communicating. In work, the quality of our personal relationships depends on the quality of the communication system.

1 The speaker must know what he or she wishes to convey.

2 He or she must find visible symbols, gestures, words, body movements, to externalise the internal thoughts.

3 The listener must be receptive to these visible symbols, know the language, terminology and understand the non-verbal symbols being demonstrated.

4 The listener must translate all these symbols into thought.

Communication requires a transmitter and a receiver, and therefore it is a shared responsibility.

Speaking in a meeting you have several potential listeners, a memo you send to staff may have multiple copies. Many staff receive messages, commands, notices etc., they don't give them. Therefore the communication system may only imply a transmitting process.

The greatest scope for quantitatively improving your communication skills is to improve your listening, observing, reading and watching abilities, as a priority over speaking and writing. The most effective transmissions are those that are able to fit into the receiving processes of the recipients.

Hearing and understanding the content of the instruction of the message is not sufficient for full communication. There has to be a match between the telling known as the 'intent' and the 'effect' – the instruction a message has on the individual.

Breakdowns in communication can be identified by looking at the 'intent' and the 'effect' as two separate realities. It is when the intent is not translated into the effect. Such breakdowns affect staff and team relationships, the attitude and views of each other. Good relationships vitally depend on good communication, awareness of the potential gap between the intent and the effect can help clarify and prevent any misunderstanding within the group.

By bridging the gap, between the intent and the effect you can begin to change the culture of the working environment, the processes become self-reinforcing in a positive direction. The staff begin to respect each other in a positive framework, they listen more carefully to each other with positive expectations, hearing the constructive intent and responding to it.

As a manager, the art is achieving results through the team, with communication being the key to exercise. A great deal of time will be taken up with communicating in one way or another.

Planning communication

Communication can be planned in a systematic way with clarity about the objectives and the methods to be used. Not every communication needs to be planned, as many trivial or routine transmissions can go through automatic channels.

The significant communication lines are those that recur frequently and or take up a great deal of time or carry substantial prizes or penalties for success or failure.

Firstly, the manager must define his or her job objectives, then he or she must identify the communication strategy to achieve these objectives.

Planning the communication will cover the subject and the method content and process.

The **content** means:

○ collecting the data;

○ getting your thoughts in order;

○ formulating information.

The process means:

○ alternative ways communication may proceed and achieve objectives.

The **medium** can be:

○ face to face   ○ meeting   ○ phone call   ○ fax   ○ email   ○ memo.

A major factor in the quality of any communication system is the climate in which it takes place. The climate refers to the prevailing attitudes and habitual behaviours of the team within which the communication is being attempted. The degree of friendliness and/or hostility that exists between the transmitters and receivers will affect the communication outcome.

The climate for communication is greatly influenced by the leader and the effect this has on the recipients. The leader sets the tone in the way he or she interacts with the team. Do not patronise the staff as this causes resentment which results in sullen silence or overt hostility. Being dogmatic with a closed mind results in others being dogmatic in return.

Accept disagreement as an interesting alternative view which is worth exploring, demonstrating how you are able to learn from it. This provides a climate of open-mindedness.

Staff very often respond to the expectations communicated to them, either directly or indirectly.

MEETINGS

Any chef manager must ask themselves what is the purpose of meetings, what are you trying to achieve by holding the meeting. The purpose needs to be expressed in specific terms.

We are able to identify the predominant communication component in each category of the meeting.

Purpose of meeting	Predominant communication components
Information exchange	Facts and opinions
Problem solving	Ideas and goal wishes
Briefing	Facts
Consultation	Opinions
Conflict resolution	Ideas and goal wishes
Morale building	Feelings and goal wishes

WORK LIFE BALANCE

It is being increasingly recognised universally by employers of all sizes and in all industry sectors that it makes good business sense to create a better work life balance for their workers. Where this has been successfully organised, it has resulted in increased morale and employee loyalty, better productivity and effectiveness at work, and improved adaptability in the face of change.

Research shows that when employees are better able to integrate their needs outside work into their daily lives with no detriment to their work, there are considerable benefits to the business.

A survey of 2,000 managers in the UK found that a third of them would change their jobs if they felt they could improve their work life balance.

57% of students consider achieving a balanced life style and having a rewarding life outside work as their top priority in their future career.

Source:

A good practice guide for the Hospitality Industry produced by the HCIMA's Managing Diversity Working Group in conjunction with the DTI's work life balance team.

Free copies are available from DTI Publications.

continued

Tel: 0870 1502 500 Fax: 0870 1502 333

Web: www.dti.gov.uk/publications

Email: dtipubs@eclogistics.co.uk reference number URN 01/1186

Leading the team

○ Look at tomorrow's problems and issues today to detect signs of changes and pitfalls.

○ Learn to adapt to change, to embrace it and turn it to positive advantage.

○ Set high standards and clear objectives.

○ Think clearly allowing intuition to influence rationality.

○ Create a sense of value and purpose in work, so that team members believe in what they do and do it successfully.

○ Provide a positive sense of direction in order to give meaning to the lives of team members.

○ Act decisively but ensure decisions made are soundly based and not just on impulse.

○ Set the right tone by your actions and beliefs thus creating a clear, consistent and honest model to be followed.

○ Choose the right time to make decisions and take action.

○ Create an atmosphere of enthusiasm in which individuals are stimulated to perform well, find fulfilment, gain self respect and play an integral role in meeting the organisation's overall goals.

○ Be sensitive to individual team needs and their expectations.

○ Define clear responsibilities and structures, so collective effort is enhanced not hindered.

○ Recognise what motivates each team member and work with these motivations to achieve standards and objectives.

○ Determine boundaries within which team members can work freely.

Most managers do one of the following:

1 Make a decision the team accepts.

2 Sell a decision before trying to have it accepted.

3 Present decisions but respond to team's questions.

4 Present a tentative decision, subject to change after team input.

5 Present problems, ask the team for input, then make a decision.

6 Define the limits within which the team can make a decision.

7 Chef and team make a joint decision.

MANAGING DIVERSITY

The work of work, especially the hospitality industry, is becoming more diverse. Increasing numbers of women ae entering the labour force who expect to progress to senior management, the ethnic mix is becoming wider and the population in Western economies is ageing. In the case of multinational companies, domestic diversity is compounded by the diversity which is introduced through the movement of people around the globe. The mobility of labour is further encouraged by regional mechanisms such as the arrangements for the free movement of people in the European Union. All these changes (and more) are affecting the nature of customers and their needs.

What is diversity?

Diversity recognises that people are different. It includes some of the more obvious and visible differences such as gender, ethnicity, age and disability and also the less visible differences such as sexual orientation, background, personality and work style. Diversity management is about recognising, valuing and celebrating these differences. It is about harnessing difference to improve creativity and innovation and is based on the belief that groups of people who bring different perspectives together will find better solutions to problems than groups of people who are the same.

Why is diversity management important?

The markets served are constantly changing (e.g. women and older people have more spending power; ethnic minorities are an important market segment, disabled people and their carers want accessible holidays) and in order to meet the needs of these diverse markets the same groups need to be represented in the workforce. By taking the proactive approach to diversity management all of the following can be achieved:

- ○ access to the best people from the widest labour pool available;
- ○ develop the creative talents of all employees;
- ○ motivate all staff;
- ○ reduce labour turnover;
- ○ improve quality and customer service.

Source: HCIMA May 1999

▌MINIMISING INTERPERSONAL CONFLICT

Interpersonal conflict is a fact of life. It starts with children in school, who in most cases are able to quickly resolve their disagreements and are often friends again. With adults this ability to resolve conflict tends to fade away as we become older. In an organisational context a whole range of things can get in the way, which makes handling conflict even more difficult. A conflict with the manager or with colleagues can easily get entangled with issues about work and status – both of which can make it difficult to approach the problem in a rational and professional way.

- ○ One of the skills of all front-line managers is the need to identify conflict, so that plans can be put in place to minimise it.
- ○ Conflict arises where there are already strained relations and personality clashes between members of your team.
- ○ Conflict often occurs in a professional kitchen when the brigade is understaffed and under pressure especially over a long period. Pressure can also come from e.g. restaurant reviews and guides where a chef is after a Michelin star or special accolade.
- ○ Conflicts damage working relationships and upset the team and eventually this will show in the finished product.

The chef and manager must also be aware of the insidious conflict that may be going on around you, in less obvious places. Covert conflicts are the ones which take place in secret and can be very harmful. This type of conflict is often difficult to detect. A new person joining the team may have no idea that the conflict is taking place. This type of conflict will also undermine the team's performance. Such conflict may happen when a person has been passed over for promotion and has never received feedback as to why? In other words, they have been ignored. The resentment, anger and bitterness can bubble away underneath the surface.

Many conflicts start with misunderstandings or a small upset that grows and develops out of all proportions. The manager or chef should attempt to:

○ stop it getting worse;

○ make the individuals confront their own problems;

○ manage the situation to avoid any escalation.

Destructive and constructive conflicts

It is important to reflect and analyse the nature of conflict and individual attitudes to it. While conflicts can be very damaging and upsetting, there can also be some positive outcomes. Conflict can also be a learning curve that a chef or manager has to enter into, this then has to be handled properly and focused to achieve the desired outcome.

Conflict is destructive when it:

○ produces name calling;

○ makes people feel angry and let down with each other;

○ causes people to close off and withdraw.

Conflict is constructive when it:

○ acts as the first stage towards negotiating;

○ clears the air;

○ helps your staff to talk to each other.

Some common physical reactions when we are threatened by conflict are:

○ sweaty palms; rise in pulse rate; dry mouth; trembling.

FLIGHT

This is an unsatisfactory way of dealing with conflict at work or in other social situations. Much of the time here, you just can't run, and if there is no escape, it can turn into a demonstration of submission, a form of passive behaviour. Don't be so intent on pleasing others that you fail to please yourself. The emotional aftermath of submitting results often in guilt and feeling that you have let yourself down.

Flight reaction and passive behaviour could be:

○ withdrawing eye contact, looking down, hiding behind hair;

○ withdrawing body language, hiding;

○ continual agreement.

FIGHT

Aggressive behaviour is equally unsatisfactory. This can be seen by:

○ a raised voice, clipped or sarcastic tone;

○ pointing a finger, clenched fist, banging the table and waving the arms;

○ staring and invasive eye contact – glaring;

○ moving closer to someone, standing up to tower over someone else;

○ not listening, talking so much, there is no space to respond.

Why does conflict arise?

The chef/manager needs to be aware within which areas interpersonal conflict can arise in order to put strategies in place to manage them. Being positive rather than simply reacting to a conflict when it breaks out.

People feeling that they do not have a chance to discuss their problems and difficulties with someone can also lead to conflict. It can also lead to

- a breakdown in trust;
- misunderstandings about standards;
- failing to communicate with one another correctly;
- dealing with complex personnel problems that should have been passed to an expert.

Other reasons for conflict can be due to

- Racism, sexism, differences in opinion
- Inappropriate personal habits, non-compliance with organisational norms/values
- Discriminatory behaviour, working conditions
- Unrealistic work expectations, personal antagonism

In some cases conflicts that arise from these issues may result in formal grievances, or even disciplinary matters.

Formal procedures can often be helpful in containing conflict to a standard approach. This depersonalises it and stops and the manager or chef taking it personally, converting it into a standard work role approach that spells out who is to do what by when.

Conflict between the chef and the manager

This can be very damaging and leads to feelings of dissatisfaction. Often it may be the result of poor communication in either direction, about activities, progress results and achievements.

The main issues include:

- failing to communicate accurately or promptly – on problems, opportunities and activities;
- going it alone – taking decisions that require approval of the manager or another party;
- coming up with problems rather than solutions and neglecting to put forward proposals for action at the appropriate level of detail;
- feeling hurt when ideas are rejected and instead of coming up with other proposals;
- allowing some disagreements to grow without limiting the damage;
- failing to do what the job requires and not meeting expectations without good reason;
- balancing the expectations of the kitchen/restaurant team and trying to live up to your manager's expectations and demands.

Therefore, there is a need to continue to find ways of improving and maintaining relationships with line managers and the team. Relationships have to be worked on, they need constant nurturing.

Turning the situation round

Nine steps to enhance working relationships with your immediate manager.

1. Keep the manager well informed on what you and the team are doing. By regular process reports clearly identifying achievements.
2. Inform him or her of problems and opportunities. Give information at the right stage.
3. Ask for advice when you need it. Use you manager as a resource.
4. Make proposals for action clearly and at the right time giving the right level of detail.
5. Not all proposals will be accepted by your line manager. If a proposal is rejected, wait for some time, then put forward an alternative proposal.
6. Deal with disagreements with your line manager in a positive way. Avoid falling out and so damaging the relationship.

7 Continue to find ways to improve your relationship.

8 Check you have completed everything you are required to do in your job.

9 Carry out your activities positively, willingly and in a helpful way.

Sometimes there may be a member of staff who keeps calm, gets everyone listening and talking sensibly and comes up with a reasonable compromise that gets everyone out of the hole. This person should be the chef or the manager.

Some references to management elsewhere in the book

Computer use	565	Organisation	215, 360
Supervision	218	Working methods	216
Conservation	262	Functions	336
Portion control	349	Cost control	355

Topics for Discussion

1 Ways in which conflict can be resolved in a kitchen.

2 The importance of acquiring management skills when working as a head chef.

3 Why trust in the management process is important.

4 Which is more important – gaining accolades and Michelin stars or operating a successful kitchen where managers and staff feel comfortable and the product is successful?

5 The importance of developing teams.

6 Why good communication in the organisation is important.

7 What are the qualities of a good manager?

8 What do employees expect of the manager?

9 What does the manager expect of the employee?

CHAPTER 14

MARKETING, SALES AND CUSTOMER CARE

MARKETING

Operating a successful business in today's competitive environment means that an establishment has to gain an advantage over its competitors. A hospitality establishment has to carefully predict customers' wants, needs and desires and to translate these into a product that people will want to purchase.

This chapter primarily focuses on promotion and selling. Marketing is not just about selling, it is the whole complex of business behaviour which identifies these customer needs and trends in buying behaviour and carefully monitors and interprets the business environment the establishment or organisation is operating in. Factors include the amount of disposable income people have, the economic environment and exchange rates. There are also political factors such as the likelihood of the introduction of a minimum wage, and other legislation such as the impact of the Food Safety Act on an establishment's hygiene costs.

Marketing is necessary for the long term survival of any business

Market research relies on a systematic approach, and there are a number of different approaches to researching a particular market. The SWOT analysis is a well known approach. SWOT stands for Strengths, Weaknesses, Opportunities and Threats. When a SWOT analysis is carried out it is useful to take into account the seven 'Ps' of marketing:

○ product;

○ place;

○ price;

○ promotion;

○ process;

○ physical environment;

○ people.

Strengths refer to the positive aspects of the establishment:

- good reputation;
- good location;
- attractive environment;
- comfortable restaurant.

Weaknesses could refer to

- declining market;
- lack of staff training;
- lack of investment;
- no parking spaces.

Opportunities could include:

- economic environment – people with high disposable incomes;
- geographical – good attractive area, good parking facilities;
- attractive area;
- good transport links;
- demographic – increasing numbers of young professional people moving in to the area;
- technological – availability of new equipment, good control systems available;
- competition – little competition in the area.

Threats could include

- technological – out-of-date equipment;
- competition;
- decline in demand for product;
- geographical – area becoming run down, poorly kept area, difficult parking;
- legislation – impact of new legislation which means more bureaucracy.

It is important for any manager to know the market, and this is done by carrying out detailed market research. Some companies will have their own market research, while others will bring in consultants. This research will assist the company in knowing the potential and current customers, the competition, the business pattern, and bring the company closer to knowing its own product, strengths, weaknesses and specific characteristics.

Pricing

Once it is clear from the research what the business is, where the profits should be coming from and what the competition is, then charging decisions on pricing can be made. There are a number of different pricing policies which can be adopted.

COMPETITIVE PRICING

This looks carefully at what the competition is charging and aims to price at the same level, or sometimes at a slightly lower price. It is vital that the prices charged and the cost structure are compatible.

BACKWARD PRICING

This requires an accurate estimate of what people are likely to spend in the future. The product and services are then designed to match what the market will bear. In other words, what the customer is prepared to pay for the product or service within that particular market segment.

COST PLUS

This is where a set mark-up or a set percentage is added to basic costs. This approach is reasonably high risk – for example if the price of the raw materials rises, then a cost plus approach will mean that the price of the product or service will also have to rise, in some cases beyond the reach of the customer. For this reason many organisations adopt the backward pricing approach.

MARGINAL PRICING

This takes into account the actual costs a customer incurs in using the product or service, and these costs include materials and energy costs. These are the *direct* costs. The customer is charged just over the direct costs, and so a contribution is made to the overhead costs. Overheads such as capital, insurance and staff costs have to be incurred whether the customer used the product or service. This pricing is used often at weekends and off season to sell hotel rooms in a hope that the customer will purchase other products at the realistic price.

DISCOUNTS

Discounting is used to sell hotel rooms and hospitality products. Discounting is used to maintain customer loyalty, increase the business, to attract repeat business, increase demand in off-peak periods and to encourage prompt settlement of accounts.

THE CATERING CYCLE

Caterers running a business should attempt to understand and apply the catering cycle principle.

Food and beverage (or food service) operations are concerned with the provision of food and a variety of beverages within business. The various elements that comprise food and beverage operations can be summarised in the catering cycle. Food and beverage operations are concerned with:

1 The markets served by the various sectors of the foodservice industry and consumer needs.
2 The range and formulation of policies and business goals and objectives of the various operations and how these affect the methods adopted.
3 The interpretation of demand and decisions to be made on the food and beverages to be provided as well as the other services.
4 The planning and design to create a convergence of facilities required for food and beverage operations and making decisions about the plant and equipment required.
5 The development of appropriate provisioning methods to meet the needs of the production and service methods used within given operational settings.
6 Operational knowledge of technical methods and processes and ability in the production and service processes and methods available to the foodservice operator, understanding the varying resource requirements (including staffing) for their operation, as well as decision-making on the appropriateness of the various processes and methods to meet operational requirements.
7 Controlling the costs of materials as well as the costs associated with the operation of production and service, and controlling the revenue.
8 The monitoring of customer satisfaction.

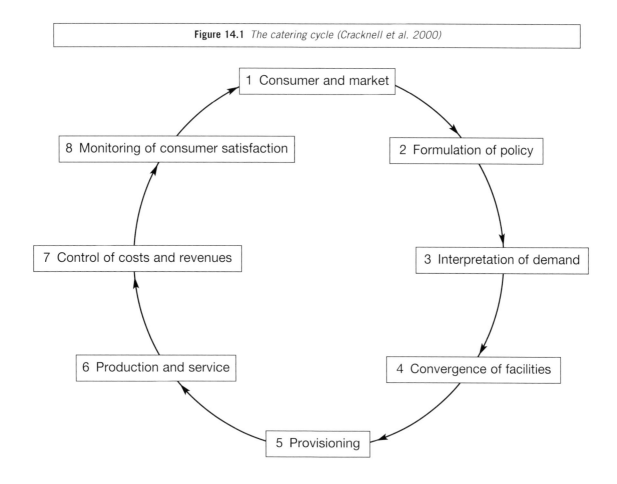

Figure 14.1 *The catering cycle (Cracknell et al. 2000)*

1 Consumer and market

8 Monitoring of consumer satisfaction

2 Formulation of policy

7 Control of costs and revenues

3 Interpretation of demand

6 Production and service

4 Convergence of facilities

5 Provisioning

ASPECTS OF PROMOTION AND SELLING

Once a catering establishment has been planned, the process has to be generated whereby the buyer and seller come together. Through *promotion*, customers are made aware of the establishment, persuaded to make a visit and encouraged to return. Promotion is concerned with the product. This product constitutes a total package on offer, and includes some of the following concepts:

- the image of the establishment;
- the prices charged;
- the quality of the product and service;
- the environment, facilities and services;
- the style of management and staff.

Promotion should inform the customer of the establishment, make them aware of its existence, persuade them to buy and convince them of the image and quality of the product. This is done through:

- personal selling;
- merchandising;
- advertising;
- public relations;
- sales promotion;
- agents.

Promotion is an activity which must be carefully planned and controlled. Usually, the main objective of the promotional campaign is to stimulate demand by using persuasive messages to attract new customers and past users of the establishment. Such messages must convince prospective customers that the product on offer is good value for money.

Defining the market

The manager or chef should establish the best potential market. This will determine the type of messages to project in order to influence customer behaviour. It will also indicate the best form of media relevant to the age, sex, social class, income level and location of the target customer. It is important for these messages to emphasise the benefits of the product to the customer.

Promotion timing

Promotion timing depends on the objectives and when the decision to purchase is to be made by the customer.

Personal selling

Personal selling is done through contacts with local organisations and committees, for example, or, more directly, through the senior restaurant staff talking to clients. All employees who are in contact with customers must be made aware of the importance of selling the products to increase profits and provide a satisfactory experience for the customer.

All staff must therefore gain a good knowledge of the company's products and services and develop good social skills with an ability to promote and sell. Showing concern for the customers not only makes them feel comfortable but also promotes sales and increases the effectiveness of the establishment.

Advertising

This should convey messages which will influence consumer attitudes and behaviour favourable to the seller. Advertising should:

- increase sales immediately;
- create greater public awareness of the location and existence of the establishment;
- persuade the public that the product and services are good value for money;
- concentrate on the benefits of using the establishment and consuming the product;
- focus on the product differences from those of competitors.

Advertising can be done via the following media:

- posters;
- magazines;
- newspapers;
- radio;
- television;
- direct mail.

The selection depends on finance and the target audience.

DIRECT MAIL

The advantages of direct mail include:

- the ability to select potential customers who are likely to buy the product: target groups can be broken down into geographical location, leisure interest and socio-economic groups, to name a few;
- the ability to express a personal message to each customer;
- the ability to time the promotion;
- the ability to gauge the level of response from various segments of the market and evaluate the cost-effectiveness of the exercise.

Sales promotion

Sales promotion is a day-to-day operation relating to discount offers, price reductions, special offers, such as a free bottle of wine with every meal for two. They are designed to appeal to a certain section of the market: weekend promoting, gastronomic evenings, gastronomic weekends, golfing weekends and food festivals.

Food festivals are held to promote cuisine and beverages of a particular region or country. A themed promotion may help the business and promote sales in the following ways:

○ increase sales during off-peak periods by attracting new customers;

○ gain publicity in local press and on local radio;

○ stimulate and keep the interest of regular customers.

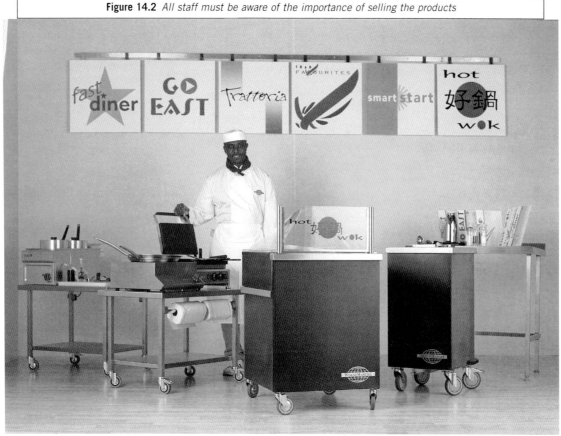

Figure 14.2 *All staff must be aware of the importance of selling the products*

Competing with other establishments and creating a new type of trade, such as conferences, are two other examples of sales promotions activities.

Merchandising

To be a successful caterer a knowledge of merchandising is important. The object of merchandising is to sell more and to reassure customers about the quality of what is being offered: for example, the quality of the cooking, fresh produce being used and persuading customers to return to the establishment.

Merchandising is the art of displaying products attractively to promote sales. This is done to great effect in supermarkets. For example, on the fresh fish counter they display a very small selection of rare or expensive fish and shellfish. This has the effect of making the fish counter interesting, drawing customers' attention and encouraging them to buy, not necessarily the specialist items but more generally the everyday species. An example of merchandising in a fast-food restaurant is the illustrated fascia above the counter showing what is available with the help of coloured photographs. Such a display may also be used in a luxury restaurant where a display of exotic fruits and vegetables helps to promote sales.

In a staff restaurant, tent cards and displays are used at various points on the counter to promote certain dishes. These areas are commonly known as hot spots where the customer is encouraged to buy either an additional item or an item which yields a higher profit margin.

Menus and wine lists are important merchandising tools and should be at the forefront of the merchandising strategy.

THE CUSTOMER

Firstly profile the groups of customers and consider their preferences. Before you decide what you are going to display, first define:

○ type of customer (age, background, social class, income groups, gender);
○ the people and organisations that use your establishment;
○ the frequency of their custom;
○ their use of other catering services;
○ how they use their time;
○ how they use their disposable income.

THE PRODUCT

Consider the product profile, this will define the context of your merchandising policy. You must consider all aspects of the product and products, particularly those aspects which relate to:

○ the appearance of food and beverage; for example, preparing dishes in front of the customer such as salads, grilling meat and fish or flambé dishes; this may be suitable in some situations but not others.
○ how customers see the service you offer;
○ how the product can be further developed with appearance in mind;
○ how the product may be promoted using posters, tent cards, illustrated menu cards.

Many of the major supermarkets can give caterers good ideas on how to develop merchandising.

WHAT AND HOW TO DISPLAY

When the marketing context has been established, the next stage is to consider how to show services and products to their best advantage and to develop aspects of them which will provide additional attractions. The caterer may like to focus on:

○ the quality and freshness of ingredients;
○ the use of fresh flowers and fruits for display;
○ using a selection of finished dishes for display; this is done to great effect when displaying a choice of plated sweets on a tray;
○ assessing how displayed food on a self-service buffet will look after customers have taken portions from the various dishes;
○ how dishes deteriorate in presentation and flavour when they have been standing for too long;

○ assessing how the smell of cooking is an advantage or disadvantage; supermarkets encourage the smell of freshly baked bread and this encourages people to buy bread products;

○ how the menu is displayed and the language which is used to describe dishes (does the layout and language encourage sales?);

○ the provision of essential information about ingredients, sources of wine, vintages and prices in menus and wine lists.

WHERE TO DISPLAY

In any restaurant thought must be given to the space required for merchandising and the strategic points where a display will give maximum effect. Consider:

○ customer flow:

○ position of check-in and cash desks;

○ entrances and exits;

○ use of lounges and bar areas;

○ use of displays outside restaurants (for example in the street or windows);

○ hotel bedrooms for a hotel restaurant;

○ the facility of agents of business associates.

WHEN TO DISPLAY

Timing is important both as an opportunity and as a means of getting the best from a merchandising project. Opportunities on many occasions present themselves at short notice and projects need not be long lasting.

Special evening events may be held where key clients or customers are invited to sample food. Major department stores including Marks and Spencers invite store card holders to special evenings, presales events or special Christmas shopping events. These account customers feel special and are encouraged to buy.

If special events are to be held, the caterer must consider:

○ the season;

○ the weather;

○ the event, whether this is to be local or national.

The meal experience

People who eat out do so because they want to satisfy a need. Reasons for eating out may be summarised as follows:

1 For convenience – at work or near home.

2 For variety – to make life more interesting.

3 To avoid preparing food at home.

4 Status – hosting business lunches, to feel important.

5 To attend social events.

6 Impulse – spur of the moment decision making.

7 Captive market – no choice for example hospital patients, prisoners.

People are however a collection of different types. While it is true that some types of food operations might attract certain types of customers, this is by no means true all the time; for example, McDonalds is marketed to the whole population and attracts customers depending on their needs at the time.

The decision to eat out may be split into two parts.

1 The decision to do so for the reasons given above.

2 The decision as to what type of experience is to be undertaken.

There are a number of factors which influence the latter decision.

The factors that affect the meal experience are as follows:

FOOD AND DRINK

The range of foods, choice availability, flexibility of the restaurant to cope with special orders, quality of the food and drink.

LEVEL OF SERVICE

Depending on the needs people have at the time, the level of service must be suitable to the needs.

For example, a romantic night out may call for a quiet table in a luxury restaurant, whereas a group of friends may well be seeking a more informal service. This factor also takes into account services such as booking and account facilities, acceptance of credit cards and also the reliability of the operation's product.

LEVEL OF CLEANLINESS AND HYGIENE

This relates to the premises, equipment and staff. People are today concerned about food safety and are prepared to pay for it.

PERCEIVED VALUE FOR MONEY AND PRICE

People have perceptions of the amount they are prepared to spend in different establishments, and in different operations.

MERCHANDISING ADMINISTRATION

Ideas have to be developed and implemented. All relevant material relating to food and drink must reflect the style and service of the product on offer.

- Descriptive terms used in menus and displays must be appropriate to the aims of the catering establishment. Accuracy and spelling is very important. Remember the menu and wine list are selling tools and should help the customer to understand what you have to offer.
- All themes should be carefully researched; ambition must not exceed capability.
- Point of sale notices should be in keeping with the overall style of the restaurant. Wording must be positive and friendly. Notices should be presented with style and confidence.
- Avoid hand-written notices, these give a very amateur impression of your establishment.
- Items displayed in generous quantities can assist sales. For example, when supermarkets have special offers on, they sometimes stack the product so it gives the impression that it is plentiful; this has the effect of encouraging the customer to buy not one but at least two of the items on special offer.
- Consider combined presentations, port with stilton, dessert wine with the sweet course.
- All display material must be maintained in good order, otherwise it will have the adverse effect of discouraging sales. For example the sweet tray should be replenished. Menus and wine lists should be replaced before they become shabby.

MAKING THE MOST OF YOUR LOCAL MEDIA TO PROMOTE YOUR HOSPITALITY BUSINESS

Introduction

Local newspapers and radio can provide excellent free publicity. The local media are interested primarily in local stories, or at least national stories to which they (or you) are able to provide a local "slant". It is also likely that their staff are hard-pressed, with limited resources, and would therefore welcome well-presented, topical local (or localised) stories.

From the public's point of view, everyone is interested in what is going on in their own locality. There are approximately 43 million local/regional newspapers published every week – enough for every adult in the country. Some 30 million people listen to local radio – more than the combined audiences of BBC Radios, 1, 2, 3, 4 and 5 Live. So, never underestimate the appeal and power of the local media.

Being featured in the mass media gives a story, an organisation, an initiative or a person credibility and authority, verification and status.

There are many opportunities available to use the media.

Remember that there are six principal "News values" – consistent elements in virtually any news story:

○ Conflict, controversy or disaster
○ Scandal
○ Something that affects (especially threatens or disrupts) the community
○ Unusualness, novelty
○ Personality, character or individualism
○ An event

Get to know your local media

Make a list of all the media outlets in your area: newspapers, free sheets and radio stations. Some will be familiar to most of you; others can be found by looking up a reference book such as **Willings** or **Benn's** in the local library.

Compile a mailing list including the News Editors of local papers, local or regional news agencies and any other sympathetic journalist known to you.

Include the names of Picture Editors for "photocalls" or "photo-opportunities". Add the News Editor of local radio station/s, as well as the producers of any programmes which may cover your activities: current affairs programmes, magazine programmes.

Specialist food/restaurant programmes, consumer affairs and news round ups.

This will form the basis of your mailing list and should be kept up-to-date and ready to use at short notice. If your list is very short, you can type the addresses each time you send out a press release, but if you have access to a photocopier and/or a computer it is much easier to print your addresses onto A4 sheets of labels.

Read your local papers, listen to your local radio stations and watch television programmes. Obvious perhaps, but too many press officers approach the producers of programmes they have never seen or heard, hoping for coverage.

Deadlines

When you send out a press release or ring up a newsroom remember the journalist's deadline. Here is a rough guide to deadlines:

Weekly newspapers	–	2/3 days before publication
Morning papers	–	up to 8pm the previous day (for a major story) but usually by about 4pm
Evening papers	–	11am the same day for the first edition
Local radio	–	one hour before the news bulletin
Weekly magazines	–	3/4 days before publication

Deadlines vary considerably and some sections of the paper close before others. It is best to ring your local newspaper and radio station to ask them to tell you the deadline.

Making contacts

There is nothing to beat having good contacts in the media. Let's assume you are starting from scratch. Compile a list of your local media as outlined above. Then ring the Editor or News Editor of the local paper and introduce yourself. Give him/her your work number and home number (and mobile number if you have one!). **MAKE YOURSELF AS ACCESSIBLE AS POSSIBLE**. Ask to meet for lunch or a drink so that you can tell them what is coming up and find out what they are interested in. However, don't be too pushy. That can make you unpopular and minimise your chances for coverage.

Each time a journalist calls you make a note of the name, the paper or programme they represent, their direct line number, the nature of the call, and your impressions, if any. Anyone interested or sympathetic you can immediately add to your mailing list. Your 'logbook' will enable you to place the journalist the moment he/she rings you again. This will avoid your having to repeat questions like '**which programme are you from?**', which will only irritate the journalist and create an impression of inefficiency on your part. Gradually, through building up information in your logbook and by reading, listening and watching, you will be able to approach the right journalist with the right story at the right time.

Scan the newspapers carefully for names (bi-lines) of journalists who may be sympathetic and add them to your list. When journalists turn up at your events, make a point of chatting to them. Avoid ringing them when they are approaching their deadlines. When you do ring, get to the point quickly. Above all, when they make it clear that they are not interested in what you have to say, give up and try the next time.

How to write a press release

Press releases should be:

○ neatly typed, using one-and-a-half or double spacing, with a wide margin on either side to allow the sub-editor to make notes;

○ written on one side of the sheet, on standard A4 paper with the logo at the top of the page. **NEWS INFORMATION** or **PRESS** (or **NEWS**) **RELEASE** should also be prominent at the top of the page;

○ preferably ONE, but not more than two, sides long.

Resist the temptation to go on at length in a press release.

Journalists scan press releases quickly, often throwing them in the wastepaper bin without reading them. The longer your release, the more likely it is to end up in the round file.

Even News Editors in local radio stations are likely to receive several hundred press releases every day, so keep them short! And aim to present them with a headline and an opening paragraph which catches their eye or makes your release stand out from the rest.

Put the address of your contact at the top of the page, including the telephone numbers of the contact at the end of your release. Put the date at the top of the first page and '**FOR IMMEDIATE RELEASE**', unless you want to embargo it.

Type, in capital letters, a short title which summarises the context of your press release '**MICHELIN STAR CHEF TO MAKE WORLD'S BIGGEST PANCAKE**'.

Keep the number of words per sentence to a maximum of 25–30, and avoid using more than three sentences per paragraph. List the items you want to include in decreasing order of importance, as the press release will be cut from the bottom up. The first paragraph should contain a summary of the whole story, so that even if all the rest is cut the first paragraph 'stands up', or makes sense on its own. The other paragraphs should provide more information in decreasing order of importance.

A good guide is to include the five W's in the first paragraph:

WHO	–	Local famous chef
WHAT	–	World's largest pancake
WHERE	–	Ealing Common
WHEN	–	Tuesday 6th March 2003
WHY	–	To raise money for local hospice

If you need to continue on to a second page type 'mf' or 'continues' centred at the bottom of the last paragraph on page one. Do not split a sentence between two pages. Stable the pages together. Make sure you include an abbreviated form of the heading on page two in case the pages do get separated, e.g. World's largest pancake.

When you finish the press release type **ENDS** at the bottom of the last paragraph, then the name and contact number. Send out your press release a week to ten days before the event, depending on the deadline you are trying to meet.

Follow-up

Sending out a press release is only stage one. The follow-up to issuing a press release is vital but often forgotten by press officers.

A few days before the event, ring round all the newsdesks to find out if they have received your press release. Do this in time for you to send another one in the post. If they say they have not received it, and there is not time to get one out in the post, fax it or deliver it by hand. When you call make sure the exact date, time and place are in the diary.

However, once again, don't make a nuisance of yourself. If the answer is '**No, we're not planning to cover your story**', back off graciously. There'll probably be other opportunities.

A follow-up phone call will give you an opportunity to offer someone for interview. This is particularly desirable with radio stations, as they will often prefer someone to come into the studio to do an interview rather than send a reporter to the event. Make sure you are happy about when the interview will be broadcast so that it does not damage your chance of getting other media coverage.

Embargoes

You will probably never need to worry about embargoes, but it is worth mentioning what they are and when they can be used. An embargo means that you do not wish the information outlined in your press release to be used before the exact time stated at the top of your press release. Embargoes can be broken, so you cannot be sure that your press release will not be printed before the stated time. Embargoes can be useful on a few occasions:

○ if you want publicity for a report or book on a certain date and you want to give the journalist time to read it;

○ if you want to issue a speech in advance of an important meeting held after the deadline of the paper, or if the journalist cannot attend for some reason;

○ if you are simply unable to issue the press release at a later date because you will be away. In this case make sure you include the phone number of someone who can be contacted during your absence.

Letter to the Editor

The Letters Page is a good place to get free publicity. The Letters Editor is looking for punchy, articulate letters which are topical and sometimes controversial. You can write letters to local, regional and national newspapers for example the *Caterer* and *Hotelkeeper*. Letters are useful for correcting inaccurate reporting of an event, but always include more information about your activities.

A letter to the Letters Page is a good way to flag up future events and to invite people to take part. Letters pages are not there to supply you with a free advertisement, so try to link your letter to something already in the news. Study the letters page and try to imitate the length and style of the letters in it. Get into a debate by writing in response to a letter which has just appeared, putting forward a different point of view.

National newspapers are unlikely to print letters about local or regional events, but will be interested in letters about national news – it is up to you to provide an angle.

Radio phone-ins

Many programmes on local radio stations are devoted wholly or partly to telephoned questions from the public. Queries and comments are invited on a particular topic and discussed by participants in the studio. Make a habit of listening in to phone-ins.

Once you have decided to call, jot down what you want to say. You will reach a programme assistant who will ask you what your comment or question is and she/he may arrange to call you back. Listen to the programme until the phone rings, then **SWITCH OFF THE RADIO**. If you don't, you will hear 'howlround' – a howling sound that will put you off your stride. Speak clearly in your normal voice to the person you wish to address. Stay on the line and don't hesitate to follow up what you have said with another point.

Telephone interviews

You may find yourself being interviewed on the telephone. **STOP AND THINK**. Are you the best person to do the interview? If not, tell the journalist immediately. Suggest another interviewee and give the journalist their number. Then ring the person yourself to warn him/her.

When you receive a call from a newspaper journalist who wants some information, your first question should always be, '**What is your deadline?**'. Make a note of it and the questions they want an answer to and say you will ring back in five minutes or an hour, depending on the deadline. There is no need for you to give an immediate response and it is better to check your information and to prepare yourself with a few facts. **ALWAYS** ring back when you said you would. Otherwise the journalist will never trust you again. And quite rightly.

If you are being interviewed by a newspaper journalist, choose your words carefully. They may end up in print. Don't fall into the old trap of answering yes to a question unless you are entirely happy with the sentiments expressed.

For example, journalist:

'*Wouldn't you say that the industry is not doing enough to tackle the skills shortage? Don't you think that government should commit more money to hospitality training*' Answer **Yes**. This could end up published as **Well known chef slams government on training**.

'The well known chef said today that more public money should be committed to training and industry is not doing enough to tackle the problem of skills shortages'.

Instead answer:

'No, but I would say that more is needed by industry and government to help solve the problem of skills shortages'.

On and off the record

The safe rule is, simply do not speak to journalist off the record. In other words, do not say anything you would not be happy to see in print. If you know a journalist very well it can sometimes be useful to go 'off the record' but even then only to give him/her more background information about a situation. You should never say anything off the record you might later regret saying. It is useful to say to journalists on occasion, **'I'll talk off the record to fill you in and give you the background, and then I'll give you a comment 'on the record'.'**

Preparing for the radio interview
EVALUATE

1   Ask for details of the programme and find out what they want to know and why.

2   Anticipate the interviewer's questions. She/he will ask – **who? what? where? when? why? and how?** – the kind of questions the listener or viewer would want to ask.

3   Time is important. Find out when and where they will want you, how long it will last, and whether the interview will be 'live' or pre-recorded. If possible, know something about the interviewer and be sure they know who you are. Then ring them back, never give spontaneous interviews. Create thinking time.

INVESTIGATE

4   Prepare by writing down the main points you want to get across – **maximum of three points** – plus their supporting arguments. Check relevant facts; be sure of what you want to say, and practice with a colleague or friend.

5   Being interviewed is a one-to-one conversation with the interviewer; but remember that an audience will be listening – eavesdropping! **Find out what you can about the audience – the chances are they will not be specialists in your subject, even if they're interested.** Target your preparation accordingly.

ELIMINATE

6   Use the opportunity for maximum benefit. Whatever questions are asked be sure to say what you want to say. **Use the subject of questions to make the points you want to make.** Remember the time constraints: focus on the most important issues and don't get involved in the abstract or theoretical.

7   If the interview is to be 'live', **find out what the first question will be**. Not only will this help you to be prepared for it; it will also give you the chance to match your first answer (your most important point) with the first question.

ILLUSTRATE

8   Listen carefully to the questions and illustrate your answers with examples and anecdotes. Concentrate on the interviewer's face, make eye contact, try to look relaxed, and smile. Do not rush in to fill natural silence: that's the interviewer's job! Personalise it, don't talk about issues.

9   Don't be intimidated. You will usually know far more about the topic than the person asking

the questions. The interviewer's only role is to draw you out, to help you tell your story. You are the expert but be prepared for the occasional personal question. Remember: people-based stories make powerful radio! Create sound pictures to illustrate.

ORCHESTRATE

10 Adopt a conversational and lively style, keep it brief, simple and avoid jargon. Cutting in is unattractive, but if you decide it is necessary, do it decisively or don't do it at all. Never get angry ... there could be a next time! What is the first question?

11 What you look like, the general impression you create, and how you sound, have much more impact on most people than anything you say. **Looking good, even for radio, will help you FEEL good!**

Public relations

Public relations is an exercise concerned with building an "image" of the establishment in the public's mind. Public relations must create a favourable impression to present and future customers, employees and investors and, therefore, is not usually directly related to a particular product or service.

Evaluation

Evaluation is a necessary part of a promotion campaign. It is achieved by:

○ monitoring the enquiries received as a result of a particular advertisement;
○ analysing sales figures;
○ measuring public awareness of a product and after promotion;
○ actual sales in 'test markets'.

AUTOMATIC VENDING

> **Figure 14.3** *Self-service restaurant: general merchandisers vending complete cook-chill dishes for reheating in an adjacent microwave oven, plus hot and cold drinks – all coin- or card-operated*

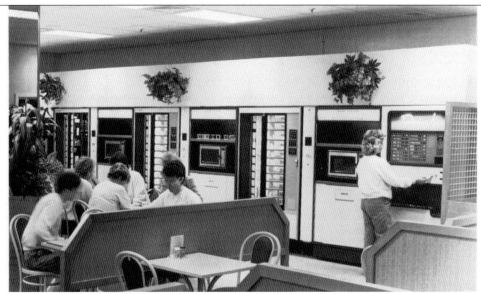

Vending has a long history. The first mention is of the Greek mathematician Hero who invented a vending machine in 215BC to dispense holy water in Egyptian Temples. Vending has moved on since then and today's machines and services are sophisticated, technologically advanced and designed to provide top-quality, hygienic and reliable service 24 hours a day.

Consumers annually spend some £1bn through the slots of the more than 450 000 refreshment vending machines in use in Britain. Every day 8 million cups of coffee and 2 million cups of tea are vended because vending is accessible, convenient and meets consumer demand to be always available.

Why vending?

○ **Convenience:** vended goods are available 24 hours a day and machines can be sited just where you want them.

○ **Time saving:** vending machines are not only convenient, they are time saving too. Research conducted by NOP showed that an average size business with 50 staff could be spending more than £85000 of its annual wages bill in time spent by employees making their own tea and coffee.

○ **Hygiene:** with vending you get a clean cup every time and avoid the chore of washing up china cups, or worse still having dirty crockery hanging around all day.

○ **Recycling:** the SaveaCup scheme provides a ready way to recycle used vending cups into durable items for the office.

○ **Variety:** vending machines offer a whole range of different products and beverages. Drinks vending machines can offer not just black and white coffee and tea but can also make the drink weak or strong according to taste. Fresh brew, cappuccino and chocolate drinks are also available. Then there is confectionery, savoury snacks, ice cream, sandwiches, snack foods and meals.

Types of equipment

The main types of refreshment machine are:

○ beverage – traditional or in-cup;
○ can or carton;
○ glass Fronted Merchandisers for confectionery and snacks;
○ refrigerated food;
○ confectionery and Ambient Foods;
○ ice Cream.

Beverage machines are available to suit all sizes of operation, from table-top machines suitable for a small office environment to fully automatic high volume machines.

Manual Dispenser-type machines are either plumbed into mains water or have a built-in water tank for filling by hand. There are two types – In-cup, where the ingredients are pre-packed in the cup, or dispenser, where customers place an empty cup under the ingredient dispensing point.

Most dispensers are mounted on cabinets and can have payment systems fitted if required.

Single product dispensers are dedicated to one drink such as leaf tea, ground coffee, hot chocolate or cappuccino. They are sited primarily at counter service areas.

Vending equipment

The type of machine and its exact location will depend on the likely demand. Before deciding on equipment consider:

○ How many people will be using the machine, during what hours?
○ What products will they want?
○ How much will they be prepared to pay for the drinks?
○ Will there be long periods when the machine is not in use (for example school holidays)?
○ What other sources of supply are available locally, what do they charge and what do they offer?
○ Where will the machine be located?
○ Is it readily accessible to all those who want to use it?
○ Is there a convenient supply of portable water and electricity nearby?
○ Do you want users to pay by cash, token, card or are you providing free drinks?
○ What is your budget for the machine?

Further information can be obtained from the Automatic Vending Association, Upper Mulgrave Road, Cheam, Surrey SM2 7AJ. Tel: 020 8661 1112. e.mail. info @ avavending.org. website: www.ava-vending.org

HARMONISATION OF QUALITY STANDARDS

The year 2000 saw the introduction by the English Tourism Council, AA and RAC of **'Harmonised Quality Standards'** for serviced accommodation. The symbols of Stars for hotels and Diamonds for guest accommodation will be common to the schemes that now inspect to the same standard. Properties are visited annually by trained, impartial assessors and inspected before being awarded a classification that is standard across all three organisations.

The English Tourism Council gives **Gold and Silver Awards** for both hotels and guest accommodation who have achieved the highest levels of quality within their rating. While the overall rating is based on a combination of facilities and quality, the Gold and Silver Awards are based solely on quality.

Accommodation Guide – England
HOTELS – STAR RATINGS ★★★★★

Hotels are given a rating of one to five Stars – the more Stars, the higher the quality and the greater the range of facilities and level of service provided.

STAR RATINGS

★ **Practical accommodation** with a limited range of facilities and services, and a high standard of cleanliness throughout (75% of rooms will have en-suite or private facilities. Friendly and courteous staff. A restaurant/eating area offering breakfast and dinner to you and your guests. Alcoholic drinks served in a bar or lounge.

★★ **Good accommodation** offering a personal style of service with additional facilities, normally including a lift. More comfortable bedrooms (all with en-suite or private facilities and colour TV).

★★★ **Often a larger establishment** with more spacious public areas and bedrooms, all offering a significantly greater quality and range of facilities and services. A more formal style of service with a receptionist. A wide selection of drinks, light lunch and snacks served in a bar or lounge. Room service for continental breakfast and laundry service.

★★★★ **Superior comfort and quality.** All rooms with en-suite facilities. Spacious and well appointed public areas, and a strong emphasis on food and drink. Experienced staff responding to your needs and requests. Room service for continental breakfast and laundry service.

★★★★★ **Spacious and luxurious** offering accommodation, extensive facilities, services and cuisine of the highest international quality. Professional, attentive staff, exceptional comfort and a sophisticated ambience.

Guest Accommodation – Diamond Ratings ◆◆◆◆◆

Guest Accommodation, which includes guesthouses, bed and breakfasts, inns and farmhouses and other establishments not eligible for hotel standard, is rated from one to five Diamonds. The scheme puts emphasis on quality with a minimum requirement of facilities applying to all Guest Accommodation covering areas such as cleanliness, service and hospitality, bedrooms, bathrooms and food quality. Progressively higher levels of quality and customer care must be provided for each of the one to five Diamond ratings.

◆ clean accommodation, providing acceptable comfort with functional decor and offering as a minimum, a full cooked or continental breakfast. Other meals, where provided, will be freshly cooked. You will have a clean, comfortable bed, towels and fresh soap. Adequate heating and hot water available at reasonable times for baths or showers at no extra charge. An acceptable overall level of quality and helpful service.

◆◆ In addition to that provided at One Diamond: **A sound overall level of quality** and customer care in all areas.

◆◆◆ In addition to that provided at Two Diamond: **Good quality, comfortable bedrooms;** well maintained, practical decor; a good choice of quality items available for breakfast; other meals provided, will be freshly cooked from good quality ingredients. A good degree of comfort and customer care.

◆◆◆◆ In addition to that provided at Three Diamond: **A very good overall level of quality** in all areas and customer care showing attention to your needs.

◆◆◆◆◆ In addition to that provided at Four diamond: **Ample space with a degree of luxury,** excellent quality bed, high quality furniture, and excellent interior design. Breakfast offering a wide choice of high quality fresh ingredients; other meals, where provided, seasonal local ingredients. Excellent levels of customer care anticipating your needs.

NATIONAL ACCESSIBILITY SCHEME

The English Tourism Council and National and Regional Tourists Boards throughout Britain types of places to stay, on holiday or business, that provide accessible accommodation for wheelchair users and others who may have difficulty walking.

The Tourist Boards recognise three categories of accessibility: Accessible to all wheelchair users including those travelling independently; Accessible to a wheelchair user with assistance; Accessible to a wheelchair user able to walk short distances and up at least three steps.

Quality standards – Scotland
HOTEL, GUEST ACCOMMODATION AND SELF-CATERING

The different types of accommodation from Hotels and Bed & Breakfasts, through to Inns, Lodges and Self-Catering, are all in keeping with a new simple system. The grading system gives you a clear indication of ambience, cleanliness, hospitality, accommodation standard and food.

The True Stars of Scottish Hospitality

★★★★★ Exceptional, World-Class

★★★★ Excellent

★★★ Very Good

★★ Good

★ Fair and Acceptable

Quality Standards – Wales

The stars are your guide to quality. The star grades apply to all serviced accommodation and places which score highly will have an especially welcoming atmosphere and pleasing ambience, with high levels of comfort and guest care, paying special attention to detail.

★★★★★ Exceptional quality, with the highest standard of furnishings flawless service and meticulous guest care

★★★★ Excellent quality, with a high standard of furnishings, service and guest care.

★★★ Very good quality in the overall standard of furnishings, service and guest care.

★★ Good quality in the overall standard of furnishings, service and guest care.

★ Fair to good quality in the overall standard of furnishings, service and guest care.

Please note that the star grade takes into account the nature of the property and expectation of the guests, therefore a farmhouse is just as entitled to five stars as a hotel, as long as the facilities are of the highest quality.

http://www.good.accommodation.guide.co.uk

http://www.a/tourism.com/uk/ratings

http://www.englishtourism.org.uk

CUSTOMER CARE

Many staff may have the opportunity of direct contact with consumer or customers in most types of establishments. For some it will be a regular aspect of their job, for others it may be for irregular events or special occasions. Waiters and waitresses and food service personnel called upon to serve customers need to be aware of how to provide consumer satisfaction.

Catering staff serving at food service counters directly to customers may be employed in canteens, refectories, dining halls, etc., in schools, hospitals, industrial establishments, offices and other establishments. Other food outlets include fast-food establishments such as crêperies, baked potato houses, McDonalds, fish and chip shops and take-aways; buffets at all kinds of functions including outdoor catering, wedding receptions and carveries. The following information is intended to assist catering employees at all levels not only to provide customer satisfaction but to obtain job satisfaction when caring for customers. The first thing to remember is that a smile puts both the customer and you off to a good start; however it is important to realise that excellent food served from the kitchen is the first essential to satisfy the customer but the finest food produced for a meal can be completely spoiled if served by uncaring staff. Technical skills and technique are very important, but equally or perhaps more important, are sincere caring attitudes and manners, with the food served in an environment which has an atmosphere making the customer feel at ease, wanted and welcome.

Customer care is, therefore, caring for customers. Remember:

○ put the customer first;   ○ make them feel good;

○ make them feel comfortable;

○ make them feel important;

○ make them want to return to your restaurant or establishment.

It is important that you adjust your behaviour to suit certain customers and to treat all customers equally as if they were special. Give them your time and full attention. Use body language to put customers at ease.

Concentrate on:

○ your appearance;

○ a clean tidy environment;

○ answering the phone within three rings;

○ achieving positive results;

○ using the phone correctly;

○ writing to customers;

○ finding out what makes customers happy;

○ ensuring that what you give is what the customer wants.

The customer needs to be kept informed. You yourself should take responsibility and not pass the buck, and achieve results if people complain. You must show the customer empathy and be able to discuss things from their point of view. They expect good *customer care*.

Customer care is now an important concept: getting customers and keeping them creates revenue (income). All other activities create costs.

Emotional factors surround the products that people buy; these include the after-sales service, speed of delivery and the ambience, especially in a restaurant. Customer satisfaction or dissatisfaction comes more and more from the way people are treated. Customers buy a total package. Customer care gives the caterer the opportunity to be "special", to stand above the competition, winning customers and keeping them loyal. When a customer comes into contact with you the caterer, your image is being exposed to the customer. The staff of the company are perceived as representing not themselves but the company that they are working for.

Customer perceptions are often emotional, idiosyncratic and sometimes irrational, often based on narrow observations. When a restaurant manager remembers a customer's name, customers are delighted, but if staff treat customers badly, they will be unhappy. Often customers then react making the staff unhappy, thus affecting the business. If staff make the customers happy they will respond in kind:

Happy staff ↔ Happy customers
↓
Good profits

Staff can benefit from good customer-care training. Dealing with people is a highly complex skill; we train people to use complicated machinery but we do not often consider training staff to deal with the most complex machinery of all, the human being.

The caterer must first:

○ set standards for customer care;

○ set up training schemes;

○ measure performance;

○ reward accordingly.

Staff must know:

○ what the company stands for, what is its mission;

○ what behaviour the company values highly;

○ that cutting costs is *not* more important than customer care;

○ that all guarantees must be honoured;

○ that the restaurant or establishment is in business to keep the customer happy;

○ that happy customers can lead to repeat business and recommendations to friends and colleagues.

HOW TO WIN COMMITMENT FROM STAFF

Staff will be happier and feel more committed by:

○ good leadership;
○ avoiding unnecessary stress; remove the causes, if they are under your control;
○ knowing the fundamental importance of the customer; seek ideas from your staff on how to improve customer care;
○ receiving good customer-care training;
○ building pride in their work performance;
○ having their training reinforced periodically.

Training aspects in customer care

When you are training staff the following can be used as a guide:

○ Identify what the staff should know in caring for the customer.
○ Know what the customer may ask them.
○ Know what's on the menu, the composition of the dishes.
○ Know what the special dishes of the day are.
○ Know what the chef's specialities are.

Examples of good customer-care phrases you may hear in a restaurant or service area include:

○ 'I'll take care of that for you right away.'
○ 'I'll go and get it for you myself.'
○ 'Is there anything else I can help you with?'
○ 'I'll be glad to help you.'
○ 'I don't know, but I'll find out now. Please take a seat for a moment.'
○ 'I'm sorry to hear about that. Let's find out what went wrong and I'll put it right.'
○ 'I'm sorry for the delay. I'll check with the kitchen to see how long your order will be.'

Good communication within the organisation assists in the development of customer care. It is important that the staff are constantly kept informed of what is going on otherwise they will feel that they are not part of the organisation. They must have a sense of 'ownership' or responsibility, since well motivated staff are good for the organisation and they will help in the progressive development of the business, helping to avoid the 'It's not my job attitude'.

If staff are expected to work hygienically and treat the staff well you must likewise treat the staff with respect and care for their well-being. Good staff welfare aids the process of customer care. Staff must have good clean changing rooms, washing or/and showering facilities, quality facilities for refreshments and medical provision.

Staff too must treat each other with respect, co-operating and supporting each other. A good team spirit will ultimately affect the customer. Remember behaviour begets behaviour so, if one member of staff treats another badly, they in turn may treat the customer badly.

Customer care is a team game: it is about all the staff working to the same aim, getting the customers on their side.

Define standards of performance

The starting point is a clear analysis of what should happen at each of the points of contact that a customer might have with the restaurant and it becomes a check list. For example:

○ A customer enters the restaurant or service area.
  – The entrance should be clean and tidy.
  – The doors could be marked 'welcome'.

○ The customer is then greeted by the head waiter, restaurant manager or receptionist.
  – The reception area is clean, tidy, perhaps decorated with fresh flowers.
  – Menu sample and drinks list on display.
  – All staff smartly dressed and well groomed.
  – Staff smile when greeting customers.
  – If possible head waiter, restaurant manager or receptionist use customer's name.
  – Customer is escorted to the table, assisted into the seating position.
  – If there is any delay, staff apologise and explanation is given to the customer.
  – Waiter introduces him/herself to the customer.

○ At the end of the meal, head waiter or restaurant manager escorts customer to the door, smiles and exchanges pleasantries: 'good day'/'good night'.

When defining standards of performance, use numbers: for example, answer the 'phone within three rings; if there is a delay, update the caller every 20 seconds with 'Sorry, the line is still engaged, do you still wish to hold?'

Staff must have a sense of identity with the company or organisation. At McDonalds, there is a 700-page Operations and Training Manual which explains every stage of the cooking process and the correct behaviour to be used when dealing with customers.

Disney gives all new staff an induction programme called 'traditions' which explains about Walt Disney, the characters, what it is like to work in Disneyland and their role. It stresses that all visitors are not 'customers' but 'guests' so they must be treated that way. Although on most days there will be more than half a million of them, they must be dealt with as individuals not as a crowd. These individuals look to the staff to help them enjoy their day, the staff therefore have a crucial role to play. Disney explains to all their staff that they:

○ are part of show business;
○ are performers in a live show;
○ must make sure that nothing spoils the perfect picture the guests see;
○ must make a clear distinction between 'on stage' and 'off stage': off stage they are able to relax, on stage they must play the perfect role; they must never be seen with their 'mask off'.

It may be said that caterers are also part of showbusiness, that waiters are performers in a live show. TGI Friday restaurants have further developed this concept where waiters and food service staff are interviewed on the basis of their personality. They become actors as part of a large show. Traditionally waiters that perform flambé dishes 'live' in front of a customer, show off their flair and skill. Such staff develop a sense of importance and pride in their job.

Measure and monitor performance

The defined standards of performance must be monitored and measured. You need to measure success in terms of your premises to customers. Measuring the right thing helps staff understand what is important to customers and how to act accordingly.

Staff who look after customers and provide the service and care they expect, deserve rewarding. Good positive feedback to staff is important; you may:

○ just say 'well done' which goes a long way or payment of a bonus;

○ make a payment of a bonus;

○ give an increment on an annual pay increase;

○ give a promotion.

Continuing customer care

Keep in touch with customers through mailshot, advertising, etc.

Customer care skills

ATTITUDE AND BEHAVIOUR

If a customer is rude or aggressive to a waiter (blames a waiter for the chef's mistake), the waiter should not be rude or aggressive in return. If the waiter can remain calm and use his/her skills of patience, the customer will often apologise for their anger. Behaviour is a choice; you should select the behaviour which is appropriate for the customer.

When dealing with customers, behaviour should be:

○ professional;

○ understanding – customers in a restaurant want a service and are paying for it; learn to understand their needs;

○ patient – learn to be patient with all customers.

○ enthusiastic – it can be contagious;

○ confident – it can increase a potential customer's trust in you;

○ welcoming – it can satisfy customer's basic human desire to feel liked and be approved of;

○ helpful – customers warm to helpful staff;

○ polite – good manners are always welcomed;

○ caring – make each customer feel special.

APPEARANCE

Remember you never get a second chance to make a first impression. What you wear and how you look is part of how potential customers judge your organisation. You are part of the company's image.

BODY LANGUAGE

Body language includes:

○ how you dress;

○ your distance from others;

○ how you sit;

○ movements;

○ gestures;

○ posture;

○ stance;

○ facial expressions;

○ eye contact;

○ eye movements.

Body language tells us what people really mean. It is the art of seeing what others are thinking. If someone is telling a lie their body language will usually give them away. By focusing on other people's body language you can discover their true feeling towards you and what they think of what you are saying. It has a clear value in business situations and is therefore very important in customer care.

Learn to:
- look for what is important;
- recognise other people so you are able to "read" them better;
- recognise how to use body language;
- control it and use it to your advantage, so that you give the right positive message to people.

Remember that body language is universal but does mean different things in different cultures.

SIGNS AND MEANINGS

- One gesture: doesn't show how the other person is thinking.
- Arms folded: may mean that:
  - they are being defensive about something;
  - they are cold;
  - they are comfortable.
- Some gestures: are open, expansive, positive.
- Leaning forward with open palms facing upwards: shows interest, acceptance, welcoming attitude.
- Leaning backwards, arms folded, head down: closed defensive and negative, disinterested, rejection.
- Plenty of gestures: warmth, enthusiasm and emotion.
- Using gestures sparsely: cold, reserved logical.

DISTANCE

Each person has around them an area that they regard as a personal space. Beware of intruding into a customer's personal space. Although some customers may regard it as friendliness you may make others feel uncomfortable.

Placing people at a table for a meeting or for lunch or dinner is an art. The way people sit round a table, sends messages.

- Formal meeting – people sit opposite each other.
- Team work – sitting people side by side is stressful.

EYES

Eye contact should be used as a way of acknowledging customers, making them feel welcome and as a foundation of building a good relationship. Eye contact should be used to show the customer you are listening.

EARS

Really listening is the highest form of courtesy:
- Look at the customer.
- Ignore any negative thoughts you have about them.
- Lean towards them.
- Think at the pace they are talking.
- Listen to every word.
- Try not to interrupt.
- Use facial expressions and body language to show you understand.

○ Stick to the subject.

○ Use their name wherever possible.

GREETING PEOPLE

If you are already dealing with another customer in the restaurant acknowledge the new customer and reassure them that you will help them as soon as possible. Try to greet people with a smile that's genuine. You may even get one in return, after all smiles are free. Remember that good manners are important.

Use peoples' names, it holds their attention. It demonstrates recognition and respect. Their name is probably the most important word in the world to them. Always use their surname until they give you permission for you to use their first name.

Asking the customer questions will demonstrate

○ you have properly understood what the customer wants;

○ you have time for them to talk;

○ interest on your part;

○ you feel the customer is important;

○ you are able to find out how they feel;

○ you can keep control of the conversation;

○ you can understand their needs, their complaints;

○ you know how to make customers feel better.

STROKING

This is defined as giving any kind of attention. Humans need stroking. A prolonged absence of it can cause serious adverse effects.

How good a customer feels about your restaurant or catering establishment is directly connected to the amount and types of strokes (attention) they have received.

Stroking can be both positive or negative, it can be physical, verbal and non-verbal.

Some examples of positive stroking include:

○ greetings; compliments; laughing.

Some examples of negative stroking include:

○ unpleasant greeting;

○ pushing;

○ sarcastic remarks;

○ absence of praise;

○ adverse criticism;

○ swearing;

○ snatching;

○ unpleasant hand gestures.

PACING

Pacing is speaking in a way that is compatible with your customers. Match their speed, tone and volume. Do not talk above their heads.

ASSERTIVENESS

Remember customers are human beings; you may have to handle them when they shout at you, interrupt you, are rude to you, criticise you or blame you for something you have not done. The answer is for you to be assertive, standing up for your rights.

Being assertive means

○ stating your views while showing that you understand their views;

○ enhancing yourself without diminishing them;

○ speaking calmly, sincerely and steadily.

Advantages of assertive behaviour

There are some advantages to be gained:

It gives you greater self confidence.

○ You will be treating others as equals, recognising the ability and limitations of others, rather than regarding them as superiors.

○ It gives greater self-responsibility.

○ It gives greater self-control; your mind is concentrated on achieving the behaviour you want.

○ It can produce a win situation; opinions on both sides are given a fair hearing, so they feel that they have won.

TELEPHONE

A badly handled telephone call can destroy the effect of good advertising. Remember: when using the telephone, give all your attention to the customer; get their name, write it down and use it. Take note of all the other details the customer is wanting. Listen and use your voice correctly. Summarise what you have agreed with the customer at the end of the conversation.

HOW TO HANDLE CUSTOMER COMPLAINTS

Some statistics on complaints:

○ 96% of dissatisfied customers do not go back and complain, but they do tell between seven and eleven other people how bad your restaurant or service is.

○ 13% will tell at least twenty other people.

○ 90% will never return to your restaurant.

○ It costs roughly five times as much to attract a new customer as it does to keep an existing one.

Therefore, encourage customers to complain on the spot. If they are unhappy about anything that is served to them, they should be encouraged to inform the member of staff who served them. This will give the establishment the opportunity to rectify the fault immediately. Ask them about their eating experience; this information will be vital for future planning. Treat any customer who complains well; offer them a free drink or a free meal. Make the complainant your ambassadors. Show them empathy, use the appropriate body language, show concern, sympathise. Always apologise. If you handle the complaint well you will make the customer feel important. Remember:

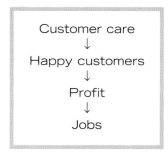

```
Customer care
       ↓
Happy customers
       ↓
    Profit
       ↓
     Jobs
```

DON'T

○ say 'it's not my fault'
○ say 'you're the fifth today to complain about that'
○ interrupt – it will only add to their wrath
○ jump to conclusions
○ accept responsibility until you are sure it's your firm's fault
○ be patronising
○ argue
○ lose your temper
○ blame others

DO

○ show empathy and use appropriate body language (e.g. show concern on your face, nod)
○ use their name, when possible
○ shut up and listen, and use body language to show that you are listening (e.g. use eye contact)
○ take notes
○ let them make their case, they will lose their head of steam
○ ask questions to clarify the details
○ recapitulate; confirm with them that you've got it right.
○ sympathise (regardless of where the blame lies).
○ gather together your version of the facts before replying.
○ phone back if necessary – on time!
○ apologise profusely if your company is at fault.
○ tell them what you propose to do.
○ give them alternatives to choose from, if your company is at fault.
○ offer more than the bare minimum (e.g. make some concession on 'future business')
○ get their full agreement that this will resolve the issue.
○ make sure that it is done properly and that they are kept fully informed.
○ contact them very soon afterwards to make sure that they are happy.
○ see it as an opportunity to cement the relationship and encourage more business.

If you handle the customer complaint well, you will make the customer feel important. They will want to praise your company to their friends. Then they may well be prepared to deal with you again. So ask open questions to discover their future wants. For example:

○ 'How often do you come to this establishment? and how often do you order this from the menu'?
○ 'How do you think your requirements will change in the future'?
○ 'What will you be looking for then?' 'What other services or meal items will you be looking for in the future?'

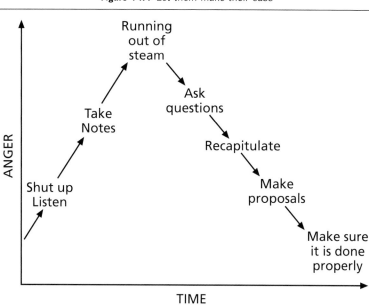

Figure 14.4 *Let them make their case*

Some references to marketing elsewhere in the book

Menu planning	316	Computer use	565
Pricing	338		

Topics for Discussion

1 Your ideas for promoting a 100-seat industrial catering restaurant in an office block.
2 Examples of advertising.
3 What you understand by good public relations.
4 The advantages of cafeteria service.
5 The popularity of take-aways and what you think the changes will be in take-away services in the future.
6 When is the use of vending machines worthwhile? Discuss where and how.
7 Can advertising increase sales? Explain how it could be used for a restaurant or any food service facility.
8 Making contact with local media to promote your business.

PART 6

Legislation

CHAPTER 15

HEALTH AND SAFETY

INTRODUCTION – ACCIDENTS

Why are health and safety important factors?

400 people are killed in accidents each year

One million workers get injured each year

Almost 30,000 workers in a year suffer major injuries at work

5% of the population suffer from ill health caused by work

Back problems are the most common form of work related ill health

The fatal injury rate in Great Britain is $\frac{1}{4}$ of what it was in 1971

Around one in five workers have been attacked or threatened by a member of the public

Self employed people at work are twice as likely to be killed at work as employees

Health and safety targets

By the year 2010 it is the intention to reduce the working days lost from injury and ill health at work by 30%.

To reduce by 10% the number of fatal and major accidents at the work place.

Cases of work related ill heath to be reduced by 20%.

By 2004 half the improvement rate should be achieved.

Significant factors for the catering industry

CAUSE	IMPORTANCE	SIGNIFICANT FACTOR
Slips, trips	30% but 75% of all major injuries	88% due to slippery floors due to spillage not cleared up, wet floors and buckets etc in passage ways and uneven floors
Handling	29%	$\frac{1}{3}$ due to lifting pans, trays, etc. $\frac{1}{3}$ handling sharp objects e.g. knives. $\frac{1}{3}$ awkward lifts from low ovens or from high positions
Exposure to hazardous substances, hot surfaces, steam	16%	61% from splashes. 13% from hot objects Causes poor maintenance. 28% or cases Steam from ovens, steamer. 23% carrying hot liquids 16% misuse of cleaning materials. 14% cleaning flat fryers. 14% equipment failure. 12% horseplay 4% hot surfaces 1%
Struck by moving articles including hand tools	10%	$\frac{1}{3}$ from most probably knives. $\frac{1}{4}$ from falling articles. $\frac{1}{10}$ from assault
Walking into objects	4%	$\frac{3}{4}$ of cases involved walking into fixed as opposed to moveable one
Machinery	3%	Slicers 30%. Mixers 16%. Vegetable cutting machines 9%. Vegetable slicing, mincing and grating attachments 10%. Pie and tart machines 4%. Dough mixers, dough moulder, mincing machine, dish washer 2%
Falls	1.8%	$\frac{3}{4}$ falls from low height (but $\frac{1}{2}$ of the major injuries) occurred on stairs
Fire and explosion	1.6%	80% during manually igniting gas fire appliances, mainly ovens
Electric shock	0.5%	25% due to poor maintenance. 25% trolley involved. 25% unsafe switching and unplugging ($\frac{3}{4}$ in wet conditions). 25% poor maintenance
Transporter	3%	$\frac{1}{2}$ involved lift trucks

RIDDOR – Reporting Injuries, Diseases and Dangerous Occurrences

RIDDOR regulations came into effect in 1996 and requires work related accidents, diseases and dangerous occurrences to be reported by employers to Incident Contact Centre, Caerphilly Business Park, Caerphilly CF 83 3GG.

Records must be kept of each occurrence.

REPORTABLE MAJOR INJURIES	
Fracture other than finger, thumb or toe	
Amputation	
Dislocation of hip, knee or spine	
Loss of sight (temporary or permanent)	
Chemical or hot metal burn to the eye or any penetration to the eye	
Injury from electric shock or burn leading to unconsciousness or requiring resuscitation or admittance to hospital for more than 24 hours	
Any other injury leading to hypothermia, health induced illness or unconsciousness or requiring resuscitation or admittance to hospital for more than 24 hours	
Unconsciousness caused by asphyxia or exposure to a harmful substance or biological agent	
Acute illness requiring medical treatment, or loss of consciousness from absorption by inhalation, ingestion or through the skin	
Acute illness requiring medical treatment where there is reason to believe that this resulted from exposure to a biological agent or its toxins or infected material	

Examples of reportable diseases include certain poisons, dermatitis, skin cancer, lung diseases such as occupational asthma, infections such as hepatitis, tuberculosis, anthrax and tetanus.

An example of a dangerous occurrence could be an overloaded electric circuit causing a major fire.

Three day injuries are not major but cause the employee to be absent for more than 3 days consecutively but not counting the day of the injury, but including days they would not normally be at work.

HSE Guidance Literature

Health & Safety in kitchens and food preparation areas (HS(G) 55.

Catering safety: food preparation machinery (HS(G) 35.

Safety in meat preparation HS(G) 45.

Manual handling. Solutions you can handle HS(G) 115.

Essentials of health and safety at work.

Food sheet No. 1 Safety pays in the catering industry.

Food sheet No. 2 Priorities for health and safety in catering activities.

THE NEED FOR SAFETY

The dual responsibility of employers and employees at work is to ensure that the premises and equipment are safe and that they are kept safe so as to prevent accidents. Employers need to assess any hazards or risks and organise procedures to deal with any accidents. Employees, full-time, part-time or temporary, need to be trained to prevent accidents, to report hazards and to comply with instructions intended to reduce risks.

Safety signs are used to inform all persons using an establishment in order to prevent accidents or what to do in the event of an accident.

The kitchen is not the safest of environments and three major areas require particular attention.

○ Safe hygienic food handling

○ Safe premises and equipment storage

○ Safe storage and use of hazardous substances

Firstly, it is essential to analyse the situation to ascertain what could be unsafe, what may cause risk or be a hazard to the chefs themselves and/or their customers, and to have a system to reduce risks.

○ Analyse potential hazard. If possible remove the hazard

↓

○ Reduce risks to a minimum having identified them

↓

○ Determine which are critical

↓

○ Implement a control system

↓

○ Review and record

HACCP or Hazard Analysis and Critical Control Points is a system intended to reduce risks and dangers at crucial points. This systematic way of determining the presence of food safety risks and deciding on controls which, when implemented, will avoid the risk.

As an example of the use of critical control points regarding high risk food, Figure 8.5, page 269 is an example of the use of critical control points regarding high risk points, in this case poultry.

Knowledge of all aspects of food hygiene, is essential so that CCP, Critical Control Points, can be pinpointed at crucial stages. See page 269.

The working environment, which includes premises and equipment both large and small, should be subjected to analysis so that critical control points can be identified. The objective is to eliminate, if possible, or reduce accidents to a minimum. Well-trained, experienced people working in the catering industry seldom have accidents – because they do not take risks. They are aware of the dangers and have regard for themselves, their equipment and those they work with.

As an example, there is always a possibility of spillage of liquid on the floor. It is essential that it is cleaned immediately because it is a hazard. Others in the area need to know of the danger, if necessary with a cone. However, a non-slip floor would reduce the risk factor and lessen accidents.

Training in the use of equipment, knives and also what to do in the event of an accident or fire is essential.

USEFUL ADDRESS

Health & Safety Executive (HSE)

Rose Court

2 Southwark Bridge

London

SE1 9HS

CONTROL OF SUBSTANCES HAZARDOUS TO HEALTH (COSHH)

Substances dangerous to health are labelled **very toxic**, **toxic harmful**, **irritant** or **corrosive**. Whilst only a small number of such chemicals are used in catering for cleaning, it is necessary to be aware of the regulations introduced in 1989 and to know of the symbols used on products.

Principles

Those persons using such substances must be made aware of their correct use and proper dilution where appropriate, and must wear protection: goggles, gloves and face masks as appropriate. Eye goggles should be worn when using oven cleaners, gloves when hands may come into contact with any chemical cleaner and face masks when using grease cutting and oven degreasers.

It is essential that staff are trained to take precautions and not to take risks. What does COSHH require? The basic principles of occupational hygiene underlie the COSHH Regulations:

○ Assess the risk to health arising from work and what precautions are needed.

○ Introduce appropriate measures to prevent or control the risk.

○ Ensure that control measures are used and that equipment is properly maintained and procedures observed.

○ Where necessary, monitor the exposure of the workers and carry out an appropriate form of surveillance of their health.

○ Inform, instruct and train employees about the risks and the precautions to be taken.

Rules of using chemicals

○ Always follow makers' instructions.

○ Always store in original containers. Decanting a chemical means you may lose its name and classification.

○ Keep lids tightly closed.

○ Do not store in direct sunlight, near heat or naked flames.

○ Read the labels. Know the product and its risk.

○ Never mix chemicals.

○ Know the first-aid procedure.

○ Always add product to water, not water to product.

○ Dispose of empty drums immediately.

○ Dispose of waste chemical solutions safely.

○ Wear the correct safety equipment.

LEGISLATION

Every year in the UK a thousand people are killed at work; a million people suffer injuries; and 23 million working days are lost annually because of industrial injury and disease. As catering is one of the largest employers of labour the catering industry is substantially affected by accidents at work.

In 1974 the *Health and Safety at Work Act* was passed with two main aims:

○ to extend the coverage and protection of the law to all employers and employees;

○ to increase awareness of safety amongst those at work, both employers and employees.

The law imposes a general duty on an employer 'to ensure so far as is reasonably practicable, the health, safety and welfare at work of all his employees'. The law also imposes a duty on every employee while at work to:

○ take reasonable care for the health and safety of himself or herself and of other persons who may be affected by his or her acts or omissions at work;

○ co-operate with his or her employer so far as is necessary to meet or comply with any requirement concerning health and safety;

○ not interfere with, or misuse, anything provided in the interests of health, safety or welfare.

It can be clearly seen that both health and safety at work is everybody's responsibility.

Furthermore the Act protects the members of the public who may be affected by the activities of those at work.

Penalties are provided by the Act which include improvement notices, prohibition notices and criminal prosecution. The Health and Safety Executive has been set up to enforce the law and the Health and Safety Commission will issue codes of conduct and act as advisers.

Responsibilities of the employer

The employer's responsibilities are to:

○ provide and maintain premises and equipment that are safe and without risk to health;

- ○ provide supervision, information and training;
- ○ issue a written statement of 'safety policy' to employees to include:
  - – general policy with respect to health and safety at work of employees;
  - – the organisation, to ensure the policy is carried out;
  - – how the policy will be made effective.
- ○ consult with the employees' safety representative and to establish a Safety Committee.

Figure 15.1 *Business protection*

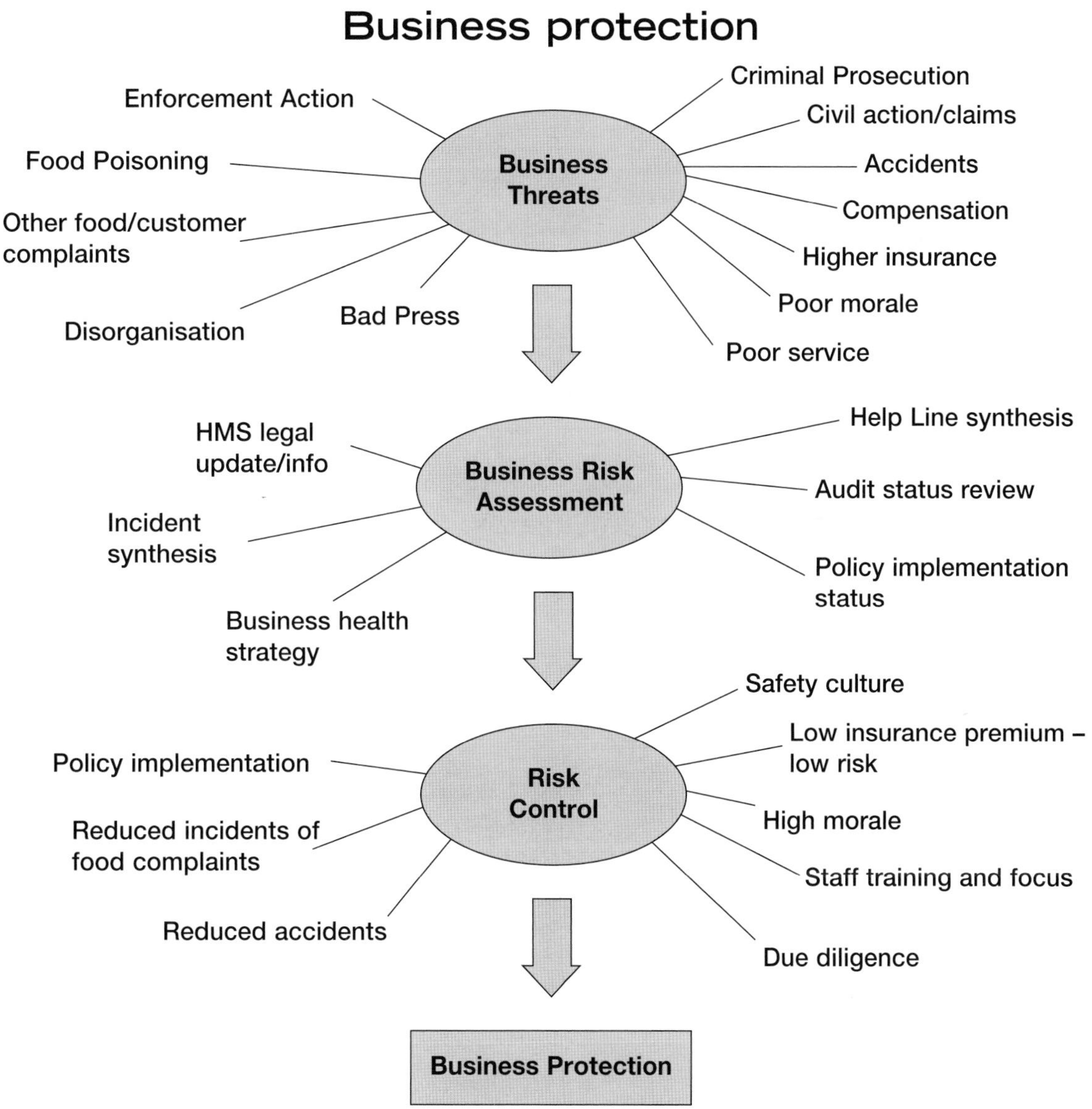

Business protection

Business Threats: Enforcement Action, Criminal Prosecution, Civil action/claims, Food Poisoning, Accidents, Compensation, Other food/customer complaints, Higher insurance, Poor morale, Disorganisation, Bad Press, Poor service

Business Risk Assessment: HMS legal update/info, Help Line synthesis, Audit status review, Incident synthesis, Policy implementation status, Business health strategy

Risk Control: Safety culture, Low insurance premium – low risk, Policy implementation, High morale, Reduced incidents of food complaints, Staff training and focus, Reduced accidents, Due diligence

Business Protection

Source: Croners Catering

SAFETY REGULATIONS

As from 1993 six health and safety at work regulations have come into force.

○ *Management of Health and Safety at Work Regulations 1992*
  – risk assessment;
  – control of hazardous substances;
  – training.
○ *Work Place (Health, Safety and Welfare) Regulations 1992*
  – floors to be of suitable construction;
  – floors free from hazardous articles or substances;
  – steps taken to avoid slips, trips and falls.
○ *Manual Handling Operation Regulations 1992*
  – reducing incorrect handling of loads;
  – preventing hazardous handling.
○ *Fire Precautions in Places of Work*
  – means of fire fighting;
  – evacuation procedures;
  – raising the alarm.
○ *Provision and Use of Work Equipment*
  – ensure correct usage;
  – properly maintained;
  – training given.
○ *Health and Safety (Display Screen Equipment)*
  – to see that staff using visual display units have suitable work place and take regular breaks.

Risk assessment and reduction

Prevention of accidents and preventing food poisoning in catering establishments is essential, therefore it is necessary to assess the situation and decide what action is to be taken. Risk assessment can be divided into four areas:

Minimal risk – safe conditions with safety measures in place.

○ Some risk – acceptable risk, however attention must be given to ensure safety measures operate.
○ Significant risk – where safety measures are not fully in operation (also includes food most likely to cause food poisoning). Requires immediate action.
○ Dangerous risk – operations of process or equipment to stop immediately. The system of equipment to be completely checked and recommended after clearance.

To operate an assessment of risks the following points should be considered:

○ assess the risks;
○ determine preventative measures;
○ decide who carries out safety inspections;
○ decide frequency of inspection;
○ determine methods of reporting back and to whom;

○ detail how to ensure inspections are effective;

○ see that on the job training in safety is related to the job.

The purpose of the exercise of assessing the possibility of risks and hazards is to prevent accidents. Firstly it is necessary to monitor the situations, to have regular and spasmodic checks to see that standards set are being complied with. However, should an incident or incidences occur, it is essential that an investigation is made as to the cause or causes and any defects in the system remedied at once. Immediate action is required to prevent further accidents. All personnel need to be trained to be actively aware of the possible hazards and risks and to take positive action to prevent accidents occurring.

The work place

The highest number of accidents occurring in catering premises are due to persons falling, slipping or tripping. Therefore, floor surfaces must be of a suitable construction to reduce this risk. A major reason for the high incidence of this kind of accident is that water and grease are likely to be spilt and the combination of these substances is treacherous and makes the floor surface slippery. For this reason any spillage must be cleaned immediately and warning notices put in place, where appropriate, stating the danger of slippery surface. Ideally a member of staff should stand guard until the hazard is cleared.

Another cause of falls is the placing of articles on the floor in corridors, passageways or between stoves and tables. Persons carry trays and containers have their vision obstructed and items on the floor may not be visible; the fall may occur onto a hot stove and the item being carried may be hot. These falls can have very bad consequences.

The solution is to ensure that nothing is left on the floor which may cause a hazard. If it is necessary to have articles temporarily on the floor, then it is desirable that they are guarded so as to prevent accidents.

Kitchen personnel should be trained to think and act in a safe manner so as to avoid this kind of accident.

Manual handling

Figure 15.2 *How to lift correctly*

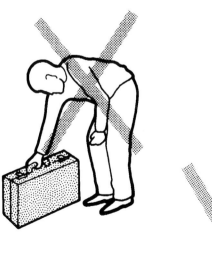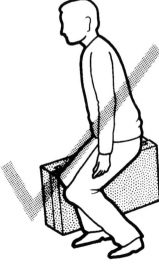

The incorrect handling of heavy and awkward loads causes accidents and staff can be off work for some time. How to lift heavy items the correct way is illustrated in Figure 15.2. The safer way to lift items is to bend at the knees rather than bend the back. Strain and damage can be reduced if two people do the lifting rather that one person.

When goods are moved on trolleys, trucks or any wheeled vehicles, they should be loaded carefully (not overloaded) and in a manner which enables the handler to see where they are going.

It is essential that heavy items are stacked at the bottom and that steps are used with care.

Particular care is needed when large pots are moved containing liquid, especially hot liquid. They should not be filled to the brim.

Warning that equipment handles, lids etc., can be hot, should be indicated by a small sprinkle of flour or something similar.

Extra care is needed when taking trays from ovens or salamanders so that the tray does not burn someone else.

Provision and use of work equipment

Figure 15.3 *Heat- and flame-resistant kitchen apparel*

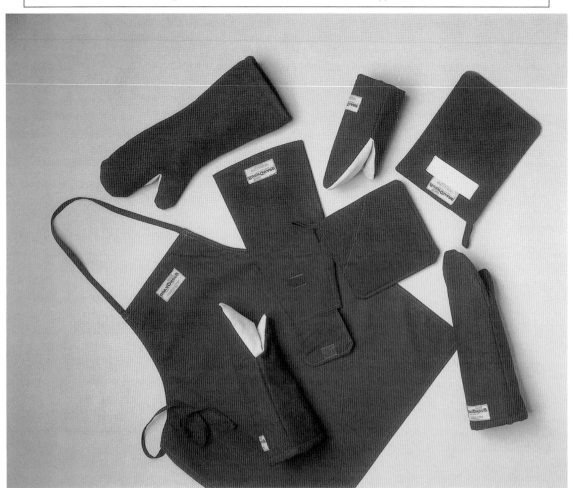

Equipment selected for use must be suitable for what it is intended. It should be of the right capacity and be sited conveniently and safely. All equipment must be properly maintained and staff using it must receive training with regards to correct usage and the safety measures which need to be taken.

Equipment must conform to EU safety directive. Since 1 January 1995, British Standards have been combined with European Standards and equipment must carry the CE mark indicating that the required safety standards are met.

Need for signage

Following risk assessment under the Management of Health and Safety at Work Regulations 1992, safety signage should only be implemented to control a hazard when all other methods to reduce the risk to employees have been exhausted. Safety signs must not take the place of other risk control methods and should significantly decrease the likelihood of an accident occurring.

The employer has a duty to:

○ provide and maintain any safety sign;

○ give employees clear information on unfamiliar signs;

○ give employees instructions and training in the meaning of the signs and what to do in connection with them.

There are two **main** types of signage:

Permanent – used for prohibitions, warnings and mandatory requirements, identifying emergency escape routes, first aid facilities and fire fighting equipment.

Occasional – including acoustic signals like fire alarms and illuminated signs such as fire escape signs which operate with emergency lighting systems.

Prohibition signs

Prohibit behaviour likely to increase or cause danger. Round with a red circular band and crossbar, featuring a black pictogram on a white background. (Red shall cover at least 35% of the area of the sign) eg *No Entry, No Exit*.

Figure 15.4 *No Smoking Sign*

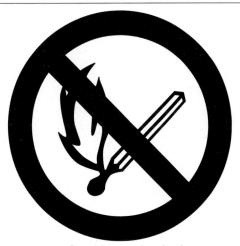

Smoking and naked
flames forbidden

Warning signs

Give warning of hazard or danger. Black triangular band with a black pictogram on a yellow background. (Yellow shall cover at least 50% of the area of the sign)

Slippery floor being cleaned – sign featuring *Danger – Slippery Surface*

Any "tricky" steps – sign featuring *Danger – Beware of Step*

Hot surfaces of equipment – sign featuring *Danger – Hot Surface*.

Figure 15.5 *Warning Signs*

Flammable material
or
high temperature

Mandatory signs

Give warning of hazard or danger. Describe a behaviour. Blue circle with a white pictogram. (Blue shall take up at least 50% of the area of the sign)

For all fire doors – *Fire door – Keep Closed*

For chemical dosing areas – *Wear Gloves, Eye Protection Must be Worn*

For dangerous machinery – *Guards Must Be In Position Before Starting*

Figure 15.6 *Mandatory Signs*

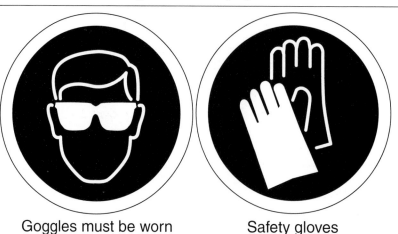

Goggles must be worn   Safety gloves
(no goggles, no job)   must be worn

Emergency Escape/First Aid Signs

Rectangular/square shape, with a white pictogram on green background. (Green part shall take up at least 40% of the area of the sign)

Emergency eye wash stations – sign featuring *Emergency Eye Wash*

For dangerous machinery, if applicable – sign featuring *Emergency Stop Push Button*

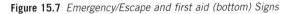

Figure 15.7 *Emergency/Escape and first aid (bottom) Signs*

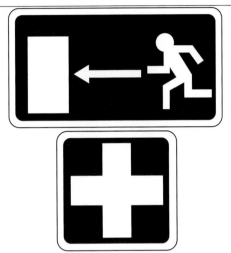

PERSONAL PROTECTIVE EQUIPMENT (PPE)

The Personal Protective Equipment at Work Regulations 1992 came into effect on 1st January 1993 and applies to all equipment designed to be worn or held by persons to protect them from one or more risks (uniforms, clothing required for hygiene purposes).

Health and Safety (Safety Signs and Signals) Regulations 1996

On 1st April 1996 these regulations completely revoked the previous Safety Signs and Signals Regulations 1986. They aim to standardise safety signing across the European Union, such that signs are seen, they will have the same meaning.

The labelling of dangerous substances and most machinery is not covered by these regulations.

Due to the hazardous nature of some of the work in the kitchens, it is necessary to assess the risks to employees. Provision of protective clothing and footwear, properly maintained, is essential to safety. Suitable storage, such as lockers, needs to be available for the storage of personal clothing.

Items such as oven cloths and heat-proof gloves need to be provided and maintained or replaced so that they are safe to use.

First-aid equipment must be readily available and replenished when necessary. There must be one trained first-aider for every 50 employees.

KITCHEN EQUIPMENT

All equipment should be safe and used correctly, properly maintained and not misused.

○ Tables must be strong, easily cleaned for hygiene reasons and never sat on.

○ Bratt pans and tilting pans should not be able to be accidentally tilted.

○ Fat fryers must not have thermostats tampered with and must never be over-filled.

○ Step ladders should only be used for reaching items stored on high shelves, not for standing on boxes or a chair.

○ Electrical equipment must have special attention particularly those listed under Dangerous Machines Order 1964:

 – worm type mincing machines;

 – rotary bowl choppers;

 – mixing machines;

 – slicing, shredding machines;

 – chipping, chopping machines.

Only trained and over 18-year-olds are allowed to use and clean such machines and warning signs and instruction in their use must be sited by the machine. Electrical Safety www.sgs.co.uk.

○ Gas equipment must have instructions for igniting any piece of gas equipment and these should be followed. In the event of a gas leak or problems with pilot lights, maintenance personnel or the gas equipment suppliers should be contacted immediately.

○ Maintenance should be regular to ensure correct function and safety of all gas and electrical equipment. This includes checking seals on microwave ovens.

○ Extraction system should function correctly and particular care is needed to see that it is regularly cleaned as fat is liable to accumulate.

○ Walk in refrigerators and deep freezers must have a door operable from the inside.

○ Records of staff trained in the use of equipment and records of maintenance need to be kept.

DISPLAY SCREEN EQUIPMENT

Persons using VDU (Visual Display Units) must operate in suitable conditions so as to reduce strain. Such units should be situated so that the working conditions are good, well ventilated, comfortable with good seating. Regular breaks are essential so as to reduce eye strain, and eye tests given and spectacles should be provided if needed.

Staff facilities and welfare

The welfare of all employees at a place of work is the responsibility of the employee. Facilities should be provided that are both safe and beneficial and include:

○ sufficient working space (minimum 11 cubic metres (14.4 cubic yards) per person);

○ easy evacuation in an emergency;

○ floors and exit routes non-slip and in good repair;

○ proper ventilation;

○ temperature comfortable (normally 16°C (61°F) never below 13°C (55°F) except when foods are to be kept cold);

○ system of maintenance put into practice;

○ system of cleaning in operation;

○ quick disposal of waste, so that is does not accumulate;

○ safe and non-obstructed, loading and unloading bays;

○ provision of adequate toilets, working facilities, drinking water;

○ changing facilities and accommodation for outdoor clothes, separate for men and women;

○ provision of a rest room, to include a non-smoking area.

Enforcement of legislation

Health and safety inspectors and local authority inspectors (Environmental Health Officers) have the authority to enforce legal requirements. They are empowered to:

○ issue a prohibition notice which immediately prevents further business until remedial action has been taken;

○ issue an improvement notice whereby action must be taken within a stated time, to an employee, employer or supplier;

○ prosecute any person breaking the Act; this can be instead of or in addition to serving a notice and may lead to a substantial fine or prison;

○ seize, render harmless or destroy anything that the inspector considers to be the cause of imminent danger.

ENVIRONMENTAL HEALTH OFFICERS

The Environmental Health Officer has two main functions: one is to enforce the law; the other aspect of the job is to act as an adviser and educator in the areas of food hygiene and catering premises. Here his or her function is to improve the existing standard of hygiene and to advise how this may be achieved. Frequently health education programmes are organised by Environmental Health Officers which may include talks and free literature. If in doubt about any matter concerning food hygiene, pests, premises or legal aspects the Environmental Health Officer is there to be consulted.

OCCUPATIONAL HEALTH

Occupational health means keeping oneself free from illnesses associated with conditions at work. Work related illnesses are a major health problem in the UK today. Hazards at work may, or may not, be obvious. For example:

EXPOSURE LIMITS

For many substances and environments established under COSHH regulations, exposure limits may be exceeded accidentally.

SUSCEPTIBILITY TO ILLNESS

This can vary from person to person.

SYMPTOMS OF ILLNESS

These may not appear for many years after the original contract, for example in the case of asbestos causing Asbestosis.

Action should be taken to protect employees from hazards at work, for example:

○ **Assessments** should be made and records kept of any hazards employees may face.

○ **Trained professionals** should be employed to eliminate or reduce potential hazards.

○ **Safety policies** should be designed to minimise the health risk to employees.

○ **Special equipment** should be used to help shield employees from danger.

The employee must display the right attitude and action to safeguard their own health and safety while at work.

The employee should co-operate with occupational health and safety programmes. They are designed to identify and control occupational health hazards.

A safety programme may include the following:

TRAINING AND INFORMATION

Such programmes instruct you on handling materials safely, using equipment correctly, detecting symptoms of illness.

MEDICAL EXAMINATIONS

Some problems can be detected early and before they become serious. Employees should have regular check-ups. This will depend on their age and position within the organisation.

EARLY TREATMENT

If any unusual symptoms appear, the employee should inform their line manager, then report to the Health and Safety Officer and seek medical advice. Early investigation and treatment can be most effective.

MONITORING ILLNESS PATTERNS

Health professionals, such as occupational health nurses, record cases of illness, take samples from contaminated areas and keep medical records.

Self protection

Always keep a healthy frame of mind. Never assume that 'it can't happen to me' – it can! The way to help prevent illness and accidents is to take proper precautions every day you work. Treat hazardous substances and working conditions with respect. Never cut corners to get work done faster. Follow the company's health and safety policies regarding exposure limits, clean up procedures, protective equipment, smoking etc.

Be aware of hazards that might exist at work, for example:

- Acids
- Alkalis
- Asbestos
- Fumes
- Resins
- Dust
- Noise
- Solvents
- Paints

Take care with substances that you use or that are used around you at work. Know the generic name of all chemicals. Check whether any substances can enter the body, for example by inhaling, swallowing or by skin contact.

Where exposure limits have been established, stick to them. Know what the potential risks are and report any health problems that are noticed.

Watch for dangerous conditions that may affect your health. These include noise, heat, radiation, vibrations, as well as leaks, spills, malfunctions in protective equipment, poor safety practices on the part of colleagues. Report any unsafe or suspicious conditions to your line manager.

ACCIDENTS

It is essential that people working in the kitchen are capable of using the tools and equipment in a manner which will neither harm themselves nor those with whom they work. Moreover, they should be aware of the causes of accidents and be able to deal with any which occur.

Accidents may be caused in various ways:

○ excessive haste – the golden rule of the kitchen is 'never run'; this may be difficult to observe during a very busy service but excessive haste causes people to take chances which inevitably lead to mishaps;

○ distraction – accidents may be caused by not concentrating on the job in hand, through lack of interest, personal worry or distraction by someone else; the mind must always be kept on the work so as to reduce the number of accidents;

○ failure to apply safety rules.

Accident prevention

It is the responsibility of everyone to observe the safety rules; in this way a great deal of pain and loss of time can be avoided.

Figure 15.8 *Sample in-house record of accidents and dangerous occurrences*

Full name of injured person:	

Occupation:	Supervisor:

Time of accident:	Date of accident:	Time of report:	Date of report:

Nature of injury or condition:

Details of hospitalisation:

Extent of injury (after medical attention):

Place of accident or dangerous occurrence:

Injured person's evidence of what happened (include equipment/items/or other persons):

Use separate sheets if necessary

Witness evidence (1):	Witness evidence (2):

Supervisor's recommendations:

Date: Supervisor's signature:

This form must be sent to the company health and safety officer

PREVENTION OF CUTS AND SCRATCHES

Knives

These should never be misused and the following rules should always be observed:

○ the correct knife should be used for the appropriate job;

○ knives must always be sharp and clean; a blunt knife is more likely to cause a cut because excessive pressure has to be used;

○ handles should be free from grease;

○ the points must be held downwards;

○ knives should be placed flat on the board or table so that the blade is not exposed upwards;

○ knives should be wiped clean with the edge away from the hands;

○ do not put knives in a washing-up sink.

Choppers

These should be kept sharp and clean. Care should be taken that no other knives, saws, hooks etc., can be struck by the chopper, which could cause them to fly into the air. This also applies when using a large knife for chopping.

Cutting blades on machines

Guards should always be in place when the machine is in use; they should not be tampered with nor should hands or fingers be inserted past the guards. Before the guards are removed for cleaning, the blade or blades must have stopped revolving.

When the guard is removed for cleaning, the blade should not be left unattended in case someone should put a hand on it by accident. If the machine is electrically operated the plug should, when possible, be removed.

Cuts from meat and fish bones

Jagged bones can cause cuts which may turn septic, particularly fish bones and the bones of a calf's head which has been opened to remove the brain. Cuts of this nature, however slight, should never be neglected. Frozen meat should not be boned out until it is completely thawed out because it is difficult to handle, the hands become very cold and the knife slips easily.

Prevention of burns and scalds

A burn is caused by dry heat and a scald by wet heat. Both burns and scalds can be very painful and have serious effects, so certain precautions should be taken to prevent them.

○ Sleeves of jackets and overalls should be rolled down and aprons worn at a sensible length so as to give adequate protection.

○ A good, thick dry cloth or gloves are most important for handling hot utensils (Figure 15.3). It should never be used wet on hot objects and is best folded to give greater protection. It should not be used if thin, torn or with holes.

○ Trays containing hot liquid, such as roast gravy, should be handled carefully, one hand on the side and the other on the end of the tray so as to balance it.

○ Hot pans brought out of the oven should have something white, such as a little flour, placed on the handle and lid as a warning that it is hot. This should be done as soon as the pan is taken out of the oven.

○ Handles of pans should not protrude over the edge of the stove as the pan may be knocked off the stove.

○ Large full pans should be carried correctly: when there is only one handle the forearm should run along the full length of the handle and the other hand should be used to balance the pan where the handle joins the pan. This should prevent the contents from spilling.

○ Certain foods require extra care when heat is applied to them, as for example when a cold liquid is added to a hot roux or when adding cold water to boiling sugar for making caramel. Extra care should always be taken when boiling sugar.

○ Frying, especially deep frying, needs careful attention. When shallow or deep frying fish, for example, put the fish into the pan away from the person so that any splashes will do no harm. With deep frying, fritures should be moved with care and if possible only when the fat is cool. Fritures should not be more than two-thirds full. Wet foods should be drained and dried before being placed in the fat, and when foods are tipped out of the frying basket a spider should be at hand. Should the fat in the friture bubble over on to a gas stove then the gas taps should be turned off immediately. Fire blankets and fire extinguishers should be provided in every kitchen, conveniently sited ready for use.

○ Steam causes scalds just as hot liquids do. It is important to be certain that before steamers are opened the steam is turned off and that when the steamer door is opened no one is in the way of the escaping steam. The steamer should be in proper working condition; the drain hole should always be clear. The door should not be opened immediately the steam is turned off; it is better to wait for about half a minute before doing so.

○ Scalds can also be caused by splashing when passing liquids through conical strainers; it is wise to keep the face well back so as to avoid getting splashed. This also applies when hot liquids are poured into containers.

EMPTYING AND CLEANING OF FRYERS

Accidents during the emptying and cleaning of fryers is a major cause of accidents.

Hazards include:
○ fire;
○ burns from hot oil;
○ contact with hot surfaces;
○ fumes from boiling cleaning chemicals;
○ danger of chemicals overflowing;
○ eye injuries from splashes;
○ strains and sprains while lifting and moving containers of oil.

Procedure for draining
○ Switch off appliance.
○ Drain only when oil is cool.
○ Do not drain until oil is below 40°C.
○ Follow any instructions. Remove debris.
○ Clean and dry.
○ Ensure that the drain-off tap cannot be accidentally turned on.
○ If appropriate, eye protection should be worn.

MACHINERY

Accidents are easily caused by misuse of machines. The following rules should always be put into practice:
○ The machine should be in correct running order before use.

○ The controls of the machine should be operated by the person using the machine. If two people are involved there is the danger that a misunderstanding can occur and the machine be switched on when the other person does not expect it.

○ Machine attachments should be correctly assembled and only the correct tools used to force food through mincers.

○ When mixing machines are being used the hands should not be placed inside the bowl until the blades, whisk or hook have stopped revolving. Failure to observe this rule may result in a broken arm or severe cut.

○ Plugs should be removed from electric machines when they are being cleaned so they cannot be accidentally switched on.

Gas Safety (Installation and Use) Regulations requires employers to maintain gas appliances and is distinctly separate from the duty of landlord to maintain gas appliances in let properties. It is vital that all gas equipment, and in particular Calor gas equipment is properly and regularly serviced and adjusted. Therefore an agreement should be in place with a properly unrelated gas installer or maintenance company.

GAS EXPLOSIONS

The risk of explosion from gas is considerable. To avoid this occurring it is necessary to ensure that the gas is properly lit. On ranges with a pilot on the oven it is important to see that the main jet has ignited from the pilot. If the regulo is low, sometimes the gas does not light at once; the gas collects and an explosion occurs. When lighting the tops of solid-top ranges it is wise to place the centre ring back for a few minutes after the stove is lit because the gas may go out; gas then collects and an explosion can occur.

BLOWTORCH DANGER HIGHLIGHTED

At its December 1999 meeting, the Health and Safety in Hospitality Liaison Committee heard of an incident involving a glass blowtorch of the sort used to caramelise crème brûlée (as opposed to glazing the brown sugar under a grill). B G Prichard, Health and Safety Enforcement Officer for Ceredigion, drew the committee's attention to the "danger that familiarity breeds contempt resulting in staff ignoring the significant risks involved in the use, storage and handling of this [now commonplace] equipment".

In spite of instructions on the gas canister stating that it should not be exposed to temperatures exceeding 50°C, the blowtorch had been left on or near the solid top gas cooker. The top blew off, gas escaped and there was an explosion. The glass roof of the kitchen was blown off, and the heavy wooden doors from their hinges. Fortunately no one was injured. For several days the kitchen was out of use.

It transpired that the blowtorch had been used to light the oven, apparently a not uncommon practice in kitchens. And evidently, an extremely dangerous one.

KITCHEN EQUIPMENT

On 1st January 1996 a significant European Union directive concerning the design and installation of **gas-fuelled catering equipment** became mandatory. All gas appliances sold after that date, new or secondhand, must be fitted with a fuel cut-out mechanism should the main pilot light be extinguished. Equipment will be withdrawn from the market place if it does not comply. This gas directive joins other European laws which have come into effect and are strict guidelines or explicit instructions. These rules set out safe practice on topics as diverse as electromagnetic compatibility, pressure in systems and the surface temperature of oven doors. They accompany the six sets of UK Health and Safety at Work Regulations (1992) which came into force in 1993, the legislation which implements European Union directives on Health and Safety at Work. These regulations have developed changes in the manufacture of existing equipment. *See further legislation on page 509.

Electrical equipment is mostly covered by a non-binding European Union directive, The Low Voltage directive. This was approved by the European Union's members in February 1973, which was passed into UK Health and Safety law in 1989, in the form of the Low Voltage Electrical Equipment Safety Regulations.

FLOORS

Accidents are also caused by grease and water being spilled on floors and not being cleaned up. It is most important that floors are always kept clean and clear; pots and pans etc., should never be left on the floor, nor should oven doors be left open, because anyone carrying something large may not see the door or anything on the floor, and trip over.

Many people strain themselves by incorrectly lifting or attempting to lift items which are too heavy. Large stock pots, forequarters and hindquarters of beef, for example, should be lifted with care. Particular attention should be paid to the hooks in the meat so that they do not injure anyone.

On no account should liquids be placed in containers on shelves above eye-level, especially when hot. They may be pulled down by someone else.

Safe kitchens are those which are well lit and well ventilated and where the staff take precautions to prevent accidents happening. But when accidents do happen it is necessary to know something of first-aid.

Further information can be obtained from the Royal Society for the Prevention of Accidents, or the Health and Safety Executive.

FIRST AID

As the term implies this is the immediate treatment on the spot to a person who has been injured or is ill. Since 1982 it has been a legal requirement that adequate first-aid equipment, facilities and personnel to give first aid are provided at work. If the injury is serious the injured person should be treated by a doctor or nurse as soon as possible.

First-aid equipment

A first-aid box, as a minimum, should contain:

- a card giving general first aid guidance;
- 20 individually wrapped, sterile, adhesive, waterproof dressings of various sizes;
- 4 × 25 g (1 oz) cotton wool packs;
- 1 dozen safety pins;
- 2 triangular bandages;
- 2 sterile eye pads, with attachment;
- 4 medium-sized sterile unmedicated dressings;
- 2 large sterile unmedicated dressings;

○ 2 extra large sterile unmedicated dressings;
○ tweezers;
○ scissors;
○ report book to record all injuries.

First-aid boxes must be easily identifiable and accessible in the work area. They should be in the charge of a responsible person, checked regularly and refilled when necessary.

All establishments must have first-aid equipment and employees qualified in first-aid. Large establishments usually have medical staff such as a nurse and a first-aid room. The room should include a bed or couch, blankets, chairs, a table, sink with hot and cold water, towels, tissues and a first-aid box. Hooks for clothing and a mirror should be provided. Small establishments should have members of staff trained in first aid and in possession of a certificate. After a period of three years trained first-aid staff must update their training to remain certificated.

All catering workers and students are recommended to attend a first-aid course run by the St John Ambulance, St Andrew's Ambulance Association or British Red Cross Society.

Shock

The signs of shock are faintness, sickness, clammy skin and a pale face. Shock should be treated by keeping the person comfortable, lying down and warm. Cover the person with a blanket or clothing, but do not apply hot water bottles.

Fainting

Fainting may occur after a long period of standing in a hot, badly ventilated kitchen. The signs of an impending faint are whiteness, giddiness and sweating. A faint should be treated by raising the legs slightly above the level of the head and, when the person recovers consciousness, putting the person in the fresh air for a while and making sure that the person has not incurred any injury in fainting.

Cuts

All cuts should be covered immediately with a waterproof dressing, after the skin round the cut has been washed. When there is considerable bleeding it should be stopped as soon as possible. Bleeding may be controlled by direct pressure, by bandaging firmly on the cut. It may be possible to stop bleeding from a cut artery by pressing the artery with the thumb against the underlying bone; such pressure may be applied while a dressing or bandage is being prepared for application but not for more than 15 minutes.

Nose bleeds

Sit the person down with the head forward, and loosen clothing round the neck and chest. Ask them to breathe through the mouth and to pinch the soft part of the nose. After 10 minutes release the pressure. Warn the person not to blow the nose for several hours. If the bleeding has not stopped continue for a further 10 minutes. If the bleeding has not stopped then, or recurs in 30 minutes, obtain medical assistance.

Fractures

A person suffering from broken bones should not be moved until the injured part has been secured so that it cannot move. Medical assistance should be obtained.

Burns and scalds

Place the injured part gently under slowly running water or immerse in cool water, keeping it there for at least 10 minutes or until the pain ceases. If serious, the burn or scald should then be covered with a clean cloth or dressing (preferably sterile) and the person sent immediately to hospital.

Do **not** use adhesive dressings, apply lotions or ointments or break blisters.

Electric shock

Switch off the current. If this is not possible, free the person by using a dry insulating material such as cloth, wood or rubber, taking care not to use the bare hands otherwise the electric shock may be transmitted. If breathing has stopped, give artificial respiration and send for a doctor. Treat any burns as above.

Gassing

Do not let the gassed person walk, but carry them into the fresh air. If breathing has stopped apply artificial respiration and send for a doctor.

Artificial respiration

There are several methods of artificial respiration. The most effective is mouth-to-mouth (mouth-to-nose) and this method can be used by almost all age groups and in almost all circumstances.

Again it is stressed that we would recommend all students to complete a first-aid course.

Further information can be obtained from the St John Ambulance Association, 1 Grosvenor Crescent, London SW1X 7EF.

SECURITY IN CATERING

Security in catering premises is a major concern, especially with the increasing rise in crime due to fraud. All establishments should endeavour to reduce the risk of temptation. Eliminating or reducing cash handling is one measure which should be encouraged. The use of credit cards and switch cards whilst costing a small amount in charges, reduces cash handling, thus minimising risk.

Encouraging the payment of employees through cheque or bank transfer instead of by cash, means that payrolls do not have to be collected and distributed. Other such measures could include notices that no money is kept in the premises or that safes are protected by time delay locks. Strict stock control can reduce levels thereby reducing the temptation and the problems of control.

A great deal of crime is of an opportunist nature. Large scale crime is generally well planned. Reducing the amount of information available to the criminal reduces the ability for the thief to plan and thus commit the crime.

In order for a business to function it is often necessary to have cash. In order to deprive the potential criminal of information make sure that only the staff that need to know actually know. For example, never have a regular routine for 'banking'. Regular and spot check stock taking is another valuable system to identify crime.

However, in order to carry out your business efficiently it is impossible to remove all temptation. Therefore all equipment should be security marked, for example computers, fax machines, photocopiers.

It is important to prevent the thief entering the premises. Reception staff need to be trained to identify suspicious individuals. Everyone reporting to reception should be asked to sign in and if they are a legitimate visitor be given a security badge. All contract workers too should be registered and given security badges. Contractors may be restricted to working in certain areas.

A good security system should also be in force at the back door, with everyone delivering goods reporting to the security officer. Good lighting is also important for security reasons. Supervisors and manager should carry out regular checks of all areas.

Some companies write into employee contracts the 'right to search', so that searches can be carried out from time to time as a deterrent against theft. However it is not legal to force a person to submit to a search even if they have signed a contract to that effect. However, by refusing to submit to a search they may be in breach of their employment contract.

Close circuit television (CCTV) cameras are also used as a deterrent against crime.

Prevention of crime should be the main objective. With regard to staff the first step is to appoint honest staff by taking up references from previous employers.

The Health and Safety at Work Regulations now require employers to conduct a risk assessment with regard to the safety of staff in the catering business. Where staff constantly come into close contact with strangers, it is advisable to train them in anti-aggression techniques which include the early recognition of volatile situations and how to defuse them. At the same time staff should be trained not to approach people who could pose a physical threat to them.

Staff who handle money should be trained in simple anti-fraud measures such as checking banknotes, checking signatures on plastic cards etc.

Security measures also include leaving lights on in some areas that can be seen by passers by, as well as locking doors, windows etc. Making sure that any suspicious person does not re-enter the building is also essential.

Each business will have its own type of risk. Overtime staff become familiar with the risks.

Security systems of all types should be carefully selected according to the needs of the business. Before purchasing into any security system agreements, seek advice from an independent security expert who will assess the needs of the establishment. Insurance companies will have stipulated criteria to be fulfilled before they will insure the business.

Management of a security system

As with other operations a security system needs to be managed. This involves:

○ developing a security policy for the establishment to cover on security threats, bomb alerts, theft by customers, or by employees, policy regarding prosecution;
○ establishing resources to cover the cost of security staff whether in house or contract;
○ developing procedures for security risk assessment, dealing with breaches of security;
○ understanding the legal implications of e.g. vicarious liability for false arrest or imprisonment;
○ seeking a proper balance between the often conflicting demands of security and safety.

The main security risks in the hotel and catering industry

○ **Theft**	–	Customers' property, employers' property particularly food, drink, equipment, employees' property.
○ **Burglary**	–	Theft with trespass of customers' property, employer's property, employees' property.
○ **Robbery**	–	Theft with assault, e.g. banking cash, collecting cash.
○ **Fraud**	–	False claims for damage.
	–	Counterfeit currency
	–	Stolen credit cards.
○ **Assault**	–	Fights between customers, staff banking cash, collecting cash.

○ **Vandalism** – Malicious damage to property by customers, by intruders, by employees.
○ **Arson** – Setting fire to property.
○ **Undesirables** – Drug traffickers, prostitutes.
○ **Terrorism** – Bombs, telephone bomb threats.

FIRE PRECAUTIONS

Fires in hotel and catering establishments are fairly common and can result in injury or loss of life to employees and customers.

Fire prevention

A basic knowledge regarding fire should assist in preventing fires and extinguishing them quickly if they do occur. Three components are necessary for a fire to start, if one of the three is not present, or is removed, then the fire does not happen or it is extinguished. The three parts are:

○ fuel – something to burn;
○ air – oxygen to sustain combustion (to keep the fire going);
○ heat – gas, electricity, etc.

Figure 15.9 *The fire triangle*

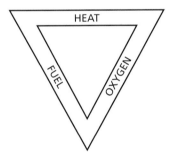

Methods of extinguishing a fire

To extinguish a fire the three principal methods are:
○ starving – removing the fuel;
○ smothering – removing the air (oxygen);
○ cooling – removing the heat.

Therefore, one of the sides of the 'fire triangle' is removed.

The fuel is that which burns, heat is that which sets the fuel alight and oxygen is needed for fire to burn. Eliminate one of these and the fire is put out. Oxygen is present in air, so if air is excluded from the fuel and the heat then the fire goes out. For example, should the clothes of someone working in the kitchen catch alight, then quickly lay them down and wrap a fire blanket round the person and place them on the floor. In so doing the flames have been cut off from the source of air. (The oxygen has been taken from the triangle.) In the event of a fire, windows and doors should be closed so as to restrict the amount of air getting to the fire.

Foam extinguishers work on the principle that the foam forms a 'blanket' thus excluding air from coming into contact with the fuel.

Should fat or oil in a pan ignite, then turn off the source of heat if it is safe to do so, quickly cover the pan with a lid, fire blanket or other suitable item to exclude the air. Turning off the source of heat will remove that side of the fire triangle.

Water extinguishes by dousing the flames, thus taking the heat out of the triangle provided the fuel is material such as wood or paper. If fat or oil is alight water must **not** be used as it causes the ignited fat to spread, thus increasing the heat.

Water extinguishers must **not** be used on live electrical equipment because water is a conductor of electricity and the person holding the extinguisher could be electrocuted.

In the event of a small fire in a store it may be possible to remove items in the store to prevent the fire from spreading; windows and doors are to be closed, if it is safe to do so. Evacuation should not be delayed if the fire is already well developed.

Fire doors are installed for the purpose of restricting an area so that, in the event of a fire, the smoke and flames do not spread to endanger the lives of people present. Fire doors must normally be kept shut.

Procedures in the event of a fire

- Raise the alarm by breaking the glass in the nearest fire alarm call point or shout 'fire'.
- Call the fire brigade.
- Turn off gas supplies, other sources of heat and the fans if it is safe to do so.
- Attempt to fight the fire with the appropriate fire extinguisher or a fire blanket but do not put yourself in danger.
- If the fire continues to grow despite your efforts, leave the building, closing doors and windows behind you if possible.
- **Do not** delay calling the fire brigade while you attempt to fight the fire.
- **Do not** extinguish gas burners with a fire extinguisher before turning off the gas supply.
- **Do not** use lifts to leave the building.
- **Do not** stop to collect your belongings before leaving.

It is important that in all catering establishments exits and passageways are kept clear and that doors open outwards. Fire doors should be clearly marked and fire-fighting equipment must be readily available and in working order. Periodic **fire drills should be held at least once a year and be taken seriously since lives may be endangered if a fire should start.**

Fire alarm sounders should be tested weekly and staff should be instructed in the use of fire fighting equipment. All extinguishers should be refilled as soon as possible after use by a competent person.

All fire extinguishers are predominantly red, with patches of colour to show the nature of the extinguishing agent. *See page 504.

Figure 15.10 *Checking fire extinguisher*

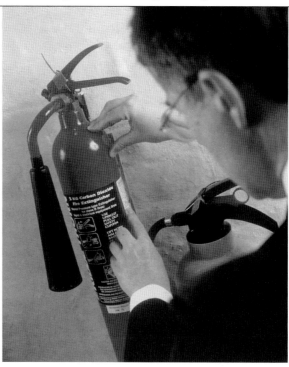

Types and use of fire extinguishers

TYPE OF EXTINGUISHER	USE	HOW USED	SPECIAL CARE
Water RED*	On paper Wood textiles General rubbish	Aim at base of fire	Do not use on electrical fires or burning liquid
Foam CREAM*	As for water and on flammable liquids	Aim at heart of the fire	Do not use on flammable liquids or electrical appliances
Powder BLUE*	Fat fires and electrical equipment and other fires	Spray across burning liquid	Beware of re-ignition
CO_2 Carbon Dioxide BLACK*	Burning liquids and fat fires Electrical appliances	Spray across the burning liquid	Beware of re-ignition

*See page 504.

Causes of fires

Cigarettes	Not fully extinguished before disposal
Electrical appliances	Faulty, not correctly maintained, overloaded
Fat fires	Overheating, overfilling of pan

F	Find	Is cause obvious?
I	Inform	Warn those in the vicinity, call fire brigade
R	Restrict	Turn off gas and electricity
E	Extinguish	Use extinguisher if safe to do so

Fire Precautions (Workplace) Regulations 1997

To ensure adequate means of escape for employees in the event of a fire, these must be provided: fire-fighting equipment, fire alarms and detectors, signs and notices, emergency lighting.

Fire Precautions (Workplace) Amendment Regulations 1999

Fire safety risk assessment must be carried out for establishments having sleeping accommodation for more than six persons, guests or staff. This applies to hotels and boarding houses and covers the risk of a fire occurring and risk to people in the event of a fire. A fire certificate states the means of safe escape, the fire-fighting equipment available and means of giving warning in the event of a fire.

References

The Fire Precautions (Workplace) Regulations 1997, Stationery Office

The Fire Precautions (Workplace) Amendment Regulations 1999, Stationery Office

Guide to Fire Precautions in the Workplace, Stationery Office

Fire Risk Management in the Workplace, Fire Protection Association

Fire fighting equipment, location and identification

Red rectangle/square shape with a white pictogram

This new legal requirement states that all fire fighting equipment (hoses, extinguishers and blankets) must be identified with a red signboard placed either around the equipment or on the place where it is stored.

The fact that the signboard has to be red could inevitably lead to confusion. To counter this, signs are available which incorporate the colour of the extinguisher, and give guidance on what types of fires it can be used on.

ELECTRICITY AT WORK REGULATIONS 1989

Extend legal protection to electrical safety in all workplaces and work activities over and above the general duty of care owed by employers to their employees.

GAS SAFETY (INSTALLATION AND USE) REGULATIONS 1998

These regulations cover any place or installation on land, the foreshore and offshore.

FIRE CERTIFICATES

Fire certificates are issued by the local fire authority.

On receipt of the application, the authority is under duty to inspect the premises to ensure that the means of escape and related precautions are what is required for that particular premises.

REQUIREMENTS OF FIRE CERTIFICATE

The fire certificate will specify

1   The particular use of the premises.

2   The means of escape in case of fire.

3   The means of securing that the way of escape can be safely and effectively used at all times (e.g. providing emergency lighting, measures to restrict the speed of fire, smoke and fumes).

4   The means of fighting fire for use by persons in the building.

5   The means for giving warning in case of fire.

6   Particulars of any explosive or highly inflammable materials which may be stored or used in the premises.

CARRYING OUT A FIRE RISK ASSESSMENT

1   **Identify** potential fire hazards in the workplace, eg use of blow lamps.

2   **Decide** who might be in danger in the event of a fire.

3   **Evaluate** the risks which could arise from the hazard.

4   **Keep a record** of the results of the risk assessment and details of action that was taken or needs to be taken as a result.

   Employees must be notified of the outcomes of the risk assessment and the control methods they should take.

5   **Review and Revise** the assessment. This should take place when there is a change in work practices or at least every six months.

CATERING SAFETY MANAGEMENT

Managers must think positively how they can sustain and improve safety if they are to comply with legislation and minimise the risk of incidents occurring.

Accidents often happen because of acts or omissions by management rather than staff neglect.

The Management of Health and Safety at Work Regulations 1999 provide the base for safety management requirements.

The legislation requires:

○   all involved in safety to think positively;

○   competence to be established;

○   risk assessment to be undertaken;

○   implementation of effective control.

Measures to reduce risk:

○   staff training on hazard awareness and control in their workplace.

Safety management involves identifying the hazards in a business and tailoring controls through physical measures, safe systems of work, the safety policy training.

OTHER EXTINGUISHERS

Fire hoses

Fire hoses are used for similar fires to those classified under water fire extinguishers. Staff should be trained in the use of hoses.

WATER SPRINKLER SYSTEMS

A sprinkler system consists of an array of sprinkler heads at ceiling level connected to a mains water supply. The distances between sprinkler heads and the water pressure required is laid down for each occupancy in the *Rules of the Fire Officer's Committee for Automatic Sprinkler Installations*, (29th edition). In the event of a fire the nearest sprinkler head above the fire operates when the temperature at ceiling level rises above a preset level, such as 68°C (154°F) and sprays an area of 12 to 20 sq m (39 to 66 sq ft). Additional heads operate later if necessary to control the fire. The heads are designed so that the heat of a fire causes the sprinkler head nearest the fire to operate, releasing water automatically. If the fire grows larger, more heads will operate to control the flames.

Further information regarding fire safety can be obtained from the Fire Prevention Branch of the local fire brigade or from the Fire Protection Association, Bestille Court, 2 Paris Garden, London SE1 8ND www.thefpa.co.uk

Some references to health and safety elsewhere in the book. See also HCIMA Technical brief No 40.

Catering for health	180	Bacteria	188, 530
Ventilation	210	Hygiene production	266
Cross-contamination	214, 530	systems	
HACCP	268	Refrigeration	247, 367
Control of Health & Safety	362, 479	Food hygiene regulations	550

Topics for Discussion

1. Discuss the causes of accidents and how they may be prevented. Are some people accident prone, others naturally clumsy and others lacking in common sense: If so how can they be 'educated' to be safe workers?

2. Do notices regarding safety have any effect? How best may people employed in the kitchen be made aware of hazards, thus making a potentially dangerous environment much safer?

3. Attendance at a first-aid course could be made obligatory for every catering employee. Do you think this would be sensible and if you do, or do not, explain why?

4. Discuss what training and the procedures following training, should be provided for every person being employed in catering establishment. Does training reduce accidents, fires etc.?

5. What provision should be made for the welfare of catering staff? Discuss this, bearing in mind costs and the fact that in the industry many employees are casual or part-time.

6. How can premises be made secure and stealing be prevented?

7. Discuss the hazards that should be prevented in the kitchen.

8. Discuss the relationship between the caterer and the Environmental Health Officer.

9. Discuss accident prevention and the responsibilities of the worker and the employer.

10. Is ample provision made for first aid?

11 What fire precautions and appropriate systems are in place for fire prevention?

12 Explain how fire extinguishers are recognised for their appropriate use.

13 If you find temperatures and food hygiene legislation complex, discuss how could it be simplified.

14 Discuss the relationship between knowing the law and implementing it.

* Note on fire legislation (contd from page 499):

Any completely new kitchen built after September 2002 must have interlocking in the ventilation system, and any replacement, new installation or modification to existing ventilation systems must incorporate interlocking.

Interlocking describes the mechanical link between sensors in the extraction system and the main valve of the gas supply to cooking equipment. Should the carbon monoxide level in the ventilation system go up, the interlocker will turn off.

CHAPTER 16

HYGIENE AND FOOD LEGISLATION

WHY IS HYGIENE IMPORTANT?

Hygiene is the science and practice of preserving health and is one of the most important subjects for all persons working in the Hotel and Catering Industry to study, understand and practise in their everyday working lives. The subject is broken down into three areas: personal, food and kitchen hygiene, all of which are of equal importance.

PERSONAL HYGIENE

Germs or bacteria are to be found in and on the body and they can be transferred onto anything with which the body comes in contact. Personal cleanliness is essential to prevent germs getting onto food.

Personal cleanliness

Self-respect is necessary in every food-handler because a pride in one's appearance promotes a high standard of cleanliness and physical fitness. Persons suffering from ill-health or who are not clean about themselves should not handle food.

BATHING

It is essential to take a bath or a shower every day (or at least two or three times a week), otherwise germs can be transferred onto clothes and so onto food, particularly in warm weather.

HANDS

Hands must be washed thoroughly and frequently, particularly after using the toilet, before commencing work and during the handling of food.

They should be washed in hot water, with the aid of a nail brush and bactericidal soap. This can be dispensed from a fixed container in a liquid or gel form and is preferable to bar soap, which can accumulate germs when passed from hand to hand. After washing, hands should be rinsed and dried on a *clean* towel, suitable paper towel or by hand hot-air drier. Hands and fingernails can be a great source of danger if not kept clean, as they can so easily transfer harmful bacteria on to the food.

Figure 16.1 *Drying hands on a paper towel.*

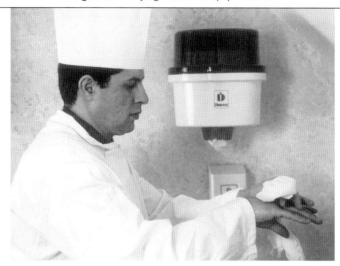

Rings (except for a plain wedding band), watches and jewellery should not be worn where food is handled. Particles of food may be caught under the ring, and germs could multiply there until they are transferred onto food.

Watches should not be worn because some foodstuffs have to be plunged into plenty of water. Apart from this, the steam in a kitchen will ruin watches that are not waterproofed anyway.

Jewellery should not be worn, since it may fall off into food, unknown to the wearer; small sleepers for pierced ears are, however, permissible.

FINGERNAILS

These should always be kept clean and short as dirt can easily lodge under the nails and be dislodged when, for example, making pastry, so introducing bacteria into food. Nails should be cleaned with a nail brush and nail varnish should not be worn.

HAIR

Hair should be washed regularly and kept covered where food is being handled. Hair that is not cared for is likely to come out or shed dandruff which may fall into food. Men's hair should be kept short as it is easier to keep clean; it also looks neater. Women's hair should be covered as much as possible. Both men's and women's hair can be kept in place using a hair net. The hair should never be scratched, combed or touched in the kitchen, as germs could be transferred via the hands to the food.

NOSE

The nose should not be touched when food is being handled. If a handkerchief is used, the hands should be washed afterwards. Ideally, paper handkerchiefs should be used and then destroyed, and the hands washed afterwards. The nose is an area where there are vast numbers of harmful bacteria; it is therefore very important that neither food, people nor working surfaces are sneezed over, so spreading germs.

Figure 16.2 *Hygiene standards being observed in good production and service*

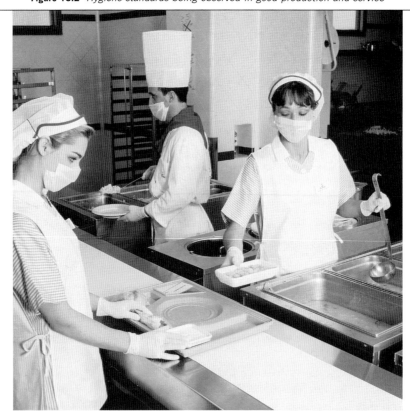

MOUTH

There are many germs in the area of the mouth, therefore the mouth or lips should not be touched by the hands or utensils which may come into contact with food. No cooking utensils should be used for tasting food, nor should fingers be used for this purpose as germs may be transferred to food. A clean teaspoon should be used for tasting, and washed well afterwards.

Coughing over foods and working areas should be avoided as germs are spread long distances if not trapped in a handkerchief.

EARS

The ear-holes should not be touched while in the kitchen as, again, germs can be transferred.

TEETH

Sound teeth are essential to good health. They should be kept clean and visits to the dentist should be regular so that teeth can be kept in good repair.

FEET

As food-handlers are standing for many hours, care of the feet is important. They should be washed regularly and the toenails kept short and clean. Tired feet can cause general fatigue which leads to carelessness, and this results in a lowering of the standards of hygiene.

CUTS, BURNS AND SORES

It is particularly important to keep all cuts, burns, scratches and similar openings of the skin covered with a waterproof dressing. Where the skin is septic (as with certain cuts, spots, sores and carbuncles) there are vast numbers of harmful bacteria which must not be permitted to get on food; in most cases people suffering in this way should not handle food.

COSMETICS

Cosmetics, if used by food-handlers, should be used in moderation, but ideally their use should be discouraged. Cosmetics should not be put on in the kitchen and the hands should be washed well afterwards; they should be put on a clean skin, not used to cover up dirt.

Figure 16.3 *Newspaper reports of hygiene breaches*

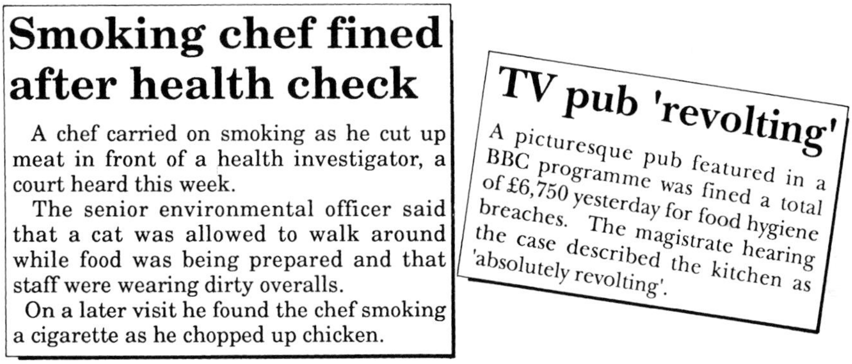

Smoking chef fined after health check

A chef carried on smoking as he cut up meat in front of a health investigator, a court heard this week.

The senior environmental officer said that a cat was allowed to walk around while food was being prepared and that staff were wearing dirty overalls.

On a later visit he found the chef smoking a cigarette as he chopped up chicken.

TV pub 'revolting'

A picturesque pub featured in a BBC programme was fined a total of £6,750 yesterday for food hygiene breaches. The magistrate hearing the case described the kitchen as 'absolutely revolting'.

SMOKING

Smoking must never take place where there is food, because when a cigarette is taken from the mouth, germs from the mouth can be transferred to the fingers and so on to food. When the cigarette is put down the end which has been in the mouth can transfer germs on to working surfaces. Ash on food is most objectionable and it should be remembered that smoking where there is food is an offence against the law.

SPITTING

Spitting should never occur, because germs can be spread by this objectionable habit.

CLOTHING AND CLOTHS

Clean whites (protective clothing) and clean underclothes should be worn at all times. Dirty clothes enable germs to multiply and if dirty clothing comes into contact with food the food may be contaminated. Cloths used for holding hot dishes should also be kept clean as the cloths are used in many ways such as wiping knives, wiping dishes and pans. All these uses could convey germs on to food.

Outdoor clothing, and other clothing which has been taken off before wearing whites, should be kept in a locker, away from the kitchen.

General health and fitness

The maintenance of good health is essential to prevent the introduction of germs into the kitchen. To keep physically fit, adequate rest, exercise, fresh air and a wholesome diet are essential.

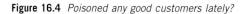

Figure 16.4 *Poisoned any good customers lately?*

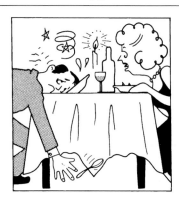

SLEEP AND RELAXATION

Persons employed in the kitchen require adequate sleep and relaxation as they are on the move all the time, often in a hot atmosphere where the tempo of work may be very fast. Frequently, the hours are long or extended over a long period of time, as with split duty, or they may be extended into the night. In off-duty periods it may be wise to obtain some relaxation and rest rather than spend all the time energetically. The amount of sleep and rest required depends on each person's needs and the variation between one person and the next is considerable.

EXERCISE AND FRESH AIR

People working in conditions of nervous tension, rush, heat and odd hours need a change of environment and particularly fresh air. Swimming, walking or cycling in the country may be suitable ways of obtaining both exercise and fresh air.

WHOLESOME FOOD AND PURE WATER

A well-balanced diet, correctly cooked, and pure water will assist in keeping kitchen personnel fit. The habit of 'picking' (eating small pieces of food while working) is bad; it spoils the appetite and does not allow the stomach to rest.

Meals should be taken regularly; long periods without food are also bad for the stomach. Pure water is ideal for replacing liquid lost in perspiring in a hot kitchen, or soft drinks may be taken to replace some of the salt as well as the fluid lost in sweating.

Kitchen clothing

It is most important that people working in the kitchen should wear suitable clothing and footwear. Suitable clothing must be:

1 protective;
2 washable;
3 of a suitable colour;
4 light in weight and comfortable;
5 strong;
6 absorbent.

PROTECTIVE

Clothes worn in the kitchen must protect the body from excessive heat. For this reason chef's jackets are double-breasted and have long sleeves; they are to protect the chest and arms from the heat of the stove and to prevent hot foods or liquids burning or scalding the body.

APRONS

These are designed to protect the body from being scalded or burned and particularly to protect the legs from any liquids which may be spilled; for this reason the apron should be of sufficient length to protect the legs.

CHEF'S HAT

This is designed to enable air to circulate on top of the head and thus keep the head cooler. The main purpose of the hat is to prevent loose hairs from dropping into food and to absorb perspiration on the forehead. The use of lightweight disposable hats is both acceptable and suitable.

FOOTWEAR

This should be stout and kept in good repair so as to protect and support the feet. As the kitchen staff are on their feet for many hours, boots (for men) and clogs (for men and women) give added support and will be found most satisfactory.

Modern industrial safety shoes with steel toecaps are to be encouraged. Sandals, training shoes etc., are insufficient protection from spillage of hot liquids.

WASHABLE

The clothing should be of an easily washable material as many changes of clothing are required.

COLOUR

White clothing is readily seen to be soiled when it needs to be changed and there is a tendency to work more cleanly when wearing 'whites'. Chefs' trousers of blue and white check are a practical colour but also require frequent changing.

LIGHT AND COMFORTABLE

Clothing must be light in weight and comfortable, not tight. Heavy clothing would be uncomfortable and a heavy hat in the heat of the kitchen would cause headaches.

STRONG

Clothes worn in the kitchen must be strong to withstand hard wear and frequent washing.

ABSORBENT

Working over a hot stove causes people to perspire; the perspiration will not evaporate in an inadequately ventilated atmosphere and so underclothes made from absorbent material, such as cotton, should be worn. The hat absorbs perspiration and the neckerchief is used to prevent perspiration from running down the body, for wiping the face and also to protect the neck, which is easily affected by draughts.

ESSENTIALS	AWARENESS
Personal cleanliness and dress. Hand washing. The need to report infections and cover cuts. No smoking, eating or drinking in food rooms. The need for temperature control i.e. keeping food either hot or cold. Keeping surfaces clean.	The organisations' policy or food hygiene. Personal hygiene. Cross contamination and food storage. Waste disposal, cleaning and disinfection. Awareness of pests.

Summary of personal hygiene

The practice of clean habits in the kitchen is the only way to achieve a satisfactory standard of hygiene. These habits are as follows:

○ hands must be washed frequently and always after using the toilet; food should be handled as little as possible;

○ bathing must occur frequently;

○ hair must be kept clean and covered in the kitchen; it should not be combed or handled near food;

○ nose and mouth should not be touched with the hands;

○ cough and sneeze in a handkerchief, not over food; people with colds should not be in contact with food;

○ jewellery, rings and watches should not be worn;

○ smoking and spitting must not occur where there is food;

○ cuts and burns should be covered with a waterproof dressing;

○ clean clothing should be worn at all times and only clean cloths used;

○ foods should be tasted with a clean spoon;

○ tables should not be sat on;

○ only healthy people should handle food.

KITCHEN HYGIENE

Hygiene scores listing law

A law compelling hotels, restaurants and other catering outlets to publish the results of their food hygiene inspections as expected within the next year or so. In the USA, restaurants have to publish the results of their food hygiene and health and safety audits alongside menus.

Cleaning and disinfection

Cleaning can be defined as the application of energy to remove dirt, grease and other soiling. Cleaning is essential to food safety as well as being a legal requirement for food businesses.

Figure 16.5 *Making sure premises are clean*

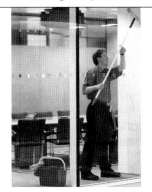

Figure 16.6 *Making sure premises are clean*

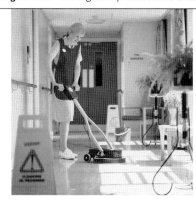

THE NEED FOR CLEANING

- It reduces the risk of food spoilage and food poisoning.
- It removes materials and food that could provide harbour and nourishment for pests.
- It helps the prompt identification of pest infestation.
- It prevents the physical contamination of food.
- It assists in maintaining a comfortable working environment which is safe and attractive, assisting in promoting economical and effective working methods.
- It reduces the risk of accidents to customers and staff affected by the work.
- It promotes a quality image to customers.
- It assists in reducing maintenance costs, reduces damage to equipment.

If cleaning is not carried out or is ineffective, various problems can arise stemming from the loss of product quality leading to:

- customer complaints;
- loss of reputation;
- food poisoning and food-borne disease;
- loss of sales;
- legal action;
- increase in food waste;
- contaminated and tainted food;
- corrosion and premature replacement of equipment;
- incorrect use of chemicals which could damage equipment, floors, walls and food preparation surfaces.

UNDERSTANDING CLEANING

Cleaning requires energy. This consists of:

- physical energy – provided by manual labour, i.e. scrubbing;

○ mechanical energy – provided by machines, i.e. floor scrubbers;
○ turbulence – used for liquids, and often used in a cleaning place, CIP systems;
○ thermal energy – provided by hot water or steam;
○ chemical energy – provided by detergents;

Usually a combination of two or more forms of energy is used.

CLEANING EQUIPMENT AND SYSTEMS

○ Clean in place for certain types of equipment, such as beer lines in a pub.
○ Sinks and tanks.
○ Cloths, brushes, mops and buckets.
○ Mechanical aids such as vacuum cleaners, dishwashers, low pressure jet washers which may be used in combination with a foam for cleaning walls and other surfaces in high risk areas.

DISINFECTANTS

The process of disinfection reduces pathogenic bacteria, but not spores or toxins, to levels that are neither harmful to human health nor to the quality of food. Disinfection may be carried out using:

○ heat, preferably moist heat at a temperature above 82°C;
○ steam
○ chemicals, either separately or in combination.

What to disinfect

Surfaces where the levels of bacteria present may have an adverse effect on the quality or safety of food should be disinfected regularly.

Examples of surfaces

○ Direct food contact surfaces – such as chopping boards, knives, work surfaces, mixing bowls, serving dishes and slicing machines.
○ Hand contact surfaces – such as taps, door handles, oven doors, refrigerator doors, light switches, telephones etc.
○ Hands – disinfection achieved by bactericidal soap, alcohol based disinfectant.
○ Cleaning materials and equipment; mops, cleaning cloths, scrapers, brushes.

Disinfection needs to be carried out carefully to ensure that it is successful and safe.

All chemicals in kitchens and food premises must be food safe. Manufacturers' instructions must always be followed. Careless use of chemicals can be dangerous. After use all detergent must be well rinsed from food surfaces before disinfecting them, otherwise the disinfectant will not be able to work properly.

Always use a fresh solution of disinfectant every time a new cleaning task is carried out. Do not top up existing solutions. Mops and cloths should not be soaked in disinfectant solutions for long periods, as the solution weakens and may allow bacteria to grow. The disinfectant must be allowed to remain on the surface for the contact time recommended by the manufacturer. Always cleanse thoroughly, unless the manufacturer's' instructions state that rinsing is unnecessary.

Six basic steps for cleaning and disinfection

1 Pre-clean: removal of loose soil by wiping, scraping, rinsing or soaking.
2 Main clean: loosening the remaining soil by use of detergents.
3 Intermediate rinse: removal of soil and chemicals.

4   Disinfection; reduction of the remaining bacteria to a safe level.

5   Final rinse: removal of the disinfectant.

6   Drying:

– natural – air drying;

– physical – using disposable paper towels or a clean dry cloth.

If the soiling is light, the pre-clean may be combined with the main clean. Disinfection may not be necessary on all surfaces; when disinfectants are used, disinfection may be incorporated in the main clean using a chemical sanitiser.

This creates a four-stage process:

Pre-clean; main clean; disinfection; rinse and dry.

Some types of equipment need to be completely or partly dismantled to allow satisfactory cleaning. Electrical safety must be checked before machines are cleaned.

CLEANING SCHEDULES

It is important for every kitchen and food premises to have a cleaning schedule. Cleaning schedules communicate standards and ensure that cleaning is carried out and managed effectively. A cleaning schedule should include:

○   all items and surfaces to be cleaned;

○   the persons responsible for carrying out the tasks;

○   when the cleaning must be done;

○   the methods of cleaning and standards required;

○   the time required for each cleaning process;

○   the chemicals, materials and equipment needed;

○   the safety precautions to be taken and the protective clothing and equipment to be worn, such as goggles and gloves;

○   the signature of the person who carries out the task;

○   the signature confirming that the work has been checked.

The cleaning process must be monitored regularly and inspected to ensure that the cleaning schedule is being followed to maintain standards. Checking should include the use of rapid bacterial tests or swabbing.

TECHNICAL TERMS

Bactericide – a substance that destroys bacteria.

Cleaning – the removal of soil, food residue, dirt, grease and other foreign matter.

Detergent – a chemical or mix of chemicals which help to remove grease and food particles so that surfaces are prepared for the action of disinfectants.

Disinfectant – a chemical or heat in the form of water or steam, used for disinfection.

Disinfection – the reduction of micro-organisms to a level that will not lead to harmful contamination or to the rapid spoilage of food. The term usually refers to the treatment of surfaces or premises but may also be applied to aspects of personal hygiene, such as disinfecting the skin.

Sanitiser – a chemical used for cleaning and disinfecting surfaces and equipment.

Sterilisation – a process that kills all micro-organisms.

Neglect in the care and cleaning of any part of the premises and equipment could lead to a risk of food infection. Kitchen hygiene is of very great importance to:

○   those who work in the kitchen, because clean working conditions are more agreeable to work in than dirty conditions;

Figure 16.7 *Newspaper report highlighting poor standards of hygiene*

Health risk at one in 10 food outlets

POOR standards of hygiene pose a serious health risk to consumers in more than one in 10 businesses where food is handled, a government-funded investigation will reveal this week.

Fast-food shops, restaurants and food manufacturers are the worst offenders, according to a survey by environmental health officers who visited 5,000 establishments in England and Wales. The investigation was ordered by the Audit Commission, which monitors the efficiency of local government services.

Results to be published on Tuesday will give a relatively clean bill of health to hospitals, schools, colleges and residential homes for the elderly or disabled. Most food shops, butchers, hotels and public houses present a moderate degree of danger, says the study.

The investigation, which led to prosecutions and closure orders, is intended to provide the first detailed comparison of standards of food-handling in different areas of the country.

○ the owners, because custom should increase when the public know the kitchen is clean;

○ the customer – no one should want to eat food prepared in a dirty kitchen.

Cleaning materials and equipment

To maintain a hygienic working environment a wide range of materials and equipment is needed. These are some of the items which need to budgeted for, ordered, stored and issued:

○ brooms
○ brushes
○ dusters
○ dustbins
○ mops
○ sponges
○ squeegee
○ scrubbing machine
○ wet suction cleaner
○ dry suction cleaner
○ ammonia
○ disinfectant
○ buckets
○ cloths
○ dustbin powder
○ floor cleaner
○ flyspray
○ oven cleaner
○ plastic sacks
○ scouring powder
○ soap
○ steel wool
○ washing powder

Kitchen premises
VENTILATION

Adequate ventilation must be provided so that fumes from stoves are taken out of the kitchen, and stale air in the stores, larder and still-room is extracted. This is usually effected by erecting hoods over stoves and using extractor fans.

Hoods and fans must be kept clean; grease and dirt are drawn up by the fan and, if they accumulate, can drop onto food. Windows used for ventilation should be screened to prevent the entry of dust, insects and birds. Good ventilation facilitates the evaporation of sweat from the body, which keeps one cool. See HCIMA Technical Brief – Kitchen ventilation.

LIGHTING

Good lighting is necessary so that people working in the kitchen do not strain their eyes. Natural lighting is preferable to artificial lighting. Good lighting is also necessary to enable staff to see into corners so the kitchen can be properly cleaned.

PLUMBING

Adequate supplies of hot and cold water must be available for keeping the kitchen clean, for cleaning food and equipment and for staff use. For certain cleaning hot water is essential, and the means of heating water must be capable of meeting the requirements of the establishment.

There must be hand-washing and drying facilities and suitable provision of toilets, which must not be in direct contact with any rooms in which food is prepared or stored.

Hand-washing facilities (separate from food preparation sinks) must also be available in the kitchen with a suitable means of drying the hands (hot air or paper towels).

CLEANING OF TOILETS AND SINKS

Toilets must never be cleaned by food-handlers. Sinks and hand basins should be cleaned and thoroughly rinsed.

FLOORS SEE HCIMA TECHNICAL BRIEF NO 3/96

Kitchen floors have to withstand a considerable amount of wear and tear, therefore they must be:

- capable of being easily cleaned;
- smooth, but not slippery;
- impervious (non-absorbent).
- even;
- without cracks or open joints;

Quarry tile floors or vinyl sheet or epoxy resin floors, properly laid, are suitable for kitchens, since they fulfil the above requirements.

Thorough cleaning is essential: floors are swept, washed with hot detergent water and then dried. This can be done by machine or by hand, and should be carried out at least once a day. As a safety precaution, suitable warning signs should be used to alert staff if the floor is wet.

WALLS

Walls should be strong, smooth, impervious, washable and light in colour. The joint between the wall and floor should be rounded for ease of cleaning. Suitable wall surfaces include ceramic tiles, heat resistant plastic sheeting, stainless steel sheeting, and resin bonded fibreglass.

Clean with hot detergent water and dry. This will probably be done monthly, but frequency will depend on circumstances.

CEILINGS

Ceilings must be free from cracks and flaking. They should not be able to harbour dirt.

DOORS AND WINDOWS

Doors and windows should fit correctly and be clean. The glass should be clean inside and out so as to admit maximum light.

FOOD LIFTS

Lifts should be kept very clean and no particles of food should be allowed to accumulate as lift shafts are ideal places for rats, mice and insects to gain access into kitchens.

Hygiene of kitchen equipment

Kitchen equipment should be so designed that it can be:

○ cleaned easily;

○ readily inspected to see that it is clean.

Failure to maintain equipment and utensils hygienically and in good repair may cause food poisoning. Manufacturers instructions must always be followed.

Material used in the construction of equipment must be:

○ hard so that it does not absorb food particles;

○ smooth so as to be easily cleaned;

○ resistant to rust;

○ resistant to chipping.

Containers, pipes and equipment made from toxic materials, such as lead and zinc, should not be in direct contact with food or drink or be allowed to wear excessively; copper pans that need retinning on the inside will expose harmful copper to food. Food must be protected from lubricants.

Figure 16.8 *Hygienic storage of equipment*

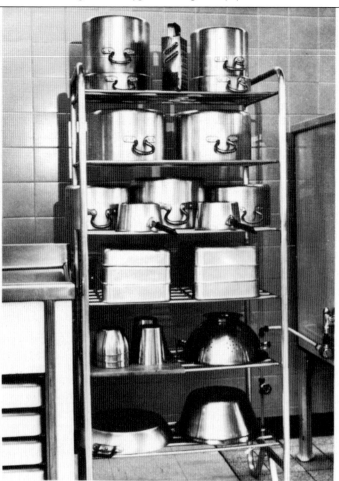

Easily cleaned equipment is free from unnecessary ridges, screws, ornamentation, dents, crevices or inside square corners, and has large, smooth areas. Articles of equipment which are difficult to clean (mincers, sieves and strainers) are items where particles of food can lodge so allowing germs to multiply and contaminate food when the utensil is next used.

NORMAL CLEANING OF MATERIALS

- *Metals:* as a rule all metal equipment should be cleaned immediately after use.
- *Portable items:* remove food particles and grease. Wash by immersion in hot detergent water. Thoroughly clean with a hard bristle brush or soak until this is possible. Rinse in water at 77°C (171°F), by immersing in the water in wire racks.
- *Fixed items:* remove all food and grease with a stiff brush or soak with a wet cloth, using hot detergent water. Thoroughly clean with hot detergent water. Rinse with clean water, disinfectant and dry with a clean cloth.
- *Abrasives:* should only be used in moderation as their constant scratching of the surface makes it more difficult to clean the article next time.
- *Marble:* scrub with a bristle brush and hot water and detergent then sanitise and leave to dry.
- *Wood:* scrub with a bristle brush and hot detergent water, rinse and dry.
- *Plastic:* wash in reasonably hot water.
- *China, earthenware:* avoid extremes of heat and do not clean with an abrasive. Wash in hot water, disinfect or sanitise and leave to dry.
- *Copper:* remove as much food as possible. Soak. Wash in hot detergent water with the aid of a brush. Clean the outside with a paste made of sand, vinegar and flour. Wash well. Rinse and dry. Alternatively, a proprietary copper cleaner may be used. Copper pans are gradually being replaced in commercial kitchens, mainly due to the expense involved in retinning.
- *Aluminium:* do not wash in water containing soda as the protective film which prevents corrosion may be damaged. To clean, remove food particles. Soak. Wash in hot detergent water. Clean with steel wool or abrasive. Immerse in very hot water 82°C. Rinse and dry.
- *Stainless steel:* stainless steel is easy to clean. Soak in hot detergent water. Clean with a brush, sanitise, rinse and leave to dry.
- *Tin:* tin which is used to line pots and pans should be soaked, washed in detergent water then immersed in very hot water (2°C) and dried. Tinned utensils, where thin sheet steel has a thin coating of tin, must be thoroughly dried, otherwise they are likely to rust.
- *Zinc:* This is used to coat storage bins of galvanised iron and it should not be cleaned with a hard abrasive.
- *Vitreous enamel:* clean with a damp cloth and dry. Avoid using abrasives.
- *Equipment requiring particular care in cleaning* (sieves, conical strainers, mincers and graters). Extra attention must be paid to these items, because food particles clog the holes. The holes can be cleaned by using the force of the water from the tap, by using a bristle brush and by moving the article, particularly a sieve, up and down in the sink, so causing water to pass through the mesh. Whisks must be thoroughly cleaned where the wires cross at the end opposite the handle as food can lodge between the wires. The handle of the whisk must also be kept clean. The use of detergents/sanitisers are recommended.
- *Saws and choppers, mandolins:* these items should be cleaned in hot detergent water, dried and greased slightly.
- *Tammy cloths, muslins and piping bags:* after use they should be emptied, food particles scraped out, scrubbed carefully and boiled. They should then be rinsed and allowed to dry. Certain piping bags made of plastic should be washed in very hot water and dried. Nylon piping bags should not be boiled.

CLEANING OF LARGE ELECTRICAL EQUIPMENT (OVENS, MINCERS, MIXERS, CHOPPERS, SLICERS)

1 Switch off the machine and remove the electric plug.

2 Remove particles of food with a cloth, palette knife, needle or brush as appropriate.

3 Thoroughly clean with hand-hot detergent water all removable and fixed parts. Pay particular attention to threads and plates with holes in mincers. Disinfect using a sanitiser or equivalent.

4 Rinse thoroughly.

5 Dry and reassemble.

6 While cleaning see that exposed blades are not left uncovered or unguarded and that the guards are replaced when cleaning is complete.

7 Any specific maker's instructions should be observed.

8 Test that the machine is properly assembled by plugging in and switching on.

All equipment once cleaned should be stored properly.

Further information

Cleaning and Maintenance Research and Services Organisation (CAMRASO) White House, Went Park Ring Rd. Leeds LS16 6Q1

Kitchen energy distribution systems

A system of this type operates from stainless steel housings (known as 'raceways') which are fastened to walls, floors, ceilings or may be island mounted. Inside the raceways are runs of electrical bus-bars or bus-wires and plumbing pipes. At intervals, appropriate for the kitchen equipment served, are switch or valve sockets, electrical, gas, water, steam, etc.

Connecting flexible cords and pipes from the kitchen equipment plug into the sockets and are designed to hang clear of the floor and are smooth plastic coated for easy cleaning.

For maximum advantage from this idea, the hygiene, safety, flexibility, ease of cleaning and maintenance, most of the kitchen equipment is mounted on castors.

Periodic cleaning is carried out by pulling the equipment out from the wall or island, unplugging all the services then moving the equipment away on its castors giving free access to all wall and floor surfaces as well as backs and sides of equipment.

Further information can be obtained from Eurocaddy Systems Ltd, Powder Mill Lane, Dartford, Kent DA1 1NN.

FOOD HYGIENE

The Food Safety Act 1990 includes:

○ increased powers for the Environmental Health Officers;

○ provision of training for food operatives;

○ registration of food premises with the local authority;

○ the defence of 'due diligence'. If the person in charge of a catering operation can show that he or she took all reasonable precautions to avoid committing an offence then this can be used in defending any presentation under the Food Safety Act 1990/95.

A law compelling restaurants, hotels and other catering outlets to publish the results of their food and hygiene inspections is expected to be passed soon.

In the USA, restaurants have to publish the results of their food hygiene and health and safety audits alongside menus.

Provision of safe food

This is a management responsibility. In order to provide safe food a safety control system should be implemented. The HACCP approach provides a means of ensuring the provision of safe food for the customers. HACCP stands for Hygiene Analysis Critical Control Point.

Hazard analysis identifies all the factors that could lead to hazards for the consumer: all ingredients, stages in the processing of foods, environmental features and human factors that could lead to unsafe food being served.

Critical Control Points (CCPs) are the points at which control is essential to ensure that potential hazards do not actually become hazardous.

- Is the food delivered at the correct temperature?
- Is the food stored and displayed at the correct temperature?
- Is cross-contamination prevented as far as possible?
- Are cleaning schedules in place for equipment?
- Are personnel correctly trained and hygienic in their work practices?

In small catering units the main principles should still apply but a modified form of HACCP is more appropriate. This is Assured Safe Catering (ASC). ASC emphasise the importance of safety precautions in the preparation, handling and temperature control of food. It is vital that catering staff are properly trained if an ASC system is to work effectively and that record sheets are kept of controls which are in place. (See defence of 'due diligence' on page 560).

The most succulent, mouth-watering dish into which has gone all the skill and art of the world's best chefs, using the finest possible ingredients, may look, taste and smell superb, yet be unsafe, even dangerous to eat because of harmful bacteria.

It is of the utmost importance that everyone who handles food, or who works in a place where food is handled, should know that food must be both clean and safe. Hygiene is the study of health and the prevention of disease, and because of the dangers of food poisoning, hygiene requires particular attention from everyone in the catering industry.

There are germs everywhere, particularly in and on our bodies; some of these germs if transferred to food can cause illness and in some cases death. These germs are so small they cannot be seen by the naked eye, and so food which looks clean and does not smell or taste bad may be dangerous to eat if harmful germs have contaminated it and multiplied.

The duty of every person concerned with food is to prevent contamination of food by germs and to prevent these germs or bacteria from multiplying.

Food-handlers must know the Food Hygiene Regulations, but no matter how much is written or read about food hygiene the practice of hygiene habits by people who handle food is the only way to safe food.

FOOD SAFETY (GENERAL FOOD HYGIENE)

Butchers shops amendment regulations 2000

Following the Pennington Group Report proposals (after the outbreak of E.coli food poisoning in Lanarkshire in 1996) a licensing scheme for butchers has now been introduced. Although the licensing scheme only applies to butchers, it is likely that a similar requirement will be placed on caterers in the future. The regulations came into force on 1st May 2000. Supermarkets meat departments and butchers now have to obtain a licence to trade issued by the local environmental health department.

The Food Labelling Regulations 1984 and the Food Labelling (Amendment) Regulations 1999

These regulations mainly affect manufacturers of food but caterers and retailers are required to comply with the requirements; most notably those relating to the labelling of genetically modified soya or maize ingredients.

There are a number of basic elements to food labelling.

1 The name of the food and the list of ingredients.

2 An indication of shelf life (minimum durability) or in the case of food which, in terms of microbiology, may have a short shelf life and therefore may become an immediate danger to human health: a 'use by' date.

3 Special storage conditions.

4 Conditions of use.

5 Name and address of the manufacturer, packer or seller.

Main shelf life indicators are 'use by', or 'best before' or 'best before end' followed by the date to which the food might be considered to remain safe with good quality and fitness. Any required storage conditions would have been properly observed.

Expected shelf lives and indicators to be used:

○ Highly perishable which may become a danger to health – 'use by' and day and month and year.

○ 3 months or less – 'best before' day and month only.

○ 3 to 18 months – 'best before' and day and month and year on 'best before end' and month and year.

○ More than 18 months – 'best before' and month and year or 'best before end' and year only.

There are a number of exempt foods including uncut fresh vegetables or high alcoholic drinks.

It is an offence to sell foods whose 'use by ' dates have expired or to alter such dates once applied.

The bread and flour regulations 1998

The principal effect of the regulations is to:

○ continue to require the fortification of most flour with certain minerals and vitamins;

○ prohibit the use of flour improvers in wholemeal bread, with the exception of vitamin c (ascorbic acid);

○ require that flour improvers are indicated in the list of ingredients of all pre-packed bread and on a label ticket or notice displayed with non-pre-packed bread;

○ prohibit use of the name 'wheatmeal' in the labelling or advertising of all sales of bread and flour;

○ prescribe names by which flour may be sold, including 'wholemeal', 'self-raising';

○ require the name of any bread made from flour derived from wheat to include the words 'wholemeal', 'brown', 'wheatgerm', 'white', 'soda' or 'aerated' as appropriate;

○ list the additives permitted to be used in bread and flour.

Catering establishments making their own bread are not exempt from these regulations.

Disposal of waste legal requirements

There is a 'duty of care' under the Environmental Protection Act 1990 which makes the catering organisation responsible for their waste. It is a legal requirement to use licensed waste contractors who must issue the caterer with a 'waste transfer notice'. Any special waste might need dealing with separately e.g. chemicals, flammable substances, potentially infectious material.

There is also a legal requirement which attempts to deal with the reduction of packaging. Large businesses must register with the Environmental Protection Agency and make efforts to reduce the amount of packaging they generate as waste.

Dealing with waste in catering premises

Waste disposal will put an increasing burden on caterers both financially and physically. There are measures that can be taken which will minimise the problems:

○ Waste minimisation schemes;
○ Recycling;
○ Segregation at source – this makes possible recycling and waste minimisation;
○ Evaluation of cohort, contractor arrangements – to ensure recycling is a practical proposition.

Food poisoning

Figure 16.9 *Extracts from a newspaper reports on food poisoning*

> ### E.coli puts ten in hospital
>
> TEN people were in hospital last night after an E.coli outbreak.
>
> Two cases have been confirmed and up to 16 are suspected. One of these involves a boy of ten.
>
> Health authorities are investigating a link with the Kwik Save supermarket in Eccleton, near Chorley, Lancashire. Yesterday the store closed its delicatessen counter and fresh fruit and vegetable stand. Customers have been asked to return all meat, dairy and fresh produce bough there since November 1.
>
> E.coli is a potentially fatal gastro-intestinal infection passed on from contaminated food.
>
> Last night an NHS spokesman said none of those in hospital was dangerously ill.

Over 100 thousand people each year have been found by doctors to be suffering from food poisoning. This represents the average number of notified cases over the last few years, and there are many thousands more who have not notified their doctor, but have suffered from food poisoning. This appalling amount of ill-health could largely be prevented. Failure to prevent it may be due to:

○ ignorance of the rules of hygiene;
○ carelessness, thoughtlessness or neglect;

○ poor standards of equipment or facilities to maintain hygienic standards;
○ accident.

Food poisoning can be prevented by:

○ high standards of personal hygiene;
○ attention to physical fitness;
○ maintaining good working conditions;
○ maintaining equipment in good repair and in clean condition;
○ adequate provision of cleaning facilities and cleaning equipment;
○ correct storage of foodstuffs at the right temperature;
○ correct reheating of food;
○ quick cooling of foods prior to storage;
○ protection of food from vermin and insects;
○ hygienic washing-up procedure;
○ food-handlers knowing how food poisoning is caused;
○ food-handlers carrying out correct procedures to prevent food poisoning.

WHAT IS FOOD POISONING?

Food poisoning can be defined as an illness characterised by stomach pains and diarrhoea and sometimes vomiting, generally developing within one to 36 hours after eating the affected food.

CAUSES OF FOOD POISONING

Food poisoning results when harmful foods are eaten, contaminated by:

Figure 16.10 *Testing for food poisoning*

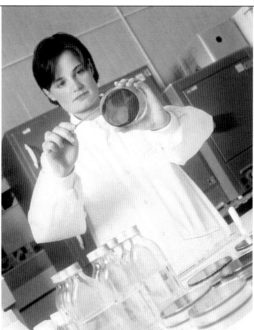

○ chemicals which entered foods accidentally during the growth, preparation or cooking of the food;

○ germs (harmful bacteria) which have entered the food from humans, animals or other sources and the bacteria themselves, or the toxins (poisons) produced in the food by certain bacteria, have caused the foods to be harmful. By far the greatest number of cases of food poisoning is caused by harmful bacteria.

CHEMICAL FOOD POISONING

Certain chemicals may accidentally enter food and cause food poisoning.

○ Arsenic is used to spray fruit during growth, and occasionally fruit has been affected by this poison.

Figure 16.11 *News reports on E Coli and Salmonella poisoning*

US DELI BEHIND BIGGEST E COLI OUTBREAK

A DELICATESSEN'S potato salad is the suspected cause of one of the biggest-ever outbreaks of E. coli poisoning.

The salad was sold over the counter and also served at more than 300 parties cat...

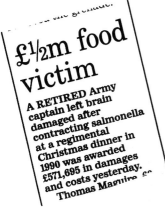

£½m food victim

A RETIRED Army captain left brain damaged after contracting salmonella at a regimental Christmas dinner in 1990 was awarded £571,695 in damages and costs yesterday.

Thomas Maguire...

Food bug hits holiday Britons

MORE than 90 British holidaymakers have been struck down with salmonella poisoning at a resort on Majorca.

Tour operator...

Salmonella is suspected as guests fall ill

Boy, 12, poisoned by cheese

A SCHOOLBOY was seriously ill in hospital last night suffering from the deadly E.coli infection.

The 12-year-old fell ill after eating an English-made gourmet cheese.

He was rushed to hospital in Bristol from his Somerset home after his family doctor was called. It

BY ANTHONY MITCHELL

was then discovered that he had eaten a Caerphilly cheese containing chives made near his home.

Last night, environmental health inspectors were set to tour specialist cheese shops and wholesalers ordering them to remove from their

shelves all cheeses made by Duckett and Co, of Walnut Tree Farm, Wedmore, Somerset.

The small cheese producer was being searched by health inspectors to trace the origins of the bacteria.

Duckett's cheeses are also used by maturers and other cheesemakers, so the

whole English cheese industry could come to a near halt during the investigation.

The Health Department said: "Among the cheeses we are appealing for retailers to stop selling is one known as Tornegus. We are also asking inspectors to sample Caerphilly and Wedmore cheeses "

○ Lead poisoning can occur from using water that has been in contact with lead pipes and then drunk or used in cooking.

○ Antimony or zinc poisoning from acid foods stored or cooked in poor quality enamelled or galvanised containers can occur.

○ Copper pans should be correctly tinned and never used for storing foods, particularly acid foods, as the food could dissolve harmful amounts of copper.

○ Certain *plants* are poisonous such as some fungi, rhubarb leaves and the parts of potatoes which are exposed to the sun above the surface of the soil.

PREVENTION OF CHEMICAL FOOD POISONING

Chemical food poisoning can be prevented by:

○ using correctly maintained and suitable kitchen utensils;

○ obtaining foodstuffs from reliable sources;

○ care in the use of rat poison, etc.

BACTERIAL FOOD POISONING

Food contaminated by bacteria (germs) is by far the most common cause of food poisoning. Cross-contamination is when bacteria are transferred from contaminated to uncontaminated foods via hands, boards, knives, surfaces, etc.

To prevent the transfer of bacteria by cross-contamination, these points should be observed:

○ ensure food is obtained from reliable sources;

○ handle foods as little as possible; when practicable use tongs, palette knives, disposable plastic gloves, etc;

○ ensure utensils and work surfaces are clean and sanitised;

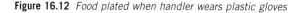

Figure 16.12 *Food plated when handler wears plastic gloves*

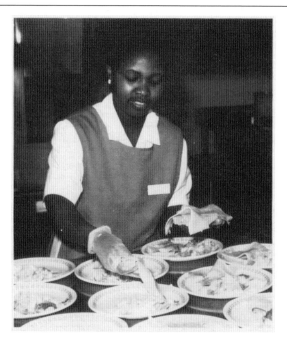

○ use cloths impregnated with a bactericide which fades in colour when no longer effective;

○ pay particular attention when handling raw poultry, meat and fish;

○ wash raw fruits and vegetables;

○ clean methodically and as frequently as necessary; clean as you go;

○ keep foods covered as much as possible;

○ have boards and knives coloured for particular foods, for example red for raw meat, blue for raw fish, yellow for cooked meat (Figure 16.18, page 536).

○ take particular care in thorough reheating of made up dishes.

Bacteria are minute, single-celled organisms which can only be seen under a microscope. They are everywhere in our surroundings, and as most bacteria cannot move by themselves they are transferred to something by coming into direct contact with it.

Some bacteria from spores can withstand high temperatures for long periods of time (even six hours) and on return to favourable conditions revert to normal bacteria again which then multiply.

Some bacteria produce toxins outside their cells so that they mix with the food; the food itself is then poisonous and symptoms of food poisoning follow within a few hours.

Other bacteria cause food poisoning by virtue of large numbers of bacteria in food entering the digestive system, multiplying further and setting up an infection.

Certain bacteria produce toxins which are resistant to heat; foods in which this toxin has been produced may still cause illness, even though the food is heated to boiling-point and boiled for half an hour. Some bacteria will grow in the absence of air (anaerobes), others need it (aerobes).

Bacteria multiplying by dividing in two, under suitable conditions, once every 10–20 minutes. Therefore one bacterium could multiply in 10 to 12 hours to between 500 million and 1000 million bacteria.

Not all bacteria are harmful. Some are useful, such as those used in cheese production; some cause food spoilage, such as souring of milk.

Some bacteria which are conveyed by food cause diseases other than food poisoning, diseases known as food-borne diseases. With bacterial food poisoning the bacteria multiply in the food.

Typhoid and paratyphoid are diseases caused by harmful bacteria carried in food or water. Scarlet fever, tuberculosis and dysentery may be caused by drinking milk which has not been pasteurised.

The time between eating the contaminated food (ingestion) to the beginning of the symptoms of the illness (onset) depends on the type of bacteria which have caused the illness.

For the multiplication of bacteria certain conditions are necessary:

○ food must be the right kind;   ○ moisture must be adequate;

○ temperature must be suitable;   ○ time must pass.

FOOD

Most foods are easily contaminated; those less likely to cause food poisoning have a high concentration of vinegar, sugar or salt, or are preserved in some special way (see page 191).

The following foods are particularly susceptible to the growth of bacteria because of their composition. Extra care must be taken to prevent them from being contaminated.

○ stock, sauces, gravies, soups;   ○ eggs and egg products;

○ meat and meat products (sausages, pies, cold meats);   ○ all foods which are handled;

○ all foods which are reheated;   ○ milk and milk products.

The bacterium *Campylobacter* causes symptoms similar to salmonella food poisoning and can be present in unpasteurised milk and undercooked chicken.

To prevent diseases being spread by food and water the following measures should be taken:

○ water supplies must be purified;

○ milk and meat products should be pasteurised or otherwise heat treated;

○ carriers should be excluded from food preparation rooms.

Figure 16.13 *Germometer*

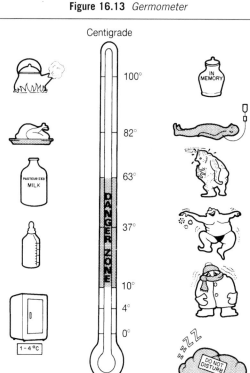

TEMPERATURE

Food poisoning bacteria multiply rapidly at body temperature, 37°C (98.6°F). They grow between temperatures of 5°C and 63°C. This is a similar heat to a badly ventilated kitchen and for this reason foods should not be kept in the kitchen. They should be kept in the larder or refrigerator. Lukewarm water is an ideal heat for bacteria to grow in. Washing-up must not take place in warm water as bacteria are not killed and the conditions are ideal for their growth, therefore pots and pans, crockery and cutlery may become contaminated. Hot water must be used for washing up.

Boiling water will kill bacteria in a few seconds, but to destroy toxins boiling for a half-hour is necessary. To kill the most heat-resistant spores, 4 to 5 hours' boiling is required. It is important to remember that it is necessary not only to heat foods to a sufficiently high temperature but also for a sufficient length of time to be sure of safe food. Extra care should be taken in warm weather to store foods at low temperatures and to reheat thoroughly foods which cannot be boiled.

Bacteria are not killed by cold although they do not multiply at very low temperatures; in a deep freeze they lie dormant for long periods. If foods have been contaminated before being made cold, on raising the temperature the bacteria will multiply. Foods which have been taken out of the refrigerator, kept in a warm kitchen and returned to the refrigerator for use later on may well be contaminated.

MOISTURE

Bacteria require moisture for growth – they cannot multiply on dry food. Ideal foods for their growth are jellies with meats, custards, creams, sauces, etc.

TIME

Under ideal conditions one bacterium divides into two every 20 minutes; in six to seven hours millions of bacteria will have been produced. Small numbers of bacteria may have little effect, but in a comparatively short time sufficient numbers can be produced to cause food poisoning. Particular care therefore is required with foods stored overnight, especially if adequate refrigerated space is not available.

Figure 16.14 *Germs multiplying on moist foods in warm temperature over time*

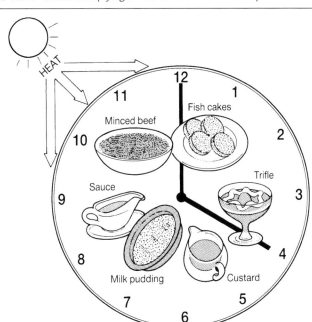

TYPES OF FOOD POISONING BACTERIA

The commonest food poisoning bacteria are:

○ the salmonella group (causing food poisoning because of large numbers of bacteria in the food);
○ *Staphylococcus aureus* (causing food poisoning due to poison (toxin) production in the food);
○ *Clostridium perfringens* (causing food poisoning due to large numbers of bacteria producing toxins in the intestines).

SALMONELLA GROUP

These bacteria can be present in the intestines of animals or human beings; they are excreted and anything coming into contact directly or indirectly with the excreta may be contaminated (raw meat at the slaughter house or the unwashed hands of an infected person). Infected excreta from human beings or animals may contaminate rivers and water to be used for drinking purposes, although chlorination of water is very effective in killing harmful bacteria.

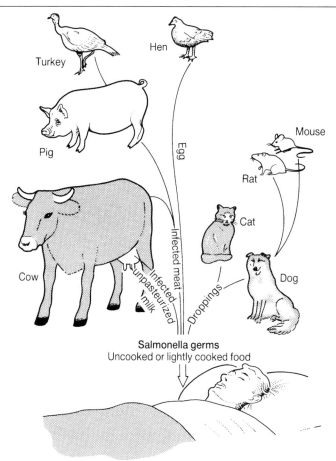

> **Figure 16.15** *Foods contaminated by Salmonella organisms if uncooked or lightly cooked may result in food poisoning*

Salmonella infection is the result of human beings or animals eating food contaminated by salmonella-infected excreta originating from human beings or animals, so completing a chain of infection. For example, when flies land on the excreta of a dog which has eaten infected dog-meat and the flies then go on to food, if that food is then left out in warm conditions for a time, the people who eat the contaminated food could well suffer from food poisoning.

Foods most affected by the salmonella group are poultry, meat and eggs (rarely processed egg products or duck eggs, although some hens' eggs have been found to be infected with salmonellae). Contamination can be caused by:

○ insects and vermin, because salmonellae are spread by droppings, feet, hairs, etc.;

○ the food itself (as, very occasionally, with duck eggs);

○ cross-contamination (if a chicken is eviscerated on a board and the board is not properly cleaned before another food (such as cold meat) is cut on the board;

○ the food infected by a human being who has the disease or who is a carrier (a person who does not suffer from food poisoning but who carries and passes on the germs to others).

Preparation of mayonnaise using raw eggs is a common practice but one which is fraught with danger. The problem is that raw eggs often contain salmonellae. To avoid the consequential high risk of food poisoning, the Department of Health (DoH) issued guidelines stating that unpasteurised eggs should not be used for preparing mayonnaise. Using raw egg products can be

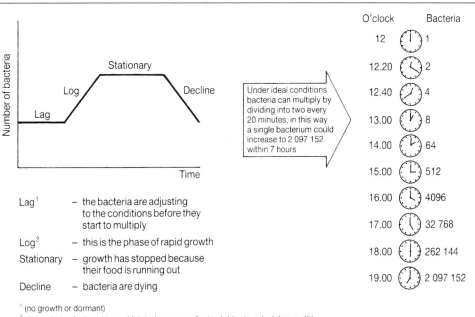

Figure 16.16 *Danger temperature at which germs can multiply*

Number of bacteria

Lag

Log

Stationary

Decline

Time

Under ideal conditions bacteria can multiply by dividing into two every 20 minutes, in this way a single bacterium could increase to 2 097 152 within 7 hours

O'clock	Bacteria
12	1
12.20	2
12.40	4
13.00	8
14.00	64
15.00	512
16.00	4096
17.00	32 768
18.00	262 144
19.00	2 097 152

Lag[1] – the bacteria are adjusting to the conditions before they start to multiply

Log[2] – this is the phase of rapid growth

Stationary – growth has stopped because their food is running out

Decline – bacteria are dying

[1] (no growth or dormant)

[2] (abbreviation for logarithm, which is the means of using tables to calculate growth)

Figure 16.17 *Reports on Salmonella food poisoning*

Food poisoning hits conference

Doctors attending a conference on diabetes at the weekend were struck down with food poisoning, believed to be salmonella.

Four hundred clinicians, nurses and health specialists had eaten cold meats, meat pies, seafood and salad at Friday lunchtime.

That evening two of the delegates were admitted to the casualty department with severe vomiting and diarrhoea. The next day a further 23 people with suspected salmonella poisoning were admitted to the hospital.

By Saturday evening 35 people had been seen, some at neighbouring hospitals and 80 people had reported symptoms of food poisoning.

VIPs food poison alert

More than 150 VIPs at two banquets in the city of London are suspected victims of food poisoning.

Salmonella is believed to be the cause and suspicion has centred on a cheese and egg savoury – Canape Roquefort – which was on both menus.

both unwise and costly. It is *not* illegal to use raw eggs to prepare mayonnaise, but the chances of food poisoning are high. In view of the Department of Health guidelines, a commercial kitchen using unpasteurised raw eggs would need to be able to show a sophisticated checking system to avoid the use of contaminated eggs and/or the use of some other factor (such as acidity) to control any food poisoning bacteria. Without being able to show these matters, it is difficult, if not impossible to rely upon a due diligence defence. The usual catering kitchen is very unlikely to have the equipment, skills and controls available to make these checks in order to satisfy the defence. The message for caterers is either to use bought-in commercially prepared mayonnaise, or to use pasteurised eggs. The alternatives are probably too expensive to contemplate.

> **Figure 16.18** *Separate chopping boards for different foods will help to prevent cross-contamination*

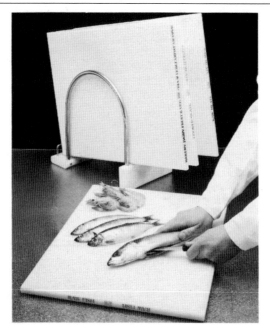

STAPHYLOCOCCUS AUREUS

These germs are present on human hands and other parts of the skin, or sores, spots etc., and in the nose and throat.

Foods affected by *Staphylococcus aureus* include foods which have been handled because the hands have been infected from the nose or throat, cuts etc. Brawn, pressed beef, pies and custards are foods frequently contaminated (either by food-handlers or air-borne infection) because they are ideal for foods for the multiplication of the bacterium.

CLOSTRIDIUM PERFRINGENS

These bacteria are distributed from the intestines of humans and animals and are found in the soil.

Foods affected by *Clostridium perfringens* include raw meat which is the main source of these bacteria, the spores of which survive light cooking.

Clostridium botulinum is another type of bacterium which causes food poisoning, but it is rare in the UK.

CAMPYLOBACTER bacteria are a common cause of diarrhoea in the UK. Large numbers are not required to cause illness; poultry and meats are the main foods infected but adequate cooking will kill the bacteria.

BACILLUS CEREUS is found in soil where vegetables and cereals, like rice, may grow. Long, moist storage of warm cooked food, especially rice, allows the spores to germinate into bacteria which multiply and produce toxin.

LISTERIA bacteria are aerobic, non-sporing organisms which can cause serious food-borne disease, particularly in the elderly, the chronically sick or babies. These bacteria are found in soil, vegetables and animal feed. They are killed by correct cooking but grow at refrigeration temperatures and in mildly acidic conditions such as that found in soft cheeses where lactic acid is present.

There is particular concern over contamination of prepacked salads and chilled raw chicken. Although it is unlikely that a small number of organisms would cause any harm to healthy people, the bacteria can cause illness in vulnerable groups, infecting babies in the womb, elderly people and the sick.

ESCHERICHIA COLI (E. COLI)

Found in the intestinal flora of man and animals, it is usually used as an indicator of faecal contamination of food or water. However, certain strains are known to be pathogenic and produce an enterotoxin in the intestine which results in symptoms of abdominal pain and diarrhoea. One group of pathogenic, E. coli, is responsible for severe infantile diarrhoea and another group causes travellers' diarrhoea. E. coli has been recorded as low as 4°C.

Found in human sewage water and raw meat, onset period 10 to 72 hours, but usually 12 to 24 hours. Symptoms are abdominal pain, fever, diarrhoea and vomiting 1 to 3 days.

Outbreaks of E. coli occurred in Scotland in 1997 from a butcher selling raw and cooked meat, resulting in 20 deaths.

SOURCES OF INFECTION

Food-poisoning bacteria live in:

○ the soil;

○ humans – intestines, nose, throat, skin, cuts, sores, spots etc.;

○ animals, insects and birds – intestines and skin etc.

Recommended reading: Technical Brief No 23/96, The Thawing of Raw Poultry and Game, HCIMA.

BOVINE SPONGIFORM ENCEPHALOPATHY (BSE)

In 1985 the first incident of a new disease of the brain was identified in a cow, althouth it was not until 1986 that this was formally recognised by the authorities. In 1990 and again in 1993 when the outbreak had reached its peak, the Chief Medical Officer assured the public that beef was safe to eat. But in 1995 the first case of vCJD was diagnosed and government and the EU took a series of actions which meant that as from 1996 no cattle over the age of thirty months were allowed to enter the food chain and exports of British beef were banned.

From November 2000 butchers shops selling cooked and raw products will be breaking the law if they do not have a licence from the local authority. Butchers are charged an annual inspection fee which provides an authorised officer from the local council to make a full compliance audit of the business. The officer will examine compliance with the Food Safety (General Food Hygiene) Regulations 1995.

PREVENTION OF FOOD POISONING FROM BACTERIA

To prevent food poisoning everyone concerned with food must:

○ prevent bacteria from multiplying;

○ prevent bacteria from spreading from place to place.

This means harmful bacteria must be isolated, the chain of infection must be broken and conditions favourable to their growth eliminated. (The conditions favourable to their growth –

Figure **16.19** *How food poisoning may be caused*

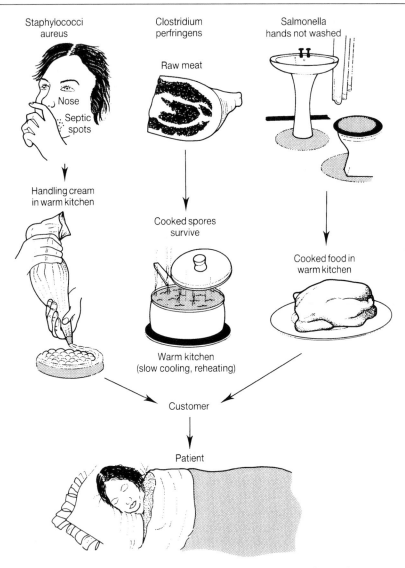

heat, time, moisture and a suitable food on which to grow – are explained on pages 528–539). It is also necessary to prevent harmful bacteria being brought into premises or getting on to food. This is achieved by a high standard of hygiene of personnel, premises, equipment and food-handling.

Chemical and metallic poisoning

Residues of drugs, pesticides and fertilisers may be present in raw materials. Pesticides sprayed onto fruit and vegetables just prior to harvesting may result in cumulative toxic effects. Two outbreaks of chemical food poisoning in 1991 resulted from the contamination of watermelons and cucumbers with the pesticide Aldicarb. In 1995 warnings were issued regarding the need to peel carrots.

Chemicals can enter foodstuffs by leakage, spillage or other accidents during processing or preparation.

Chemical additives of food have to undergo rigorous tests before they are allowed to be used and are usually harmless

Chemical poisoning may also occur because of the waste, such as mercury compounds, polluting river water used for drinking or food production.

Several metals are toxic and if ingested in sufficient quantities can give rise to food poisoning. The symptoms, mainly vomiting and abdominal pain, usually develop within an hour. Diarrhoea may also occur. Metals may be absorbed by growing crops or contaminate food during processing.

Acid foods should not be cooked or stored in equipment containing any of the following metals:

Antimony – used in the enamel coating of equipment. Under certain conditions antimony poisoning can occur.

Cadmium – is used extensively for plating utensils and fittings for electric cookers and refrigeration apparatus. It is attacked by some acids including fruit and wines. Foods, such as meat, placed directly on the refrigerator shelves containing cadmium may become poisonous.

Copper – poisoning can occur when the interior lining of saucepans becomes worn and the copper is exposed.

Lead – is a very poisonous metal if ingested. Fruit and leafy vegetables can become contaminated by lead through airborne lead from petrol and incinerators.

Tin and iron – Most cans used for the storage of food are constructed of tin plated iron sheet. Occasionally, due to prolonged storage, certain acid foods such as pineapples, rhubarb, strawberries, citrus fruits and tomatoes react with the tin plate and hydrogen gas is produced. Iron and tin are absorbed by the food which may become unfit for human consumption.

Zinc – is used in the galvanising of metals. Galvanised equipment should not be used in direct contact with food, particularly acid foods.

Aluminium – There has been for some time some concern over the use of aluminium in kitchens. Some evidence exists that there is a link between pre-senile dementia and aluminium.

KITCHEN HYGIENE

Infection can be spread by:

○ humans: coughing, sneezing, by the hands;
○ animals, insects, birds: droppings, hair etc.;
○ inanimate objects: towels, dishcloths, knives, boards.

Human

People who are feeling ill, suffering from vomiting, diarrhoea, sore throat or head cold must not handle food.

As soon as a person becomes aware that he or she is suffering from, or is a carrier, of typhoid or paratyphoid fever, or salmonella or staphylococcal infection likely to cause food poisoning or dysentery, the person responsible for the premises must be informed. He or she must then inform the Medical Officer for Health.

Standards of personal hygiene should be high at all times (see Personal cleanliness, page 510).

Animal

Vermin, insects, domestic animals and birds can bring infection into food premises.

RATS AND MICE

Rats and mice are a dangerous source of food infection because they carry harmful bacteria on themselves and in their droppings. Rats infest sewers and drains and, since excreta is a main source of food-poisoning bacteria, it is therefore possible for any surface touched by rats to be contaminated.

Rats and mice frequent warm dark corners and are found in lift shafts, meter cupboards, lofts, opening in walls where pipes enter, under low shelves and on high shelves. They enter premises through any holes, defective drains, open doorways and in sacks of food-stuffs.

Signs to look for are droppings, smears, holes, runways, gnawing marks, grease marks on skirting boards and above pipes, clawmarks, damage to stock and also rat odour.

Rats spoil ten times as much food as they eat and there are at least as many rats as human beings. They are very prolific, averaging ten babies per litter and six litters per year, so that under ideal conditions it is theoretically possible for one pair of rats to increase to 350 million in three years. To prevent infestation from rats and mice the following measures should be taken:

○ food stocks should be moved and examined to see that no rats or mice have entered the store-room;

○ no scraps of food should be left lying about;

○ dustbins and swill-bins should be covered with tight-fitting lids;

○ no rubbish should be allowed to accumulate outside the building;

○ buildings must be kept in good repair;

○ premises must be kept clean.

If premises become infested with rats or mice the environmental health inspector or a pest control contractor should be contacted.

Figure 16.20 *Pests and the damage they cause*

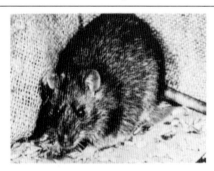
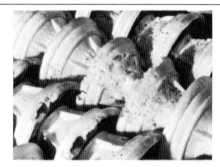
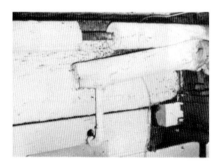
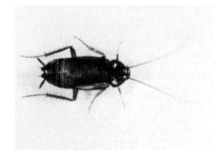

INSECT INFESTATION

House flies are the foremost of the insects which spread infection. Flies alight on filth and contaminate their legs, wings and bodies with harmful bacteria, and deposit these on the next object on which they settle; this may well be food. They also contaminate food with their excreta and saliva.

Cockroaches like warm, moist, dark places. They leave their droppings and a liquid which gives off a nauseating odour. They can carry harmful bacteria on their bodies and deposit them on anything with which they come into contact.

Silverfish are small silver-coloured insects which feed on starchy foods (among other things) and are found on moist surfaces. They thrive in badly ventilated areas and improving ventilation will help to control them.

Beetles are found in warm places and can also carry harmful germs from place to place.

Insects are destroyed by using an insecticide, and it is usual to employ people familiar with this work. The British Pest Control Association has a list of member companies.

Further information: Technical Brief No 35, Pest Control, HCIMA.

CATS AND DOGS

Domestic pets should not be permitted in kitchens or on food premises as they carry harmful bacteria on their coats and are not always clean in their habits. Cats also introduce fleas and should not be allowed to go in places where food is prepared.

BIRDS

Entry of birds through windows should be prevented as food and surfaces on which food is prepared may be contaminated by droppings and food poisoning bacteria.

DUST

Dust contains bacteria, therefore it should not be allowed to settle on food or surfaces used for food. Kitchen premises should be kept clean so that no dust can accumulate. Hands should be cleaned after handling dirty vegetables.

Further information HCIMA Technical brief No. 35.
British Pest Control Association
1 Glencages House
Vernon Gate, South St. Derby
DE1 1UP
www.bpca.org.uk

To control flies, the best way is to eliminate their breeding place, As they breed in rubbish and in warm, moist places, dustbins in summer are ideal breeding grounds; correct control and disposal of waste is paramount.

Figure 16.21 *Electrical equipment to attract, kill and collect winged insects*

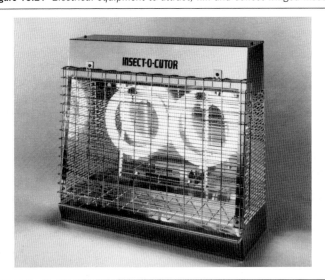

This is what happens when a fly lands on your food.

Flies can't eat solid food, so to soften it up they vomit on it.

Then they stamp the vomit in until it's a liquid, usually stamping in a few germs for good measure.

Then when it's good and runny they suck it all back again, probably dropping some excrement at the same time.

And then, when they've finished eating, it's your turn.

Control of waste and recyclable materials

Waste material is a potential threat to food safety because it is a source of contamination which can provide food for the variety of pests.

In today's ecological climate it is in everyone's interest to be aware of the issues which affect the environment and take steps to reduce waste. The catering industry has a responsibility by being environmentally friendly by recycling as much as possible. The reputation of the industry could be enhanced by those employed in it if they have the right attitude to the environment. It could be jeopardised if the catering industry neglected to implement recycling measures.

It is necessary to know the policy of the establishment regarding waste and to ensure that management and staff ensure that everything possible is done to encourage conservation and to practice the salvaging of as much as is possible. This includes the practice of not wasting gas, electricity or water. Staff, and customers, need to be made aware and reminded tactfully of this important issue. Hygiene and Safety is of paramount importance, but measures such as suitable notices asking persons using electricity or water not to waste is also important.

There may be initial costs in introducing an anti-waste policy but there could also be a saving of fuel bills and perhaps an income from sale of waste products. However this would depend on the quality involved, the area in which the establishments are situated or other factors.

Items which may be salvaged include

paper	tin foil	bottles; glass
cardboard	aluminium cans	spectacles
plastic bottles	used stamps	
clothing and footwear	Plastic wrappings, hard and soft	materials etc.

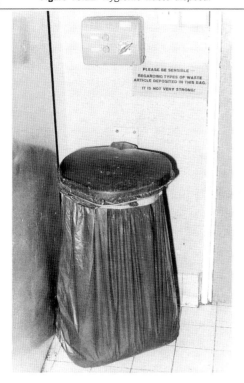

Figure 16.22 *Hygienic waste disposal*

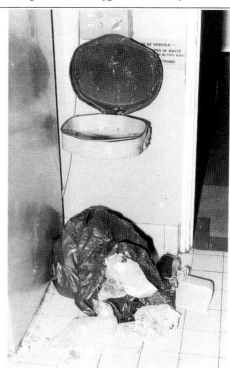

Figure 16.23 *Unhygienic waste disposal*

Disposal of waste may be through
○ Commercial firms; Local Councils; Charities.

Storage of waste and recyclable materials

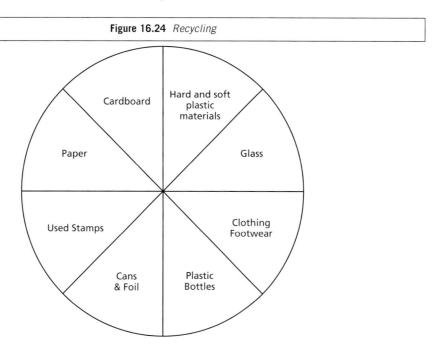

Figure 16.24 *Recycling*

Cardboard

Hard and soft plastic materials

Paper

Glass

Used Stamps

Clothing Footwear

Cans & Foil

Plastic Bottles

Most establishments will have an area for 'pure' or unusable waste in dustbins and bins for pig swill. Provisions in such an area can be provided for accumulating recyclables bearing in mind the need for safety and hygiene. Separation of green, brown and clear glass and paper from cardboard is necessary. Regular collections by reliable collectors is essential and a member of the staff needs to be responsible for the storage, tidiness and correct usage by staff members as well as the disposal of all materials salvaged.

The object is to reduce the unusable waste to a minimum, to utilise all that can be recycled or used.

Management need

○ to provide facilities for storage;
○ organise collections on the premises;
○ to educate and encourage staff to use the facilities correctly;
○ to control the situation;
○ to have the salvage materials regularly collected.

This entails the regular inspection of the 'waste' area and if necessary to remedy any misuse. To control the financial aspect and to keep staff informed of the success of recycling especially if any charities benefit from it.

Staff should be made aware that it is:

○ economically necessary;
○ environmentally sensible;
○ it creates a good image of the establishment in the community.

The Environment Protection (Duty of Care) Regulations 1991 create four main responsibilities for the producers of waste.

1 To prevent any other person committing the offences of disposing of 'controlled waste' or treating or storing it:
   – without a waste management licence; or
   – breaking the conditions of a licence; or
   – in a manner likely to cause pollution or harm to health.

2 To prevent the escape of waste, that is, to contain it.

3 To ensure that, if the waste is transferred, it goes only to an 'authorised person' on to a person for 'authorised transport purposes'.

4 When waste is transferred, to make sure that there is also transferred a written description of the waste, a description good enough to enable a person receiving it:
   – to avoid committing an offence;
   – to comply with the law to prevent the escape of waste.

Waste can be divided into five groups.

○ **Dry non-food waste**. This comes mainly from packaging wood, cardboard, plastic some of which can be sorted for resale. Cardboard and paper can be compacted by a waste compactor machine.

○ **Dry food waste**. This can either be a) disposed of at source in a waste disposal unit which grinds the waste into small particles, mixed with water and flushed into the drainage system or b) stored in galvanised steel bins with close fitting lids for disposal to swill collectors. The Disease of Animals (Waste Food) Order 1973 requires all swill collectors to be licensed by the local authority. The operator will arrange for cleaned and sterile bins to be delivered and collected on a regular basis.

○ Unsavoury or offensive food waste. This should be disposed of immediately where possible using a waste disposal unit.

○ Waste cooking oils and fats. Large quantities have a resale value, small quantities can be absorbed into dry food waste.

○ Bulky waste. This can be disposed of by either a) incineration (only by using specific equipment or in isolated areas) or b) by compaction. The advantages of compaction are:

– small, compact bulks easier to handle;

– less accessibility to pests;

– saving in refuse collection charges which are often charged by volume.

The refuse site should be a clean, easy to clean area with a water supply for washing down and adequate drainage. The site should be well lit and ventilated.

For general internal rubbish, plastic or paper lined bins which can be destroyed with the rubbish are preferable to other types of bin.

Other ways to control flies are to:

○ screen windows to keep flies out of kitchens;

○ install ultra-violet electrical fly-killers (Figure 16.21, page 542);

○ use sprays to kill flies (only where there is no food);

○ employ a pest control contractor.

Washing up

The correct cleaning of all equipment used for the serving and cooking of food is of vital importance to prevent multiplication of bacteria. This cleaning may be divided into the pan wash (plonge) or scullery and the china wash-up.

SCULLERY

For the effective washing up of pots and pans and other kitchen equipment the following method of work should be observed:

○ pans should be scraped and all food particles placed in a bin;

○ hot pans should be allowed to cool before being plunged into water;

○ pans which have food stuck to them should be allowed to soak (pans used for starchy foods, such as porridge and potatoes, are best soaked in cold water);

○ frying-pans should be thoroughly wiped with a clean cloth; they should not be washed unless absolutely necessary;

○ trays and tins used for pastry work should be thoroughly cleaned with a clean dry cloth, while warm;

○ pots, pans and other equipment should be washed and cleaned with a stiff brush, steel wool or similar article, in hot detergent water;

○ pan scrubbers are electrically driven with a hydraulic or flexible drive transmission. Brush type heads can be varied to suit differing surfaces or types of soiling. Pan scrubbers can either be wall mounted near the pot wash or free standing mounted on mobile dollies to assist with equipment cleaning;

○ the washing-up water must be changed frequently; it must be kept both clean and hot;

○ the cleaned items should be rinsed in very hot clean water to sterilise;

○ pans which have been sterilised (minimum temperature 82°C)) dry quickly; if it has not been possible to rinse in very hot water they should be dried with a clean cloth;

○ equipment should be stored on clean racks, pans should be stacked upside down.

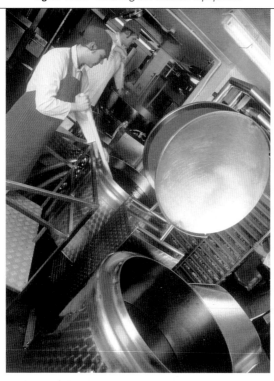

Figure 16.25 *Cleaning the kitchen equipment*

CHINA WASH-UP

The washing up of crockery and cutlery may be by hand or machine.

HANDWASHING

- Remove scraps from plates with a scraper or by hand.
- Wash in water containing a detergent as hot as the hands can bear (whether gloves are worn or not).
- Place utensils in wire baskets and immerse them into water thermostatically controlled at 82°C for at least two minutes.
- The hot utensils will air-dry without the use of a drying cloth.
- Both the washing and sterilising water must be kept clean and at the correct temperature.

MACHINE WASHING-UP

There are several types of machines which wash and sterilise crockery. In the more modern machines the detergent is automatically fed into the machine, which has continuous operation.

To be effective the temperature of the water must be high enough to kill any harmful bacteria and the articles passing through the machine must be subjected to the water for sufficient time to enable the detergent water to cleanse all the items thoroughly. The detergent used must be of the correct amount and strength to be effective. Alternatively low temperature equipment is available which sterilises by means of a chemical, sodium hypochlorite (bleach).

Where brushes are used they must be kept free from food particles.

Further information can be obtained from Lever Industrial, Lever House, St James's Road, Kingston-upon-Thames, Surrey KT1 2BA.

Hygienic storage of foods

One of the most important ways to prevent contamination of food is the correct storage of food (see also Chapter 10). Foodstuffs of all kinds should be kept covered as much as possible to prevent infection from dust and flies. Foods should be kept in a refrigerated cold room or refrigerator where possible.

Hot foods which have to go into a refrigerator must be cooled quickly. This can be done in several ways: by dividing large quantities of food into smaller containers; by cooling in a draught of air using fans or by raising the container and placing an article underneath, for example, a triangle or weight, so that air can circulate; or by placing the container in a sink with running cold water. If large quantities of food, such as minced beef, are left in one container the outside cools but the centre is still warm. When reheated the time taken to bring such a large quantity to the boil is sufficient to allow the bacteria to continue to multiply. If the food is not boiled long enough food poisoning can occur (see the section on Temperature, page 532).

Particular care must be taken to store foods correctly in the warmer months; food not refrigerated in hot weather does not cool completely and, furthermore, flies and bluebottles are numerous in the summer. It is not by chance that the vast majority of food poisoning cases occur in the summer months in the UK.

Following consultations, the Government announced proposals which will considerably simplify food storage temperature. The main features of the Temperature Control Regulations are:

○ a general requirement to keep foods at temperatures which will not result in a risk to health;

○ to store such foods at or below 8°C (46°F); there will be exemptions for foods where chill control is not necessary;

○ flexibility for certain food businesses to store at higher temperatures where this can be justified by a safety assessment;

○ a hot holding requirement of at least 63°C (145°F) for foods which could provide a risk to health;

○ tolerances for limited periods outside the chill and hot holding controls.

The main differences from the previous regulations are the removal of the detailed list of foods subject to control. The current two-tiered chill controls of 5°C (41°F) and 8°C (46°F) are replaced by the single 8°C (46°F) control. These relaxations place more responsibility on food businesses to be able to conduct effective risk analysis – proof of 'due diligence' becomes even more important.

These proposals came into effect in September 1995, so anyone considering changing their refrigeration equipment should bear these proposals in mind.

Foods requiring special attention (See also Food Hygiene Regulations 1990, page 550)

MEAT

- All made-up dishes, such as cottage pie, need extra care. They must be very thoroughly cooked.
- Reheated meat dishes must be thoroughly reheated.
- Pork must be well cooked (this is because pork may be affected by trichinosis, which is a disease caused by a minute roundworm).
- Poultry which is drawn in the kitchen should be cleaned carefully; boards, tables and knives must be thoroughly cleaned and sanitised afterwards, otherwise there is a danger of contamination from excreta.
- Meat should be handled as little as possible. Minced and cut-up meats are more likely to become contaminated because of infection from the food-handler. Boned and rolled joints require extra care in cooking as inside surfaces may have been contaminated.
- Sausages should be cooked right through.
- Tinned hams are lightly cooked, therefore they must be stored in a refrigerator.

FISH

Fish is usually washed, cooked and eaten fresh and is not often a cause of food poisoning, except in reheated fish dishes. Care must be taken to reheat thoroughly such dishes as fish cakes, fish pie, coquilles de poisson, etc.

Some shellfish, such as oysters and mussels, have caused food poisoning because they have been bred in water which has been polluted by sewage. They are today purified before being sold. All shellfish should be used fresh. If you buy them alive, there is no doubt as to their freshness.

EGGS (see page 120)

Both hens' eggs and ducks' eggs have been implicated in causing food poisoning, and Department of Health guidelines now suggest that it would be prudent to avoid eating raw eggs or uncooked foods made from them, such as home-made mayonnaise, home-made mousses, etc. If dried eggs are used they should be reconstituted and used right away, not left in this condition in a warm kitchen as they may have been contaminated in or after processing. Bulk liquid egg undergoes pasteurisation but may be contaminated after the container is opened. Hollandaise sauce which is made with eggs is an example of a food which should not be kept in a warm kitchen for long. If not used in the morning it should not be used in the evening.

MILK DISHES

When used in custards, trifles and puddings unless eaten soon after preparation, milk should be treated with care. Two hours is the maximum for keeping, then it should be discarded.

WATERCRESS AND OTHER GREEN SALAD

Watercress must be thoroughly washed as it grows in water which could be contaminated by animals. All green salads and other foods eaten raw should be well washed.

SYNTHETIC CREAM

Synthetic cream can be a cause of food poisoning if allowed to remain in warm conditions for long periods. It is easily contaminated by handling and from the air. Particular care is required in the handling and holding at the correct temperature of soups, sauces and gravies because bacteria multiply rapidly in these foods.

REHEATED FOODS

In the interests of economy a sound knowledge of handling left-over food is necessary. Many tasty dishes can be prepared, but care must always be taken to see that the food is thoroughly and carefully reheated. If care is not taken then food poisoning can result. Only sound food should be used ('if in doubt, throw it out').

Surplus prepared food

Some caterers as a matter of policy, and in the interests of safety, dispose of all unused prepared foods after set times, and always at the end of service. While this may be an ideal solution for some, for many it is not an option. In practical terms all reasonable steps must be taken to avoid overproduction. Caterers and consumers are most vulnerable when surplus prepared food is offered for consumption again. The best way of reducing the problem of what to do with surplus prepared food is to tighten the production planning process, and so reduce the amount of surplus prepared food.

Surplus prepared foods include:

○ items displayed but not sold during a meal service;

○ overproduction.

This brief offers some help in dealing with the safe handling of food suitable for resale.

PRINCIPLES

Surplus food should be considered fit for consumption only if, after normal preparation and display, it has not suffered excessive handling or prolonged exposure at serving temperatures above 8°C and has been returned to and kept in chilled storage at or below 5°C.

Surplus hot food to be served again hot, must be cooled as rapidly as possible and kept at or below 5°C until it is to be re-heated for service. It must then be re-heated thoroughly to temperatures in excess of 75°C and subsequently kept above 63°C until served.

Food should only be re-heated once.

Surplus hot food cooled rapidly and kept at or below 5°C can be served as cold food over the following 48 hours. Roast joints to be used for sandwiches and salads should be sliced, cooled and kept at or below 5°C until required for service.

Care must be taken at all stages to avoid introducing contamination. Examples of how this can occur; by slicing joints of meat on unsanitised chopping boards or using dirty knives or utensils.

Partially used products on display such as coleslaw should not be 'topped up' with fresh. A fresh replacement container should be used.

The assessment of safety should consider whether the surplus food was likely to have been subject to poor temperature control or contamination during handling or display. These issues should be critical to any decision on reuse.

PROCEDURES

○ Surplus food should be sorted into its various categories and placed under refrigeration as quickly as possible.

○ It is desirable to use a blast chiller to cool hot food rapidly.

○ Examine items in each category for damage and possible signs of contamination. Special attention should be given to short-life products particularly those which support bacterial growth, particularly meat, fish, poultry and egg dishes, rice, pasta, mousses and fresh cream products.

○ Examine perishable items such as bread rolls, biscuits and fresh fruit for obvious signs of damage or contamination and dispose of any suspect foods.

○ Items returned to cold storage must be carefully covered and stored separately from fresh and raw foods to avoid possible risks of cross contamination.

○ Comply with any relevant 'use by' or date codes.

RESPONSIBILITIES

It is the responsibility of management to develop and implement:

○ A firm policy detailing procedures for dealing with surplus prepared products. This must be available for inspection and regularly reviewed.

○ Relevant staff must be fully trained in these procedures and made aware of the potential hazards involved. The necessary controls must be in place at critical points.

○ All surplus prepared food must be clearly labelled showing the date of production and the 'use by' date before it is returned to cold storage.

SAFETY FIRST

When deciding whether or not to use 'Leftovers', if in doubt – throw it out.

FURTHER READING

Food Safety (General Food Hygiene) Regulations 1995 HMSO
ISBN 0 11 053383 6
Food Safety (Temperature Control) Regulations 1995 HMSO
ISBN 0 11 053227 9
Industry Guide to Good Hygiene Practice: Catering Guide
Chadwick House Group Ltd
Chadwick Court, 15 Hatfields, LONDON SE1 8DJ
Tel: 020 7827 5882
Fax: 020 7827 9930
Managing Hygiene 1999 HCIMA
Hazard Analysis and Critical Control Points (HACCP) HCIMA Technical Brief No. 5
Preventing Food Poisoning HCIMA Technical Brief No. 12
Cooling Cooked Joints of Meat HCIMA Technical Brief No. 14
Food Safety (General Food Hygiene) Regulations 1995 HCIMA Technical Brief No. 21
HCMP Technical Brief No. 9/2000

FOOD HYGIENE REGULATIONS

These regulations should be known and complied with by all people involved in the handling of food. A copy of the full regulations can be obtained from HMSO and an abstract can be obtained which gives the main points of the full regulations.

These points are as follows:

The Food Safety General Food Hygiene Regulations 1995

PROPRIETORS OF FOOD PREMISES ARE REQUIRED

1 To operate hygienically:
   (a) analyse food hazards;
   (b) identify where hazards may occur;
   (c) decide which points are critical to food safety;
   (d) implement control and monitoring procedures, review periodically and change when necessary.

2 Premises must be kept clean and in good repair:
   (a) designed to permit good hygiene practices;
   (b) adequate washbasins, toilets and cleaning disinfecting facilities;
   (c) satisfactory standards of lighting and ventilation.

3 Walls, floors and food-contact surfaces must be easy to clean and where necessary, to disinfect.

4 Conveyance and containers used for transporting food must be kept clean and in good repair.

5 Food equipment must be kept clean and in good repair.

6 Food waste and refuse must not be accumulated in food rooms. Adequate provision must be made for its storage and removal.

7 An adequate supply of drinking water must be provided

8 Food handlers:
   (a) must keep themselves clean;
   (b) wear suitable clean, and where appropriate, protective clothing;
   (c) if they know or suspect they are carrying a food borne disease, or have an infected cut or skin condition, their manager **must** be advised;
   (d) they must not be allowed to work if they are likely to contaminate food.

9 Food, including raw materials, must be fit for human consumption, stored and protected to minimise risk of contamination.

10 Food handlers must be trained and supervised in food hygiene matters.

11 Offences are punishable on conviction:
   (a) fines of up to £5,000 for each offence;
   (b) in serious cases up to 2 years in prison;
   (c) and unlimited fines.

Equipment

This must be kept clean and in good condition.

Personal requirements

○ All parts of the person liable to come into contact with food must be kept as clean as possible.
○ All clothing must be kept as clean as possible.
○ All cuts and abrasions must be covered with a waterproof dressing.
○ Spitting is forbidden.

○ Smoking is forbidden in a food room or where there is food.

○ As soon as a person is aware that he is suffering from or is a carrier of such infections as typhoid, paratyphoid, dysentery, salmonella or staphylococcal infection he must notify his employer, who must notify the Medical Office of Health.

Requirements for food premises
TOILETS

○ These must be clean, well lighted and ventilated.

○ No food room shall contain or directly communicate with a toilet.

○ A notice requesting people to wash their hands after using the toilet must be displayed in a prominent place.

○ The ventilation of the soil drainage must not be in a food room.

○ The water supply to a food room and toilet is only permitted through an efficient flushing cistern.

WASHING FACILITIES

○ Hand basins and an adequate supply of hot water must be provided.

○ Supplies of soap and hand drying facilities must be available by the hand basins.

OTHER FACILITIES

○ *First Aid:* bandages and waterproof dressings must be provided in a readily accessible position.

○ *Lockers:* enough storage space must be available for outdoor clothes.

○ *Lighting and ventilation:* food rooms must be suitably lit and ventilated.

○ *Sleeping room:* rooms in which food is prepared must not be slept in. Sleeping rooms must not be adjacent to a food room.

○ *Refuse:* refuse must not be allowed to accumulate in a food room. Waste bins must be lidded.

○ *Buildings:* the structure of food rooms must be kept in good repair to enable them to be cleaned and to prevent entry of rats, mice, etc.

○ *Food storage temperatures.*

○ *Storage:* foods should not be placed in a yard lower than 0.5m (18in) unless properly protected.

PENALTIES

Any person guilty of an offence shall be liable to a heavy fine and/or a term of imprisonment. Under the latest Food Safety Act, unhygienic premises can be closed down by a local authority immediately, on the advice of the Environmental Health Officer.

The Environmental Health Officer when visiting premises will probably check for:

○ grease in ventilation ducts and on canopies;

○ long-standing dirt in less accessible areas;

○ cracked or chipped equipment;

○ provision for staff toilets and clothing;

○ 'now wash your hands' notice;

○ adequate and correct storage of food (cooked food stored above raw food if there is not separate refrigerated provision);

○ correct storage temperature of foodstuffs;
○ signs of pests and how they are prevented;
○ any hazards;
○ cleaning, training records and proper supervision.

CHECKLIST FOR CATERING ESTABLISHMENTS

○ Entrances and exits unobstructed.
○ Fire doors undamaged and in operating position.
○ Escape routes clearly indicated.
○ Fire-fighting equipment visible and accessible.
○ Lighting good.
○ Suitable supply of hot and cold water.
○ Good ventilation.
○ Separate hand-washing basin.
○ Soap, nail-brush (if provided) and towels by basin.
○ Floors in good repair, clean and dry.
○ Equipment operating correctly.
○ Guards on machines.
○ All surfaces undamaged and clean.
○ Staff trained to use machines.
○ Notice concerning use of machine close to it.
○ Suitable protective clothing worn.
○ Food, equipment and cleaning materials stored properly.
○ Rubbish bins covered and emptied regularly.
○ Staff work in accordance with safety guidelines.

Food Safety Act 1990

The Food Safety (General Food Hygiene) Regulations 1995
The Food Safety (Temperature Control) Regulations 1995
The Food Premises (Registration) Regulations 1997
Food safety is achieved provided you:
○ keep yourself clean;
○ keep the workplace clean;
○ wear suitable clean clothing;
○ protect food from contamination;
○ store, prepare, serve and display food at the correct temperature;
○ inform manager if you have an illness;
○ do not work with food if you have food poisoning symptoms.
You will have complied with the Food Safety Act 1990.
Food poisoning is an illness acquired from eating contaminated food. This usually means contaminated with bacteria, viruses or a chemical poisonous plant or an actual physical item.

Contamination

Bacterial and virus contamination comes from people, animals, insects, raw food, rubbish, dust, water and the air.

Chemical contamination may come from pesticides or cleaning fluids.

Physical contamination may be from dirty clothing or from touching the food or from a used plaster lost from a finger.

Cross contamination

To avoid cross contamination it is important that the same equipment is not used for handling raw meat and milk products without being disinfected. To prevent the inadvertent use of equipment for raw and high risk foods it is recommended that where possible different colours and shapes are used to identify products.

Yellow   Food preparation areas
Green   Food and beverage service
Blue   General purpose
Red   Toilet areas

Cutting boards and knives:

White   Dairy products
Grey   Bread
Green   Fruit
Brown   Vegetables
Red   Raw meat
Yellow   Cooked meat
Blue   Raw fish

Personal habits

- ○ Avoid touching hair, ears, nose, mouth and spots when preparing food.
- ○ Never use handkerchief, use disposable tissues.
- ○ Do not sneeze or cough over food.
- ○ Do not bite your nails.
- ○ Use utensils to handle food whenever possible, not your fingers.

Always wash hands after:

- ○ visiting the toilet;
- ○ blowing your nose;
- ○ handling money;
- ○ disposing of rubbish;
- ○ cleaning.

Temperature control

For bacteria to multiply, they need:

- ○ food;
- ○ moisture;
- ○ time;
- ○ warmth.

By removing warmth from the presence of bacteria we can control or stop the growth of bacteria.

The temperature danger zone is between 5°C and 63°C. The ideal temperature for bacteria to multiply is the same as our body temperature, 37°C.

Keeping food frozen and chilled restricts growth.

Freezer unit minus 18°C
Ice cream unit minus 15°C
Chilled unit 0–5°C

Always close the refrigerator door after use. Heating food to a hot temperature kills bacteria. Ideally the cooking temperature should be 70°C or above.

Heat must penetrate all the food and a probe used to ensure that the temperature is hot enough. Once food has been served it is very important that the minimum temperature for hot food is monitored at all times. The minimum temperature is 65°C. If it does not achieve or maintain the required temperature, it should not be served.

Illness

The manager must be informed if you are suffering from diarrhoea, cold, sore throat, sickness or skin infection.

Cleaning

Clean as you go protects the food from contamination, bacteria, chemical and physically deters pests.
Use hot water with detergent or a sanitiser to breakdown grease and remove dirt.
Rubbish should be disposed of frequently.

Control of substances hazardous to health

A number of cleaning substances are regarded as hazardous to health. Therefore, a number of precautions have to be taken to control their use.

Firstly, read the label and identify the substance and its potential hazards.
Secondly, use only the right substance for the appropriate job.
Thirdly, check to see if any protective clothing is required.

Good industrial hygiene practice

○ Do not eat, drink or smoke when using chemicals.
○ Use protective clothing as appropriate.
○ Wash hands and exposed skin after using chemicals.

Practical implications of the Temperature Control Regulations

○ On receipt of deliveries goods should be cooled to the proper temperature as soon as possible.
○ To account for defrost cycle or breakdown of refrigeration an allowance of 2°C (3°F) is permitted.
○ A maximum time of two hours for cold food preparation in the kitchen is tolerated provided there is no more than 2°C (3°F) rise above the 5°C (41°F) or 8°C (46°F) specified temperature.
○ Food intended to be served hot at 63°C (115°F) or above can be held at a temperature below 63°C (115°F) but for no more than two hours.
○ Exception is made for foods served warm (hollandaise sauce). They may be kept for no more than two hours and any remaining must be discarded.

○ Foods intended to be served cold 5°C (41°F) or 8°C (46°F) may be held at a higher temperature but for no longer than four hours; it must then be brought back to 5°C (41°F) or 8°C (46°F).

○ Displayed foods (sweet trolley, cheese board, self-service display, 'counter display with assisted service') need not be maintained at the required temperature provided displayed food is kept to a minimum and does not exceed four hours.

The main food hygiene regulations of importance to the caterer are the following:

○ Food Safety (General Food Hygiene) Regulations 1995;

○ Food Safety (Temperature Control) Regulations 1995.

These implemented the EC Food Hygiene directive (93/43 EEC). They replaced a number of different sets of regulations including the Food Safety (General) Regulations 1970.

THE 1995 REGULATIONS are similar in many respects to earlier regulations. However, as with the Health and Safety legislation, these regulations place a strong emphasis on owners and managers to identify the safety risks, and to design and implement appropriate systems to prevention contamination. These systems and procedures are covered by Hazard Analysis Critical Control points, and/or Assured Safe Catering.

The regulations place two general requirements on the owners of food businesses:

1 To ensure that all food handling operators are carried out hygienically and according to the 'Rules of Hygiene'.

2 To identify and control all potential food safety hazards, using a systems approach either HACCP or Assured Safe Catering.

In addition there is an obligation by any food handler who may be suffering from or carrying a disease which could be transmitted through food to report this to the employer, who may be obliged to prevent the person concerned from handling food.

Catering establishments have a general obligation to supervise, instruct and provide training in food hygiene commensurate with their employees' responsibilities. Details with regard to how much training is required are not specified in the regulations. However the HMSO Industry Guide to Catering provides guidance on training which can be taken as a general standard to comply with the legislation.

The HMSO guide suggests three categories of food handler, all of which need training.

Category A – Support and front of house staff including: storekeeper, waiter/waitress, bar staff, counter staff, servery assistant, cellar person etc.

Category B – These involved in the preparation of high risk (unwrapped) foods including: chefs, cooks, catering supervisors, kitchen assistants and bar staff who prepare food.

Category C – Managers or supervisors who may handle food including all such persons based on site.

Before any food handler starts work they must be given written and verbal instructions in the essentials of food hygiene.

The second stage of training is hygiene awareness instruction.

Formal training

Formal food hygiene training as suggested by the industry guide, going beyond essentials and awareness, is recommended to comply with the law.

A guide to the training of individuals in food handling

CATEGORY OF STAFF	ESSENTIALS OF FOOD HYGIENE	HYGIENE AWARENESS INSTRUCTION	FORMAL TRAINING LEVEL	FORMAL TRAINING LEVEL 2 AND/OR 3
A Storekeeper Waiting Staff Bar Staff Catering Assistants	Yes before starting work.	Yes within 4 weeks (8 weeks for part-time staff.	No	No
B Chefs Cooks Supervisors Food Preparation Assistants	Yes before starting work.	Yes within 4 weeks or 3 months for part-timers.	Yes	No
C Managers Supervisors	Yes before starting work.	Yes within 4 weeks.	Yes within 3 months.	Yes but only good practice not essential.

FORMAL TRAINING BEYOND ESSENTIALS AND AWARENESS

Level 1

The overall aim of this training is to provide a firm foundation of basic knowledge in the following disciplines:

○ food poisoning micro-organisms – sources and types together with simple microbiology;
○ common food hazards – physical, chemical and microbiological;
○ personal hygiene – responsibilities;
○ pest prevention and control;
○ cleaning and disinfection;
○ food storage and preparation including temperature control;
○ legal requirements.

The duration of such a course is suggested to be at least six hours.

Level 2

This is more advanced training than level 1 and should cover more detail especially about management and food safety monitoring systems. Recommended duration around 12–24 hours. This is known as the intermediate level.

Level 3

This would be aimed at the most advanced food hygiene training and would provide management with the ability to manage and evaluate hygiene systems such as HACCP and Assured Safe Catering.

Recommended duration of training 24–40 hours. This is known as Advanced Hygiene for Managers, and is an essential qualification for those who wish to train employees in essential food hygiene. It is also strongly advised that those who wish to deliver in essential hygiene training take a trainer skills qualification as well.

*See further note on legislation.

THE FOOD SAFETY (TEMPERATURE CONTROL) REGULATIONS 1995

These regulations came into force on 15 September 1995 and replace earlier and quite complex regulations.

Foods which may be subject to microbiological multiplication must be held at no more than 8°C or 63°C. There are a few exceptions which include food on display, which can be displayed for up to four hours, and also low risk and preserved foods which can be stored at ambient temperatures. Manufacturers can vary upward the 8°C ceiling if there is a scientific basis to do so.

Food which is to be served hot should be held at over 63°C.

Food reheated in Scotland must retain a temperature of 82°C unless this will adversely affect the food.

This requires that any food which is likely to support the growth of pathogens, micro-organisms or the formation of toxins must be kept at or below 8°C. In other words high risk foods, these which are ready for consumption without further heat treatment, must be stored under temperature control. These exceptions include food which has been cooked or re-heated or is for service on display for sale and needs to be kept hot. It also applies to food where there is no health risk if it is kept at ambient temperature. Any preserved foods, including dehydrated, canned or perhaps where sugar or vinegar is added, fall into this category, providing that these containers have not been opened. If the containers of such foods are open it may be necessary to store the food using temperature control.

Foods which require ripening or maturing such as cheese may be kept outside of temperature control, however once the process has been completed they should then be refrigerated.

Recommended reading: Technical Brief No 21/95, Food Safety, HCIMA. Technical Brief No 33, Food Safety, Temperature Control, HCIMA.

Registration of premises

Under the Food Premises (Registration) Regulations 1991 as amended by the Food Premises (Registration) Amendment Regulations 1993 all existing food premises in England, Wales and Scotland, have to register with their local authority.

Anyone starting a new food business must register 28 days before doing so. It is an offence not to be registered.

SUMMARY OF FOOD HYGIENE
Dangers to food

○ Chemical (copper, lead, etc.).
○ Plant (toadstools) and fungi.
○ Bacteria (cause of most cases of food poisoning).

Bacteria

- ○ Almost everywhere; not all are harmful.
- ○ Must be magnified 500–1000 times to be seen.
- ○ Under ideal conditions, they multiply by dividing in two every 20 minutes.

Sources of food-poisoning bacteria.

- ○ Human – nose, throat, excreta, spots, cuts, etc.
- ○ Animal – excreta.
- ○ Foodstuffs – meat, eggs, milk, from animal carriers.

Method of spread of bacteria

- ○ Human – coughs, sneezes, hands.
- ○ Animals – excreta (rats, mice, cows, pets, etc.), infected carcasses.
- ○ Other means – equipment, china, towels.

Factors essential for bacterial growth

- ○ Suitable temperature, time.
- ○ Enough moisture; suitable food.

Methods of control of bacterial growth

- ○ Heat – sterilisation, using high temperatures to kill all micro-organisms;
  - – pasteurisation using lower temperatures to kill harmful bacteria only;
  - – cooking.
- ○ Cold – refrigeration at 3–5°C (37–41°F) stops growth of food poisoning bacteria and retards growth of other micro-organisms;
  - – deep freeze at 218°C (0°F) stops growth of all micro-organisms.

Foods commonly causing food poisoning

- ○ Poultry, made-up meat dishes, trifles, custards, synthetic cream, sauces, left-over foods.

Common causes of food poisoning

- ○ Food prepared too far in advance, storage at ambient temperature.
- ○ Inadequate cooling, inadequate reheating.
- ○ Contamination processed food, undercooking.
- ○ Inadequate thawing, cross-contamination.
- ○ Improper warm holding, infected food handlers.

Food poisoning prevention

- ○ Comply with the rules of hygiene.
- ○ Take care and thought.
- ○ Ensure that high standards of cleanliness are applied to premises and equipment.
- ○ Prevent accidents.

Specific points to be applied:

- ○ High standards of personal hygiene.

○ Attention to physical fitness.
○ Maintaining good working conditions.
○ Maintaining equipment in good repair and clean.
○ Use separate equipment and knives for cooked and uncooked foods.
○ Ample provision of cleaning facilities and equipment.
○ Correct storage of foods at the right temperature.
○ Safe reheating of foods.
○ Quick cooking of foods prior to storage.
○ Protection of foods from vermin and insects.
○ Hygienic washing up procedure.
○ Food handlers knowing how food poisoning is caused.

Due diligence defence

Every food handler, whether they prepare, manufacture, serve or transport the food, has a responsibility to make sure the food is safe to eat. If the food is found to be unfit to eat, the person responsible can be prosecuted unless he or she can prove they took all responsible precautions, that he or she exercised all due diligence to avoid causing the offence. This defence can be established if a food handler can prove that it was the fault of another person, or someone that they trusted carried out all the necessary checks, that he or she had no reason to believe that their omission or action which they had taken would result in an offence.

A due diligence can be claimed if a caterer was supplied with ready prepared meals which after consumption caused food poisoning. The caterer would have to prove that he or she had taken all reasonable precautions to avoid the situation occurring by carrying out all the necessary checks on the method of production and by obtaining details of storage and transportation temperatures of the food before delivery.

Written records which show dates and the types of checks made are very important and would form a crucial part of the evidence.

TAKING SERVICES FORWARD

○ Managing the operation
○ Food hygiene

Managers must know:

○ Food Safety (General Food Hygiene) Regulations 1995
○ Food Safety (Temperature Control) Regulations 1995
○ Hazard Analysis Critical Control Point (HACCP)

HACCP enables the:

1 Evaluation of the operation.
2 Locate possible points of contamination.
3 Determine the severity of the hazard.
4 Take preventative measures to protect against a food borne illness outbreak.

The HACCP system is more suited to food manufacturing and not food production and as a result the Department of Health requires consideration to be given to the ASC (Assured Safe Catering).

This is an assessment of all the hazards associated with each step of a catering organisation. Staff need to know the hazards, the degree of risk involved and that they apply the controls which have been introduced to reduce and eliminate the risk.

Food Hygiene Training Areas

Knowledge of temperature control and recording of temperatures

Awareness of current legislation

Protective clothing

Personal cleanliness

Cross contamination

Bacteria triangle

Promote and maintain a high sense of awareness to food hygiene and safety

○ Ensure products are stored at correct temperature.

○ The frequency of taking and recording temperature readings are carried out.

○ Any unfit food is disposed of.

Food Labelling

Council Directive 2000/13/EC on labelling, presentation and advertising of foodstuffs to the final consumer is the main piece of EU legislation regarding the labelling of footstuffs. This Directive is based upon the principle of functional labelling. Its aim is to ensure that the consumer gets all the essential/objective information as regards the composition of the product, the manufacturer, methods of storage and preparation, etc. Producers and manufacturers are free to provide whatever additional information they wish, provided that it is accurate and does not mislead the consumer. Furthermore, this Directive prohibits the attribution to any foodstuff of the property of preventing, treating or curing a human disease, or reference to such properties.

In 1997 Quantitative Ingredients Declaration (QUID) has been introduced. Labels are to indicate the quantity of certain ingredients expressed as a percentage of the final product. The **Guidelines for Quantitative Ingredient Declaration** aim to clarify QUID requirements.

In the **White Paper on Food Safety** (paragraph 100, Action 16), the Commission announced that it intends to propose changes to the existing legislation by December 2000, to introduce additional requirements for labelling of components of compound ingredients where they form less than 25% of the final product. Furthermore, for some consumers who suffer from allergies to certain substances, a lack of detailed information is a serious handicap. In order to assist those suffering from food allergies, certain substances, recognised scientifically as being the source of allergies, should be included in the list of ingredients and not qualify as exceptions under Direct 2000/13/EC.

The Food Standards Agency

On 1st April 2000 the Food Standards Agency took over the UK responsibility for food safety and food quality from the Department of Health and the Ministry of Agriculture, Fisheries and Food, and the equivalent organisations in Wales, Northern Ireland and Scotland.

The Agency was established by the Food Standard Act 1999. The Agency's main objective is:

○ to protect public health from risks which may raise in connection with the consumption of foods, and otherwise to protect the interests of consumers in relation to food.

As such, the Agency has assumed the UK government's responsibilities relating to:

○ the implementation of legislation on food safety, hygiene, composition and labelling;

○ diet and nutrition issues and related consumer labelling.

Agency Priorities

These include:

○ better communication, with a commitment to working in an open way;

○ putting the consumer first;

○ promoting healthy and safe eating;

○ developing a food chain strategy from farm to fork, including the provision of advice on food safety and quality;

○ improving research and surveillance;

○ strengthening links with local authority enforcement services to improve the effectiveness and consistency of food law enforcement.

Agency Structure

A 14 member Board is responsible for the strategic direction of the Agency. The Board's role is to ensure that the Agency fulfils its legal obligations, and takes proper account of scientific advice in the interest of consumers.

Board members have a wide range of experience, and have been appointed to act in the public interest.

| DEFINITION OF TERMS

Antibiotic	Drug used to destroy pathogenic bacteria within human or animals bodies.
Antiseptic	Substance that prevents the growth of bacteria and moulds, specifically on or in the human body.
Bactericide	Substance which destroys bacteria.
Carrier	Person who harbours, and may transmit, pathogenic organisms without showing signs of illness.
Cleaning	Removal of soil, food residues, dirt, grease and other objectionable matter.
Contamination	Occurrence of any objectionable matter in food.
Danger zone of bacterial growth	Temperature range within which multiplication of pathogenic bacteria is possible (from 5°–63°C).
First-aid materials	Suitable and sufficient bandages and dressings, including waterproof dressings and antiseptic. All dressings to be individually wrapped.
Food handling	Any operation in the production, preparation, processing, packaging, storage, transport, distribution and sale of food.
Gastroenteritis	Inflammation of the stomach and intestinal tract that normally results in diarrhoea.
Germicide	Agent used for killing micro-organisms.
Incubation period	Period between infection and the first signs of illness.
Mildew	Type of fungus similar to mould.
Moulds	Microscopic organisms (fungi) that may appear as woolly patches on food.

Optimum	Best.
Pathogen	Disease-producing organism.
Pesticide	Chemical used to kill pests.
Residual insecticide	Long-lasting insecticide applied in such a way that it remains active for a considerable period of time.
Sanitiser	Chemical agent used for cleansing and disinfecting surfaces and equipment.
Spores	Resistant resting-phase of bacteria protecting them against adverse conditions, such as high temperatures.
Sterile	Free from all living organisms.
Sterilisation	Process that destroys all living organisms.
Steriliser	Chemical used to destroy all living organisms.
Toxins	Poisons produced by pathogens.
Viruses	Microscopic pathogens that multiply in living cells of their host.
Wholesome food	Sound food, fit for human consumption.

Further information

The Royal Society for the Promotion of Health, 13 Grosvenor Place, London SW1X 7EN.

Royal Institute of Public Health and Hygiene, 28 Portland Place, London W1N 4DE.

The Institution of Environmental Health Officers, Chadwick House, Rushworth Street, London SE1 0QT.

Local Environmental Health Departments.

Health and Safety Executive, Rose Court, 2 Southwark Bridge, London SE1 9HS.

Health Education Authority, Trevelyan House, 30 Great Peter St., London SW1P 2HW.

Royal Society of Health, 38A St George's Drive, London SW1V 4BH.

Food Hygiene Bureau Ltd, Long Hanborough, Oxford OX8 8LH.

Chartered Institute of Environmental Health, Chadwick Court, Hadfields, London SE1 8DJ

Some references to hygiene and food legislation elsewhere in the book

Topics for Discussion

1 The implications of the Food Safety (Temperature Control) Regulations 1995 for the Catering Industry.

2 The importance of regular food hygiene training for all staff.

3 The advantages and disadvantages of the Food Standards Agency.

4 The importance of good and accurate record keeping as a preparation to prove 'due diligence'.

5 Why should waste and recycling occur in every establishment?

6 Explain how food should be stored hygenically.

7 Does personal hygiene matter? Discuss this topic.

8 Why is a system or recording necessary to maintain higher standards of hygiene.

9 Discuss the food hygiene regulations, do you consider there are any omissions, if so what are they?

*[note from page 558] May 2002 EU, first reading of the food hygiene regulations, a significant change was made to the rule on training. Food business operators should ensure that food handlers are regularly supervised and annually undergo appropriate training by experts of food hygiene as well as general legislation on protection of health and prevention of infection.

CHAPTER 17

COMPUTING IN THE HOSPITALITY INDUSTRY

COMPUTERS IN HOSPITALITY

The most valuable commodity for any business is reliable up-to-date information, hence the need for computers and the advances they provide in information storage and manipulation. Like any other well-run business the Hospitality Industry cannot afford to ignore the many advantages that the developments in information technology have made possible regarding the efficient and effective operation of their business. Today cheap and powerful computers are within reach of even the smallest business.

Computer operations in the industry

Complete computer packages designed especially for the hospitality industry are readily available over a wide price range, the most commonly found being:

○ Point of Sale Systems.

○ Food & Beverage Management Systems.

○ Property Management Systems.

Most catering businesses also use general purpose (generic) systems which offer the speedy solution to a range of business tasks such as the production of text and graphic based materials, data storage, financial modelling and forecasting. User-friendly interfaces now mean that these products are easy to use and set up. This section of the book will give an overview of the systems in use.

Figure 17.1 *Computing a food order*

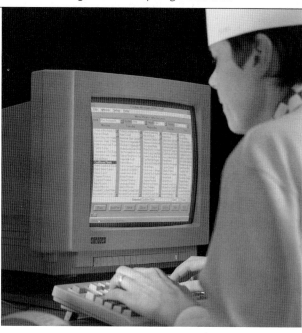

Reservations systems

There are four principle types of system in use:

Single property based system, which will usually be part of a Property Management Systems (PMS) (see below). These deal with the recording of accommodation sales for a single property.

For hotels that belong or are affiliated to a group, Central Reservation Systems (CRS) are run by the group or on their behalf by consortia. These provide a single point of contact for a prospective guest and ensure that sales are maximised. Increasingly these systems are directly linked with the individual property's reservations system but in some cases there is still a manual transfer of data between the systems at the individual property.

Global distribution systems (GDS) are based on airline reservations systems; these in turn are linked to the CRS and travel agents (and sometimes other large users) and thus allow direct selling and reservation of accommodation to take place.

Currently there are a number of agencies offering the industry the opportunity to market their hotel on the World Wide Web of the Internet. These systems also offer the facility to make a direct reservation of hotel accommodation. The benefit of this approach is that they are available to anyone having access to the Internet (see below).

Property management systems

Property Management System (PMS) is the name given to the systems found in hotels which manage reservations and guest billing. There are a wide range of PMSs available and these range from simple systems to cover basic reservations and billing to sophisticated systems with many additional facilities, which through appropriate interfaces are able to monitor and control all activities within a hotel.

This means that whilst in small hotels PMSs can simply look after reservations and guest billing, in large hotels they are usually used as top level systems. Data and reports from other systems such as event management, point of sale, food and beverage management, telephone management, security stems and in-room guest services will be incorporated into their own billing and reporting systems. Increasingly frequently PMSs feature an interface into central reservation systems and direct on-line booking services via the Internet.

Data regarding past guests stored in these systems (the guest history) is now increasingly being regarded as a valuable asset by the business and is frequently used as the basis for sophisticated sales and marketing operations, allowing hotels to target potential guests whose preferences are known. This data is also valuable in building up information to support forecasting with respect to future patterns of business, which in turn allows effective room rates and discounts to be calculated. This information provides the basis for Yield Management systems that are increasingly being used by larger establishments. The introduction of Yield Management (YM) techniques allows the business to maximise the financial return from bedroom sales, although not in itself a computer package, the use of computer data greatly simplifies the operation and improves the effectiveness of the YM process.

Electronic point of sale systems

These are systems which take the place of the traditional cash register. At the simplest level they take the form of a single cash register with a processor, memory and printer which are usually supplied in a single case. Although relatively simple to use they offer greatly enhanced facilities over a traditional cash register. Typical facilities offered include multiple total storing to enable sales to be analysed as required by the end user, price look up which enables the user to press a key labelled with the name of a dish or a drink and the correct price will be added to the transaction and multi-level pricing to cope with special offers or 'happy hour' arrangements.

The most sophisticated systems offer a large range of features and usually consist of a number of machines linked together (networked) in the restaurant and bar and sometimes to a central computer. These large systems offer an extremely sophisticated control process, which reduces work for the staff and supplies detailed information about the business to the management. For example orders keyed in by the bar staff when a guest arrives in a restaurant may be transferred to the restaurant account giving the guest one consolidated account at the end of the meal. Waiting staff entering the guest's order, often via a touch screen terminal, into the system will find that it will automatically print out in the correct preparation department, saving a great deal of time and work. As this process proceeds the guest account is automatically prepared ready for presentation at the end of the meal.

With this type of system all orders to kitchen and bar are printed and show the time the order was processed, they also eliminate errors and arguments between staff due to badly handwritten cheques. As the account is developed by the system as the meal progresses there is no danger that items will be omitted from the bill or items will be incorrectly charged as not infrequently happens with manual systems and thus simplifying the control systems which need to be in place.

Management reports are very comprehensive, giving details such as sales of each dish or drink item. Sales breakdown by each outlet, by each member of staff and for each session are also easy to obtain. Most systems will also give the profit on each item sold and may also be linked to stock control systems. When waiting staff are responsible for their own guest bills then the system will not allow them to log off duty until all accounts are cleared and the cash paid into a central point.

Information of this type intelligently used can assist the management to ensure that the business operates to maximum effectiveness.

Stock control systems

At the simplest level these systems allow the user to enter stock received and issued, extract details of consumption and calculate the value of stock in hand. More sophisticated systems provide these basic facilities plus a considerable range of other features such as details of suppliers, the automatic issue of orders when stocks drop to a pre-defined level, detailed records of issues and current prices of all stock items.

Stock control is relatively easy to operate on bar stock but dealing with food items, especially fresh foods, is far more complex as food items are rarely used in the quantities in which they are supplied and there is a wide range of measurements in use which require accurate conversion tables. There is also the need to allow for and deal effectively with wastage. If we take what at first glance may seem the relatively simple stock item of fresh eggs; these may be supplied by the dozen or a multiple of a dozen or by the case or multiple or fraction of a case or in some instances by the tray or multiple of a tray. They may be used in recipes as single eggs or by weight in ounces or grams or by volume by the fluid ounce or by the pint or litre. Recipes calling for just egg yolk or egg white or by different quantities of each may further compound this and in this example further complications may be made by the use of pasteurised egg and dried egg in certain recipes.

Figure 17.2 *Using computer software*

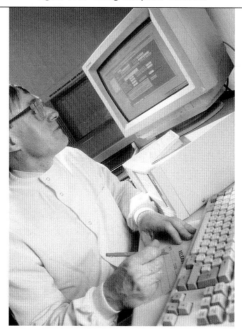

Food and beverage management systems

Food and beverage management systems take the concept of stock control one stage further. They add a control framework which, when correctly implemented, gives greatly improved levels of management control. With this type of system a database is created with all the recipes in use in the business, together with a further database containing the ingredients that are used to support those dishes.

Typical information stored about each ingredient is:

○ ingredient code;
○ ingredient name;
○ ingredient description;
○ category

- purchase unit;
- unit of use;
- unit of measure;
- content weight;
- price;
- supplier(s);
- tax rate;
- shelf life;
- re-order level;
- percentage usable.

Typical information stored about each recipe is:

- recipe code;
- quantity of production;
- selling unit;
- tax code;
- re-order level;
- profit required (%);
- for each ingredient in recipe:
  ingredient code;
  ingredient unit of measure.

Using this information as a base it is possible for kitchen staff to order goods from the stores by recipe and to automatically scale for the quantity required and effectively cost those dishes. The system will then give the required selling price to achieve the required profit.

Food and beverage management systems, because of their cost and complexity, still tend to be used by large-scale users, particularly where tight control of costs and adherence to pre-set budgets is important. For example, large production cook and chill units in hospitals. Add-on modules allow for differing user requirements such as cyclic menus and nutritional analysis.

Comprehensive reporting is offered which give, a high level of management information and thus control. For example, it is easy to check purchase levels and to track high cost ingredients. These systems are frequently being linked to point of sale systems to take the control process one stage further.

Menu engineering

This is a technique utilising computer modelling of data, originally developed in the USA (See page 323). The system holds data about sales volume and the costs and profits of each dish on the menu. By changing the ratio of the areas it is possible, in theory, to create a menu offering the optimum balance between popularity and maximum profit. The technique can be carried out with pencil and paper but it is far more effective when using a computer system. Using such a system to build up a reliable store of trading information it becomes possible over a period of time to develop a 'computer model' of the performance of each of the dishes on the menu. This type of activity is frequently carried out using a 'model' created on a spreadsheet, such as Microsoft Excel, rather than in a stand-alone commercial package.

Dietary analysis

As we become more selective about what we eat, customers require more dietary information about the dishes on our menus. Dietary analysis works from large databases of dietary information and will give details of the composition of individual foods or complete dishes at the touch of a button. Again there is a range of systems available, from simple ones which give a relatively crude breakdown which may be suitable for the basic information required by the average restaurant guest, to the more complex breakdowns which are linked to government food tables and give extremely accurate and comprehensive data. These are suitable for calculating detailed nutritional profiles.

Simple dietary analysis systems are often available as and-on modules to food and beverage management systems whilst the more comprehensive systems are usually available as 'stand alone' systems available from specialist suppliers.

Event management

Targeted at hotels and conference centres these systems are designed to deal with all the elements of taking a booking and managing one-off events such as conferences, meetings, weddings and banquets. The range of facilities that they offer vary but one would expect to find a booking diary together with a comprehensive costing and billing section. Many systems have modules which allow the allocation of equipment to specific events thus ensuring that it is not possible to inadvertently double book equipment. The costing of food from pre-designed menus is another feature commonly found. Modules which allow the physical planning of the room layout on the screen are also available with some products. In some cases these also have the ability to give graphic views of how the room will appear from specific angles. As with any modern computer management system comprehensive management reporting is a major feature.

Generic software

This is the term we give to software which we use to support the operation of a business but which does not have a purpose which is unique to any specific industry. The most common types found are: Word Processing, Spreadsheets, Databases, Presentation Tools and Internet Browsers. When buying business PCs these systems are often supplied with the computer as added value items. When purchasing independently there is a wide range of systems across a wide price band and offering a great variety of facilities. The best known and widest used is Microsoft Office which is offered in a number of versions.

The Internet

The merging of information technology and communications is having and will in the future continue to have a significant impact on society, the way we live our lives and how we conduct our businesses. The most obvious manifestation of this is the Internet: a global network of networks. This worldwide network of computers allows anyone connected to it access to a virtually limitless database of information and almost instantaneous communication with anyone else connected.

For most businesses the Internet is used to send and receive e-mail and to access information via the world-wide-web. Technically the Internet is the name for the system and the world-wide-web is the software of its most popular element.

Although it is possible to be directly connected to the Internet, for most users the most practical method is to be connected when required via a phone line to an Internet service provider (ISP). These are specialist web sites that exist to provide a connection into the Internet for users. Each service provider offers alternative add-on facilities and will make charges for their services; all will offer access to the Internet and an address for E-mail.

Most computers are now supplied Internet ready and all that is necessary is to connect the system to a telephone line. To use the Web a piece of software called a Web Browser is required, this software allows you to move around the Internet once you are connected. Today Web Browsers are usually supplied with the computer. The best known is Microsoft Explorer, which is part of

Microsoft Windows, and the other main browser, Netscape Explorer, is provided free as part of the Netscape Communicator package which can be downloaded directly from the Internet.

The Web is made up of Web Sites; it is possible to visit any Web Site and view its contents. In addition to text and graphics many sites offer video and sound images. It is possible for anyone to set up a Web Site but most small business users contract this out to a specialist company who will maintain and monitor the site on their behalf.

The major area of impact within hospitality to date is in the area of selling and reservation of hotel accommodation. Many hotels now have their own Web Site, which acts as an electronic brochure and usually offers the opportunity to reserve accommodation. This is already having an impact on global distribution companies and travel agents and the way they do business.

By setting up their own page on the web a business can have, for a relatively low cost, a versatile promotional tool which can be used for marketing and direct selling. A Web presence allows the smallest operator to compete with the largest company in terms of attracting business; an important consideration in an industry with a large percentage of small operations.

Whilst marketing currently provides the major use of the internet for the industry it should not be overlooked that it offers an unrivalled source of information on current developments and legislation, particularly useful in the food and catering technology area. Increasingly new information on major developments is being published on the Internet in addition to the more traditional forms of distribution. Most professional bodies and trade associations now operate Web Sites for their members, giving access to impressive data sources targeted for the industry. For all hospitality industry businesses the potential offered by the Internet is unlimited; it can provide them with access to a vast range of global data and expertise that can be used in the operation of the business.

COMPUTERS & HOSPITALITY MANAGEMENT

Computers are a valuable tool in the management of a business. Correctly operated and controlled they are virtually indispensable to the well-run business that wishes to keep a step ahead of the competition. However, the best systems will only give maximum effectiveness if well managed and if the management make effective use of the information the systems provide. The management of computers ideally needs to be focused into two general areas; firstly the selection, set up and day-to-day operation of the equipment and secondly the application of management information obtained from the systems.

Management structure

In large hospitality businesses, especially large hotels, there may be a member of the management team, usually known as the Systems Manager, with responsibility for the operation of all IT systems within the business. Reporting to the General Manager or Chief Accountant this role is usually at head of department level. The post holder must understand the operation of the business very thoroughly and have a good all round knowledge of applied information technology. In addition to being responsible for the smooth operation of the IT systems on a day-to-day basis the Systems Manager will also be responsible for the selection of and the updating of systems, the training of new and existing staff for the IT systems in use and for compliance with all relevant legislation. In smaller businesses these responsibilities will usually be taken over by the manager or owner of the business or by an assistant manager or department heads. Whatever structure is in place it is important that the management ensure that all staff are aware of their responsibilities with respect to the use of IT. In some cases it may be a criminal offence if systems are not correctly implemented and controlled. In any case, poor management of the IT systems and the information which they are able to provide will ensure that the business is not benefiting from its investment.

Choice of systems

The costs involved in setting up and running the computer over its lifetime will be far more expensive than the purchase price. When considering the computerisation of an element of the business it is good practice to remember that computers are good at repetitive tasks with large volumes of data to process, they can provide information to help you make effective decisions but they cannot in themselves take decisions for you.

The first task is to identify the areas of the business which could potentially benefit from computerisation. The most effective way to do this is to undertake a feasibility study of the existing task(s) involved to identify exactly what happens and what volume of activity takes place. On reviewing this process it may prove that you only need to revise the existing systems and that a computer is not strictly necessary. If the decision is to go ahead, then you must identify what information the system must provide for the management of the business. From this it is fairly easy to identify what data must go into the system to give that information as output; for example if you expect a stock control system to advise you when to re-order it must hold details of minimum stock levels. Once you have identified these features together with volume and critical operational constraints such as speed, types of printer and methods of output, you are ready to go shopping.

The software, which will actually carry out the task required, is the most important element to consider. Apart from a detailed check list drawn up on the above principles, when choosing software a purchaser will need to consider the following issues:

- Does the software cover all the major requirements of the system specification?
- What hardware configuration is required? Relative costs?
- Is costly supporting equipment or software required?
- Does the software cover all the detailed requirements of the system specification?
- What are the performance standards required (i.e. speed, capacity, number of users)?
- What level of customisation is possible?
- Is the product supported by regular updates? What are the costs of this?
- System expandability?
- How easy is it to use?
- What is the available level of support?
- Supplier background and expertise?
- Financial arrangement available?

Whilst the hardware must, at a minimum, be capable of running the required software, you should spend as much as possible on the processor and internal memory, known as Random Access Memory (RAM) and external memory, the hard disk. Memory capacity especially is relatively low cost if specified at the time of purchase. Software takes more space with every upgrade or development and a system running at capacity is generally unhappy and will run slowly and give problems in operation.

The following gives some of the areas a prospective purchaser will need to consider when purchasing equipment (hardware):

- Is the speed of performance adequate?
- Is the memory capacity adequate?
- What is the physical size and space requirement?

- ○ Can the equipment be expanded to meet increased software demands?
- ○ Reliability/backup support?
- ○ Ease of use/ergonomics?
- ○ Comparative operating costs?
- ○ Maintenance support?

Sources of supply

If a straightforward system for a general office, using generic business software, then it may initially appear cost effective to purchase from the direct mail suppliers who advertise in most computing magazines or from one of the large specialist discount stores or high street shops. Through bulk buying capacity these are often able to offer attractive financial deals. Some caution is required however, as generally a level of pre-knowledge is expected (even if not stated) and levels of user support are often more in line with the needs of a hobbyist user than that of a business which is relying on the systems. Some of these large suppliers offer support for the business user, which may be worth considering where the systems are non-critical to the operation of the business.

In most cases a specialist dealer/distributor will offer a higher level of personalised support, but this is at a cost. For a non-technical user it is often much more cost effective in the long term to build up a relationship with a good local dealer who will get to know individual requirements and can offer good, although it should be noted not always impartial, advice.

Specialist companies supply most catering IT systems. Frequently these companies provide a complete service including hardware, software, installation and training. Again, although not offering impartial advice, they will be only too happy to discuss your specification and advise accordingly. Prices, facilities and the range of services provided vary widely and it is essential to shop around. Normally with these large 'turnkey' systems once the decision is made the business is committed to the supplying company for the life of the system, so it is important that all factors are considered before completing the purchase.

For impartial advice it is possible to use the services of a consultant. For a fee they will investigate possible solutions for a specific problem or task and then will offer or recommend a number of systems from which to choose. It is important to bear two things in mind when dealing with consultants:

- ○ they must be impartial; that is, not taking commission from hardware or software suppliers;
- ○ the final choice of system will be left to the establishment.

Consultants can be extremely useful but do not make up for a lack of knowledge of information technology and of its application to a business on the part of the user.

Operation

Once the business has selected and purchased a system, it will need to ensure the maximum effectiveness from its investment. A computer system must give a competitive edge, no matter how well matched the system is to the needs of the business this will only happen if the systems are correctly implemented and operated.

The strategic concerns of operating computers will of course rest with the management of the business but it is also important that the management ensure that all users understand their contribution to the effective operation of the system. For example, a stock control system will not give the correct information in its reports if the storekeeper is careless when entering delivery notes and invoices. It should be ensured that all members of staff using the systems or preparing data for entry to the systems are correctly trained, that working conditions are comfortable and comply with legislation and that regular monitoring of system performance takes place.

System reporting

Most software systems available today have extremely comprehensive reporting facilities. In addition many systems also have a built in report generator to allow the user to develop reports which suit their own operation. With the high levels of compatibility found today it is possible to export data from specialist systems into spreadsheets and databases for further analysis. Whilst a business will expect a system to give reports on the level of activity and performance against agreed targets, the area where a computer system can really help to give competitive advantage is in the strategy development of the business. Businesses frequently export performance data from their operational systems, e.g. point of sale, food and beverage management and use this data for the basis of computer modelling, forecasting future business performance.

LEGISLATION

This is an area which rapidly expanded from the mid 1980s, reflecting the increasing use of IT and the corresponding need to offer legal protection to suppliers, users and people on whom data is held in computers.

The principle areas for legislation which have a major impact on the way that information technology is used in businesses are data protection, health and safety and copyright protection.

The Data Protection Act of 1988 updated and expanded the scope of the original act of 1984. The Act defines the basic principles that must be followed if anyone wishes to store data about living identifiable individuals on a computer system. It gives the person whose data is stored right of access to that data and lays down principles for secure storage of that data. The act makes it an offence to hold personal data, as defined in the act, unless the holder is registered with the Data Protection Register.

The Screen Display (VDU) Regulations of 1992 lay down very strict guidelines about the way computers are operated and the environment in which they are located. For example there should not be glare from windows or artificial light and the working environment must be ergonomically correct to ensure that there are no long-term health hazards for staff using the systems. The legislation also covers the actual design of the appearance of the software on the screen and also states that training must take place on a regular basis. It covers issues with respect to extended use by an operative which includes such issues as regular eye tests. The Management of Health & Safety at Work Regulations (as amended 1992) also lay down specific conditions that must be followed when expectant mothers operate VDUs. This area of legislation is currently under review.

The Copyright Design and Patent Act of 1988 protects the copyright of the software owner, amongst its provisions this law makes it an offence to buy a piece of software for use on a single computer and then load it on further computers without additional payment.

There is also the Computer Misuse Act of 1990. This act makes it a criminal offence to access a computer without permission or to corrupt data stored in a computer. As more and more computers are now becoming linked so that remote access is common then this piece of legislation will become of more benefit to smaller businesses.

FUTURE DEVELOPMENTS

Catering was the first industry to make commercial use of computing. It is increasingly important that users within the industry, whatever the size of their business, make use of applied information technology if they wish to remain effective and gain a lead over their competitors.

Computing is a fast advancing area of technology and it is perhaps unwise to look too far into the future where developments may take us. It seems certain that the integration of computer systems will lead to a single point of data capture and more effective use of that data once captured. The increasingly common use of computers as communication links, for example to external suppliers using electronic data exchange and the widespread use of the Internet, will continue to have a significant impact on the way that we do business.

Further Reading

O'Connor, P, Using Computers in Hospitality (2nd ed) (2000), Continuum, London ISBN 0 826453589.

Grant, D & McBride, P; Caterer & Hotelkeeper Guide to the Internet (2000), Butterworth-Heinemann, Oxford ISBN 0 750648961.

Websites

- Ask a Chef – http://www.askachef.com
- BBC Food Pages –http://www.bbc.co.uk/food
- Beverage Net – http://www.beveragenet.net
- British Dietetic Association – http://www.bda.com.uk
- British Hospitality Association – http://www.bha-online.org.uk
- British Institute of Inkeeping – http://www.bii.org
- British Nutrition Foundation – http://www.nutrition.co.uk
- Caterer and Hotelkeeper – http://caterer.com
- Catering Net – http://www.cateringnet.co.uk
- Culinary Resource Centre UK – http://www.culinary-resource.co.uk
- ehoteliercom – http://www.ehotelier.com
- Electronic Food News – http://www.eFoodNews.com
- European Catering Association – http://ecagb.co.uk
- Food Standards Agency – http://foodstandards.gov.uk
- Foodlines – http://www.foodlines.com
- Foodservice World – http://www.FoodserviceWorld.com
- Foodservice.com – http://www.foodservice.com
- Hospitality Net – http://hospitalitynet.org
- Hospitality Traning Foundation – http://htf.org.uk
- Hotel and Catering, International Management Association – http://www.hcima.org.uk
- Into Wine – http://www.intowine.com
- Restaurant Association of Great Britain – http://www.rafb.co.uk
- Restaurants and Institutions – http://www.rimag.com
- Simply Food – http://www.simplyfood.co.uk
- The Wine Line – http://www.the-wine-line.co.uk
- The Wine School – http://www.wine-school.com
- UK Brewers and Licensed Retailers Association – http://www.blra.co.uk
- UK Food Law – http://www.fst.rdg.ac.uk/foodlaw
- Webtender – online bartender – http://www.webtender.com
- Wine and Dine E-zine – http://dine-online.co.uk

○ Wine Spectator – http://winespectator.com
○ Wine.com – http://www.wine.com
○ Yahoo Food Websites – http://www.yaho.co.uk/Society and Culture/Food and Drink

ABBREVIATIONS

ACAS	Advisory Conciliation and Arbitration Service	40
ASC	Assured Safe Catering	525
BEd	Bachelor of Education	Title Page
(Hons)	Honours	
BSc	Bachelor of Science	225
BEPA	British Egg Producers Association	120
BHA	British Hospitality Association	10
BHT	Butlated Hydroxy Toluene	187
BSE	Bovine Spongiform Encephalopathy	561
CO_2	Carbon dioxide	199
CEMA	Catering Equipment Manufacturers Association	237
CPA	Chevalier Dans L'ordre des Palmes Académique	Title Page
CCTV	Closed Circuit Television	502
CAP	Common Agricultural Policy	50
CAD	Computer-Aided Design	205
CJD	Creutzfeldt-Jakob Disease	537
COSHH	Control of Substances Hazardous to Health	483
CCP	Critical Control Points	483
DfES	Department of Education and Skills	18
DEFRA	Department of Environment Fisheries and Rural Affairs	5
DNA	Deoxyribonucleic acid	422
DMS	Diploma Management Studies	V
DSO	Direct Service Organisation	19
EPOS	Electronic Point of Sale	324
EHO	Environmental Health Officer	
ECA	European Catering Association	23
EFTA	European Free Trade Association	37
ETSU	Energy Technology Support Unit	249
EU	European Union	35
F & B	Food and Beverage	VIII
GMO	Genetically Modified Foods	20
GNP	Gross National Product	8
GDS	Global Distribution System	566
GMS	Glycerol Monosteorate	187
HSE	Health and Safety Executive	482
HSEO	Health and Safety Enforcement Officer	498
HACCP	Hazard Analysis and Critical Control Point	268

LEGISLATION

INDEX